The People of South Asia

The Biological Anthropology of India, Pakistan, and Nepal

The People of South Asia

The Biological Anthropology of India, Pakistan, and Nepal

Edited by
JOHN R. LUKACS
University of Oregon
Eugene, Oregon

SPRINGER SCIENCE+BUSINESS MEDIA, LLC

Library of Congress Cataloging in Publication Data

Main entry under title:

The People of South Asia.

Includes bibliographies and index.

1. Anthropometry—South Asia—Addresses, essays, lectures. 2. Physical Anthropology—Addresses, essays, lectures. 3. South Asia—Antiquities—Addresses, essays, lectures. I. Lukacs, John R.

GN58.S64P46 1984 573.'.0954 83-27058

ISBN 978-1-4899-5003-1 ISBN 978-1-4899-5001-7 (eBook)

DOI 10.1007/978-1-4899-5001-7

Originally published by Plenum Press, New York in 1984

Softcover reprint of the hardcover 1st edition 1984

For my parents
JOHN ANDREW LUKACS, M.D.
and
ANN RHINEHART LUKACS
with love and appreciation

Contributors

Z. D. Ansari Department of Archaeology, Deccan College, Pune 411 006, India

Catherine Badgley Peabody Museum, Harvard University, Cambridge, Massachusetts 02138

Amitabha Basu Human Adaptability Programme, Biological Sciences Division, Indian Statistical Institute, Calcutta 700 035, India

Cynthia M. Beall Department of Anthropology, Case Western Reserve University, Cleveland, Ohio 44106

Peggy C. Caldwell Department of Anthropology, National Museum of Natural History, The Smithsonian Institution, Washington, D.C. 20560

Robert S. Corruccini Department of Anthropology, Southern Illinois University, Carbondale, Illinois 62901

P. Dash Sharma Department of Physical Anthropology, University of Ranchi, 834 001, India

M. K. Dhavalikar Department of Archaeology, Deccan College, Pune 411 006, India

Pratap C. Dutta Anthropological Survey of India, 27 Jawaharlal Nehru Rd., Calcutta 700 016, India

Madhav Gadgil Indian Institute of Science, Center for Theoretical Studies, Bangalore 560 012, India

Ranjan Gupta Human Adaptability Programme, Biological Sciences Division, Indian Statistical Institute, Calcutta 700 035, India

Samvit S. Kaul Department of Anthropology, Punjab University, Chandigarh 160 014, India

John Kelley Peabody Museum, Harvard University, Cambridge, Massachusetts 02138

Kenneth A. R. Kennedy Ecology and Systematics, Division of Biological Sciences, Cornell University, Ithaca, New York 14853

John R. Lukacs Department of Anthropology, University of Oregon, Eugene, Oregon 97403

Kailash C. Malhotra Biological Sciences Division, Indian Statistical Institute, Calcutta 700 035, India

S. L. Malik Department of Anthropology, University of Delhi, Delhi 110 007, India

Barun Mukhopadhyay Human Adaptability Programme, Biological Sciences Division, Indian Statistical Institute, Calcutta 700 035, India

David Pilbeam Peabody Museum, Harvard University, Cambridge, Massachusetts 02138

A. K. Roychoudhury Biometry and Population Genetics Unit, Bose Institute, Calcutta 700 009, India

Russell M. Reid Department of Anthropology, University of Louisville, Louisville, Kentucky 40292

H. D. Sankalia Department of Archaeology, Deccan College, Pune 411 006, India

Jim G. Shaffer Department of Anthropology, Case Western Reserve University, Cleveland, Ohio 44106

Indera P. Singh Department of Anthropology, University of Delhi, Delhi 110 007, India

P. S. Sundar Rao Department of Biostatistics, Christian Medical College, Vellore 632 002, India

Subhash R. Walimbe Department of Archaeology, Deccan College Postgraduate and Research Institute, Pune 411 006, India

Steven Ward Departments of Anthropology and Biology, Kent State University, Kent, Ohio 44242

Charles A. Weitz Department of Anthropology, Temple University, Philadelphia, Pennsylvania 19122

Preface[*]

The people of South Asia have long fascinated the serious traveler and research scholar with their biological and cultural diversity. Early descriptions of ascetic holy men and physical features of the "monstrous" races of India appear in the works of Herodotus (484–425 B.C.). Progressively more fantastic descriptions of the physical appearance of monstrous races of South Asia can be found in the works of Ktesias, Megasthenes, and Pliny the Elder (Malfijt, 1968). Detailed illustrations of these varieties of *Homo monstrosus* (Linnaeus, 1758) accompany the numerous encyclopedias and bestiaries published during the Middle Ages (Hodgen, 1964; Kennedy, 1973, 1976).

Given the antiquity of Western intellectual interest in the cultures and biological features of South Asian people, it is surprising that a scholarly scientific approach to this diversity developed so slowly. Perhaps the great geographical distance involved and the cultural differences that separate Europeans and South Asians are partly responsible. Nevertheless, the discipline of physical anthropology, whose goal is the elucidation and explanation of biological and cultural interactions, did not become established in the subcontinent until early in the 20th century.

Today, anthropologists regard Herbert H. Risley's (1908) *People of India* as a landmark publication that established the discipline of physical anthropology in South Asia. However, until recently, physical anthropology in the subcontinent consisted of grand anthropometric surveys, which were often conducted in conjunction with the Indian census (Guha, 1935). The goal of these surveys was to

[*]Editorial work and preparation of this introduction were completed during the 1981–1982 academic year, during which the editor received support from the American Institute of Indian Studies, the Fulbright-Hays Program, and the Smithsonian Institution (Special Foreign Currency Program). The continuing support of these institutions is deeply appreciated.

determine the racial composition of the people of India. Since the 1950s similar objectives have been pursued but with greater emphasis on data provided by serology and dermatoglyphics.

Physical anthropologists working in South Asia have recently adopted a problem-oriented research focus, and they have demonstrated a commitment to analyzing biological problems in a broader cultural context. The prime objective of this volume is to reflect these recent developments by bringing together original research and review articles about the biological anthropology of living and prehistoric South Asians.

Another message conveyed by this volume is that the *unity-in-diversity* concept, so often repeated with respect to South Asia's rich biocultural variations, also applies with equal force to the discipline of physical anthropology. As a physical anthropologist with research interests in the skeletal biology of prehistoric South Asians, I was surprised to find a clear dichotomy among my colleagues. Paleoanthropologists and archaeologists appeared to form a natural group that was distinct from human biologists and geneticists. A second purpose of this volume, therefore, is to emphasize that paleoanthropologists and human biologists must collaborate in order to solve problems of human adaptation and evolution. The biological diversity exhibited by living South Asian populations is a consequence of repeated and successful biological and cultural adaptations by their ancestors to changing ecological conditions. The holistic view of human biological adaptation provided by physical anthropology requires an understanding of adaptational processes, past and present. Though different analytical techniques and research designs are employed by paleoanthropologists and human biologists, interpretive frameworks in evolutionary biology and ecology are shared.

A book about the biological adaptations of living and prehistoric South Asians should reflect the contributions of both indigenous and Western scholars. This volume is unique in its equal balance of Western and South Asian authors. The editor regards this balance of authorship as a valuable feature of the volume because it exposes the reader to important differences in research methodology and design. Also, it indicates the range of topical interests regarded as important by scholars from different cultures and therefore may help to foster international cooperation in research on the biological anthropology of South Asia.

Literature on the physical anthropology of South Asian populations is found with considerable difficulty because it is widely dispersed in the professional journals of many disciplines and because many of the journals and anthologies are published in India and are sometimes difficult of access to European and American scholars. The brief review of selected anthropology anthologies provided here should serve as a useful guide to relevant sources on the physical anthropology of South Asian people. This review will be especially valuable to those for whom South Asia is a new and unfamiliar area of academic interest.

Anthropological anthologies of the 1960s consisted primarily of papers on the prehistoric archaeology and sociocultural anthropology of South Asia. Contributions in the area of physical anthropology, comprising about 37% of the papers in these volumes, were few, and they focused on the racial classifications of living and prehistoric peoples of the subcontinent (Madan and Sarana, 1962; Ratnam, 1963). In more recent anthologies such as *Indian Anthropology Today,* for example, papers on physical anthropological topics constitute a similar proportion (39%) of the contributions. Published in commemoration of the 50th anniversary of the founding of Calcutta University's Department of Anthropology, this volume includes three contributions on human paleontology and five on the biology of living South Asians (Sen, 1974).

Edited volumes on human paleontology in South Asia are rare, possibly because of the absence of a Pleistocene skeletal record of early man, but also because of the lack of synthetic interpretive analyses of post-Pleistocene skeletal series. Chopra's (1979) *Early Man in North West India* focuses more on paleoenvironmental reconstruction than on the analysis and interpretation of the hominoid fossil evidence from northwestern India. The geographically and topically diverse selection of articles included by Ghosh (1974) in *Perspectives in Paleoanthropology* limits the usefulness of that volume. Only two contributions in it treat topics in human paleontology: Simons (1974), on the discovery and interpretation of *Gigantopithecus,* and Kennedy (1974), on the paleodemography of Ceylon.

The skeletal record for human evolution and the biological diversity of the living peoples of Africa (Hiernaux, 1975), America (Stewart, 1973), and the Pacific islands (Howells, 1973) have been described in a concise and informative manner in Scribner's People of the World series. The *People of Asia* volume in this series is disappointing, partly because of the great breadth of focus it adopts (Bowles, 1977). The seven chapters that comprise the third part of that volume are devoted to the "human pageantry of greater India." Bowles documents the cultural history of the subcontinent well, but the absence of a biological focus is disappointing to the physical anthropologist. When an assessment of South Asia's biological diversity is provided—later in the volume—it conforms to traditional methods and objectives of morphological classification of racial groups. A thorough historical and interpretive analysis of the paleoanthropology of South Asia was prepared by Kennedy (in press), and it promises to be a valuable addition to the literature on human paleontology.

Frequently, anthologies in physical anthropology published in India have a broad geographic scope that extends far beyond the borders of the subcontinent. The Professor S. S. Sarkar memorial volume, for example, contains only five contributions on the physical anthropology of Indian populations, with the remainder devoted to the human biology of African and Eurasian peoples or to problems of methodology (Basu, Ghosh, Biswas, and Ghosh, 1973).

The most comprehensive compendia of physical anthropological research in India were published by the Anthropological Survey of India (Rakshit, 1975, 1976). These dates of publication obscure the fact that the volumes consist of papers written for seminars held in 1970, and consequently they reflect the status of research during the late 1960s rather than the early or mid-1970s. Nonetheless, these volumes include numerous contributions that are primarily by Indian physical anthropologists on a wide range of topics. Papers on human genetics, dermatoglyphics, and demography comprise the bulk of these volumes and, though few in number, articles on paleoanthropological topics are contained in each.

A special issue of the *Journal of Human Evolution* (1978, Vol. 7, No. 1) was devoted to papers on the prehistory and physical anthropology of India. Six of the 11 articles in this issue are on physical anthropological topics; several of these nicely complement papers that appear in the present volume (Malhotra, 1978; Sanghvi, 1978). Specific problems regarding the demography of Indian populations are addressed by the wide selection of articles appearing in *Biosocial Studies in India* (Pakrasi, Banerjee, and Das, 1976). The results of the joint Indo-Soviet research expedition provided abundant new data on anthropological variation in genetics and on the morphology of North Indian populations (Abdushalishvili and Malhotra, 1980).

The journal *Anthropologischer Anzeiger* devoted a recent issue to topics in South Asian physical anthropology in honor of Professor Ilse Schwidetsky's 75th birthday. It contains pertinent reviews of the relationship of Indian and German physical anthropology (Schwidetsky, 1983), population structure and genetics (Chopra, 1983; Walter, 1983), somatology (Hauser and Wytek, 1983), maturation and senescence (Sidhu, Singh, and Kansal, 1983), anthropometry of Himachel Pradesh (Singh and Bhasin, 1983), and the ethnogenesis of South Asian populations (Bernhard, 1983). This collection of papers reflects well the main areas of activity of German–Indian research in the physical anthropology of South Asia, and provides valuable alternative perspectives and supplemental data to the papers contained in the present volume.

Several recent publications provide an excellent introduction to problems in human population genetics in India. The proceedings of the first conference of the Indian Society of Human Genetics offers a well-balanced introduction to current areas of research in population genetics in India (Sanghvi, Balakrishnan, Bhatia, Sukumaran, and Undevia, 1974). The anthropometric, anthroposcopic, and genetic variations of the people of Tamil Nadu are analyzed by Sanghvi, Balakrishnan, and Karve (1981) to determine the biological relationships among several sociocultural groups in this region of southeastern India.

A series of important papers on human genetics and adaptation of Indian and non-Indian populations were presented at the Golden Jubilee Conference of the Indian Statistical Institute. These papers were recently published under the editorship of A. Basu and K. C. Malhotra (1984).

The present volume is divided into two main sections: Part I, Paleoanthropology, and Part II, Biological Anthropology of the Living. Neither of these sections can exist independently and adequately reflect the topical diversity and theoretical unity of physical anthropology. Contributions to Part I are organized in a roughly chronological order. Badgley and colleagues discuss the Miocene hominoid fossil record from the Potwar Plateau of northern Pakistan, and they provide data regarding the environments these primates inhabited. Pleistocene hominid fossils are unknown for the South Asian subcontinent, although a prolific artifactual record of the presence of early man is present (Kennedy, 1980). Biological characteristics of two very important skeletal series from Mesolithic sites in the Ganga Plains of North India are described by Kennedy. The large body size, robust skeletal morphology, and megadonty of these early occupants of northern India are described by Kennedy as being similar to other terminal Pleistocene/early Holocene populations of Africa, Asia, and Europe.

In his reanalysis of the human remains from Harappa, Dutta finds evidence for biological continuity between these protohistoric inhabitants of the Indus Valley and the people living there today. Sankalia, Ansari, and Dhavalikar provide an insightful perspective on settlement patterns and socioeconomic variations at Inamgaon, an early farming village in western India. This work is based on a house-by-house analysis of artifacts and is the first overview of this evidence since the completion of excavations at Inamgaon in 1982. Consequently, it provides a current contextual framework for an analysis of paleodemography at Inamgaon by Lukacs and Walimbe.

The concept of an Indo-Aryan invasion of the South Asian subcontinent frequently appears in the literature of physical anthropology and, perhaps more often, archaeology. The contribution by Schaffer considers the archaeological evidence for such an invasion and presents an alternative hypothesis of sociocultural evolution that he finds more consistent with the evidence.

A reference compendium of prehistoric human skeletal remains and burial practices is provided by Kennedy and Caldwell. This contribution contains a wealth of information regarding human skeletal samples from South Asia and includes data on (1) geographic location, chronology, and cultural context of the sites yielding human remains; (2) the burial practices as evidenced by archaeological data and skeletal remains; and (3) the size, condition, and current status of each osteological sample.

Part II, Biological Anthropology of the Living, includes contributions on the morphology, genetics, demography, and ecology of South Asian populations. Occlusal variation among urban and rural children in northern India is evaluated comparatively by Kaul and Corruccini. More frequent and more severe malocclusion is found among urban children whose diets are softer than those of their rural age-mates.

Dermatoglyphics has figured prominently in the physical anthropology of South Asian populations. Dash Sharma provides a thorough review of the history of dermatoglyphic studies in the subcontinent and presents the major research conclusions derived from this field of study.

Four contributions on genetic topics provide a sample of the kinds of genetic research currently being conducted in South Asia. Sundar Rao carefully defines the terms and concepts essential to understanding the significance of inbreeding, and then proceeds to discuss the nature of inbreeding and its consequences for South Indian populations.

Genetic methods of estimating taxonomic distance are discussed by Reid, who applies these methods to determine genetic relationships between certain Indian populations. The genetic distance between Indian populations and their neighbors to the southeast and northwest is the focus of Roychoudhury's contribution. He finds strong genetic ties between certain Indian groups and their northwestern neighbors in Iran and Afghanistan. The genetic consequences of population structure are discussed by Malhotra who reviews matrimonial distance, marriage rules, and levels of inbreeding among the Dhangar caste-cluster of Maharashtra.

Are changes in rate of population growth the result or the cause of changes in subsistence? Population data for the Peshawar Basin before and after the introduction of irrigation is presented by Weitz to show that increased agricultural productivity does not always result in immediate population growth. Demographic data from northeastern India and eastern Nepal are examined by Basu, Gupta, and Mukhopadhyay, who find broadly similar rates of population growth in different study areas. Differences in growth rate are attributed to variations in sociocultural response to a range of high altitude stressors.

The biological processes of growth and aging are affected by a variety of factors, one of which is life in high altitude environments. Using the "lifespan approach," Beall describes growth, development, and aging for several biological variables in the resident high altitude population of Upper Chumik, Nepal. These data are then compared with parallel data from appropriate high and low altitude populations.

Though widely known because of their success as guides for international mountaineering expeditions, the Sherpas of eastern Nepal's Khumbu region have only recently been subjected to scientific study. Weitz provides a valuable summary of settlement patterns, demography, nutrition, and disease among the Sherpas of Khumbu and discusses in detail their adaptations to hypoxia. Malik and Singh describe the biological and cultural adaptations of the Ladakis of the western Himalaya Mountains to their barren, high altitude environment.

A more ecological perspective is adopted by Malhotra and Gadgil in their analysis of subsistence strategies among the pastoralists of Maharashtra. Traditional subsistence patterns of two nomadic groups are described, and recent changes in their subsistence patterns are discussed and explained.

This volume will be considered a success by the editor if it does the following: (1) opens new vistas for students of human evolution and biological adaptation who are unfamiliar with the evidence from South Asia; (2) enlightens and intellectually stimulates South Asian scholars in fields of study that are peripheral to physical anthropology; (3) results in a reappraisal of current research foci; and (4) engenders greater international cooperation in the study of the physical anthropology of South Asia.

The greatest vote of thanks is given to the authors, whose dedication and commitment to quality research in physical anthropology and archaeology are reflected by their contributions to this volume. It is regrettable but perhaps unavoidable that several solicited papers were unable to appear in this volume because of the heavy research, writing, and administrative obligations of the authors.

ACKNOWLEDGMENTS

This volume developed from a session on biological anthropology of South Asia held at the Ninth Wisconsin Conference on South Asia (Madison; November, 1980). The focus of this volume and a list of potential contributors were discussed in detail with Dr. K. C. Malhotra during his visit to the University of Oregon in November, 1980. The editor is indebted to Dr. Malhotra for his valuable advice and assistance and to the Smithsonian Institution (Special Foreign Currency Program) for providing Dr. Malhotra's travel funds.

References

Abdushalishvili, M. G., and Malhotra, K. C., 1980, *New Anthropological Data for Northern India: Results of the 1971 Joint Indo–Soviet Expedition,* Academy of Sciences of U.S.S.R., Moscow. (In Russian.)

Basu, A., and Malhotra, K. C. (eds.), 1983, Human genetics and adaptation, *Proc. of the Indian Statistical Institute's Golden Jubilee Conference, Calcutta, 1982.*

Basu, A. (ed.), 1973, *Physical Anthropology and Its Expanding Horizons,* (Prof. S. S. Sarkar Memorial Volume), Orient Longman, Bombay.

Basu, A., Ghosh, A. K., Biswas, S. K., and Ghosh, R., 1973, *Physical Anthropology and its Extending Horizons.* Orient Longman, New Delhi.

Bernhard, W., 1983, Ethnogenesis of South Asia with special reference to India. *Anthropologischer Anzeiger.* **41**(2):93–110.

Bowles, G. T., 1977, *The People of Asia,* Charles Scribner's Sons, New York.

Chopra, S. R. K., 1979, *Early Man in North West India,* Allied Publishers, Bombay.

Chopra, V. P., 1983, Population structure of the Indian people: Some microevolutionary aspects. *Anthropologischer Anzeiger.* **41**(2):111–117.

Ghosh, A. K. (ed.), 1974, *Perspectives in Paleoanthropology,* Firma K. L. Mukhopadhyay, Calcutta.

Guha, B. S., 1935, The racial affinities of the people of India, in: *Census of India: 1931,* Volume 1, Part 3a, Government of India, Simla.

Hauser, G., and Wytek, R., 1983, Somatovariants of females from Northern India. *Anthropologischer Anzeiger*. **41**(2):129–135.
Hiernaux, J., 1975, *The People of Africa*, Charles Scribner's Sons, New York.
Hodgen, M. T., 1964, *Early Anthropology in the Sixteenth and Seventeenth Centuries*, University of Pennsylvania Press, Philadelphia.
Howells, W. W., 1973, *The Pacific Islanders*, Charles Scribner's Sons, New York.
Kennedy, K. A. R., 1973, Race and Culture, in: *Main Currents in Cultural Anthropology*, (R. Naroll and F. Naroll, eds.), Prentice-Hall, Englewood Cliffs.
Kennedy, K. A. R., 1974, Paleodemography of Ceylon: A study of the biological continuum of a population from prehistoric to historic times, in: *Perspectives in paleoanthropology* (A. Ghosh, ed.). K. L. Mukhopadhyay, Calcutta, pp. 95–112.
Kennedy, K. A. R., 1976, *Human Variation in Space and Time*, Wm. C. Brown, Dubuque.
Kennedy, K. A. R., 1980, Prehistoric skeletal record of man in South Asia, *Annu. Rev. of Anthropol.* **9**:391–432.
Kennedy, K. A. R., 1983, *God-apes and Ape-men: The Paleoanthropology of South Asia*, Cornell University Press, Ithaca. (In press.)
Madan, T. N., and Gopala, Sarana (eds.), 1962, *Indian Anthropology: Essays in Memory of D. N. Majumdar*, Asia Publishing House, Bombay.
Malefijt, A. de Wall, 1968, *Homo monstrosus*, *Sci. Am.* **219**(4):112–118.
Malhotra, K. C., 1978, Morphological composition of the people of India, *J. Hum. Evol.* **7**(1):45–54.
Pakrasi, K. B., Banerjee, A. R., and Das, A. K. (eds.), 1976, *Bio-social Studies in India: A Reading in Collected Papers, 1961–1970*, Editions India, Calcutta.
Rakshit, H. K. (ed.), 1975, Bio-anthropological research in India, *Proc. of the Seminar in Physical Anthropology and Allied Sciences*, Anthropological Survey of India, Calcutta.
Rakshit, H. K. (ed.), 1976, *Anthropology in India. Physical Anthropology*, Volume 2, Anthropological Survey of India, Calcutta.
Ratnam, B. (ed.), 1963, *Anthropology on the March*, Social Sciences Association, Madras.
Risley, H. H., 1908, *The People of India*, Thacker, Spink and Company, Calcutta and Simla.
Sanghvi, L. D., 1978, Nature of genetic variation in the people of western India, *J. Hum. Evol.* **7**(1):55–66.
Sanghvi, L. D., Balakrishnan, V., Bhatia, H. M., Sukumaran, P. K., and Undevia, J. V. (eds.), 1974, Human population genetics in India, *Proc. First Conf. Ind. Soc. Hum. Genet.*, Orient Longman, New Delhi.
Sanghvi, L. D., Balakrishnan, V., and Karve, I., 1981, *Biology of the People of Tamil Nadu*, Indian Society of Human Genetics, Bombay, and Indian Anthropological Survey, Calcutta.
Schwidetsky, I., 1983, Short History of Indian–German relations in physical anthropology. *Anthropologischer Anzeiger*. **41**(2):85–92.
Sen, D. (ed.), 1974, Indian anthropology today, *Proc. of the All-India Seminar on Indian Anthropology*, Anthropology Department, Calcutta University.
Sidhu, L. S., Singh, I. P., and Kansal, D. K., 1983, Processes of maturation and senescence in two communities of Punjab (India) as studied from morphological measures. *Anthropologischer Anzeiger*. **41**(2):149–159.
Simons, E. L., 1974, On the discovery of *Gigantopithecus* in north India, in: *Perspectives in paleoanthropology* (A. Ghosh, ed.). K. L. Mukhopadhyay, Calcutta, pp. 1–7.
Singh, I. P., and Bhasin, M. K., 1983, Anthropological studies among Pangwalas and Gaddis of Himachel Pradesh, North India. *Anthropologischer Anzeiger*. **41**(2):137–148.
Stewart, T. D., 1973, *The People of America*, Charles Scribner's Sons, New York.
Walter, H., 1983, Population genetical investigations on Indian tribals: preliminary report. *Anthropologischer Anzeiger*. **41**(2):119–128.

Contents

Part I. Paleoanthropology

Chapter 1

The Paleobiology of South Asian Miocene Hominoids

Catherine Badgley, John Kelley, David Pilbeam, and Steven Ward

Chapter 2

Biological Adaptations and Affinities of Mesolithic South Asians

Kenneth A. R. Kennedy

Chapter 3

Biological Anthropology of Bronze Age Harappans: New Perspectives

Pratap C. Dutta

Chapter 4

The Indo-Aryan Invasions: Cultural Myth and Archaeological Reality

Jim G. Shaffer

Chapter 5

Excavations at the Early Farming Village of Inamgaon, 1968–1982

H. D. Sankalia, Z. D. Ansari, and M. K. Dhavalikar

Chapter 6

Paleodemography at Inamgaon: An Early Farming Village in Western India

John R. Lukacs and Subhash R. Walimbe

Chapter 7

Dental Anthropology of South Asian Populations: A Review

John R. Lukacs

Chapter 8

South Asian Prehistoric Human Skeletal Remains and Burial Practices

Kenneth A. R. Kennedy and Peggy C. Caldwell

Part II. Biological Anthropology of the Living

Chapter 9

The Epidemiological Transition in Dental Occlusion in a North Indian Population

Samvit S. Kaul and Robert S. Corruccini

Chapter 10

Current Status of Dermatoglyphic Studies in South Asia

P. Dash Sharma

Chapter 11

Inbreeding in India: Concepts and Consequences

P. S. Sundar Rao

PART I

Paleoanthropology

CHAPTER 1

The Paleobiology of South Asian Miocene Hominoids

CATHERINE BADGLEY, JOHN KELLEY, DAVID PILBEAM, AND STEVEN WARD

1. Introduction*

Our knowledge of hominoid paleobiology has expanded dramatically in the past 10 years. Many new hominoid fossils have been recovered, principally from middle and late Miocene deposits in Europe and Asia. They are between 17 and 5 million years old. Comparative molecular studies on living hominoids have established a clear pattern of similarities and differences that almost certainly reflects a branching sequence. Broader "historical geological" research in many areas has enriched our knowledge of paleogeography, paleoclimates, and past faunas and floras considerably.

Understanding the adaptations of past hominoids involves a mixture of what can be called *direct* and *indirect evidence*. Direct evidence comes from the fossil hominoids themselves. Given our ability to select from an array of anatomical attributes in fossils clusters that can be characterized as adaptations (sometimes a relatively large "given"), we proceed to interpret the adaptations using rules or principles derived from an understanding of similar systems in living species. Inasmuch as living systems can be understood, plausible inferences can be made about past adaptations. The indirect evidence consists of the features of past

*This section prepared by D. Pilbeam.

CATHERINE BADGLEY • Museum of Paleontology, University of Michigan, Ann Arbor, Michigan 48109. ***JOHN KELLEY AND DAVID PILBEAM*** • Peabody Museum, Harvard University, Cambridge, Massachusetts 02138. ***STEVEN WARD*** • Department of Anthropology and Biology, Kent State University, Kent, Ohio 44242.

communities in which hominoids lived that might limit the possible range of inferences about their niches.

Various kinds of data can be synthesized into a generally consistent story of hominoid evolution. The initial split of "western" (African apes plus humans) and "eastern" (the Asian orangutan *Pongo*) larger hominoids and their ancestors probably occurred at least 14 million years ago—perhaps earlier. This interpretation is based on anatomical similarities between the Asian middle and late Miocene hominoid genera *Sivapithecus* and *Ramapithecus* and the living orangutan *Pongo* in features plausibly viewed as derived relative to other hominoids (Andrews, 1982; Pilbeam, 1982; Ward and Pilbeam, 1982). The oldest specimen with such features is a *Sivapithecus* from Pakistan, which is some 12 to 13 million years old (n.d.). The adaptive radiation of Eurasian Miocene hominoids, from which the living orangutan *Pongo* is probably ultimately derived, is now moderately well documented (Pilbeam, 1982). Six areas have yielded particularly significant material: Salonika in Greece, Yassioren in Turkey, the Potwar Plateau of Pakistan, Ramnagar in Kashmir, Hari Talyangar in India, and Lufeng in China. Among these, Pakistan possesses an unusually long, informative record of Miocene hominoids and their environmental contexts.

The later divergence of African apes and hominids is essentially undocumented by fossils. It can be estimated, on the basis of molecular comparisons (Sarich and Cronin, 1975), to fall between 6 and 10 million years ago, if we accept that the initial western-eastern split is 14 to 18 million years old. Unfortunately, the hominoid fossil record in East Africa is very poor between 4 and 14 million years ago, and that for western and central Africa is nonexistent.

Over the last nine years in the Potwar Plateau in Pakistan, the Geological Survey of Pakistan–Harvard Peabody Museum (GSP–HPM) research project has essentially "drilled" the equivalent of a long deep-sea core, continuous from 15–16 million to 1–2 million years ago (Pilbeam *et al.*, 1979; Barry *et al.*, 1982). It is quite well calibrated, the basic paleontological work is now nearing completion, and almost all the many new hominoid fossils found have been described (Pilbeam *et al.*, 1980; Pilbeam, 1982). In addition, tentative inferences about paleoecology have been made (Badgley and Behrensmeyer, 1980), and there have been considerable advances in approaches to paleoecology. The new information from this Siwalik research is very significant; for example, biostratigraphic documentation is now detailed enough so that we can consider the distribution of hominoid fossils through time in relation to the temporal distribution of many other mammals. Still, much fieldwork and synthesis remain to be completed.

Our research in Pakistan has been made possible through close collaboration with the Geological Survey of Pakistan. The joint GSP–HPM project led by Dr. S. M. Ibrahim Shah and David Pilbeam has concentrated mostly in Siwalik Group rocks of the Potwar Plateau. These sediments are fluvial, consisting of alternating sandstones and conglomerates, silts, and clays. They span approximately the last 15 or 16 million years with few major breaks in deposition.

We have collected more than 15,000 fossils from over 500 localities on the Plateau, and these have been tied to local and then to composite regional stratigraphic columns. These columns are calibrated by a few radiometric age estimates and by a comprehensive suite of paleomagnetic determinations.

Elsewhere in Pakistan, brief field surveys at Dera Bugti in Baluchistan and near Lake Manchar in the Sind, also in fluvial rocks, have added older fossils, enabling us to extend our biostratigraphic columns back into the early Miocene. Pakistan thus provides a composite South Asian sequence spanning the last 20 million years; this sequence documents some significant faunal changes. These are presumably in response to paleogeographical and paleoecological changes that affected migration, faunal mixing, competition, and other factors, as well as to even less well-understood phenomena.

Although appearances and disappearances occur throughout the sequence, there are some periods of more marked change. One of these at ca. 17 million years ago documents the first appearance in South Asia of bovids, suids, possibly hominoids, and other mammals of perhaps ultimately Afro-Arabian origin. This may correspond to the (? temporary) closure of the eastern Tethys. Nearly 10 million years ago the region experienced a substantial turnover of large mammals, although a number of groups, including hominoids, endured and were apparently unchanged. Some 7 million years ago a third period of flux began. This is less well sampled than is the preceding one, and it may have continued until 3 million years ago. It probably documents a phase of faunal exchange with Africa and perhaps Europe. During this period, hominoids became locally extinct in this part of southern Asia.

2. Siwalik Hominoid Material*

The GSP–HPM Siwalik fossil collection includes approximately 135 hominoid specimens. Approximately 50 additional specimens from the Potwar Plateau collected over the last 100 years are in the collections of the American Museum of Natural History, the Yale Peabody Museum, the British Museum of Natural History, and the Geological Survey of India. Several specimens collected by G. H. R. von Koenigswald are at the Forschungsinstitut in Senckenberg. The earlier Potwar specimens are, for the most part, of uncertain provenance, which limits their usefulness for taxonomy. Siwalik hominids from Ramnagar and Hari Talyangar are mostly housed with the Geological Survey of India. Approximately two thirds of the GSP–HPM specimens come from only

*This section prepared by J. Kelley.

Table I
Potwar Hominoid Fossils by Locality[a]

Locality	Hominoid fossils		Systematics			Lithology
	Cranial or dental	Postcranial	Large	Small	Indet.	
137	1	—	1	—	—	indeterminate
182	16	1	3	9	5	Sand & gravel
191	1	—	1	—	—	Sand & gravel
207	1	—	1	—	—	Sand; Sand/Silt
211	1	—	—	—	1	Sand & gravel
221	2	1	1	—	2	Sand & gravel; Sand/Silt
224	4	1	1	2	2	sandy Silt
226	1	—	—	1	—	Sand; Silt
227	2	—	—	—	2	Sand
230	1	—	1	—	—	indeterminate
251	1	—	—	—	1	Sand & gravel
259	1	—	—	—	1	Sand & gravel
260	26	9	18	9	8	sandy Silt
261	1	—	1	—	—	Sand & gravel
309	3	—	2	1	—	Sand; silty sand; silt
310	—	1	—	1	—	Sand & gravel
311 Nagri	16	9	16	1	8	Sand & gravel; sandy Silt
314	1	—	1	—	—	Sand & gravel
317	12	2	7	4	3	Sand & gravel; Sand/Silt
327	1	—	—	—	1	silty Clay
328	1	—	1	—	—	?
350	2	—	1	—	1	Sand & gravel
409	1	—	—	1	—	Sand & gravel
410	1	—	1	—	—	Silt
414	2	—	1	1	—	Sand & gravel
416	2	—	1	—	1	Sand & gravel
442	1	—	—	—	1	Sand
463	1	—	1	—	—	Sand & gravel
494[b] Chinji	1	—	1	—	—	sandy Silt
495[b] Chinji	—	1	—	—	1	Sand & gravel
496[b] Chinji	3	—	2	1	—	sandy Silt
498[b] Chinji	1	—	—	1	—	Sand
499[b] Chinji	1	—	1	—	—	Sand
500[b] Chinji	1	1	1	—	1	Sand

[a]Each hominoid locality is described in terms of skeletal parts present (cranial/dental, or postcranial), systematics of hominoid material (large, small, or indeterminate), and the lithology of fossiliferous horizons. All localities are from Middle Siwalik sediments in the Khaur area, unless otherwise indicated. Locality numbers followed by "Nagri" or "Chinji" signify that the locality occurs in the type section of the formation. The predominant lithology is indicated by a capital letter; hence, "sandy Silt" means that the lithology is sand with a substantial portion of silt present. "Sand/Silt" signifies interbedded sand and silt. For some localities (e.g. 207, 221), more than one lithology is fossiliferous.

[b]For all these localities, the information is a personal communication from S. Mahmood Raza.

four localities near the U level—the label given to a prominent sandstone (Table I). A large portion of the remaining hominoid localities, none of which has produced more than a few specimens, also cluster near the U level (Barry *et al.*, 1980; Pilbeam *et al.*, 1980) (Figure 1). Thus, our knowledge of Potwar Siwalik hominoids that occupied the region at least intermittently from more than 12 million years ago to around 7.5 million years ago derives almost exclusively from a period of time that is probably no more than a few hundred thousand years in duration. Adding the Indian localities improves the sampling density only slightly.

The collection consists mostly of maxillary and mandibular fragments and isolated teeth (Tables II and III). This sample was augmented recently by the discovery of a partial face and associated mandible, GSP 15000 (Pilbeam, 1982; Pilbeam and Smith, 1981). There are also an increasing number of postcranial elements, mostly fragmentary, from which we can now make some tentative functional statements with implications for positional behavior and substrate preference (Pilbeam *et al.*, 1980). At present, association between cranial and postcranial elements can be made only on the basis of size because no associated material has been found yet. The following discussion of sorting and taxonomy will concern only craniofacial remains.

Table II
Potwar Hominoid Sample, Excluding Teeth

Craniofacial	Specimen number
Maxillae (3)	GSP 9977, 16075, 15000
Maxillary fragments (5)	GSP 9897, 11708, 11786, 11704, 15557
Mandibles (3)	GSP 4622, 9564, 15000
Mandibular fragments (20)	GSP 4230, 9563, 13165, 11706, 11705/07, 7619, 6153, 6160, 13445, 13444, 13566, 15629, 15397, 14951, 15556, 13808, 13873, 16082, 17125, 16077
Juv. mandibular fragments (2)	GSP 11536/7, 12709
Postcranial	
Humeral fragments (3)	GSP 12271, 13606, 6663
Radius (1)	GSP 7611
Capitate (1)	GSP 17119
Pollical phalangeal fragment (1)	GSP 6664
Femoral head (5)	GSP 6178, 15782, 13929, 11867, 9894
Femoral fragments (2)	GSP 13420, 12654
Talar fragment (1)	GSP 10785
Calcaneal fragments (3)	GSP 4664, 17606, 17152
Intermediate cuneiform (1)	GSP 6454
Lateral cuneiform (1)	GSP 17118
Hallucial metatarsal fragment (1)	GSP 14064
Hallux (1)	GSP 14064
Phalangeal fragments (5)	GSP 15784, 15783, 6666, 13168, 17152

2.1. Mandibles and Mandibular Fragments

There are 23 adult mandibles and mandibular fragments in the collection. Most of these consist of a single fragment of corpus, which is usually broken posteriorly near the root of the ascending ramus and anteriorly in the canine/premolar region. Two of these preserve both left and right corpora with an intact symphysis, whereas only GSP 15000 has significant portions of the ascending rami, including a portion of a condyle. Eight of the mandibular fragments are edentulous; the others preserve one or more postcanine teeth. GSP 15000 has a complete dentition and is the only mandibular specimen with complete, associated canine crowns. It is also the only specimen preserving erupted incisors. There are two juvenile mandibles, one with the symphysis, three deciduous molars, and a deciduous canine.

2.2. Maxillae and Maxillary Fragments

There are eight maxillae and maxillary fragments. GSP 15000 preserves a complete, intact palate that includes complete dentition. The left side of the face is nearly complete, lacking only a portion of the maxilla near the zygomatico-maxillary suture, part of the alveolar process, and a segment of the inferior orbital margin. The zygomatic process and mandibular fossa of the left temporal bone are also present. Most of the right side is missing, with the exception of nasal and alveolar processes of the maxilla and most of the nasal bones. There are two other nearly complete palates, and both preserve much of the premaxillary region. One lacks only the incisors and the other is nearly edentulous. Two half maxillae preserve a portion of the zygomatic process, the canine juga and fossa, the palate to the midline, and the naso-alveolar clivus. Four maxillae have associated canines that preserve at least part of the crowns.

2.3. Dentition

Table III summarizes the dental sample. Because it is often difficult to distinguish between isolated first and second molars, these are combined for the total sample of associated and isolated teeth.

2.4. Sorting and Taxonomy

2.4.1. Methodological problems. Difficulties in sorting a fossil sample into taxa center on the problem of correctly partitioning the total sample variation resulting from intraspecific variation, including sexual dimorphism, and interspecific differences. For estimates of these components of variation we look to extant species for standards of maximum and minimum intraspecific variation,

TABLE III
Dental Sample. Associated Teeth Are Those Still Implanted in the Maxilla or Mandible, (Total Sample Includes Isolated Teeth)

	I1		I2		C		P3		P4		M1		M2		M3		dm1		dm2		dC	
	U	L	U	L	U	L	U	L	U	L	U	L	U	L	U	L	U	L	U	L	U	L
Associated	2	2	2	2	5	2	7	6	8	7	9	9	6	15	5	15	0	2	0	1	0	1
Total	11	5	3	2	16	7	7	7	13	10	33[a]	29[a]	33[a]	29[a]	11	24	0	2	1	1	0	1

[a]These entries denote M1 and M2 combined.

patterns of sexual dimorphism, and amounts of overlap among sympatric species, assuming that fossil taxa conform to these ranges or patterns of variation. However, this assumption may not be warranted. For example, certain Miocene hominoid samples considered by some to represent a single dimorphic species based on canine size and morphology exceed the limits of intraspecific variation that is seen in extant species in postcanine tooth size. Such conflicts between different modern analogies cannot be easily resolved.

Even with these modern standards, attempts to sort fossil samples are limited by several factors. Important among them are small sample size, the time-averaged nature of fossil accumulations, the kinds of skeletal parts preserved, and their state of preservation. Small sample size often precludes satisfactory statistical analysis of variation, which is necessary when dealing with characters such as dental metrics whose distributions are continuous rather than discrete. The time-averaged nature of fossil samples means they are not strictly comparable to samples of extant species, which essentially represent a single point in time. A single fossiliferous horizon may represent thousands of years. It would not be surprising if a species sample from even a single locality showed a range of variation near the upper limit of that seen in extant species. There is also no reason to assume that a modern species that is sampled over its entire range will more closely approximate in variability a time-averaged sample. Preservational conditions and bias limit the comparisons with extant species to a relatively few skeletal parts. As is evident from Tables II and III, dental and gnathic elements are disproportionately represented. These are not always useful for making species-level distinctions, particularly when they are fragmentary and few in number. Additionally, most Siwalik specimens are unassociated. Many characters must be treated independently so that it is difficult to build up an inventory of associated character states—that is, a number of characters that appear in association on many specimens and that sort the specimens identically. This makes for apparent noncongruence of states, such as the extremely large teeth associated with a very small mandible seen in GSP 13566, which is particularly confusing.

The difficulty of sorting fossil samples can be illustrated by doing the same with extant and closely related sympatric species, using only the skeletal parts that are typically preserved in fossil assemblages. Here, degrees of intraspecific variation, sexual dimorphism, and mean interspecific difference would be known. Sorting errors would still occur (even with a reasonable sample size), and the number of species represented would not likely be unambiguous. Without knowing *a priori* the relative contribution to total variation of each of these factors, particularly with inadequate samples, sorting specimens into species and sex classes is difficult indeed.

Sorting and taxonomy of Siwalik hominoids. There is some morphological heterogeneity in the Potwar sample, but the implications of this with respect to intraspecific variation, sexual dimorphism, and interspecific differences are unclear and may not be resolvable given the sample sizes and dissociated state of most of the material. There are at least two distinct upper and lower canine morphs. There are also both mandibular and maxillary specimens with canine roots or alveoli for which all known canines are too large. The latter may be indicative of a low-crowned canine like those in Miocene hominoid samples from Lufeng in China and Ravin de la Pluie in Greece. There are at least two different upper, central incisor morphs. There also appears to be differential development of the maxillary sinus in large and small specimens, which may be an expression of sexual dimorphism. Finally, among dentally large specimens there may be two distinct mandibular morphologies with some, as represented by GSP 9564, having relatively deep and extremely thickened corpora and perhaps very narrow incisor regions. A larger sample size may show variation in these mandibular features to be continuous, but that would necessitate an extreme amount of intraspecific, intrasexual variation.

Kay (1983) has recently attempted a taxonomy of all Siwalik hominoids. He sorted the specimens and diagnosed the taxa entirely on the dimensions of the postcanine teeth, implying that in other features the samples was homogeneous. He recognized four taxa (listed in order of decreasing size): *Gigantopithecus giganteus, Sivapithecus indicus, S. sivalensis,* and *S. simonsi*. The hypodigm of *G. giganteus* and *S. simonsi* included two and three specimens respectively; the remainder of the specimens were assigned to *S. indicus* and *S. sivalensis*. Excluding the size extremes represented by *G. giganteus* and *S. simonsi,* larger specimens were assigned to *S. indicus* and smaller specimens to *S. sivalensis,* with both species showing low to moderate sexual dimorphism. *S. sivalensis* included specimens attributed by others to *Ramapithecus* (Pilbeam *et al.*, 1977). Kay assumed that the coefficients of variation for a fossil species sampled over time do not exceed the maximum seen in extant species, and that there was no geographic variation or phyletic evolution over time within species in the sample. We do not feel that either of these assumptions is justified; nor, as noted, is it accurate to characterize the sample as morphologically homogeneous in features other than postcanine dental metrics.

Regarding the first assumption, it is unwarranted to assume that a sample spread over several million years is comparable in terms of coefficients of variation to samples of extant species. Regarding the second assumption, there is some indication that there is either geographic or temporal variation (or perhaps a separate species) present in the sample from Hari Talyangar; the large specimens are uniformly larger than all but the largest Potwar specimens. Hari Talyangar may be as much as a million years younger than the U sandstone level and is faunally distinct (J. Barry, personal communication). Excluding these hominoid fossils from Kay's *S. indicus* dental sample might allow for quite different interpretations of the clustering of specimens.

A further weakness in Kay's methodology is his reliance upon dental metrics in sorting. The problem is the noncongruence of different character states. Clusters derived from a single tooth size sometimes include specimens that vary greatly in other characters, such as mandibular depth and morphology or the size and morphology of other associated teeth. There is no reason to expect that any one character (tooth dimensions) should fall within the ranges of variation of extant species while others exceed those ranges. These discrepancies may reflect only normal intraspecific variation, including sexual dimorphism, although in some cases it would again appear to require extreme amounts of variation. Unfortunately, species variability in many characters of interest, particularly nonmetric characters, has not been systematically investigated.

There are several other ways in which the Siwalik hominoids from the Potwar Plateau could be sorted, with taxonomy depending upon the results of the sorting. We will discuss only a few alternatives that we view as being somewhat more plausible than others. These opinions could change after a more rigorous examination of the Potwar material that is now in progress; alternatives that seem less likely now may no longer be considered so, and there may be several equally probable alternatives.

One alternative would be to recognize two species with most of the specimens belonging to one species, highly dimorphic in size, and with only the smallest specimens belonging to a second (possibly rare) species. This scheme is quite plausible if the large Hari Talyangar specimens are not included in the sample. The first species would include material previously assigned by Pilbeam and others (1977) to *S. indicus* and *Ramapithecus punjabicus*. It would include most of the Potwar material in Kay's *S. sivalensis* hypodigm and the Potwar specimens assigned by him to *S. indicus*. *S. sivalensis* has precedence over *S. indicus;* therefore the species would be named *S. sivalensis*. Naming the second species would be more problematic, and it would depend upon comparisons with material from Hari Talyangar. This species would include only the smallest of Kay's *S. sivalensis* specimens and probably those placed in *S. simonsi*. In this case, *S. sivalensis* (the larger species) would have canines that are very dimorphic morphologically but that are only slightly dimorphic in size. Canine and body-size dimorphism in the second, smaller species would be unclear because of the small sample size.

A second alternative would be similar to that proposed by Kay but with individual specimens sorting differently between the two middle-sized species of his taxonomy. Naming the two species would depend on the sorting of the type of *S. sivalensis*. In this case, the smaller species (*S. sivalensis? Ramapithecus* sp.?) would probably have relatively larger canines; the degree of canine dimorphism in the two species would probably be quite low; and body-size dimorphism would be low in each.

A third alternative would recognize two species among the larger specimens, based on mandibular morphology, with the smaller specimens representing females of both, the sorting of the latter being unclear, and with still the possibility of a very small species.

There are further possibilities. The situation becomes more complex when time is added to morphology as an associated variable, and even more so when the remaining non-Potwar, Siwalik hominoid material is added to the sample. Perhaps the most certain statement that can be made at this time regarding the Potwar sample is that more than one species is needed to account for the observed variation. For the moment, we prefer to divide the specimens into large- and small-sized groups and to retain *S. indicus* for the former and *R. punjabicus* for the latter.

3. Hominoid Functional Morphology*

With the accumulation of many new hominoid fossils from the Siwaliks, we are becoming more confident in our ability to reconstruct some elements of their natural history. However, we know far more detail about the dental mechanism of *Ramapithecus*† and *Sivapithecus* than we do about postcranial parts. Consequently, we are now in a position to formulate testable hypotheses concerning chewing and feeding behavior, but we can say little as yet about locomotor activities and substrate preferences.

3.1. The Dental Mechanism

Although the Siwalik hominoid dental and gnathic remains suggest a wide range of body sizes, most of the specimens share a common morphological pattern. As was first recognized by Simons and Pilbeam (1972) and frequently noted since, these hominoids possessed molars with thick enamel caps, implanted in robust jaws. Both features also characterize Pliocene *Australopithecus* species. This similarity in the composition of molar and jaw structure, coupled with patterns of canine implantation and the disposition of maxillomandibular buttressing systems, is believed by some to indicate shared affinity between at least some of the Asian Miocene ramamorphs (*Ramapithecus*) and the African hominids. Until recently, this was a reasonable interpretation, but with the recovery of fairly complete maxillae, some of which are associated with mandibles, it is an opportune time for a complete review of the "ramamorph" (Ward and Pilbeam, 1982) dental mechanism. While this process is still underway, we can offer some alternatives to earlier reconstructions of hominoid phylogeny that

*This section prepared by S. Ward.

†*Ramapithecus*, as used here, includes smaller Siwalik hominoid specimens that are traditionally included in this genus.

posit a direct ancestor–descendant relationship for *Ramapithecus* and *Australopithecus*.

3.1.1. The maxilla. Most of the Miocene hominoid maxillae that have been collected in the Siwaliks (since Lydekker's first report in 1879) have been attributed to *Sivapithecus*. Very few maxillae attributable to *Ramapithecus* have been recovered. The two best specimens, YPM 13799 and GSI 185, both from Hari Talyangar, are similar to each other in many respects but are incomplete. A composite picture of *Ramapithecus* can be reconstructed, however. Such a reconstruction suggests that despite a considerable difference in size, *Ramapithecus* and *Sivapithecus* were similar in maxillary structure. The central incisors of both taxa were much larger than the laterals. The subnasal alveolar process in which the incisors were implanted is distinctive among Miocene hominoids. It is a long curving element in *Sivapithecus*, when measured from the interdental point between the central incisors to its termination at the incisive fossa with the nasal cavity. The fossa itself is very small and much obstructed mediolaterally. From what we can observe in YPM 13799, *Ramapithecus* shares with *Sivapithecus* a tiny incisive canal and therefore a subnasal alveolar process that is not set off from the hard palate. The subnasal configuration preserved in the Siwalik ramamorphs is basically similar to that of the Asian pongid *Pongo pygmaeus*, but it is considerably different from the condition presented by the early Miocene hominoids in East Africa and the earliest known hominids from the Hadar Formation and Laetoli (Ward *et al.*, 1983).

Additional information about the structure of the ramamorph maxilla is provided by the size and axial alignment of the canine teeth. It has long been known that the maxillary canine of YPM 13799 was transversely rotated (Lewis, 1934; Simons, 1976). The rotational geometry of the canine of *Ramapithecus* has been interpreted as a feature shared with the earliest hominids, which also possessed rotated canines. However, *Sivapithecus* maxillae also contain transversely rotated canines (Ward and Pilbeam, 1982). The only substantive difference between *Sivapithecus* and *Ramapithecus* involves the absolute size of the canine teeth, which are massive in the former genus. At present, the functional basis of canine rotation is unclear, but a rotated configuration can be seen to augment the space available for the postcanine dentition (Ward and Pilbeam, 1982). This would be advantageous to an animal that incorporated thick enamel as part of its dental adaptation. As enamel became thicker (and the premolars and molars more voluminous), the critical constraining dimension would be the anteroposterior one. Lengthening the face would accommodate increasingly megadont molars, but this would be likely to confound another element of the ramamorph gnathic adaptation—the anteriorly situated cranio-mandibular muscle attachments. Further difficulties would be encountered in the region of the sphenomaxillary union, involving the pterygoid process and maxillary tuber. By simply rotating the canine root, there is a minimum 5% increase in the length of the postcanine segment and, in most cases, more.

With the recovery of several new *Sivapithecus* palates (Pilbeam *et al.*, 1980; Pilbeam, 1982), the maxillary postcanine dentition and supporting structures are now fairly well known. The new specimens confirm that premolars and molars have thick enamel caps and low obtuse cusps. A curious fact that was recently noted in the postcanine segments of the Siwalik hominoid sample concerns the robusticity of the maxillary alveolar processes. The smaller specimens—those that are conventionally attributed to *Ramapithecus*—appear considerably more robust than many of the larger *Sivapithecus* maxillae. This is due to the topographic relationships of the maxillary sinus that is situated above the molars and occasionally the premolars of all hominoids. If the sinus deeply excavates the alveolar process, it creates what appears to be a lightly constructed maxilla. If its floor does not encroach upon the molar roots, the maxilla is considerably more robust. At present, the biomechanical correlates of these differences are unclear. The application of computational stress analysis models to this question may clarify this issue. At the moment, at least two patterns of maxillary pneumatization can be identified in the Siwalik hominoid sample.

3.1.2. The mandible. The mandibular anatomy of *Ramapithecus* has been reviewed by Simons (1976). Except for obvious size differences, most of the observations on mandibular morphology reported by Simons apply to both *Ramapithecus* and *Sivapithecus*. The incisors are implanted in a constricted region between the two canines. The anterior premolar is sectorial but shows some reduction in the length of its shearing edge when compared to most of the early Miocene apes. In addition, there is considerable variation with respect to development of a metaconid. Thus, in a strict sense, some Potwar anterior premolars can be considered *bicuspid*.

All molars possess thick enamel caps and low, blunt cusps. An interesting fact that has emerged from our X-ray studies of the Siwalik hominoid dental mechanism is that there is a pronounced size differential in the crown–root lengths of the postcanine teeth. The first molar and the two premolars have roots of similar length. An abrupt shift in root length occurs at the second molar. This tooth as well as the third molar has roots that extend into the mandible considerably farther than their more anterior counterparts. It is interesting to note that this pattern also occurs in baboons, macaques, and guenons. At present, we can offer no functional explanation for molar root heteromorphy, but it appears likely that two morphogenetic fields are operating in the postcanine segment of the Siwalik hominoids.

The mandibular corpus itself diverges posteriorly. The corpus of *Ramapithecus* tends to be broad and, in some specimens, almost circular in section. However, in disagreement with Kay (1981), "ramapithecine" mandibular corpora are not uniformly shallow and broad. In the Siwalik hominoid collection, the mandibular corpus has at least three patterns. Two are indeed relatively shallow, but the third is quite deep. If we include *Gigantopithecus* in the "ramapithecines," then the corpus can be deeper still.

3.2. Postcranial Elements

Although the sample of Siwalik hominoid postcranial remains is limited (see Table II), sufficient materials have been collected to make some preliminary assessments of locomotor function. At the outset, however, it is necessary to state some assumptions concerning the affinities of the postcranial specimens. Not one of these fossils was found in direct association with dental remains, but we believe that they are attributable to *Ramapithecus* or *Sivapithecus,* according to their size.

3.2.1. The forelimb. The pectoral limb is represented in the Potwar sample by a partial humeral shaft, a pair of fragmentary distal humeri, an almost complete radius from a juvenile individual, and a portion of a pollical phalanx. Pilbeam *et al.* (1980) sorted these materials into three size categories—large, medium, and small. The distal shaft of the humerus is similar to that of the living pongids, especially with respect to the size of medial and lateral supracondylar crests. The two distal articular specimens (GSP 6663, GSP 12271) provide some information on humero-ulnar and humero-radial articulation. The capitulum and trochlea appear to be clearly separated. Especially notable is the inflation of the capitulum into a bulbous, spheroid structure. This, in conjunction with a deep olecranon fossa, suggests a wide range of flexion and extension, with pronation–supination capabilities throughout this range and the possibility of "locking" the elbow joint in full or hyperextension (Pilbeam *et al.,* 1980). Of the pollical phalanx, little can be said except that it may have been less restricted in some movements than is the case for living hominoids.

The radius, although lacking its proximal and distal epiphyses, provides useful information. It is gracile, and its muscle markings are not well pronounced. This, of course, could be due to the age of the specimen, but we suspect that the gracility of the radius may reflect the adult condition. The oval, tilted head is similar to some New World monkeys, but a functional reconstruction is difficult without the articular surfaces.

Finally, a fairly complete capitate is now known from the Siwaliks. Analysis of this specimen is currently in progress. The spherical head of this specimen resembles *Ateles* and implies considerable mobility in the midcarpal joint complex (Rose, 1983).

3.2.2. The hindlimb. Portions of the hindlimb that have been attributed to Siwalik hominoids include several femoral heads, a proximal femur, femoral shafts, a talus, three calcanei, intermediate and lateral cuneiforms, part of a hallux, and several fragmentary phalangeal elements. Of these, it is possible that some femoral parts are not from primates.

GSP 13420, a femoral shaft, is broken above the condyles, and Pilbeam *et al.* (1980) speculate that the bicondylar breadth was probably rather low. Inspection of this specimen also suggests that there was little, if any, bicondylar angle.

The talus is from a small individual and is clearly hominoid. It presents a combination of features, including angulation of the trochlear surfaces and axial alignment of the subtalar articulating surfaces, suggesting that the foot was capable of a fairly wide range of inversion and of longitudinal rotation. The calcanei also support a functional reconstruction of the foot as being capable of considerable mobility. The cuboid facets are deep and funnel-shaped, indicating longitudinal rotation in the calcaneo–cuboid joint. The sustentaculum tali is large, and there is a strongly developed groove for the flexor hallucis longus. The tuber calcanei is either poorly preserved or missing altogether. However, it is clear that the posterior process is short, as in *Pongo* and *Proconsul major,* rather than long as in *Gorilla.* Collectively, the calcanei can be interpreted as components of feet that are capable of extensive eversion and inversion as well as longitudinal rotation.

The partially preserved hallux is notably robust. The proximal phalanx is especially robust and somewhat curved with moderate lateral flanging. Pilbeam *et al.* (1980) have suggested that the great toe was capable of a wide range of movement and also of powerful gripping.

It is the consensus viewpoint that the Siwalik hominoid postcranials, especially the foot elements, resemble in some ways those of the larger hominoids from early Miocene localities in East Africa. With the paucity of material, it is not possible to reconstruct substrate preferences or aspects of positional behavior. From what we know of their range of body size and postcranial morphology, it is unlikely that we can exclude the Siwalik hominoids from any specific pattern of substrate use—including the ground. However, it is plausible that *Sivapithecus* and *Ramapithecus* were fully capable of positional activities in large- and small-branch zones, given the inferred mobility of the forearm and foot.

4. Paleoecology*

After a consideration of what the hominoid fossils themselves indicate about hominoid adaptations, we shall turn to the environment of hominoid evolution in the Siwaliks. Ideally, *environment* signifies both the organic and inorganic setting which we separate here into the concepts of *climate, physiography, vegetation,* and *vertebrate community.* It is essential to document as much of the

*This section prepared by C. Badgley.

original setting as possible in order to place the origin, diversification, spread, and extinction of hominoids into a biological context.

The primary basis for paleoenvironmental reconstruction in Neogene sediments of the Potwar Plateau is the long mammalian fossil record itself. There, Siwalik deposits are unusually extensive, both in time and space, for terrestrial sedimentation. Within each local Siwalik section there are no major depositional discontinuities (Barry *et al.*, 1980). Most of the local sections have been dated by paleomagnetic stratigraphy (Tauxe and Opdyke, 1982), thus providing access to global climatic information that can be correlated with events in the faunal record. Botanical remains are nonexistent and invertebrates are uncommon. Among the vertebrate fossils, mammals predominate; and it is upon the taxonomic affiliations, inferred feeding habits, and other ecological attributes of Siwalik mammal remains that the following interpretation of hominoid environments primarily rests.

The results of field research by the GSP-HPM project permit a twofold approach to hominoid paleoecology. The first is a biostratigraphic approach. Mammalian biostratigraphy has been documented for the Potwar Siwalik sequence in considerable detail (Barry *et al.*, 1982). Thus, the abundance and distribution of hominoid fossils through time can be related to changes in composition of a diverse mammalian community. The second approach is taphonomic. Preservational features of fossil assemblages and their associated depositional environments are the basis for assessing how fossil assemblages reflect the composition of the living populations from which they were drawn. In addition, it is appropriate to review biostratigraphic changes from a taphonomic perspective: Changes through time in faunal composition can result either from changes in the composition of the living populations or from changes in preservational processes (or both). It is important to estimate the relative contribution of these two effects on that part of the Siwalik sequence under consideration.

4.1. The Biostratigraphic Approach

Within the Potwar Plateau, the most extensively documented statigraphic sequence occurs in the Khaur area. Khaur-area deposits have been traced laterally for over 30 km and measure about 4000 m in thickness. The GSP-HPM research group has collected over 10,000 fossils from the Khaur area, mostly from middle Siwalik deposits (Barry *et al.*, 1982). Figure 1 indicates the distribution of hominoid localities in the Khaur area. Most of these localities lie at the U level—a stratigraphic interval about 200 m thick. On the basis of the most recent paleomagnetic stratigraphy, the U sandstone is considered to be about 8 million years old (Tauxe and Opdyke, 1982). Individual paleomagnetic reversals have been traced laterally above and below the U sandstone for over 30 km (Behrensmeyer and Tauxe, 1982), indicating that most of the hominoid fossil

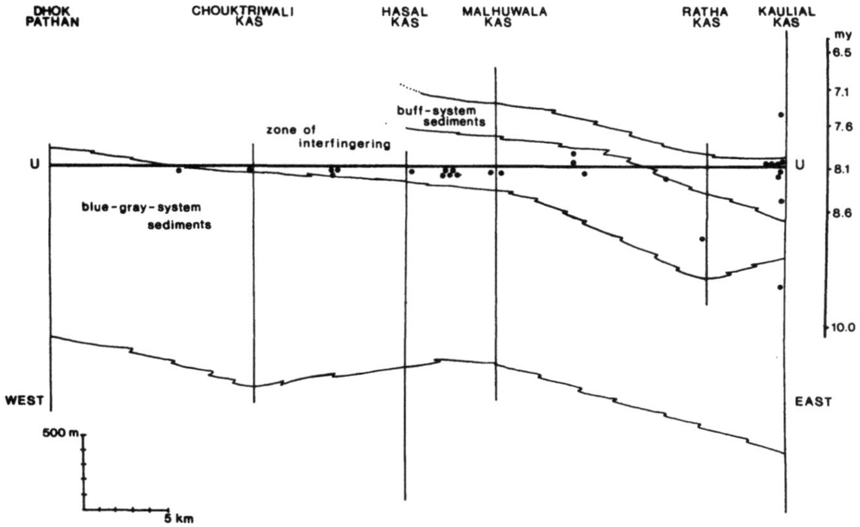

Figure 1. Hominoid localities from the Khaur area are plotted on a simplified geologic cross-section. Hominoid localities occur mainly within the sediments of the buff-sand system and the zone of interfingering of buff- and blue-gray-sand systems. Most of the localities cluster near the U sandstone which is about 8 million years old. Vertical lines indicate the positions of long measured stratigraphic sections. The names across the top of the diagram are local valley names.

localities are grouped within a narrow time interval, estimated as from 0.3 to 0.5 million years, relative to the total stratigraphic section.

It is striking that about 95% of the hominoid fossils found thus far occur within a stratigraphic interval representing only about 9% of the total Khaur section. Outside the Khaur area, hominoid remains from the middle and upper parts of the type Chinji Formation (S. M. Raza, personal communication) indicate the presence of hominoids in the Potwar area from about 12 million years ago until their final appearance in the Khaur area at about 7.5–8.0 million years ago. We will now examine the stratigraphic distribution of hominoid fossils in relation to the distribution of other mammals.

The distribution of mammal fossils in middle and upper Siwalik deposits of the Potwar Plateau has recently been organized into a novel biostratigraphic scheme by Barry *et al.* (1982). This scheme was constructed on the basis of three independently established sequences representing time (paleomagnetic stratigraphy) sediments (lithostratigraphy), and fossils (biostratigraphy). The basic unit of this scheme is the biostratigraphic *interval zone*—the stratigraphic interval between two distinctive biostratigraphic events. The boundaries of these zones, although presently assigned to precise lithostratigraphic and chronostratigraphic positions, are not immutable: New fossil discoveries may alter these boundaries

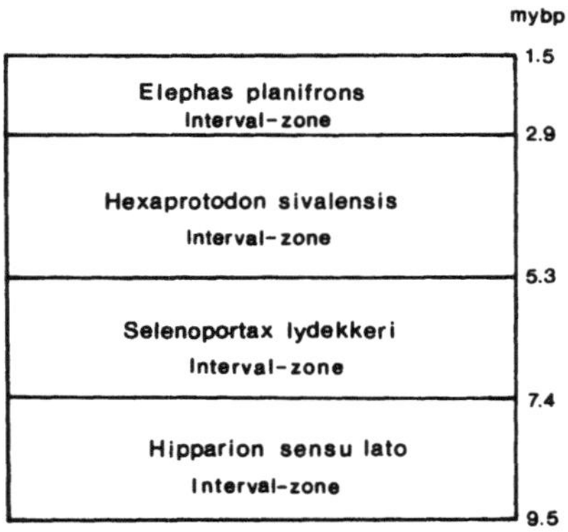

Figure 2. The biostratigraphic interval-zone scheme of Barry *et al.* (1982) with approximate age estimates, based on paleomagnetic stratigraphy for the Potwar Plateau.

within unchanged lithostratigraphic and chronostratigraphic frameworks. The faunal events marking the boundaries of the interval zones have been chosen so that they can be readily documented in fossiliferous Siwalik deposits throughout the Indian subcontinent. That is, the marker taxa are easily identifiable and relatively common as fossils in the area where they occur.

Figure 2 illustrates the interval-zone scheme of Barry *et al.* (1982), spanning the last 10 million years of the South Asian record. The U level falls within the upper third of the *Hipparian sensu lato* interval zone. In addition to hominoids, the taxa characteristic of this interval zone include the following: rodents — *Kanisamys nagrii, K. sivalensis, Brachyrhizomys nagrii, B. punjabiensis, Progonomys* sp., *Karnimata* sp.; carnivores — *Amphicyon palaeindicus, Percrocuta* sp.; proboscideans — *Choerolophodon* sp., *Stegolophodon* sp.; the rhinoceros — *Chilotherium intermedium;* several equid taxa (*Hipparion sensu lato*); suids — *Tetraconodon magnus, Hippopotamodon sivalense, Propotamochoerus hysudricus;* tragulids — *Dorcabune nagri, Dorcatherium majus, Dorcatherium* 2 spp.; and the giraffid — *Bramatherium* sp.

Taxa present that are also characteristic of the succeeding interval zone include the following: the carnivores *Sivaonyx bathygnathus* and *Eomellivora* sp.; the deinothere *Deinotherium* sp.; the rhinoceroses *Brachypotherium perimense, Gaindatherium* sp., and *Aceratherium* sp.; the peccary-like *Schizochoerus gandakasensis;* and the bovids, *Elachistoceras khauristanensis* and *Miotragoceras punjabicus.*

Barry *et al.* (1982) recognize two periods of major faunal turnover within this biostratigraphic record. The older one occurs at the base of the sequence. There the first appearance of equids coincides with the appearances of immigrant giraffids, suids, and probably bovids from diverse regional sources and the extinction of the commonest herbivore taxa from the older fauna. The later episode of faunal turnover occurs at the base of the *Elephas planifrons* interval zone. The extinction of various local taxa (the suids—cf. *Potamochoerus* and *Sivahyus,* anthracotheres, the tragulid *Dorcatherium*) coincides with the arrival of taxa with African affiliations eg., the suids—*Sivachoerus prior* and *Hippohyus* spp.) and of *Equus* and cervids from Eurasia. The modern fauna of the Indian subcontinent has its origins in this second faunal turnover.

These episodes of marked faunal change include mammals from a wide range of body sizes (rodent to elephant) and of diverse herbivorous capabilities ranging from the high-crowned teeth of the hipparionines to the relatively low-crowned bovid, suid, and giraffid dentitions. In addition, these changes involve both the disappearance of local taxa and the appearance of immigrants. This pattern suggests the influence of global environmental events involving climate and physiography, such as changes in sea level that resulted in new land bridges in Tethys or across the Bering Strait.

In contrast, between the base of the *Hipparion s.l.* interval zone and the base of the *Elephas planifrons* interval zone, there are sporadic local extinctions and immigrations and periods of taxonomic stability. These more diffuse changes in faunal composition result in a gradual change in character of the mammalian herbivores. The disappearance of hominoids above the U level is one component of this diffuse change.

The difference in pattern between abrupt and gradual faunal changes may reflect a difference in *timing* of the causes of such changes (climatic, tectonic, accompanied by possible immigrations) rather than different causal agents. Abrupt episodes of faunal turnover may be triggered by sudden tectonic or oceanographic changes, creating rapid alterations in local climates and physiography (e.g., elevation above sea level). These "physical" environmental changes may facilitate the sudden influx of foreign faunal and floral elements, resulting in relatively rapid changes in faunal composition and ecological character. The more diffuse changes probably reflect climatic, tectonic, and biological changes of an equal magnitude but at a slower rate.

As is presently documented, hominoids disappear at a time of moderate biostratigraphic change. Other faunal changes include the local extinction of deinotheres, the tragulids *Dorcatherium* and *Dorcabune,* the appearance of *Selenoportax lydekkeri* in the Khaur area, and species changes among rhizomyid rodents (Flynn and Jacobs, 1982). These events are spread over an interval representing about 0.5 million years in the fossil record. Whether these events were more synchronous or more diachronous among the actual populations is difficult to judge. Here, problems of preservation enter in. The probability that a taxon is represented in the fossil record is a function of original population size, body-size range and taphonomic history. Before attempting an interpretation of the biochronological record, we will consider the taphonomy of fossil assemblages from the U level, where hominoids are most abundant.

4.2. The Taphonomic Approach

The 200-m interval known as the U level is one of the few places in the Khaur section in which no extinctions or appearances occur. The stratigraphic-range data suggest that mammalian taxonomic composition was constant. Variations in faunal composition from one locality to another reflect both taphonomic processes and original community composition. If it is assumed that relative abundance of living populations fluctuated little and if taphonomic processes can be considered to have acted upon all skeletal remains with equal probability, then the relative abundances of taxa from fossil assemblages can serve as estimates of original community composition. With certain modifications based on taphonomic work, this model is appropriate for community reconstruction at the U level.

An examination of fossil distribution in relation to sedimentary environments indicates that fluvial transport has exerted a significant influence on the composition of fossil assemblages at the U level. The sediments can be divided into six lithologies (Behrensmeyer and Tauxe, 1982). The relative contribution of each lithology to the total section is given in Figure 3. Fossil localities are not distributed evenly through these lithologies; a representative sample of localities from the U level indicates that the lithologies most productive of fossils, both in terms of numbers of localities and of specimens, are sandstone and conglomerates. These lithologies correspond to a fluvial channel facies.

This preservational pattern has several important consequences for the interpretation of the Miocene faunal assemblages. Most collected fossils come from channel deposits—a depositional environment that is characterized by fluvial transport and winnowing of sedimentary particles (including fossils). Fossil localities from the floodplain facies (lithologies of silt and silty clay) are uncommon, and they are typically of low sample size; thus, there is little information about death assemblages undisturbed by transport. Entrainment of bone into river channels probably occurred by sheetwash floods over the contemporaneous floodplain and by erosion of channel banks consisting of earlier floodplain deposits (Badgley and Behrensmeyer, 1980). The latter may have acted as a major delivery of bones to channel-bone assemblages, because the clasts—nodular precipitates, silt, and clay fragments—of conglomerate lenses within these channel deposits are derived almost entirely from soil deposits.

In addition, the bone assemblages themselves consist primarily of fragmentary mammal remains, ranging in size from small bovid teeth to giraffe limb ends. Except for isolated teeth and podials, there are few complete skeletal elements of large mammals. We feel that the observed skeletal-element size distributions reflect the winnowing effects of the fluvial system on bones that originally entered channels. The result is that the faunal composition of channel assemblages is dominated by mammals that weighed between 20 to 200 kg. Within this size range, skeletal remains were probably preserved at random (Badgley and Behrensmeyer, 1980).

The typical hominoid locality at the U level contains one or two gnathic or dental specimens in a fossil concentration of relatively large sample size (the average number of identifiable specimens from hominoid localities is about 150) (see Table 1). As with all fossil concentrations, most hominoid localities occur in sand or gravel (Table 1 and Figure 3c). Four hominoid localities (182, 260, 311, 317) are notably prolific, with hominoid remains of high skeletal-element diver-

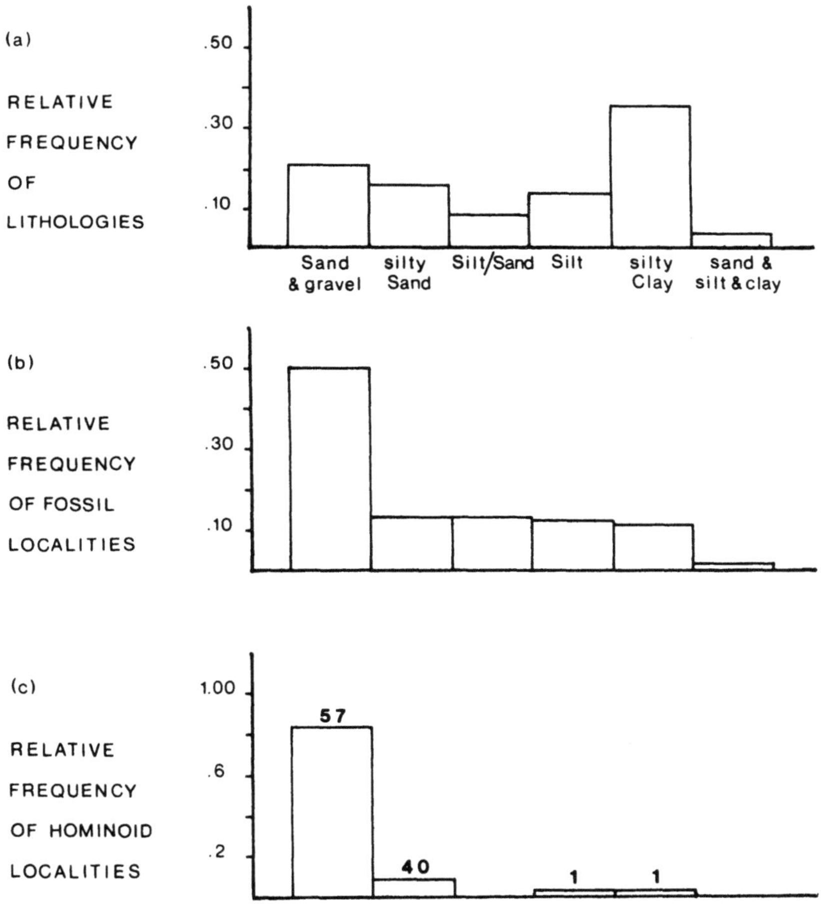

Figure 3. (a) Sediments at the U level can be divided into six major lithologies (Behrensmeyer and Tauxe, 1983). The predominant lithology is indicated by the term beginning with a capital letter; hence, "silty Sand" means that the lithology is mainly sand with substantial silt present. "Silt/Sand" means interbedded sand and silt layers. In the category "sand & silt & clay," the lithology is a heterogeneous mixture. (b) The relative frequency of fossil localities at the U level, as they occur in the six lithological categories. (c) The relative frequency of hominoid localities in different lithologies. The numbers above each histogram indicate the number of hominoid specimens from each lithology. Most localities and most specimens are from conglomerate (gravel) lenses and sandstones.

sity and representative of several individuals. The sediments at these localities suggest that the bone assemblages experienced little fluvial transport and rapid burial. Thus, the abundance of hominoid and other mammalian remains may reflect in part a local biological concentration instead of a long-term, fluvial accumulation.

A further consequence of this taphonomic history is that bones from a single channel assemblage may have been harvested from diachronous living assemblages. Behrensmeyer and Tauxe (1982) have proposed that the fluvial system in whose deposits most of the fossils occur, exhibited an alternation of floodplain buildup and then re-erosion. If so, channel bone assemblages contain skeletal remains from contemporaneous land surfaces mixed with skeletal remains eroded from older deposits of the channel banks. The time span represented by a single assemblage such as this could encompass thousands of years.

These inferred taphonomic processes have several important implications for community reconstruction. The disposition of channels across the paleolandscape suggests that no portion of the ancient floodplain went unaffected by fluvial processes that brought bones into channels; that is, no microhabitats were altogether unsampled. The approximate ''hydraulic equivalence'' of skeletal elements with other sedimentary clasts in the channel suggests that the remains of medium-sized mammals were concentrated preferentially (to larger or smaller mammals) in channel bars and channel gravels (Badgley and Behrensmeyer, 1980). But, it is plausible that the remains of medium-sized mammals were selected at random. If so, then it is possible to estimate directly the abundances of the populations from which these fossil assemblages were derived.

If bones from one fossil locality were derived at irregular intervals from a time span ranging from one to thousands of years, then the fossil assemblage cannot be considered as being representative of a synchronous fauna. The time-averaged fossil assemblage *can* serve as an estimate of original community composition only if we assume that this did not change over the period of bone accumulation. We will tentatively make this assumption with the understanding that we cannot test it in the Siwaliks. [We could possibly test this assumption by examining long-term records of faunal composition, but such records do not exist for modern communities (Badgley, 1982). Therefore, it must be regarded as a tentative assumption.]

With this caveat, a plausible description of the relative abundance of ''medium-sized'' mammal groups from channel assemblages follows: Bovids and equids are the most common, followed by suids and tragulids, then by rhinos, giraffes, and proboscideans (gomphotheres). The less-common taxa include carnivores, hominoids, and anthracotheres. It is difficult to resolve the relative abundance of fossils at the level of genus and species because lower-level taxonomic identifications are based on a small fraction of skeletal elements recovered. Therefore, these estimates are most reliable at the family level; they are useful for ecological interpretations of community organization and habitat only insofar as these mammalian families are ecologically homogenous.

Most of the ungulate herbivores were browsers, according to both macroscopic studies of dental morphology and microscopic studies of wear on occlusal surfaces (Solounias, personal communication). Possible exceptions to this pattern are the hipparionines with their high-crowned postcanine tooth row. The predominance of browsing herbivores and their wide range of body size suggests that leafy forage was present through a considerable vertical range. Thus, we infer that vegetation contained considerable areas of shrub and woodland or forest. It is difficult to estimate the density of forest from faunal remains because most fossils represent nonarboreal mammals.

The significance of these tentative paleoecological inferences for the biology of *Ramapithecus* and *Sivapithecus* is as follows. Hominoids were a minor component of the medium-sized mammal fauna at the U level. They were probably the only medium-sized mammals that inhabited an arboreal substrate, although they may have shared the arboreal realm as a food source with other large mammals such as giraffes and elephants. Occasional remains of birds, bats, and lorisids suggest that a diverse small-bodied arboreal assemblage may have existed there.

The results of this taphonomic work at the U level also provide certain plausible constraints on the interpretation of the local extinction of hominoids in the Potwar Plateau during the next million years. Postcranial hominoid elements suggest that *Ramapithecus* and *Sivapithecus* may have had considerable locomotor capabilities in an arboreal setting. Because not many of the faunal remains from any stratigraphic level can be considered arboreal, we have no basis for implicating faunal changes *within* the arboreal assemblage (e.g., the advent of a competitor for some arboreal resources) as a cause of hominoid extinction.

Above the U level, the fossil productivity of sediments declines. Since the presence of hominoids and other uncommon mammals at the U level is, in part, a function of sample size, it is plausible that hominoids persisted for another 0.5 million years without becoming preserved (or found). (In fact, intensive collecting during the 1982 field season in sediments estimated at between 7.0 to 7.5 million years ago, produced another hominoid tooth (J. Barry, personal communication). This fossil extends the biostratigraphic range of hominoids upward by about 0.5 million years in the Potwar Plateau. Thus, the decrease in hominoid fossils occurs partly because of taphonomic reasons that affected other uncommon mammals as well.

The other mammals that became extinct soon after the hominoids—deinotheres and the tragulids *Dorcabune nagrii* and *Dorcatherium* cf. *D. Nagrii* are interpreted as forest herbivores. Members of rhizomyid (rodent) lineages show an increase in hypsodonty after about 7.0 million years (Flynn and Jacobs, 1982). Taken together with the disappearance of hominoids, these faunal changes suggest that substantial changes in vegetational composition and/or seasonality occurred about 7.0 to 7.5 million years ago. Such changes may have been part of a long biogeographic transition in climate, flora, and fauna, because, as we have noted earlier, between about 9 million years and 3 million years ago, the mammalian herbivores experienced a gradual ecological shift. This shift may have marked the eastward retreat of the South Asian tropical forest that today occupies the Malayan region.

5. Conclusions*

The hominoid fossil record from South Asian has expanded considerably in the past decade—enough to permit tentative conclusion about hominoid paleobiology. The first appearance of apes in South Asia was at least 13 million years ago and was probably closer to 16 million years ago. They were part of a forest–woodland fauna, significant parts of which came from Afro-Asia. Hominoids flourished in South Asia until around 7 million years ago as part of mammal communities that occupied a mosaic of more to less wooded habitats. They became locally extinct, perhaps as a consequence of habitat change following significant geological changes such as Himalayan uplift.

Several hominoid species are documented in South Asia, and they share a number of basic features. They had robust jaws with thickly enameled cheek teeth and postcranial skeletons indicating arboreal and apelike behaviors. Overall, these species are different from both earlier Miocene and living apes. In several characters they resemble other middle and late Miocene hominoids, particularly those of Asia and eastern Europe, suggesting that all were part of an adaptive radiation of "thickly enameled" apes.

In a few characters, the South Asian hominoids resemble specifically the living orangutan *Pongo,* and we tentatively suggest that these characters can be treated as shared derived features. If so, the earliest appearances of such Miocene species documents the latest possible divergence time of the orangutan lineage. New data suggest 13 million years, perhaps more likely 16 million, as a current best estimate for that divergence. This will help in estimating tentatively the divergence dates for other hominoids.

If the middle and late Miocene South Asian hominoids are related to orangutans, then this living ape has changed markedly since the Miocene. Perhaps this is also the case for the African hominoids, including the hominids. If so, hominoid evolution has been more complex than many of us supposed. The South Asian record is, and will be crucial in unraveling that evolutionary story.

*This section prepared by D. Pilbeam.

References

Andrews, P., 1982, Hominoid evolution, *Nature* **295:**185–186.

Badgley, C., 1982, How much time is represented in the present? The development of time-averaged assemblages as models for the fossil record, in: *Proc. Third N. Am. Paleont. Conv.* **1:**23–28.

Badgley, C., and Behrensmeyer, A. K., 1980, Paleoecology of Middle Siwalik sediments and faunas, *Palaeogeogr., Palaeoclimatol., Palaeoecol.* **30:**133–155.

Barry, J. C., Behrensmeyer, A. K., and Monaghan, M. C., 1980, A geologic and biostratigraphic framework for Miocene sediments near Khaur Village, northern Pakistan, *Postilla* **183:**1–19.

Barry, J. C., Lindsay, E. H., and Jacobs, L. L., 1982, A biostratigraphic zonation of the Middle and Upper Siwaliks of the Potwar Plateau of Northern Pakistan, *Palaeogeogr., Palaeoclimatol., Palaeoecol.* **37:**95–130.

Behrensmeyer, A. K., and Tauxe, L., 1983, Isochronous fluvial systems in Miocene deposits of northern Pakistan, *Sedimentology* **29:**331–352.

Flynn, L. J., and Jacobs, L., 1982, Effects of changing environments on Siwalik rodent faunas of northern Pakistan. *Palaeogeogr., Palaeoclimatol., Palaeoecol.* **38:**129–138.

Kay, R. F., 1981, The nut-crackers—A new theory of the adaptations of the Ramapithecinae, *Am. J. Phys. Anthropol.* **55:**141–151.

Kay, R. F., 1982, *Sivapithecus simonsi,* a new species of Miocene hominoid, with comments on the phylogenetic status of the Ramapithecinae, *Intl. J. Primatol.* **3:**113–174.

Lewis, G. E., 1934, Preliminary notice of new man-like apes from India, *Am. J. Sci.* **27**(159):161–181.

Lydekker, R., 1879, Further notices of Siwalik mammalia. *Geol. Survey of India, Records* **12**(1):33–52.

Pilbeam, D., 1982, New hominoid skull material from the Miocene of Pakistan, *Nature* **295:**232–234.

Pilbeam, D., and Smith, R., 1981, New skull remains of *Sivapithecus* from Pakistan, *Mem. Geol. Surv. Pakistan* **2:**1–13.

Pilbeam, D., Meyer, G. E., Badgley, C., Rose, M. D., Pickford, M. H. L., Behrensmeyer, A. K., and Shah, S. M. I., 1977, New hominoid primates from the Siwaliks of Pakistan and their bearing on hominoid evolution, *Nature* **270:**689–695.

Pilbeam, D. R., Behrensmeyer, A. K., Barry, J. C., and Shah, S. M. I., 1979, Miocene sediments and faunas of Pakistan, *Postilla* **179:**1–45.

Pilbeam, D., Rose, M. D., Badgley, C., and Lipschutz, B., 1980, Miocene hominoids from Pakistan, *Postilla* **181:**1–94.

Rose, M. D., 1983, Miocene hominoid postcranial morphology: Monkey-like, ape-like, neither, or both?, in: *New Interpretations of Ape and Human Ancestry* (R. L. Ciochon and R. F. Corruccini, eds.), Plenum Press, New York.

Sarich, V. M., and Cronin, J. E., 1975, Molecular systematics of the primates, in: *Molecular Anthropology* (M. Goodman and R. E. Tashian, eds.), Plenum Press, New York, pp. 141–169.

Simons, E. L., 1976, The nature of the transition in the dental mechanism from pongids to hominids, *J. Hum. Evol.* **5:**511–528.

Simons, E. L., and Pilbeam, D. R., 1972, Hominoid paleoprimatology, in: *The Functional and Evolutionary Biology of Primates* (R. Tuttle, ed.), Aldine-Atherton, Chicago, pp. 36–62.

Tauxe, L., 1979, A new date for *Ramapithecus, Nature* **282:**399–401.

Tauxe, L., and Opdyke, N. D., 1982, A time framework based on magnetostratigraphy for the Siwalik sediments of the Khaur area, northern Pakistan, *Palaeogeogr., Palaeoclimatol., Palaeoecol.* **37:**43–61.

Ward, S., and Pilbeam, D., 1983, Maxillofacial morphology of Miocene hominoids from Africa and Indo-Pakistan, in: *New interpretations of ape and human ancestry* (R. L. Ciochon and R. F. Corruccini, eds.), Plenum Press, New York.

Ward, S. C., Kimbel, W. H., and Pilbeam, D., 1983, Subnasal alveolar morphology and the systematic position of *Sivapithecus, Am. J. Phys. Anthropol.* **61:**157–171.

CHAPTER 2

Biological Adaptations and Affinities of Mesolithic South Asians

KENNETH A. R. KENNEDY

1. Orientation of the Study

The earliest reported discovery in South Asia of human skeletons associated with Mesolithic cultural materials occurred in 1880–1881 at Mahara Pahar, Uttar Pradesh, India (Allchin, 1958; Carlleyle 1883, 1885). In the full century that has elapsed since the date of Carlleyle's survey, the Mesolithic skeletal record has increased considerably (Kennedy 1980). Today skeletal biologists may turn to research materials from South Asia that are commensurate in size and preservation quality with Mesolithic series from Europe, Africa, and the Levant. South Asian collections are datable within a temporal range extending from the terminal Pleistocene times of *ca.* 12,000 years B.P. (before present) to the periods of establishment of Neolithic communities in the northwestern sector of the subcontinent by the seventh millennium B.C. and by some 4000 years later in peninsular India. Thus, they are contemporary with other Mesolithic skeletal series recovered from sites outside of South Asia. Also, certain economic and technological aspects of the hunting–gathering Mesolithic life-style persisted until historic times in some tribal areas in India. Distribution of the Indian Mesolithic is attested to by the archaeological evidence scattered across the South Asian landmass from Afghanistan in the west and eastward to Assam, from the Kashmir Valley of the Himalayan ranges southward to island Sri Lanka.

KENNETH A. R. KENNEDY • Ecology and Systematics, Division of Biological Sciences, Cornell University, Ithaca, New York 14853. The research program was sponsored by the National Science Foundation (Grant No. BNS 8014293) and by the American Institute of Indian Studies (Smithsonian Award No. 00613900) during the year of the author's sabbatical leave from Cornell University.

Scientific research has focused upon this Mesolithic artifact record and its interpretation. However, with increasing attention being given to palaeodemography, prehistorians are recognizing the value of the unique kinds of data that only come from the skeletal record itself. It is no longer assumed that the primary reward of a scientific investigation of skeletal remains is earned by faithfully following traditional models of racial palaeontology. Explanations for biological diversity and genetic affinities of prehistoric populations do not lie necessarily in simplistic theories of ethnic migration or abrupt genetic changes, although these mechanisms may be significant in specific circumstances. Today, new models are proposed that give greater consideration to processes affecting human adaptability, the capacity of the individual to attain a particular level of ontogenetic development in the course of the growth period, and the effects of natural selection and genetic drift upon populations. The role of evolutionary parallelism is important in contemporary model building, and its effects may be significant in cases where genetic affinity between ancient and living populations has been hypothesized.

In 1980–1981, I, with the assistance of Mr. C. B. Burrow, examined two skeletal series recovered from the Mesolithic sites of Sarai Nahar Rai and Mahadaha on the Gangetic plains of Uttar Pradesh. These are the most ancient representatives of anatomically modern *Homo sapiens* known at the present time from India that have been thoroughly described by skeletal biologists. The radiocarbon dates associated with the specimens indicate an antiquity of 10,000 to 12,000 years B.P., that is, terminal Pleistocene and early Recent times. In the course of our morphometric analysis of both series at Allahabad University and subsequently at Cornell University, where statistical analysis of the data was conducted, the following questions were considered.

1. What are the biological characteristics of the Sarai Nahar Rai and the Mahadaha skeletal series?
2. Do the results of morphometric analysis support the current archaeological thesis that these geographically adjacent, culturally similar, and temporally coexisting populations were regional enclaves of a single macropopulation of Mesolithic hunters and gatherers? What is the degree of biological affinity between the two groups?
3. To what degree are the Sarai Nahar Rai and Mahadaha populations phenotypically similar or dissimilar with respect to later Mesolithic and other prehistoric populations of South Asia?
4. To what degree are the Sarai Nahar Rai and Mahadaha populations phenotypically similar or dissimilar with respect to Upper Paleolithic and Mesolithic populations of regions outside the Indian subcontinent?
5. How are the data of biological characteristics and measures of biological affinity of the two Gangetic plains series to be interpreted with respect to evolutionary processes and adaptability responses?

The comments which follow are summations of results of morphometric and statistical analyses obtained by the date of preparation of this paper. Detailed reports of various aspects of the study are in process of publication or, when cited, appear in print.

2. Archaeological Record of the South Asian Mesolithic

European prehistorians of the last century faced the problem of fitting certain assemblages of artifacts of disputed status within the chronological framework marking the transition from Paleolithic to Neolithic cultures. Small stone blades, or microliths, were a diagnostic feature of these enigmatic collections. De Mortillet (1883) defined the Azilian as the final Paleolithic phase and the Tardenoisian as the earliest phase of the Neolithic in a context he called the *ancien hiatus*. This scheme was accepted by Foote (1916) in the course of his prehistoric investigations in India, and he assigned the microliths he found to an early phase of the Indian Neolithic. In 1892, Brown suggested that the term *Mesolithic* be used to define the transition period from food-gathering to food-producing cultures in Europe, but for the next 30 years debate continued over the classification and nomenclature of the post-Pleistocene prehistoric sites. The Mesolithic was firmly established by Macalister in 1921. His views found support from Clark's (1932, 1936) work in the 1930s that demonstrated the stratigraphical evidence of a succession of diverse Mesolithic cultures in Europe.

Once accepted as a distinct prehistoric period falling between the Paleolithic and Neolithic, the term *Mesolithic* began to be applied to artifact assemblages in Africa and Asia, although new terminologies were invented in efforts to distinguish regionally different tool industries from those characteristic of the diverse and successive Mesolithic cultures of the European sequence. An agate flake of possible Mesolithic affinity was found as early as 1865 by Wynne (1866) in the Godavari alluvium near Paithan, but serious investigation of microlithic artifacts did not commence in South Asia until the 1930s. Burkitt classified a large collection of artifacts found by Cammiade in the Krishna Basin into major industrial phases of which the last, Series 4, was the category for microlithic tools. His scheme was adapted to chronological sequences of climatic cycles already worked out for African prehistoric studies (Cammiade and Burkitt 1930), and in a paper published with Richards (Burkitt *et al.*, 1932) the effort was made to set South Asian prehistory against a background of palaeoclimatological changes. Burkitt's fourfold classification of successive cultural stages based upon lithic typology, technology, and stratigraphy found support from Todd's (1932) work at Khandivli near Bombay, from the investigations conducted along the Narmada River near Hoshangabad by De Terra and Paterson (1939), and from other surveys carried out by Gordon (1938) in central India, Aiyappan

(1945) and Zeuner (1956) on the Madras coastal plain, and by Sankalia (1946) in Gujarat. Some of the difficulties inherent in the system were overcome by Subbarao who proposed in 1958 a three-stage division of the Indian Paleolithic into early, middle and late periods. The last stage included the so-called "geometric" and "nongeometric" industries of post-Paleolithic and pre-Neolithic periods. Subbarao was aware of certain parallels of Indian and African tool types and methods of manufacture; hence, his adoption of a classification already in use in African prehistory. This nomenclature was valued for its independence from the terminologies and conceptual models of the European Mesolithic. Furthermore, Subbarao appreciated the unique features of the Indian lithic assemblages. However, within recent years the term *Mesolithic* has come into common usage among South Asian prehistorians, replacing Subbarao's late Stone Age and Burkitt's Series 4.

The hallmarks of the Mesolithic are ubiquitous in South Asia, although exploratory research is urgently needed for eastern India and Pakistan where the archaeological record is meager. Technologically, the Indian Mesolithic is distinguished by the manufacture of microlithic tools of geometrical and non-geometrical shapes and with associated fluted cores, scrapers, points and small blades, and chipped pebbles. The preferred medium of manufacture was quartz. These replaced Middle Paleolithic or Upper Paleolithic tools that were shaped as borers and scrapers, along with some larger blades that were manufactured on a wide variety of lithic materials. There is evidence of the use of the bow and arrow and domestication of the dog that were important components of a Mesolithic hunting–gathering life-style that was concerned with successful predation upon large game. More permanent settlements and a hunting–gathering life-style that was combined in some areas with incipient pastoralism all reflect greater regionalization in the exploitation of new and varied ecological settings for the support of a population of relatively high density. Large sedentary sites are rare in the Indian Mesolithic, and social organization may have been characterized by localization of communal bands with close ethnic and cultural ties. It appears that the Indian Mesolithic was a vibrant period of population expansion and cultural innovation because new sites are encountered in a variety of habitats: the loessic hills of Gujarat, islands off the coast of Bombay, atop fossil sand dunes along the Madras coast, in both cave and open-air camps in dry-zone jungles of Sri Lanka, in the rockshelters of the Vindhyas, and on the shores of oxbow lakes on the Gangetic plains. Rockshelters and caves were used extensively as year-round and seasonal shelters, a habitat preference that is in marked contrast to the Palaeolithic inhabitants' favoring open-air camps. The artistic creativity of the Indian Mesolithic has been established by the recent investigations of the cave paintings and engravings of the Bhimbetka caves near Bhopal in central India (Wakankar 1973), but cave art appears in many other places as well. The more we learn of the Mesolithic period in South Asia, the more it becomes clear that this was not the "dark age" of prehistory, as this period has been interpreted by many scholars based upon their perceptions of European data and theoretical models. Rather, in India this was the dawn of a way of life containing the embryonic elements of the shift to food production and the establishment of settled farming villages that became the nuclei of urban life by the seventh millennium B.C. in the northwestern sector of the subcontinent. This final period of the food-gathering economy of South Asian prehistory has been the subject of a number of general and regional archaeological studies (Allchin, 1959; Misra, 1965; S. Deraniyagala, 1981).

3. Skeletal Record of the South Asian Mesolithic

Once accepted as a valid archaeological concept, the Mesolithic of Europe earned an undeserved reputation as a drab and inelegant phase of human prehistory — a degenerative phase following the glories of the Upper Paleolithic with its magnificent cave art, aesthetic tools manufactured from a diversity of raw materials, and other features that contributed to a romantic image of tall, blond, and "clean-limbed" Cro-Magnon hunters who were worthy ancestors of European man. A consequence of this attitude was the universal underrating of the significance of the Mesolithic cultures outside of Europe, as was noted previously. Within the past decade a change in attitude has taken place as biological anthropologists recognize the European and Near Eastern Mesolithic as that time of transition from food gathering to food producing in which complex biological and cultural adjustments were made in the cultural areas of tool technology, food acquisition and preparation, and social organization. The increase in population, which is a major feature of the post-Paleolithic period, demanded new procedures for obtaining nutrients. Adaptations to postglacial environments affected Mesolithic habitat preferences, even among populations that were geographically far removed from northern latitudes and high altitudes where cold-stress adaptation had persisted as a survival factor for millennia. In assessing the biological cost demanded of human populations in their continuous adjustments to unique stresses imposed by changes of both natural and cultural ecological circumstances, skeletal biologists recognized a dependency upon the archaeological record of the Mesolithic as a critical supplement to their own biological data.

Most intensive investigation of Mesolithic archaeological and skeletal data has been conducted in the Near East (Newell, 1973; Redman, 1978; Meiklejohn, 1979) and in Africa (Rightmire, 1975). Laboratory examination of the skeletal specimens observed by Carlleyle at Mahara Pahar a century ago was not conducted, nor do we have good analytical data concerning a human skull uncovered at Jalampura, Gujarat, by Foote (1916) in 1892. Some human remains collected by Hunter (1935, 1936) from Pachmarhi, Madhya Pradesh, in the 1930s were lost before they had been properly described. Serious study of the skeletal biology of Mesolithic man in South Asia did not get underway until 40 years ago with the excavations at Langhnaj, Gujarat, by Sankalia and his associates (Sankalia and Karve, 1949; Karve-Corvinus and Kennedy, 1964; Ehrhardt and Kennedy, 1965). Since 1941, additional skeletal specimens from Mesolithic contexts have been obtained and examined by qualified experts, with important collections coming from Bagor, Rajasthan in 1968–1970 (Misra 1976; Lukacs *et al.*, 1982), from Bhimbetka, Madhya Pradesh, since 1971 (Wakankar, 1975; Misra *et al.*, 1977); and from sites in the Kaimur Hills since 1963 (G. R. Sharma, 1965). The Kaimur rockshelter site of Lekhahia ki Pahari yielded 19 skeletons, and a single specimen was collected from the neighboring Baghai Khor rockshelter. Other Mesolithic burials have been observed at Harli-Bhituli, Karka, Sarai Nahar Rai, and Mahadaha in the lake country of the Ganga Valley by archaeological teams under the direction of G. R. Sharma (1973). Mesolithic cultures extended into island Sri Lanka where, in 1939, human skeletons were excavated at the cave of Batadomba lena, Sabaragamuva, in an archaeological context that P. E. P. Deraniyagala christened the *Balangoda culture*. Additional burials were recovered from the cave of Ravan Alle, Uva, in 1945, and from the cave of Alu Galge in the same province in 1954. Some 15 skeletons were collected from the open-air site of Bellanbandi Palassa, Sabaragamuva, which was discovered in 1956 and excavated in 1957, 1961, and 1970. These Sri Lankan sites have been discussed in works by P. E. P. Deraniyagala (1963), S. Deraniyagala (1981), and by me (Kennedy, 1965). Pakistan has not yet yielded a Mesolithic skeletal record, nor have human remains of this period been recovered from archaeological sites in eastern and peninsular India.

The most ancient Mesolithic skeletons known thus far are from the Gangetic plains. A radiocarbon date of 10,050 ± 110 years B.P. was obtained from a sample of unburnt and highly calcified bone from Sarai Nahar Rai (Agrawal, 1971; Agrawal and Kusumgar, 1974). This date may find support in recently examined radiocarbon samples from cemented gravels in Mahadaha, another Gangetic Mesolithic site that is without human remains. These samples are dated to 12,190 ± 410 years B.P. and 9350 ± 130 years B.P. (G. R. Sharma *et al.*, 1980, pp. 232–233). While Mahadaha has not yielded radiocarbon-dated materials, the archaeological evidence from the site as well as paleogeographical information support the view that the occupation of Mahadaha was relatively contemporary with that of Sarai Nahar Rai. Thus, the Gangetic fossil hominids appear to be relatively contemporary with other terminal Pleistocene specimens discovered at the Australian sites of Kow Swamp, Talgai, Nitchie, and Mosgiel (9000–13,000 years B.P.), from China's Upper Cave (15,000 years B.P.), from Iwo Eleru in Nigeria (11,000 years B.P.), and from the New World sites of Marmes (10,000 years B.P.) and Guitarrero cave (12,500 years B.P.).

The Gangetic skeletal specimens are separated by a temporal hiatus of four to eight millennia from later Mesolithic specimens from Bagor, Lekhahia ki Pahari, and Langhnaj that have yielded radiocarbon focal dates of 5800 years B.P., 4290 years B.P., and 3925 years B.P., respectively. The Sri Lankan site of Bellanbandi Palassa has been dated to 6500 ± 700 years B.P. on the basis of thermoluminescence of fired rock crystal that was associated with one of the skeletons.

4. Sarai Nahar Rai Skeletal Series

The Mesolithic site of Sarai Nahar Rai (long. 81°51′E; lat. 25°48′N) is 15 km southwest of the town of Pratapgarh in the district of the same name in Uttar Pradesh and within the central Ganga Valley. (See the Mesolithic site maps for localities of Sarai Nahar Rai and Mahadaha that appear elsewhere in this volume in the chapter written by Kennedy and Caldwell.) The skeletons were found on the shore of a dried oxbow lake that is an isolated meander of the Ganga of terminal Pleistocene times before the river shifted to its present course some 55 km to the south. When the lake bed held water, it provided an attractive environment for an open-air camp and burial ground for nomadic hunters. Today, the area of ancient occupancy is about 1800 m^2 and is marked by microliths, hearths, and graves eroding out of a saline and highly compact soil of heavy calcium and black kankar content. G. R. Sharma (1973) classified the cultural associations as belonging to a geometric prepottery microlithic horizon of the early Mesolithic phase, as attested by the small finely retouched stone tools of symmetrical points, lunates, blunted-backed blades, scrapers, and triangles fabricated from chalcedony, carnelian, and other fine-grained stones. The human burials were observed in shallow oblong graves that were exposed by surface erosion, but the east-west orientation of the supine extended bodies had not been disturbed. Skulls were at the western end of each grave of single and multiple interments (Figures 1 and 2).

Although Sarai Nahar Rai was discovered in 1968 by officers of the Archaeological Department of Uttar Pradesh, its excavation by Allahabad University, in collaboration with the State Department of Scientific Research and Cultural Affairs, did not commence until 4 years later. Eight skeletons were removed with the assistance of staff members from the Anthropological Survey of India, and in 1973 six more skeletons were recovered. The significance of the human skeletons from Sarai Nahar Rai was recognized by some affiliates of the survey who removed one skeleton from the site in 1970. A brief report of this specimen with a photograph of the skull appeared the following year in *Nature* (Dutta, 1971), and the survey subsequently published other reports (Dutta *et al.*, 1971; Dutta *et al.*, 1972; Dutta and Pal, 1972; Dutta, 1973). Discussion of the condition of preservation and morphology of the series of skeletons from Sarai Nahar Rai was

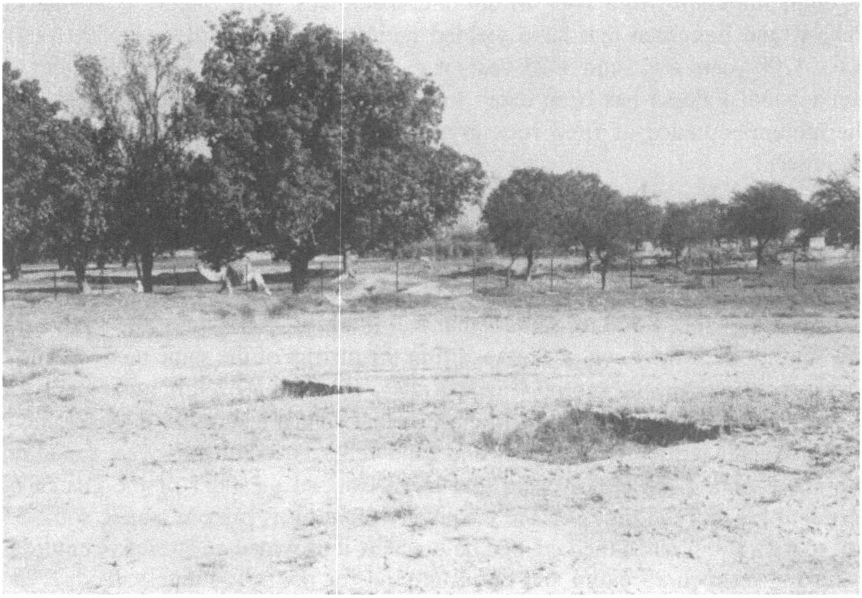

Figure 1. Site of Sarai Nahar Rai.

noted in *Indian Archaeology—A Review* in the issue for the years 1969–1970 and in G. R. Sharma's (1973, 1975) publications.

Of the total of 14 skeletons removed from Sarai Nahar Rai in the 1972 and 1973 field seasons, 9 were suitable for morphometric analysis. There was a single skeleton suitable for morphological analysis only. The remaining 4 skeletons not included in the study conducted by me in 1980 were either absent from the existing Sarai Nahar Rai series at Allahabad University, were too fragmentary to merit meaningful morphometric analysis, or, as was the case with one specimen, it was preserved as a fragmentary skeleton still embedded in solidified soil matrix and is presently retained in this form as a display specimen in the Museum of the Department of Ancient History, Culture, and Archaeology at Allahabad University. The skeleton removed from Sarai Nahar Rai by officers of the Survey in 1970 is housed at the present time in their headquarters in Calcutta where it was examined by me after completion of the research on the entire series in Allahabad. Bones of Sarai Nahar Rai skeletons are completely fossilized and, until cleaned in the laboratory, they were coated with heavy calcareous concretions. The condition of preservation of bones and teeth is extremely good.

Ten specimens from Sarai Nahar Rai were described. Of these, 7 have been identified as males, 3 as females. All are adults with an age range of 16 to 34 years for males and 15 to 35 years for females. With respect to cranial architecture, these ancient people have large and robust skulls that range from low mesocrany to hyperdolichocrany. Cranial vaults are tapeinocranic. There is one case of chamaecrany present for a male specimen. Among males, these long and moderately elevated vaults are surmounted by prominent supraorbital tori, moderately large to very large mastoid processes with prominent supramastoid crests, and sharp temporal lines. Development of the nuchal lines ranges from slight to pronounced among specimens identified as males. Like the female skulls, males have parietal eminences that are very large. Faces of both sexes are hypereuryprosopic and hypereuryne with nasal forms ranging from low leptorrhiny to chamaerrhiny. Orbits are rectangular, chamaeconchic, and have dull margins. When skulls are viewed in *norma lateralis,* the vaults reveal exceedingly low foreheads that are either slightly bulbous or vertical. Frontal bosses are moderately developed. Nasal notches are deep, except in the case of one female specimen, and the profile of the nasal root is concave. Total facial prognathism is slight, but upper facial and alveolar prognathism is pronounced for some specimens. Malars are robust and vary in size. Canine fossae are shallow. Mandibles are massive and have well-formed mental eminences and everted gonia on which the impressions of the pterygoid muscles are well marked. Dentitions are characterized by moderate to pronounced occlusal wear, especially of the anterior teeth. There is an apparent absence of the Y-5 cusp pattern for lower molars as well as absence of caries, abscess, crowding, malocclusion, and other common dental abnormalities of later prehistoric populations. The molar teeth are mesodont and megadont. Postcranial bones are consistently massive and robust for specimens of both sexes. Femora are eurymeric. Tibiae range from leptocnemia to mesocnemia. The single case of an articulated pelvic girdle of a female has an indicial value for the pelvic inlet that is platypellic. The humerus–radius index for one skeleton is mesotikerkic. These were tall people; the range of estimated statures for males is from 173.93 cm to 192.08 cm on the basis of limb-bone lengths (Trotter, 1970) (Figure 5–10).

With the exception of osteocartilaginous exostosis observed on the right radius and left first metatarsal of one male skeleton and a single case of dental enamel hypoplasia of the anterior teeth of a female specimen, all other observed pathological features of the Sarai Nahar Rai series are attributed to degenerative arthritic bone modification, or osteoarthritis. What is most striking in this latter condition is the early age at which these osteoarthritic changes begin in the Sarai Nahar Rai series; for some it was as early as the beginning years of the third decade of life. The apparent absence of dental pathologies combined with excessive occlusal surface wear are characteristic features of later Mesolithic skeletal series from India and Sri Lanka. Some investigators who have observed one or two of the Sarai Nahar Rai skeletons prior to the time of the present study have suggested the presence of other pathological conditions (A. K. Sharma 1980). This author would assign some of these conditions to anatomical anomalies rather than classify them as pathologies. In the category of anomalies, the Sarai Nahar Rai series contains three examples of squatting facets on the distal ends of tibiae; all of these cases were found with male specimens. Olecranon fossae are perforated in the humeri of another individual. More common, but not associated exclusively with males, is the hyperdevelopment of the attachments of the *Anconius* and *Supinator* muscles at the proximal ends of ulnae. When this stress mark is observed, it is most pronounced on right ulnae. Since the function of *Anconius* is to assist *Triceps* in hyperextension of the arm, whereas *Supinator* is the muscle of supination, it is reasonable to assume that here is an habitual stress indicator having to do with activities such as spear throwing, use of the bola or slingshot, hurling stones, or similar practices. It is interesting that the specimens that exhibit this ulnar feature do not possess the other common anatomical stress markers of the upper extremity—namely, the hyperdevelopment of the tendinous attachments along the palmar surfaces of the manual phalanges. However, there is a paucity of stress markers on bones and teeth that are diagnostic of episodes of fluctuations of nutritional resources or temporary cessation of nutrient acquisition due to disease. The tall statures and robust body builds of the Sarai Nahar Rai population are important factors in ascertaining that these individuals attained a high potential of ontogenetic development (Kennedy, 1983).

5. Mahadaha Skeletal Series

Also in Pratapgarh District and 31 km northeast of the town of Pratapgarh is the Mesolithic site Mahadaha (long. 82°11′E; lat. 25°20′N). (See Figure 3.) Once situated on the shore of an oxbow lake, the deposit today is dissected by a branch of the Sharda Sahayak canal and its culverts. Human skeletal remains were disturbed in the course of engineering operations, and in 1978 this situation was brought to the attention of G. R. Sharma who immediately launched an excavation that continued into a second season of work in 1979. Results of the first season's work have been published (G. R. Sharma *et al.*, 1980). The site of Mahadaha encompasses 3937.5 m^2 and is covered with surface scatter of microliths, fragments of human and animal bones, pit hearths, and burnt lumps of clayey soil. A cemetery with a habitation area and a separate butchering plot of Mesolithic cultural association is traceable in this deposit. Four stratigraphic layers are superimposed upon a compact yellow soil of high-calcium-carbonate content at a depth of 60 cm. In 1978, some 15 graves containing 17 skeletons were encountered within a 24 × 9 m rectangular excavation section. Only two of the graves contained double burials; an east–west orientation of the supine extended bodies was consistent for the series.

These burial practices parallel those at Sarai Nahar Rai and at many other Mesolithic sites in central India. Sharma recognizes four phases of interment.

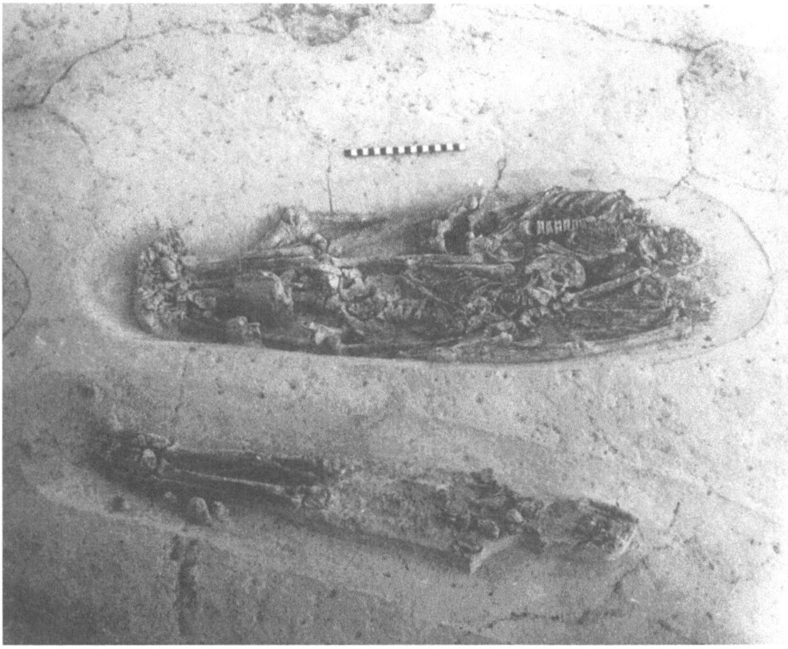

Figure 2. Single and double burials, Sarai Nahar Rai.

Additional human skeletons were collected during the 1979 season at Mahadaha under similar circumstances of burial position and cultural association (Figure 4). A total of 26 individuals were described from the Mahadaha skeletal series collected over the 2-year period of excavation, thus constituting a total sample of 35 individuals from the site. Of the 26 specimens described, 18 are identified as males, 6 as females, 1 is of uncertain sex, and there is a single child. The age range for males is from 17 to 40 years, and from young adulthood to 60 years for females.

Similarities of the Mahadaha site that are shared with Sarai Nahar Rai are most obvious with respect to burial customs, faunal associations, pit hearths, microlithic typologies, general cultural content, and degree of preservation of the human fossil remains. The two sites are only some 30 km apart and share essentially identical ecological settings today. This presumably was the case in terminal Pleistocene times as well. These parallels go far to support Sharma's suggestion that the occupants of these temporary camps and burial grounds on the shores of oxbow lakes were close contemporaries. This opinion has gained reinforcement from the archaeological reports published to date that note a resemblance of several morphological features, tall stature, and robust postcranial

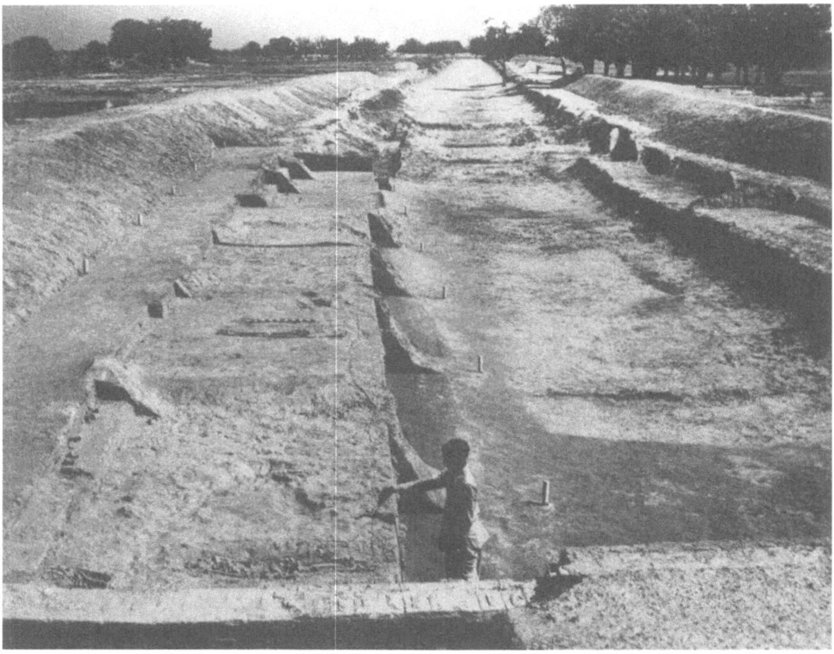

Figure 3. Site of Mahadaha.

and cranial bones between the two skeletal series. However, this was an impression that could not be judged until a more detailed analysis of these skeletal data had been completed by the research carried out in 1980 in the laboratory at Allahabad University.

Our analysis defines a skeletal series marked by cranial-shaped features of dolichocrany and hyperdolichocrany, metriocrany, tapeinocrany (there is one acrocranic female), orthocrany, and hypsicrany. Orbits are mesoconchic and hypsiconchic on euryne, euryprosopic faces. Midfacial and alveolar prognathisms are moderate. Nasal form is variable. Palates are leptostaphyline. Other morphological features of the cranium and mandible are like those of the series from Sarai Nahar Rai, especially in the pattern and degree of pronounced cranial robusticity. However, in the Mahadaha specimens, the frontal regions are lower, and the brow ridges tend to be somewhat reduced in size and they support a large median glabella. The dentition is megadont and exhibits the severe attritional features and low pathological profile of other Mesolithic skeletal series, including the series from Sarai Nahar Rai. Postcranial bones are robust and stature is tall. Height ranges for males are from 168.70 cm to 190.52 cm. The female stature ranges from 162.80 cm to 176.08 cm, as has been estimated from limb-bone lengths (Trotter, 1970). Pathological conditions are restricted to four cases

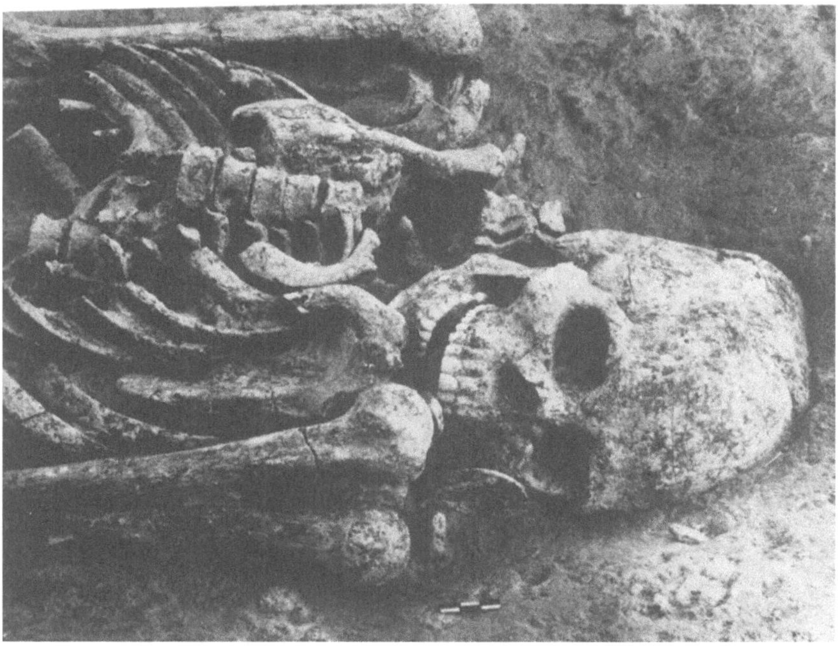

Figure 4. Skeleton with ornament, Mahadaha.

that are particular to four individuals: osteosarcoma or chondrosarcoma of the right ilium, osteophytosis of the lumbar vertebrae accompanied by osteoarthritic lipping, dental hypoplasia, and bowing of the femoral diaphysis. Anomalies are represented by an accessory maxillary tooth in one dental set and disharmony in the depths of the canine fossae on the right and left sides of the face of another individual. Hyperdevelopment of the attachments of the *Anconius* and *Supinator* muscles appears with the highest frequency in the right ulnae of Mahadaha males (Figures 11–14).

6. Comparative Analysis

The first comparative study of the Gangetic Mesolithic specimens with Mesolithic specimens from other sites in India was published by Dutta in 1973. He compared the cranium of the single specimen removed from Sarai Nahar Rai in 1970 with seven specimens from Langhnaj—the Mesolithic site in northern Gujarat that has yielded a radiocarbon date of 3925 ± 110 years B.P. Dutta noted that there are similarities with respect to cranial length, the form of the frontal area, pronounced supraorbital tori, alveolar prognathism, chamaerrhine nasal

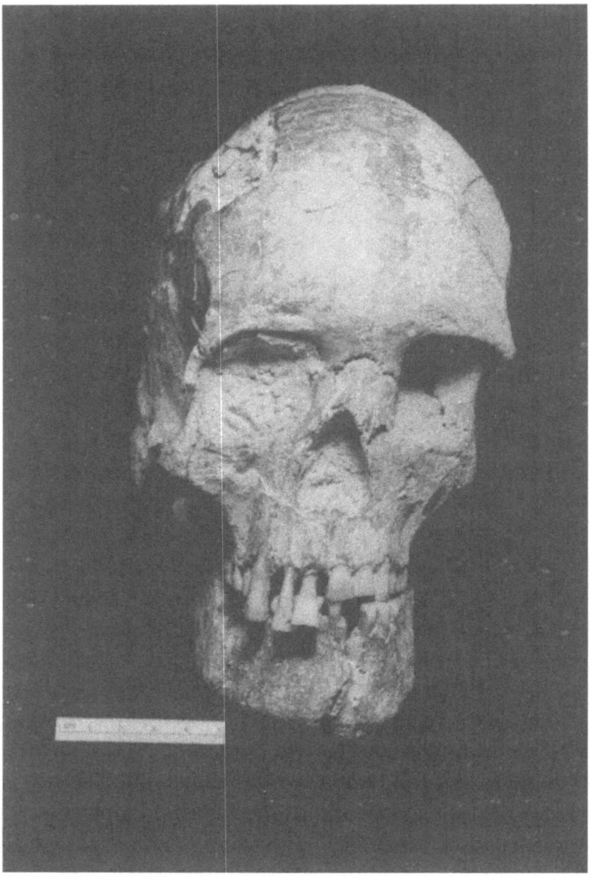

Figure 5. Skull of Sarai Nahar Rai Specimen 1972-III, frontal aspect.

form, and some other features. Differences appear in cranial and facial size-and-shape features, orbital form, dental dimensions, and stature estimates. Although the Langhnaj skeletons are moderately robust in cranial and postcranial features, the stature is lower than that encountered in the single specimen from the Gangetic site that Dutta examined. These comparisons are confirmed by our more recent study of the entire series from Sarai Nahar Rai and the Langhnaj specimens. However, we are extending this analysis by including other Mesolithic skeletal series from South Asia as well as examples from certain series from Upper Paleolithic and Mesolithic sites in Europe, Africa, and Near East, southeastern Asia, and Australia.

The statistical measures employed in this two-phase comparative analysis

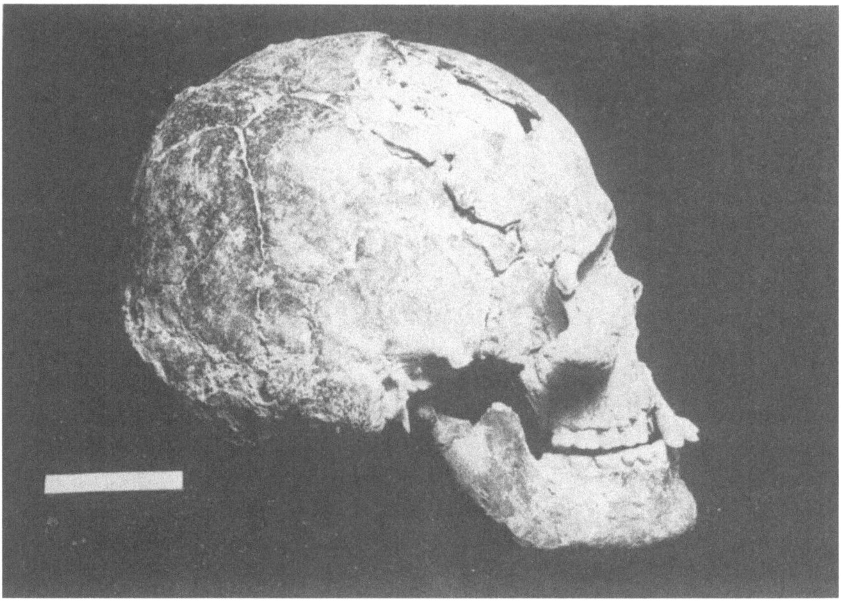

Figure 6. Skull of Sarai Nahar Rai Specimen 1972-III, right lateral aspect.

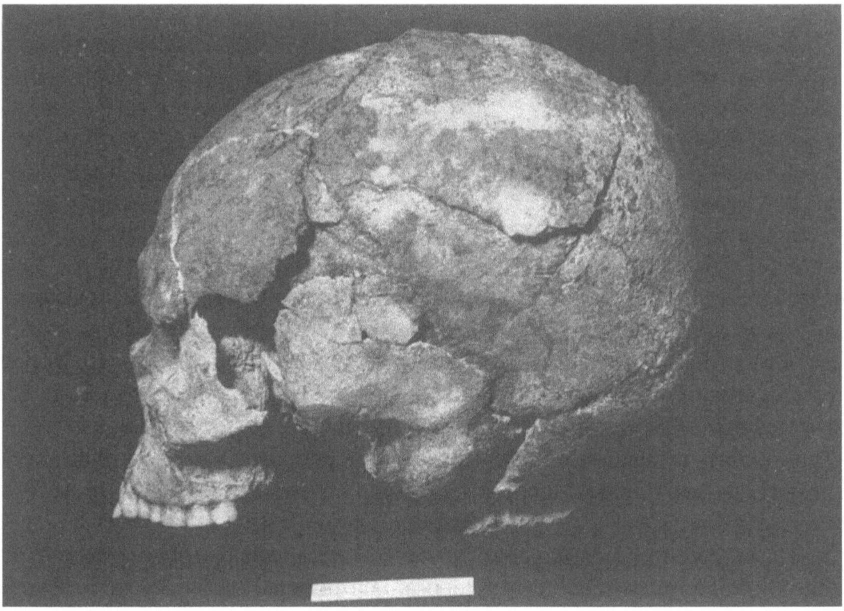

Figure 7. Cranium of Sarai Nahar Rai Specimen 1972-III, left lateral aspect.

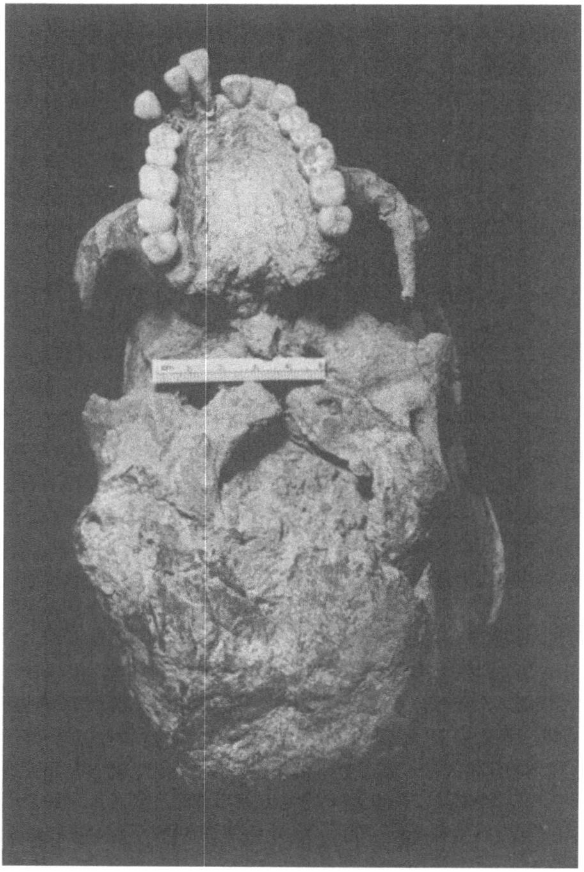

Figure 8. Cranium of Sarai Nahar Rai Specimen 1972-III, basalar aspect.

include univariate and multivariate discriminant analysis of identified clusters in addition to several clustering procedures that are programmed and assessed by the Biomed. MBDP7M set of computer programs available at Cornell University. (Results of a Principal Components Analysis are now in press.) Statistical measures that assist in the examination of trends or clines in spatial distribution or morphometric features to allow for the perception of variations that have a temporal and geographical tendency are among those that are the most useful in the present study.

During preliminary stages of analysis, certain results have emerged that relate to problems of measuring temporal and regional variations of body sizes and degrees of skeletal robusticity, dental size-and-shape variables, pathological features, markers of habitual stress, and estimations of degrees of biological

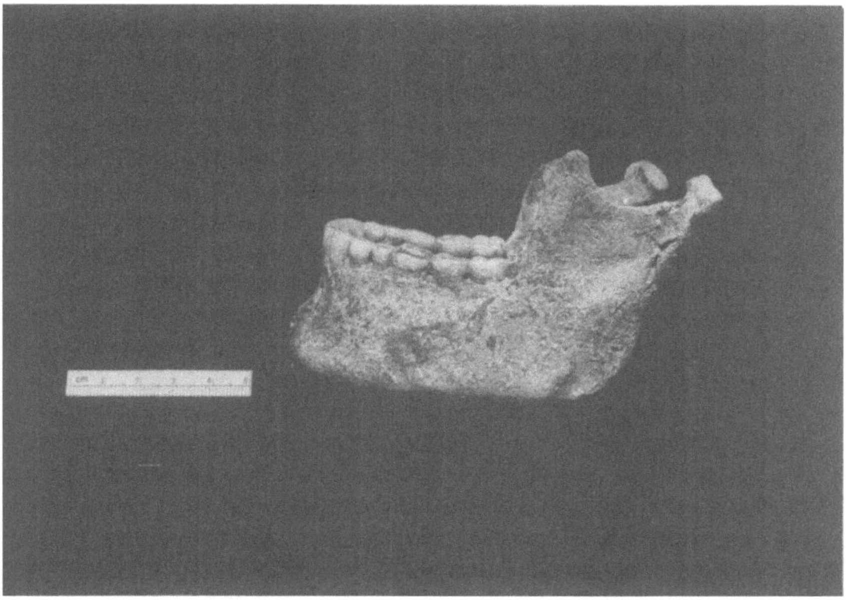

Figure 9. Mandible of Sarai Nahar Rai Specimen 1972-III, left lateral aspect.

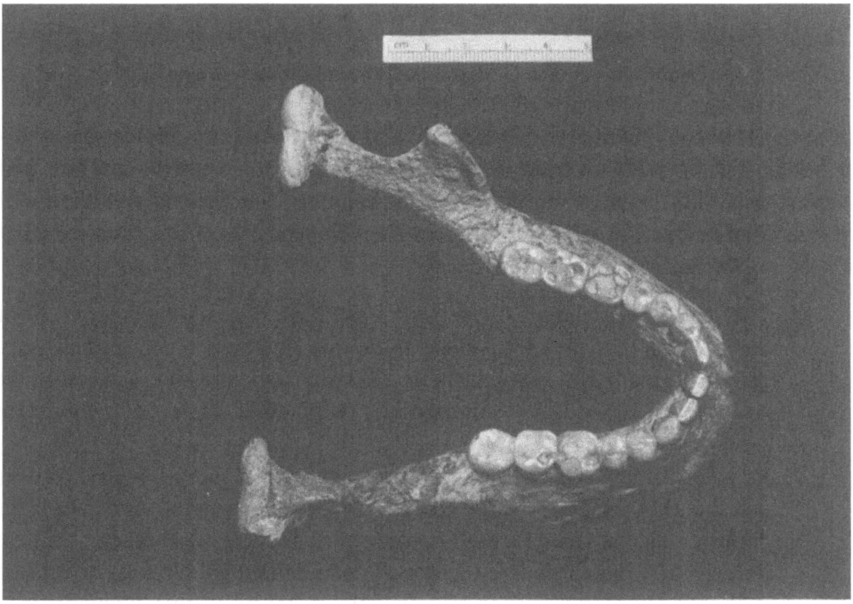

Figure 10. Mandible of Sarai Nahar Rai Specimen 1972-III, superior aspect.

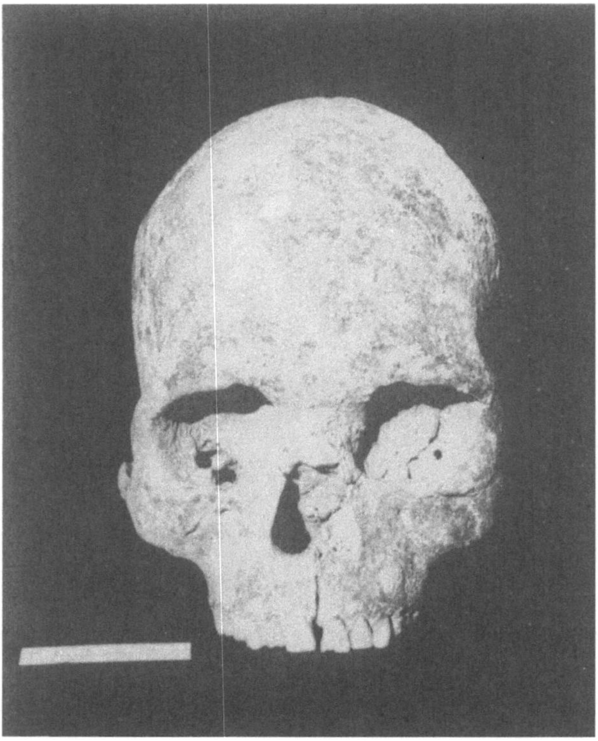

Figure 11. Cranium of Mahadaha Specimen 24, frontal aspect.

distances between a number of Mesolithic and later prehistoric populations within South Asia as well as from outside the subcontinent. Further analysis will support or modify some of the following preliminary conclusions, and these will be described in detail in the monograph on the Gangetic Mesolithic hominids that is now in preparation for publication.

1. The phenotypic pattern of the terminal Pleistocene skeletal series from Sarai Nahar Rai and Mahadaha is unique in South Asia, as has been demonstrated by morphometric descriptions and statistical analyses that have been followed by comparisons with other prehistoric mortuary series.
2. Results of univariate and multivariate analysis of morphometric studies indicate that the Sarai Nahar Rai and Mahadaha skeletal series are from populations that shared a high frequency of phenotypic characters. Close genetic ties rather than evolutionary parallelism or random effects of drift are strongly suggested as the major cause of this phenomenon. Indeed, it is possible that these Mesolithic skeletons are remains of

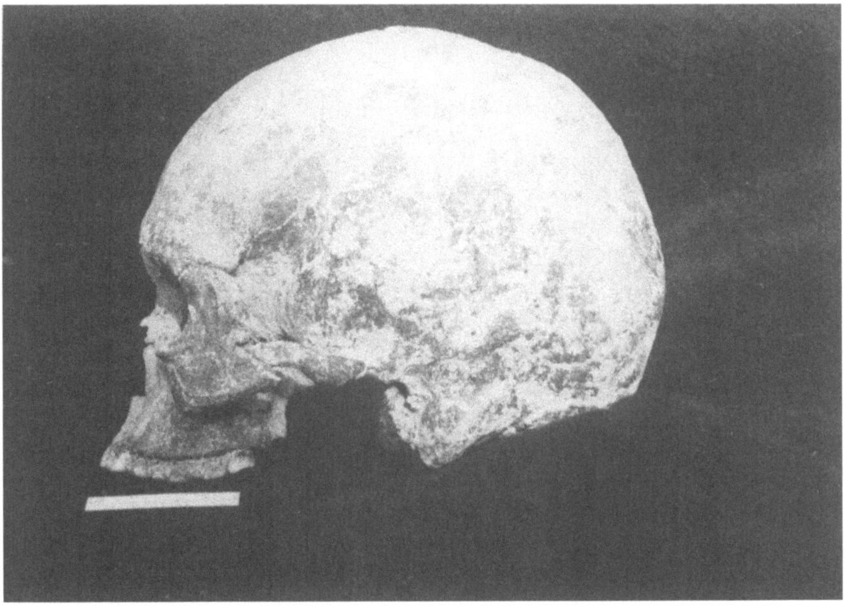

Figure 12. Cranium of Mahadaha Specimen 24, left lateral aspect.

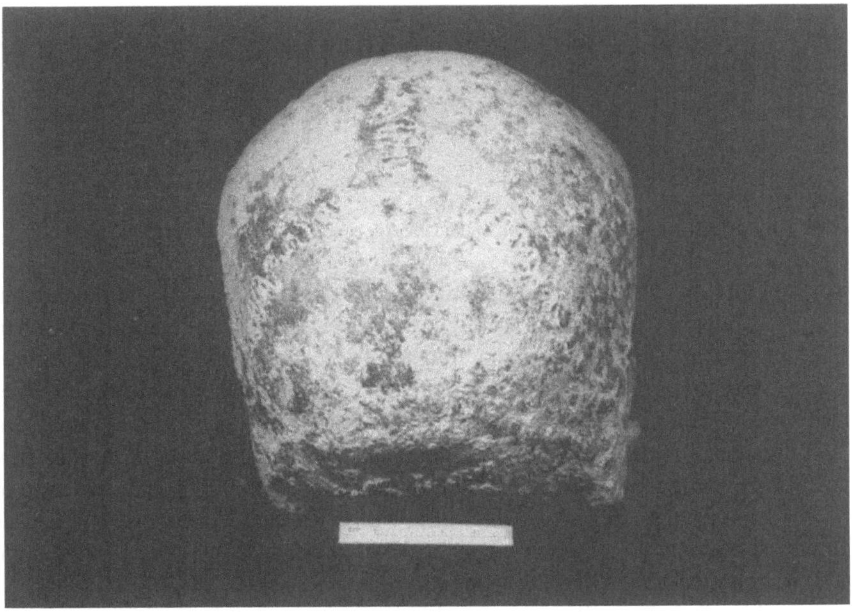

Figure 13. Cranium of Mahadaha Specimen 24, occipital aspect.

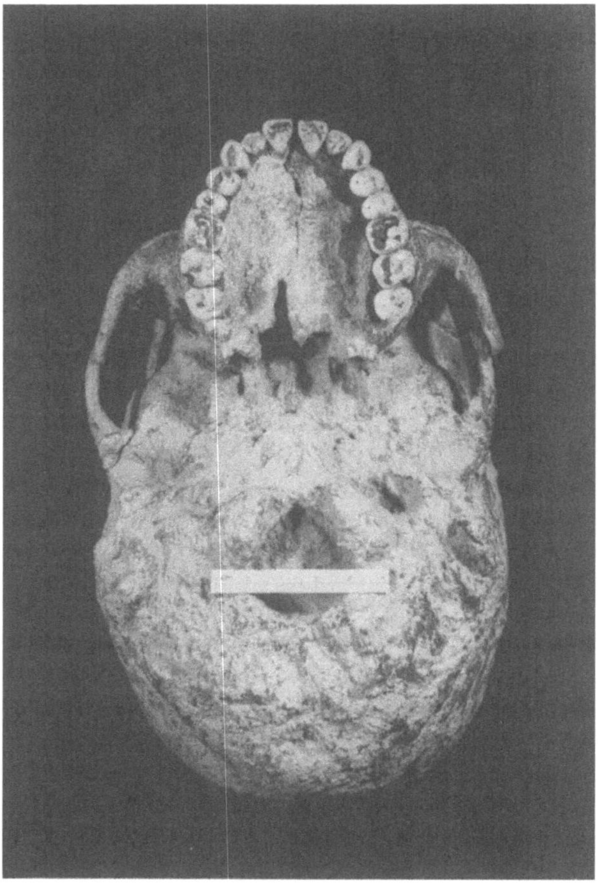

Figure 14. Cranium of Mahadaha Specimen 24, basalar aspect.

individuals from regional enclaves of the same macropopulation and that they were "contemporaries" in the sense of a few generations from one another. The following shared features are the most obvious: tall stature, robust cranial and postcranial characters, megadonty, and relative freedom from osseous and dental pathologies. But there are, as well, unusually high frequencies of identical discrete or nonmetrical traits that are shared by specimens from both series. The biological evidence of close genetic affinity of the Sarai Nahar Rai and Mahadaha populations supports the archaeological thesis of their cultural unity and relative contemporaneity in the Gangetic region.

3. Absence of a well-documented Paleolithic-context hominid fossil record from this part of South Asia precludes comparative analysis with skeletal

remains that date earlier than ca. 12,000 years B.P. (Kennedy, 1977). However, it is possible to compare the Gangetic series with those that occur in Mesolithic contexts at 6500 years B.P. and into later prehistoric times in other parts of South Asia. In this apparent hiatus of some four millennia, considerable modifications of body size and cranial and postcranial robustness took place, along with increasing incidence of pathologies that have left their traces on bones and teeth. Examination of Indian Mesolithic series from other sites in Uttar Pradesh, Madhya Pradesh, Gujarat, and Rajasthan reveals a trend toward reduced stature and skeletal strengthening that are characteristics of anatomically modern *Homo sapiens* living in South Asia today. This tendency is reflected also in reduction of tooth size and attrition of occlusal surfaces and increase of dental pathologies and anomalies (Lukacs, 1982). It is interesting that the Sri Lankan Mesolithic skeletons dating to 6500 years B.P. reveal a retention of robust skeletal features, albeit with some reduction in stature. In other features, their phenotypic pattern is quite distinct from that represented by earlier Mesolithic skeletal series. The ecological setting of a tropical forest in which these southernmost Mesolithic populations lived is different from that that prevailed in terminal Pleistocene times in the more open country of the Ganga Valley, and such differences have a bearing upon biological adaptations and diversity of phenotypic patterns.

4. A superficial inspection of the Gangetic fossil hominids may leave one with the impression that South Asia has yielded a regional variant of European and Near Eastern Cro-Magnon-like individuals. However, resemblances to European Upper Paleolithic specimens are found principally in the following features: tall stature, robusticity of cranial and postcranial muscular attachments and stress-bearing structures, and large teeth. Analysis of morphometric data by a number of statistical measures indicates that whereas the Gangetic hominids have some cranial traits that fall within the range of variation for the contemporaries of Cro-Magnon populations, these are limited to dolichocrany, euryny, chamaeconchy, and moderately well-developed supraorbital tori. There remains a broad spectrum of cranial features that are not shared by prehistoric Indian and European populations. The most obvious differences are in the greater variability of nasal form among the Gangetic series, in their high incidence of alveolar prognathism that is reduced or absent in the so-called Cromagnids, their reduced frontal elevation, and in a number of shape variables of the parietal, nuchal, and basalar areas. Even in a shared feature such as dolichocrany, the Gangetic skulls are much narrower than those of the Aurignacians and Perigordians, and they are closer to the indicial values for Magdalenians and Solutreans. These differences are most striking in comparison of the Gangetic specimens

with Upper Paleolithic hominids of Europe as described by Riquet (1970) and from our study of nonmetrical variables that include a high incidence of features under recognized genetic control.

Even more striking differences of phenotypic patterns appear when the Gangetic fossils are compared with European and Near Eastern series from Mesolithic cultural contexts. These latter populations are characterized by smaller stature, reduced cranial and postcranial robusticity, smaller teeth, and the sporadic occurrence of mesocrany and brachycrany. These features do not appear in high frequencies in South Asia until later Mesolithic times, and they continue thereafter into the historic period. Other differences can be seen in comparative analyses with skeletal series from Africa, China, southeastern Asia, and Australia. Where similarities are noted, they appear consistently in the variables of stature, body size, skeletal robusticity, and tooth size. Other phenotypic characters are discordant and do not indicate close degrees of biological affinity with the Mesolithic populations of the Gangetic plains.

It appears at this point in our research that the Sarai Nahar Rai and Mahadaha series represent a regional, area-specific, phenotypic pattern. Skeletal resemblances to certain non-Indian populations are limited to polygenic and developmental features of tall stature, skeletal robusticity, and megadonty. This constellation of features survives among certain hunting–gathering populations of both prehistoric and modern times who inhabit geographically separate regions. It is reasonable to conclude that there are evolutionary mechanisms other than those of gene migration and regional gene mutation that were operative among wide-ranging human populations living at the end of the Pleistocene that best account for these striking parallelisms in body size and form. What were these mechanisms of adaptive change that led to selection for large body size? What were the evolutionary mechanisms that allowed for reduction of body size in later Mesolithic times, that continued into the present historic periods in South Asia and in many other parts of the world?

7. Mechanisms of Adaptive Change in Mesolithic Populations

A broad view of hominid evolution reveals that many changes in selection began in *Homo sapiens* as early as 150,000 years ago, and these changes were accelerated throughout the late Pleistocene period. A trend toward reduction of postcranial strengthening, buttressing features of the skull in the regions of the supraorbital tori and nuchal muscular attachments, thinning of the bones of the vault, and reduction of facial prognathism and tooth size are all anatomical constituents of a tendency toward gracilization of the body with consequent reduction of sexual dimorphism. With the appearance of anatomically modern *Homo sapiens* some 40,000–60,000 years ago, these anatomical features distinguished human beings from their earlier Pleistocene ancestors who were anatomically archaic *Homo sapiens*. This evolutionary development is ably discussed by Wolpoff (1980) who hypothesizes that reduction of body strengthening was correlated directly with increasing improvements in technology through the invention and use of special-purpose tools, particularly after the initiation of the Levalloisian technique of stone tool manufacture in middle Pleistocene times. As a consequence of rapid cultural changes at the close of the Pleistocene, evolutionary rates of anatomical change accelerated as well. Thus, it was cultural behavior, according to Wolpoff, that became the mode and object of adaptation to life-styles in which a more advanced food-gathering and hunting economic pattern was achieved by technology rather than by an evolutionary trend toward the ever-increasing body strength of the hunter. More sophisticated weapons, such as the spear thrower (atlatl) and bow and arrow, increased the contact distance between the hunter and his or her prey, thus reducing selection for more powerful muscular development.

A parallel trend toward tooth-size reduction has been described for Upper Paleolithic and Mesolithic European skeletal series by Frayer (1978) and for Australasia and the Far East by Brace and Mahler (1971). Brace (1978) hypothesizes that the refinement of food-preparation technology led to relaxed selection for large teeth in regions where food production had been carried out for long periods of time. This is one of several theories to account for the evolutionary mechanisms of tooth reduction in *Homo sapiens*, as has been noted by Lukacs (1982) in his valuable study of tooth-size reduction in South Asian dentitions. Dental reduction is one aspect of facial reduction, and continued decrease in the use of the mouth as a tool came about as a result of technological innovations. An example of oral stress is anterior tooth loading, which involves pulling an object gripped in the mouth. This kind of activity selects for larger anterior teeth and has the developmental effect of greater alveolar prognathism and greater muscularity of the nuchal region. Lukacs (1978) has noted the relationship of biocultural factors operating upon incidence of dental disease in South Asia.

Terminal Pleistocene hominids responded in parallel ways to selective pressures towards gracilization as a consequence of widespread culturally diffused technological specializations relating to new methods of food procurement and preparation. Although the effects of migration are difficult to distinguish from the effects of selection, this hypothesis of the evolution of area-specific features as a result of widespread selective pressures (or perhaps relaxation of selection in the case of reduction of tooth size) better accounts for the phenotypic pattern of the Gangetic Mesolithic people than does a theory of population migration or equally unsubstantiated theses of extensive and abrupt genetic modification.

Wolpoff (1980) speculates that localized regionalization of variation appeared late in the evolution of *Homo sapiens* and is a characteristic feature of Upper Paleolithic and Mesolithic populations. Accumulating differences between regions were due less to selection than to different and effective responses to the same selective pressure for gracilization operating on diverse gene pools. Also, rates of change were variable in different areas, and some trait clusters covered immense geographical expanses. The Mesolithic hominids of Sarai Nahar Rai and Mahadaha may represent a regional adaptation to these selective pressures, but with considerable retention of the larger body size and megadonty characteristic of terminal Pleistocene populations that were their contemporaries in Europe, Africa, and the Near East.

By 6500 years B.P. the trend toward smaller stature and greater gracilization of body form had become apparent in the later Mesolithic populations living in India, a tendency that continued into the Neolithic, Chalcolithic, Harappan, Iron Age, and Historic periods. With these skeletal modifications there was a reduction in tooth size and degree of attritional stress at the cost of a higher incidence of dental pathologies and anomalies. If Wolpoff's model reflects what really happened in the course of recent hominid evolution, then it is possible to isolate the causes of stress as the nutritional effects of higher carbohydrates and lower protein foodstuffs, greater population density, sedentary habitats associated with farmlands and herds, and susceptibility to new pathogens and nutritional stresses associated with communal and urban life. Certainly these and related stresses would enhance selection for reduced body size and reduction of the biomass of larger communities. As Stini (1975) has argued in his studies of changing nutritional patterns, small body size is an adaptive response in circumstances of chronic protein deprivation. This phenomenon appears to be a continuing evolutionary factor in the adaptive success of most contemporary populations of South Asia that exist under nutritional pressures that stem from the transition of economic life-styles from hunting and gathering to food producing around 6500 years ago in some parts of the subcontinent.

Because skeletal changes are partially developmental and responsive to different nutritional levels, health status, and activity patterns, there is expected diversity of body size and form in cultural and economic groups within the Indian macropopulation today. Tall stature and skeletal robustness appear sporadically in the subcontinent, but there are no contemporary human groups there that possess the total phenotypic pattern of the Mesolithic people of the Gangetic plains. Even surviving tribal populations that retain certain aspects of the hunting–gathering life-style obtain a high proportion of their nutrients in the form of grains and luxury foods from neighboring settled agriculturalists using ancient customs of barter. Such tribal enclaves have long been incorporated as symbiotic subcultures within the economic patterns of the sedentary macropopulation surrounding them, and due to this relationship gene exchange has served for centuries to tie the hunting peoples of the forests to the food producers of the valleys and plains. Effective adaptations allow these somewhat differently organized groups to occupy adjacent areas, and random differences may accumulate locally.

Climatic and ecological factors in South Asia have played some role in the adaptations of Mesolithic populations, especially with respect to drift. Allchin and her colleagues (Allchin *et al.*, 1978) have described the paleogeographical and climatological changes of the Thar Desert of northwestern India during the Pleistocene when a once habitable open forest and grassland environment was altered to a harsh arid expanse that was inhospitable to human settlement and to large game animals. Cut off from most of the rest of Asia by the Himalayas and the desert, the prehistoric inhabitants of peninsular India lived in isolation from communities to the north and northwest, although communication remained open along an eastern corridor into southeastern Asia. Under these conditions, the Upper Paleolithic peoples of western and northern Asia were isolated from the inhabitants of the Ganga Plains. Thus, optimum circumstances would have existed for the effect of drift to appear at Sarai Nahar Rai and Mahadaha. Indeed, some discrete phenotypic features unique to these Mesolithic people may be attributed to this or analogous factors of geographical isolation. By 10,000 years ago substantially more humid conditions developed in the arid region that, being habitable once more, attracted populations from surrounding areas, as is attested to by the proliferation of habitat and factory sites with the microlithic tools of Mesolithic tradition. Gene flow from other areas would have been restored in this climatic phase. It is not possible at this point in our investigations to assess the significance of these paleogeographical and climatic factors upon the ecological conditions of the Gangetic plains in terminal Pleistocene times.

Allchin notes that this was a period when "some sort of missile with a fairly long range would have been an essential part of the hunter's equipment" and "the advent of lighter hunting equipment may have been associated with the introduction of other techniques of hunting in relatively dry, open country, such as the spear thrower, the boomerang, and the bow and arrow" (Allchin *et al.*, 1978, pp. 330, 325). Such technological innovations, along with the practices of hunting small game animals that was so prevalent in postglacial times in South Asia, have important implications for the thesis of evolution or modification of body size and form due to the transformation of cultural and ecological settings. The Gangetic Mesolithic skeletal series is important because it is the first paleontological evidence that these particular kinds of biological, cultural, and ecological changes took place in South Asia.

In conclusion, the Sarai Nahar Rai and Mahadaha skeletal series constitute a population that was extremely successful in its adaptations to the Mesolithic lifestyle that was carried out in an ecological setting of abundant food resources. Only in this way can we explain the particular physical responses of this population as are indicated by the apparent realization of full ontogenetic growth potentials combined with a low incidence of diseases related to nutritional stress. This pattern of adaptive success, or fitness, is not unique in prehistoric cultures antedating the invention of agriculture and pastoralism. It occurs also in some populations today. But for each one of these cases of successful adaptation among contemporary hunters and gatherers, there are myriad cases where this economic strategy has failed, has persisted as a marginal form of existence, or has undergone rapid acculturation to the influences of neighboring food-producing communities. The successful biological adaptation of Mesolithic peoples to their economic pattern in South Asia is documented by the rich archaeological record attesting to the development of some fairly sophisticated regional cultures in this part of the world. Certainly the exploitation of new ecological settings allowed populations of the Mesolithic period to occupy a wide range of natural habitats and pioneer areas that were only sparsely settled by their Paleolithic forebears. The Mesolithic hominids of the Gangetic plains retained the large body size, robustness and megadonty that is characteristic of terminal Pleistocene populations from other parts of Europe, Africa, and Asia prior to the onset of the trend toward gracilization and microdonty that is associated with the economic life-style of later Mesolithic and Neolithic populations. For these reasons, the Mesolithic period merits intensive investigation by archaeologists and skeletal biologists, because this was the moment of cultural transition and concomitant biological and demographic readjustments that mark the end of the once-universal life-style of humankind as the supreme predator and anticipate the technologically oriented and food-producing economy of the modern world. A part of this evolutionary development is now clearly documented in the skeletal record of Mesolithic people in South Asia.

Acknowledgments

The laboratory analysis of the Sarai Nahar Rai and Mahadaha skeletal series was undertaken by the author with the assistance of Mr. Christopher B. Burrow of the University of Arizona in the autumn of 1980 at Allahabad University. I am deeply grateful to Dr. G. R. Sharma, head of the Department of Ancient History, Culture and Archaeology, Allahabad University, for permission to examine these specimens and for conferring the appointment of Visiting Fellow of the Centre of Advanced Study at this institution. The single specimen from Sarai Nahar Rai that is housed with the Anthropological Survey of India in Calcutta was made available for study through the courtesy of the survey's director, Dr. H. Rakshit. Special thanks are expressed to Dr. John Yellen and to Dr. P. R. Mehendiratta, officers of the granting agencies, to Mrs. Margaret Carrick Fairlie Kennedy whose assistance in cleaning the fossil specimens in the laboratory was invaluable, and to Mr. Burrow without whose highly professional, cheerful, and enthusiastic participation in the laboratory and in subsequent analytical phases of the project, this preliminary report would not have been available for publication at this time. The author is grateful to Dr. John R. Lukacs for his invitation to include this study in the present volume as well as for his reading of the manuscript, and to Mrs. Beth Marks who typed the manuscript. Photographs in this chapter were made available by Dr. G. R. Sharma. Thanks is given for permission to publish them.

References

Agrawal, D. P., 1971, *C14 Date List, March 1971,* Tata Institute of Fundamental Research, Bombay.

Agrawal, D. P., and Kusumgar, S., 1974, *Prehistoric Chronology and Radiocarbon Dating in India,* Munshiram Manoharlal, New Delhi.

Aiyappan, A., 1945, Mesolithic artifacts from Swyerpuram in Tinnevelly District, South India, *Spolia Zeylanica* **24**(2):145–154.

Allchin, B., 1958, Morhana Pahar: A rediscovery, *Man* **58:**153–155.

Allchin, B., 1959, The late Stone Age of Ceylon, *J. R. Anthropol. Inst.* **88:**179–201.

Allchin, B., Goudie, A., and Hegde, K., 1978, *The Prehistory and Palaeogeography of the Great Indian Desert,* Academic Press, London.

Brace, C. L., 1978, Tooth reduction in the Orient, *Asian Perspectives* **19:**203–252.

Brace, C. L., and Mahler, P. E., 1971, Post-Pleistocene changes in the human dentition, *Am. J. of Phy. Anthropol.* **34:**191–203.

Brown, A., 1892, On the continuity of the Palaeolithic and Neolithic periods, *J. R. Anthropol. Inst.* **22:**66–98.

Burkitt, M. C., Cammiade, L. A., and Richards, F. J., 1932, Climatic changes in southeast Asia during early Palaeolithic times, *Geological Magazine* **69:**193–204.

Cammiade, L. A., and Burkitt, M. C., 1930, Fresh light on the Stone Age in southeast India, *Antiquity* **4:**327–339.

Carlleyle, A. C., 1883, Notes on lately discovered sepulchral mounds, cairns, caves, cave-paintings, and stone implements, in: *Proc. of the Asiatic Society of Bengal,* **February 1883:**49.

Carlleyle, A. C., 1885, Report of tours in Gorakpur and Ghazipur, *Rep. Archaeol. Surv. of India* **22.**

Clark, G., 1932, *The Mesolithic Age in Britain,* Cambridge University Press, Cambridge.

Clark, G., 1936, *The Mesolithic Cultures of Northern Europe,* Cambridge University Press, Cambridge.

Constandse-Westerman, T. S., 1974, L'Homme Mesolithique du Nord-Ouest de L'Europe, Distances biologiques, considerations genetiques, *Bulletins et Memoires de la Société d'Anthropologie de Paris,* Series 13, **1:**173–199.

Dawkins, B., 1893, On the relation of the Palaeolithic to the Neolithic period, *J. R. Anthropol. Inst.* **23:**242–247.

Deraniyagala, P. E. P., 1963, Prehistoric archaeology in Ceylon, *Asian Perspect.* **7** (1–2)**:**189–192.

Deraniyagala, S. U., 1981, Prehistoric Sri Lanka: A review, in: *Deraniyagala Commemorative Volume* (E. P. Paul). Colombo, Lake House Investments.

De Terra, H., and Paterson, T. T., 1939, *Studies on the Ice Age in India and Associated Human Cultures,* Carnegie Institution of Washington, Washington, D.C.

Dutta, P. C., 1971, Earliest Indian human remains found in a late Stone Age site, *Nature,* **233:**500–501.

Dutta, P. C., 1973, The earliest skeletal remains of a Late Stone Age man from India, *Anthropologie* **11** (3)**:**249–251.

Dutta, P. C., and Pal, A., 1972, The earliest Indian human skeletal find and the estimation of stature, *Cur. Sci.* **9:**334–335.

Dutta, P. C., Pal, A., and Dutta, B. C., 1971, Sarai Nahar Rai: A late Stone Age site in the plain of the Ganga, *J. Indian Anthropol. Soc.* **6**:15–28.

Dutta, P. C., Pal, A., and Biswas, J. N., 1972, Late Stone Age human remains from Sarai Nahar Rai: The earliest skeletal evidence of man in India, *Bull. Anthropol. Surv. of India* **21** (1–2): 114–138.

Ehrhardt, S., and Kennedy, K. A. R., 1965, Excavations at Langhnaj: 1944–63, Part 3: The human remains, *Deccan Coll. Build. Centen. and Silver Jubilee Ser.* **27.**

Foote, R. B., 1916, *The Foote Collection of Indian Prehistoric and Protohistoric Antiquities: Notes on Their Ages and Distribution.* Madras Government Museum, Madras.

Frayer, D. W., 1978, The evolution of the dentition in Upper Palaeolithic and Mesolithic Europe, *Univ. Kansas Publ. Anthropol.* **10.**

Gordon, D. H., 1938, The microlithic industries of India, *Man* **38**:91–100.

Hunter, G. R., 1935, Interim report on excavation conducted by Dr. G. R. Hunter, by permission of the government, in a rock shelter, herinafter called Dorothy Deep Shelter No. 1, situated in the valley known as Dorothy Deep about 2 miles W.N.W. of Pachmarhi in the Mahadeo Hills, Central Provinces, India, *Nagpur Univ. J.* **1**:28–57.

Hunter, G. R., 1936, Final report on the excavation in the Mahadeo Hills, *Nagpur Univ. J.* **2**:127–144.

Karve-Corvinus, G., and Kennedy, K. A. R., 1964, Preliminary report on Langhnaj: A preliminary report of the 1963 archaeological expedition to Langhnaj, northern Gujarat, *Bull. Deccan Coll. Res. Inst.* **24**:44–57.

Kennedy, K. A. R., 1965, Human skeletal material from Ceylon, with an analysis of the island's prehistoric and contemporary populations, *Bull. Brit. Mus. (Nat. History)* **11** (4):135–213.

Kennedy, K. A. R., 1977, Fossil man in India: The "missing link" in our knowledge of human evolution in Asia, *Bull. of the National Speleological Society* **39** (4):99–103.

Kennedy, K. A. R., 1980, Prehistoric skeletal record of man in South Asia, *Annu. Rev. Anthropol.* **9**:391–432.

Kennedy, K. A. R., 1983, Preliminary report on the Mesolithic human remains from Sarai Nahar Rai, India: Their skeletal biology and evolutionary significance, in: *History and Archaeology,* Volume 2 (G. R. Sharma, ed.), Allahabad University, Allahabad.

Kennedy, K. A. R., 1983, Morphological variation in ulnar *Supinator* crests and fossae as identifying markers of occupational stress, *Journal of Forensic Sciences* **28**(4):871–876.

Lukacs, J. R., 1978, Bio-cultural interaction in prehistoric India: Culture, ecology and the pattern of dental disease in Neolithic-Chalcolithic populations, in: *Am. Stud. Anthropol. India* (S. Vatuk, ed.), Manohar Publishers, New Delhi, pp. 425–444.

Lukacs, J. R., 1982, Cultural Variation and Dental Reduction: Evolutionary Mechanisms and Evidence from South Asia, Paper presented at the Indian Statistical Institute Conference on Human Genetics and Adaptation, February 1–5, 1982, Calcutta.

Lukacs, J. R., Misra, V. N., and Kennedy, K. A. R., 1982, *Bagor and Tilwara: The Late Mesolithic Cultures of Northwest India: Human Skeletal Remains,* Deccan College, Pune.

Macalister, R. A. S., 1921, *Textbook of European Archaeology,* Cambridge University Press, Cambridge.

Meiklejohn, C., 1979, Ecological aspects of population size and growth in late-glacial and early postglacial North-Western Europe, in: *The Early Post-Glacial Settlement of Northern Europe: An Ecological Perspective* (P. A. Mellars, ed.), Duckworth, London, pp. 65–79.

Misra, V. N., 1965, Mesolithic phase in its prehistory of India, in: *Indian Prehistory 1964* (V. N. Misra and M. S. Mate, eds.), *Deccan Coll. Build. Centen. Silver Jubilee Ser.* **32**:57–85.

Misra, V. N., 1976, Ecological adaptations during the terminal Stone Age in western and central India, in: *Ecological Backgrounds of South Asian Prehistory* (K. A. R. Kennedy and G. L.

Possehl, eds.), South Asia Occasional Papers and Theses, South Asia Program, Cornell University, Ithaca, pp. 28–51.
Misra, V. N., Mathpal, Y., and Nagar, M., 1977, *Bhimbetka: Prehistoric Man and His Art in Central India,* Sakal Press, Pune.
Mortillet, L. L. G. de, 1883, *Materiaux: Le Préhistoire,* Paris.
Newell, R. R., 1973, The post-glacial adaptations of the indigenous populations of the northwest European plain, in: *The Mesolithic of Europe* (S. K. Kowlowski, ed.), Warsaw University Press, Warsaw, pp. 399–440.
Redman, C. L., 1978, *The Rise of Civilization: From Early Farmers to Urban Society in the Ancient Near East,* Freeman, San Francisco.
Rightmire, G. P., 1975, Problems of the study of later Pleistocene man in Africa, *Am. Anthropol.* **77** (1):28–52.
Riquet, R., 1970, La Race Cro-Magnon, Abus de Langage ou Réalité Objective? in: *L'Homme de Cro-Magnon* (G. Camps and G. Olivier, eds.), Arts et Métiers Graphiques, Paris, pp. 37–58.
Sankalia, H. D., 1946, *Investigations into Prehistoric Archaeology of Gujarat, Being the Official Report of the First Gujarat Prehistoric Expedition 1941–42,* Baroda State Press, Baroda.
Sankalia, H. D. and Karve, I., 1949, Early primitive microlithic culture and people of Gujarat, *Am. Anthropol.* **51** (1):28–34.
Sharma, A. K., 1980, Some palaeo-pathological observations on skeletal remains from Mahadaha and Sarai Nahar Rai, in: *Beginnings of Agriculture* (G. R. Sharma, V. O. Misra, D. Mandal, B. B. Misra and J. Pal, eds.), Abinash Prakashan, Allahabad, pp. 231–232.
Sharma, G. R., 1965, Comments, in: *Indian Prehistory 1964* (V. N. Misra and M. S. Mate, eds.), *Deccan Coll. Build. Centen. Silver Jubilee Ser.* **32**:76–79.
Sharma, G. R., 1973, Mesolithic lake culture in the Ganga valley, in: *Proc. of the Prehistoric Society* **39**:129–146.
Sharma, G. R., 1975, Seasonal migrations and Mesolithic lake cultures of the Ganga Valley, in: *K. C. Chattopadhyaya Memorial Volume* (G. R. Sharma, ed.), K. K. Dubey, Allahabad, pp. 1–20.
Sharma, G. R., Misra, V. O., Mandal, D., Misra, B. B., and Pal, J. (eds.), 1980, *Beginnings of Agriculture,* Abinash Prakashan, Allahabad.
Smith, P. E. L., and Young, T. C., 1972, The evolution of early agriculture and culture in greater Mesopotamia: A trial model, in: *Population Growth: Anthropological Implications* (B. J. Spooner, ed.), M.I.T. Press, Cambridge, Mass., pp. 1–59.
Stini, W. A., 1975, Adaptive strategies of human populations under nutritional stress, in: Biosocial Interrelations in Population Adaptation (E. S. Watts, F. E. Johnston, and G. W. Lasker, eds.), Mouton, The Hague, pp. 19–41.
Subbarao, B., 1950, *The Personality of India,* University of Baroda, Baroda.
Todd, K. R. U., 1932, Prehistoric man around Bombay, in: *Proc. Prehist. Soc.* **7**:35–42.
Trotter, M., 1970, Estimation of stature from intact limb bones, in: *Personal Identification in Mass Disasters* (T. D. Stewart, ed.), National Museum of Natural History, Washington, D.C., pp. 71–83.
Wakankar, V. S., 1973, Bhim-Betka excavations, *J. Indian Hist.* **51**:23–32.
Wakankar, V. S., 1975, Bhimbetka—the prehistoric paradise, *Prachya Pratibhi* **3** (2):7–29.
Wolpoff, M., 1980, *Paleoanthropology,* Knopf, New York.
Wynne, A. B., 1866, Remains of prehistoric man in central India, *Geological Magazine* **3**:283–284.
Zeuner, F. E., and Allchin, B., 1956, The microlithic sites of Tinnevelly, Madras State, *Anc. India* **12**:4–20.

CHAPTER 3

Biological Anthropology of Bronze Age Harappans: New Perspectives

PRATAP C. DUTTA

1. Paleoanthropological Background of the Indian Subcontinent

1.1. The Hominoid Fossil Record

The Indian subcontinent occupies the major landmass of South Asia. Considering its vastness, varied physiography, and mosaic of ecological conditions suitable for adaptive radiation, the scores of early hominoid fossils are not very illuminating. The situation is an unimpressive one when compared to that of the other fossil-bearing countries. But whatever hominoid primate fossil records are available in the subcontinent, the sole credit goes to the Siwaliks.

The Siwalik Hills of Northern India and Pakistan are the most important and promising source where search for possible human ancestors is being actively continued. These hills were formed by the accumulation of mountain-worn silt, which deposited layered sediments at the lower slopes of the Himalayas during the period from 14 million to nearly 500,000 years ago. The hills are being eroded, exposing fossil records of hominoids from the first half of the sequence, which is composed of several Miocene–Pliocene deposits. And by now some 130-odd fossil specimens have been recorded (Pilbeam *et al.*, 1977; Ghosh and Sen, 1981) from the later part of the Miocene beds, during the period from 9 to 8 million years ago.

The fossil specimens, which represent roughly 50 individuals, belonged to a

PRATAP C. DUTTA • Anthropological Survey of India, Calcutta 700 016, India.

number of genera, including *Sivapithecus*, and *Gigantopithecus*. They all flourished in the Siwaliks, more or less at the same time. *Gigantopithecus* is a fossil pongid, whereas *Sivapithecus* could be a reasonable model from which to deduce the orangutan. The hominoids, however, disappeared from the Siwaliks when the region experienced a cooler climate during the time from 8 to 6 million years ago.

1.2. The Hominoid Skeletal Record

After a brief blossoming of the hominoids in the Siwaliks, there is a long gap in the hominid fossil record in the subcontinent during the vast span of the Pleistocene. Although cultural evidence attesting to the existence and activities of the hominid populations is abundant throughout the subcontinent during the middle and late Pleistocene, no fossil record of any Paleolithic person has yet been recovered. Factors responsible for either the complete lack or the low rate of recovery of fossils in South Asia has been accounted for by Kennedy (1975) very cogently. Incidentally, it may be of interest to note that the adjoining country of Afghanistan has provided a broken right temporal bone of a Neanderthal person from Darra-I-Kur. Its deposit has been radiometrically dated from 30,000 ± 1200 years B.P. (Dupree, 1972).

It is only in the late Stone Age in India that smaller, human skeletal series representing Mesolithic people have been recorded. The most important—the oldest skeletal record of people in India—is a subfossil burial complex discovered at Sarai Nahar Rai in Pratapgarh District of Uttar Pradesh in the middle Ganga Valley (Dutta, 1971, 1973; Dutta *et al.* 1972).* Radiometrically it has been dated to 10,345±110 years B.P. The deposit of the complex is composed of gray sticky clay mixed with coarse sand and irregular nodules (*kankars*) formed by the accumulation of calcium carbonate. Analysis of the lithostratigraphy and pollen assemblage of the deposit gives a picture of open grasslands characteristic of the very arid climate where *Chenopodium* had grown (Gupta, 1976).

Other series, mostly smaller and of more recent date, have also been recorded from all the prehistoric cultural phases of India. These represent Neolithic, Chalcolithic, Harappan, and the Iron Age inhabitants.

In South Asian paleoanthropology, however, the human osseous record recovered from the prehistoric city site of Harappa in the Indus Basin is of paramount importance. This is indeed so, because of two pragmatic reasons that are far-reaching. First, it is the only extensive prehistoric human skeletal series discovered to date from South Asia. And, second, because of its workable sample size (in the context of chance discoveries of archaeological material) and also for its well-documented record of cultural identity. The series can be programmed fruitfully for investigations seeking answers to questions relating to

*(See also Kennedy, Chapter 2.—Ed.)

biocultural interrelationships and evolutionary dynamics of earlier human-population groups in South Asia. This chapter discusses some aspects of our present understanding of the biological anthropology of the Harappans who lived in the Indus Valley during the third millennium B.C.

2. The Harappa Civilization and Its Domain

2.1. Type Site and the Distribution of Settlements

The Harappa civilization arose toward the end of the third millennium before Christ in the Indus Basin, and it flourished there for nearly 1000 years. This highly developed, fully urbanized—the most extensive civilization that bloomed in the Indo-Iranian borderlands, beyond the limits of the lands that comprise the Fertile Crescent—is currently named the *Harappa civilization* instead of the *Indus civilization*. The ancient city site of Harappa (lat. 30°38′ N and long. 72°52′ E), near modern Lahore in Pakistan is located beside the Ravi River—a tributary of the Indus. It is the type site of the Harappa civilization.

Prolonged research and systematic excavations at the Indo–Iranian borderlands as well as in parts of western India during the past two decades have been most rewarding. Sustained investigations have brought to light the existence and distribution of a large number of Harappa civilization sites that are located outside the nuclear area in the Indus Valley. The culture, as revealed at the two great urban centers—Mohenjo-Daro and Harappa—in the Indus basin is also seen to have been widely spread, either in its pure state or in the regional variations thereof. Remains of the culture have been recorded from Baluchistan on the west to beyond Delhi into the interfluve on the east and from the eastern foot of the Sulaiman Mountain range (Gumla and Rahman Dheri in the Gomal Valley) in the north to the Tapti estuary in the south.

The ruins of Harappa were first visited by Charles Masson as early as 1862: his visits were followed by those of Alexander Burnes around 1831. The first archaeological report on a settlement of the Indus civilization came from Sir Alexander Cunningham (1875) who made several excavations at Harappa in 1853 and 1856. But it was not until January, 1921, that systematic excavation at the site could be undertaken by the archaeology department of the Government of India. The first phase of digging, initiated by Sir John Marshall (the man responsible for unfolding the story of Mohenjo-Daro), was carried out by Rai Bahadur Daya Ram Sahni during the years from 1921 to 1925 (Marshall, 1931). Excavations at the site—uncovering the city plan with a citadel recalling the general layout of Mohenjo-Daro—were most fruitful during subsequent major excavations conducted by Madho Sarup Vats and K. N. Sastri from 1926 to 1937 (Vats, 1940). In 1946, Sir Mortimer Wheeler revealed new dimensions by excavating huge mud-brick fortifications at Harappa (Wheeler, 1947).

It is important to note that more than 200 Harappan settlements have since been identified in this area. More than 60 of these sites unmistakably attest to a mature phase of the Harappan culture. However, all these sites are not coeval. Most of the southern sites represent later dates than those in the Indus Valley proper. A time span of 2300–1750 B.C. for this culture has been obtained from radiocarbon determinations that are available from several Harappan sites in this region (Agrawal, 1971, p. 96).

Although the number of mature Harappan sites is fairly moderate, only nine sites (including Harappa) have thus far provided human skeletal remains: Harappa, Rupar, and Chandigarh in Punjab; Kalibangan and Tarkanwala Dera in Rajasthan; Lothal and Randal Dawa in Gujarat; and Mohenjo-Daro and Chanhu-Daro in Sind. Of these, the first three sites and the last two sites are in the Indus Valley; the rest are located well outside the valley. Except for Harappa, Mohenjo-Daro, and Chanhu-Daro, which are in Pakistan, the other six skeletal-bearing sites are in India.

2.2. Culture and Society

Excavations have revealed that the Harappa culture evolved to a mature and developed form. It can be said that the culture was a highly urbanized and disciplined one; there was sufficient economic wealth to support a large population. Well-planned cities, public buildings, fortifications, granaries, and standardization of material equipment by means of mass production reflect the existence of interrelated, highly developed sociopolitical and religious institutions (Mughal, 1979, p. 92).

The people possessed resources to engage in long-distance trade and in the exchange of products. They depended primarily upon farming. They also domesticated humped buffalo and short-horned bulls as well as other animals. In their daily lives, they used tools and other objects made of stone and copper and bronze objects. Most of the pots were wheel turned, pinkish in color with a bright red slip. These were normally decorated in black, either by plain horizontal lines or by pictorial motifs. The most notable artifacts are the seals made of steatite. On the basis of primary archaeological evidence, Wheeler (1947, p. 59) observed that the Harappa civilization was a centralized type, comparable to the contemporary civilizations of Sumer and Egypt.

3. Bioanthropology of the Harappans

3.1. Skeletal Biology

The Harappan skeletal series is composed of the remains of 260 individuals. Some of them are, however, represented only by tiny bits of bones. Technical information on age, sex, anatomical description, other observations, measurements, and the context of discovery of each skeleton has been published previously by Gupta, Dutta, and Basu (1962). In this pioneering work, the physical makeup of the Harappans was inferred, following the methods of classical morphology and anthropology. Using the modern genetic concept of *population,* the material was recently reexamined, resulting in a series of investigations comparing variations in the skeletal biology at the population level (Dutta, 1972, 1974, 1975a, 1975b).

The skeletons were recovered from three major skeletal-bearing deposits at Harappa. Notwithstanding the differences of provenience investigations clearly show that (1) skeletons from different deposits of Harappa constitute a single, morphologically homogenous series, and (2) the people of the Harappa can be considered as belonging to a population representing the Bronze Age Harappan race. Further analysis suggests that the male and female Harappans were of the same phenotype, although certain characteristics of the population are quite conspicuous in their distinctive sexual dimorphism (Dutta, 1983a, 1983b, 1983c). Some of the essential cranial measurements are shown in Table I. The inferences arrived at, with respect to bioanthropology, may, in brief, be outlined as follows.

The people were, on the average, moderately long headed (dolichocephalic: male, 73.71±0.78; female, 74.13±0.81), having an average cranial capacity

TABLE I
Means and Standard Deviations (S.D.) of the Harappa Series (in mm)

	Male			Female		
Character	*n*	Mean	S.D.	*n*	Mean	S.D.
Cranial length (1)[a]	28	186.11	6.03	32	178.23	7.22
Cranial breadth (8)	27	136.31	5.40	25	131.40	5.73
Minimum frontal breadth (9)	25	96.32	4.21	31	92.06	4.22
Basion–bregma height (17)	26	134.00	4.15	25	127.34	5.92
Horizontal circumference (23)	24	521.00	12.91	26	500.58	17.88
Upper face height (48)	25	69.18	4.29	25	63.94	4.67
Bizygomatic breadth (45)	13	130.92	5.39	16	121.41	4.98
Nasal height (55)	27	51.57	2.80	33	46.98	3.63
Nasal breadth (54)	26	26.17	2.15	32	24.64	1.83
Orbital breadth (L) (51)	24	41.50	2.20	30	39.98	2.36
Orbital height (L) (52)	25	33.42	2.28	29	33.05	2.86
Palatal length (62)	24	47.29	3.53	17	45.38	3.05
Palatal breadth (63)	26	40.52	4.04	18	38.28	2.70
Bigonial breadth (66)	13	88.92	9.08	6	78.92	5.04
Mandibular length (68)	15	81.87	5.72	10	77.55	6.41

[a]Numbers in parentheses refer to definitions in Martin and Saller (1956, pp. 453–481).

(euencephalic: male, 1415.99±14.02 cc; female, 1260.23±19.95 cc), average medium-high vault of head (orthocephalic: male, 72.08±0.67; female, 71.32±0.79) in relation to the length of the head, and a relatively high vault (acrocephalic: male, 97.94±1.00; female, 98.45±1.12) in relation to the breadth of head. The calvarium shapes were mostly ellipsoids to spheroids in males and ellipsoids to ovoids in females. The forehead was moderately broad and highly receding to slightly receding in males, whereas it was fairly narrow and vertical to slightly receding in females.

The upper face of the Harappans was medium or low mesen shaped (male, 51.35±1.16; female, 52.60±0.86) with varying degrees of alveolar prognathism. The noses were highly mesorrhine or moderately platyrrhine (male, 50.50±0.77; female, 52.82±1.06), and the bridge of the nose was frequently concave, depressed at the base. Orbits were medium high (mesoconchic: male, 80.89±1.44; female, 82.66±1.20). These people had moderately broad hard palates (brachystaphyline: male, 84.94±2.26; female, 85.77±1.94) with paraboloid dental arcades. Though the lower-jaw width was short in both sexes (male, 88.92±2.52 mm; female, 78.92±2.06 mm), the jaw itself was relatively robust and larger in males than in females.

The Harappans were above average in body height: Males had an average stature of 1691.87 mm (about 5 ft 6½ in.) and females 1555.59 mm (about 5 ft 1¼ inches). They were a low eurymeric (male, 80.35; female, 80.24) and mesocnemic (male, 65.17; female, 69.67) people, but neither platymeric nor platycnemic. The humero-radial index suggests that the males were mesocercic and the females dolichocercic, thus indicating relatively longer female forearms. The femoro-humerus index shows that both the male and female Harappans had shorter arms in relation to thighs.

The preceding illustrates some of the essential parameters of the skeletal biology of the Harappans. The series is adequately homogeneous with reference to a standard homogeneous series—the Egyptian E. Although Cappieri (1970) has defined the Harappans as the Indian proto-Mediterraneans, it is not really useful to classify them into the classical morphological "races" and "subraces." The classical typological concept is a sterile concept because it is not consonant with the realities of human evolutionary biology that shape and determine the courses of natural groupings of people (see discussion in Dutta, 1975b).

3.2. Anthropological Status

An anthropological problem concerning the evaluation of status is the core problem of biological taxonomy, which aims at classifying the taxons. The classification is at several hierarchical levels, and is represented by samples drawn from various populations that are considered to have different genetic origins. It necessitates the use of a statistical investigation that is essentially multivariate in approach. The multivariate analysis will utilize a conjoint investigation of quantitative variates obtained from a set of characters of the given number of populations.

The classification and ordering may be achieved by evaluating numerically the morphological affinities or differences between the Harappans and other culturally relevant contemporary groups. This can be done by analyzing the overall distance differences and ascertaining mutual relationships between all possible pairs of population groups, utilizing a suitable measure of taxonomic distance.

3.2.1. Measure of group divergence. There are three main measures of taxonomic distance available for use in anthropometric work. These are the following: (1) Durchschnittliche Differenze (DD) formulated by Czekanowski (1909); (2) Coefficient of Racial Likeness (CRL) by Pearson (1926); and (3) Generalized Distance (D^2) by Mahalanobis (1936; see also Rao, 1952).

The D^2, the most powerful and elegant of all, undoubtedly offers the best possible methods of discrimination between groups on the basis of a set of metric characters. Of course, some assumptions have to be satisfied (notably, the homogeneity of the variances and correlations and normality of the multivariate distribution). It differs fundamentally from the other two measures in that it eliminates redundant variables. And the distances of both the DD and CRL increase when a variate is added, but D^2 remains unaltered. However, the D^2, which involves a formidable process of different variate intercorrelations and matrix inversion, has not been used here due to the smaller magnitude of sample sizes of different metric characters of the Harappa series.

Huizinga (1962) has shown that there exists a high correlation between the three measures; therefore, he recommends the use of DD because it is most simple to calculate. And, on the other hand, Penrose (1954) has shown that D^2 is linearly related to CRL when all intercorrelations of variables are constant.

Two more simplified measures of generalized distance, using symbols C_H^2 for *CRL* and δg, have been proposed by Penrose (1954) and Hiernaux (1965), respectively. C_H^2 is highly correlated with D^2, and needs only the observed variable means and standard deviations; δg, which is very close to CRL and has a high correlation with D^2, requires variable means (or frequencies) and population (or sample) ranges.

Using Penrose's measure, it is possible to approximate a generalized distance between any two p variate statistical populations by mC^2_H, which is the sum of size and shape distances multiplied by the number of characters considered. The measure, denoted here as D^2_p (the suffix refers to Penrose), is easy to calculate as it is with computing CRL but reportedly with almost the same accuracy as D^2. The D^2_p assumes a common intercorrelation, ρ, between the p variables, leading to a simple function of distance closely approximating D^2. Of course, to pool correlations and assume a common value for them would involve errors that could sometimes be hazardous, as has been pointed out by Mulhall (Talbot and Mulhall, 1962, p. 122).

3.2.2. Taxonomic situation. To investigate the problem, six male cranial series have been considered. These are the following: Harappa, Tepe Hissar III, Badarian, Naqada A, Abydos, and Sakkara (see Figure 1). The last-named four prehistoric series are from Egypt, whereas Tepe Hissar is from Iran. Other appropriate comparable series, namely, Kish, al-'Ubaid, and Alishar from southwestern Asia as well as Mohenjo-Daro from the Indus Valley, which should have also been important, could not be utilized due to the smaller number of observations available concerning their metrical traits. For estimating group divergence, a battery of seven craniofacial measurements for each of the series has been programmed. Mean values and standard deviations of characters for the compared series are shown in Tables II and III, respectively.

The computed values of interpopulation D^2_p estimates obtained are arranged in decreasing order of magnitude in Table IV. A careful study of distance values immediately brings into sharper focus the general pattern of the taxonomic situation. The most relevant fact is that the Harappans and the series from Tepe Hissar and Sakkara are correlated closely in all six columns.

The values obtained from averaging the distance estimates within and between clusters are shown in Table V. The computation, based on the values of distance estimates, as in Table IV, is given in Table VI. To have a visual perspective of the whole situation, Figure 1 is useful. From all these data, it becomes reasonably clear that the Harappan, Tepe Hissar, and Sakkaran series constitute a cluster of a single unit, suggesting close similarity or affinity. On the other hand, the Naqada and Badarian series are seen to be fairly close to each other. The Abydos series apparently does not fit in the two clusters, but remains distinctly apart.

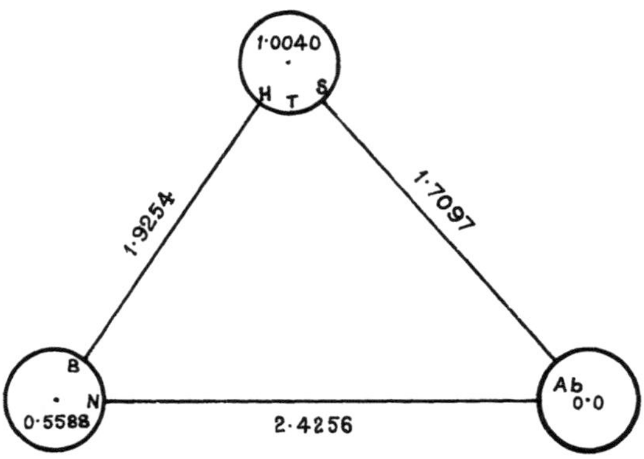

Figure 1. Schematic diagram showing the intra- and interrelationships of clusters (H = Harappa, T = Tepe Hissar, S = Sakkara, B = Badarian, N = Naqada A, and Ab = Abydos).

Table II
Mean of Male Cranial Characters[a] (in mm)

Series	Cranial length	Cranial breadth	Minimum Frontal breadth	Basilo-bregma height	Nasal height	Nasal breadth	Upper face height
Harappa	186.11(28)	136.31(27)	96.32(25)	134.00(26)	51.57(27)	26.17(26)	69.18(25)
Tepe Hissar	188.25(103)	134.09(102)	95.56(103)	134.72(91)	50.56(99)	25.45(95)	69.77(100)
Badarian	182.58(80)	131.68(80)	91.18(80)	134.27(76)	48.70(76)	24.91(75)	68.00(76)
Naqada A	183.98(90)	133.73(89)	91.21(90)	134.99(78)	49.32(63)	24.94(62)	68.06(64)
Abydos	184.93(36)	136.25(37)	93.42(34)	132.10(35)	53.95(32)	25.53(33)	74.70(31)
Sakkara	186.91(41)	138.72(43)	96.46(36)	135.38(32)	51.17(29)	25.37(30)	71.93(30)

[a]Respective sample sizes are given in parentheses.

Table III
Standard Deviations of Male Cranial Characters

Series	Cranial length	Cranial breadth	Minimum frontal breadth	Basilo-bregma height	Nasal height	Nasal breadth	Upper face height
Harappa	6.03	5.40	4.21	4.15	2.80	2.15	4.29
Tepe Hissar	6.14	5.12	4.23	5.25	3.46	1.85	5.37
Naqada A	6.03	4.96	5.40	5.68	3.02	2.01	4.19
Badarian	6.26	5.38	3.94	3.94	3.16	1.77	4.22
Abydos	5.52	3.99	4.08	6.15	3.44	1.68	4.10
Sakkara	5.23	3.95	3.78	5.73	4.07	1.73	4.39

Table IV
Values of D^2_p between Male Harappa and Five Prehistoric Series

	Harappa (H)		T. Hissar (T)		Badarian (B)
T	0.6989	H	0.6989	N	0.3123
S	0.9463	S	1.3791	T	2.9520
Ab	2.9297	N	2.0262	H	4.2371
N	2.9818	B	2.9520	S	5.9266
B	4.2371	Ab	3.3943	Ab	6.5516
	Naqada A (N)		**Abydos (Ab)**		**Sakkara (S)**
B	0.3123	S	2.4452	H	0.9463
T	2.0262	H	2.9297	T	1.3791
H	2.9818	T	3.3943	Ab	2.4452
S	4.1188	N	5.2154	N	4.1188
Ab	5.2154	B	6.5516	B	5.9266

Table V
Intra- and Intercluster Average D^2_p

Clusters	Groups	X	Y	Z
X	B,N	0.3123	3.7071	5.8835
Y	H,T,S	3.7071	1.0081	2.9231
Z	Ab	5.8835	2.9231	—

Table VI
Computational Scheme for Finding Clusters

Series added to a cluster	D_p^2	Number of terms (n)	Increase in D_p^2/ increase in n	Average D_p^2 ($\Sigma D_p^2/n$)	Cluster
B,N	0.3123	1	—	0.3123	
T	5.2905	3	2.4891	1.7635	B,N
H,T	0.6989	1	—	0.6989	
S	3.0243	3	1.1627	1.0081	H,T,S
Ab	11.7935	6	2.9231	1.9656	
Ab	—	—	—	—	Ab

4. Discussion

The investigation, using seven selected craniofacial measurements and six series, clearly brings into sharper focus the fact that the people of Harappa are biometrically close to those of the Tepe Hissar and Sakkara series. Using the result of a statistical nature, these populations from different regions, namely, the Indus Valley, Iran, and Egypt, could be fitted into a cluster of a single unit.

It is most crucial at this stage to remember that whatever information of a statistical nature could thus be abstracted cannot be used immediately for drawing inferences about problems of biological anthropology. This is especially true in addressing questions that specifically pertain to the biological affinities of ancient human population groups inferred from skeletal samples. Rather, there is a likelihood of being in a *cul-de-sac,* if the aforementioned information is not critically read, understood, and interpreted on the basis and in the context of at least two other different categories of information. The categories should be concerned generally with (1) historical and cultural backgrounds, and (2) geographical propinquity of the given prehistoric populations.

4.1. Cultural Affinities

The Indus Basin is a vast alluvial plain. It covers an irregular triangle and receives water from the Indus and its tributaries. The area was once, and still is, very fertile and capable of supporting a very large population. The valley has yielded a number of sites that are equivalent to the pre-Harappan cultural phase. In the perspective of recent archaeological knowledge gathered from all these sites, one is tempted to believe that there is cultural continuity, that is, the pre-Harappan phase evolves into the Harappan culture (Dutta, 1981).

What is notable in this context is the discovery of ceramics of non-Harappan character and building materials of a fortification wall from the predefense levels at Harappa. Out of a total of 191 potsherds, 35 came from two clearly stratified layers beneath the defense wall. The ceramics were considered to be the product of a variant or even alien culture (Wheeler, 1947). But the excavations at Kot Diji in the mid-1950s by Khan (1965) suggest that the pottery actually represented a pre-Harappan cultural settlement beneath the Harappan citadel mound.

On the left bank of the Indus, opposite Mohenjo-Daro, is Kot Diji. Today this site is located 32 km from the river, but still near one of its ancient flood channels. The site has a citadel and an outer town of Harappan style, even in the pre-Harappan phase. Below an occupation level containing mature Harappan cultural materials, an accumulation of occupational debris yielded ceramics that are identical to those found in the predefense levels at Harappa. Although the pottery forms do suggest a difference in ceramic tradition, some forms and decorative designs, such as fish scales and intersecting circles, are considered to be traits that belong to the mature Harappan culture. Many other characteristic Harappan features, terra-cotta toy-cart frames, wheels, and triangular "cakes," also appeared in the middle levels of the Kot Dijian occupation. The upper and lower Kot Diji levels are dated between 2605 ± 145 and 2090 ± 140 B.C., or between 3155 and 2599 B.C. as adjusted by applying the correction factor supplied by Museum for Applied Science Center for Archaeology (MASCA) at the University of Pennsylvania. Two other C-14 determinations from the first occupation in the area beyond the wall, corresponding to the middle levels of the citadel, are available; these give dates of 2335±155 and 2255±140 B.C., or 2885 and 2805 B.C. after MASCA correction (Ralph *et al.*, 1973, pp. 1–20).

The Kot Dijian occupation was not an isolated phenomenon at Kot Diji only, but was widespread throughout the greater Indus Valley. Detailed investigation further suggests that generally the Kot Dijian occupational sites were later dominated by people of the mature Harappan culture (Mughal, 1979, pp. 93–94).

Excavations at another pre-Harappan occupation site at Amri (160 km south of Mohenjo-Daro) revealed significant evidence of gradual development and a continuity of culture without any break in the sequence (Casal, 1964). As a result, we have not only evidence of a pre-Harappan development but also three distinct phases of the Harappan occupation together with further evidence of a post-Harappan period. It may be noted that two C-14 dates from the middle levels of Amrian occupation are available that are between 2670±113 and 2900±113 B.C., or, after adjustment, 3320 and 3600 B.C. The Kot Dijian ware was found in the earliest level of Amri.

A similar sequence, identical to that at Kot Diji, was also found at another Harappan site at Kaligangan (located on the dry course of the Ghaggar River about 192 km southeast of Harappa and some 480 km east-northeast of Kot Diji). Here, the earliest levels occurring below the mature Harappan culture yielded pottery comparable to that of the predefense levels at Harappa and Kot Diji. In the same levels, a new white-and-black or red pottery known as "Sothi" appeared. The C-14 dates of the Sothi level (Kalibangan I) fall between 2370±115 and 1825±110 B.C., or between 2920 and 2125 B.C. (adjusted).

Pottery from the early levels of Mohenjo-Daro revealed a type that is identical to Damb Sadaat I and II and is comparable to the Kot Dijian and related cultures. Again, at Gumla (Gomal Valley) in levels II and III, below the mature Harappan occupation, Kot Dijian ware was obtained and dated to 2248±74 B.C., 2798 B.C. (adjusted).

All this evidence leads us to believe rather firmly that the Harappan culture was not without contacts with the pre-Harappan communities, such as the Kot Dijians, Amrians, and Sothians. These groups must have contributed to generating the early formative phase of the Harappan culture. Purposive research is still being continued by the discovery of new sites in the Indus Valley. And, at a future date, when more abundant data are gathered on the process of urbanization, the idea of attributing Harappa Culture as a whole to any outside source may prove unjustified. Even at the present moment, with many gaps in our knowledge, one might consider the currently available archaeological indications as favoring an evolutionary model and postulate an indigenous ancestry for the Harappa culture, despite its contacts with the west. For example, there is evidence of trade contacts between the pre-Harappans of the Indus Valley and the populations of the Middle East, especially with those of Baluchistan on the Iranian Plateau. Certain features were common to both the Harappa civilization and Sumer in southern Mesopotamia. Cultural links and international trade existed between the two civilizations, but there was no direct relationship between the Indus Valley cultures and those of Egypt. In terms of geographical propinquity, Egypt is the farthest from the Indus Valley, whereas Iran, with its borderlands, lies close to the Indus.

4.2. Biological Affinities

Let us now turn to the consideration of biological affinities. The analysis, as has already been noted, classifies the Harappans with the Tepe Hissar and Sakkara populations. Although the geographical situations are diverse, the three groups constitute a cluster of a single unit, thus suggesting a close affinity. Physical classification is essentially objective; and, at the same time, it must be admitted that all anthropological conclusions do not necessarily follow the conclusions drawn from the objective assessment of metrical features. This is because anthropometric features or characters are—needless to say—complex, both in terms of material and manifestation. And, in the present instance, the geography and cultural backgrounds of the three population groups stand in high contrast, necessitating a rethinking.

Despite their morphological similarities, a more profitable line of investigation into the problem would be to study critically the estimated mean values of cranial characters of the compared groups, as was indicated earlier (Dutta, 1983a). The study suggests that the Harappans were definitely and relatively small headed but broad faced when compared to the al-'Ubaid, Tepe Hissar, and Sakkara series. The differences, though small in magnitude, are of immense value. They suggest that the Harappans should be regarded as occupying a distinct status—a status that was unique. The uniqueness does not, at any rate, indicate that they came from the west and settled at Harappa.

On the basis of the archaeological information gathered, it is clear that the Indus Valley was inhabited by the pre-Harappan communities before the advent of the Harappans. Their exact relationships are, however, not clear enough. It is unfortunate that no human skeletal remains representing these earlier communities have been discovered and recorded to date. However, considering the uniqueness of physique of the Harappans in the context of the reference population groups and also the cultural sequence of the region, it would be reasonable to conclude that there might have been biological links and genetic continuities between the pre-Harappans and the Harrapans. And because the pre-Harappan communities inhabited the same region and preceded the Harappans chronologically, the immediate ancestors of the Harappans probably are the pre-Harappans.

4.3. A Genetic Recipe

It still remains a puzzle how the Harappa civilization, which had already reached its zenith, came to an abrupt end. And it also remains a mystery where the people of Harappa relocated. Some scholars are inclined to believe that the Harappans moved in a south and southeastern direction away from Harappa.

The idea of investigating the genetic continuity of the Harappans led me to

Table VII
Means and Standard Deviations (S.D.) of the Ludhiana Series (Males)

Character	*n*	Mean	S.D.
Cranial length	16	184.12	6.72
Cranial breadth	15	131.33	5.89
Basion–bregma height	14	134.50	7.45
Upper facial height	14	65.14	5.83
Bizygomatic breadth	14	129.21	6.51
Nasal height	14	50.36	3.41
Nasal breadth	13	25.08	2.69

Table VIII
Values of t-Test between Cranial Traits of Harappa and Ludhiana Series

Character	d.f.	*t*
Cranial length	42	1.01
Cranial breadth	40	2.77[b]
Basion–bregma height	38	0.27
Nasal height	39	1.22
Nasal breadth	37	1.37
Upper facial height	37	2.47[a]
Bizygomatic breadth	25	0.74

[a]Significant at 5% level.
[b]Significant at 1% level.

examine a smaller series of modern crania at the anatomy department of the Christian Medical College at Ludhiana. Ludhiana (lat. 30°55′ N, long. 75°54′ E) is a town in Punjab, located about 160 km east-southeast from Harappa. The series represents the Punjabi population of North India.

An examination of the series was made in July, 1975, with the assistance of Mr. S. S. Datta Chaudhuri (a colleague in the survey) and through the kind courtesy of Professor J. C. Saha (head of the anatomy department). Detailed discussion of the series is not intended here, but for our present purpose, seven essential craniofacial characters of the Ludhiana series have been analyzed and compared with those of the Harappa series.

Table VII gives the character means and standard deviations for the Ludhiana series, whereas Table VIII gives the results of the *t* test between the observed character means of the two series. It could be seen that out of the seven characters compared, five pairs of character means of the two series do not differ, thus suggesting equality between the series. Only two character means, namely, cranial breadth and upper facial height, yield statistically significant differences.

On the whole, the results presently available suggest a genetic continium between the Harappans and the present-day people of the region. This speculation remains tentative and can only be substantiated through further investigations of the larger skeletal collections.

References

Agrawal, D. P., 1971, *The Copper Bronze Age in India,* Munshiram Monoharlal, New Delhi.
Cappieri, M., 1970, The population of the Indus civilization, *Occ. Pap.* **11,** Field Research Project, Miami, Florida.

Casal, Jena-Marie, 1964, *Fouilles d' Amri,* Commission des Fouilles Archéologiques, Paris [Fresh digging at Amri, *Pakistan Archaeology,* Karachi **1**:57–65].

Cunningham, Sir Alexander, 1875, Harappa, Archaeol. Surv. India Rep. 1872–1873, pp. 105–108.

Czekanowski, J., 1909, Zur Differentiadiagnose der Neandertalgruppe, *Korr. bl. Dtsch. Ges. Anthropol. Ethnol., Urgesch* **40**(6/7):44–47.

Dupree, L., 1972, Prehistoric research in Afganistan: 1959–1966, *Trans. Amer. Phil. Soc.* **62**(4).

Dutta, P. C., 1971, Earliest Indian human remains found in a late Stone Age Site, *Nature* **233**(5320): 500–501.

Dutta, P. C., 1972, The Bronze Age Harappans: A re-examination of the skulls in the context of the population concept, *Am. J. Phys. Anthropol.* **36**:391–396.

Dutta, P. C., 1973, The earliest skeletal remains of a late Stone Age from India, *Anthropologie, Brno* **11**:249–253.

Dutta, P. C., 1974, Non-metrical variation in the Bronze Age cranial material from Harappa, in: *Indian Anthropology Today* (D. Sen, ed.), University of Calcutta, Calcutta, pp. 103–113.

Dutta, P. C., 1975a, Harappa people and the contemporary world, in: *Bio-anthropological Research in India* (H. K. Rakshit, ed.), Anthropol. Surv. of India, Calcutta, pp. 20–27.

Dutta, P. C., 1975b, Race concept and palaeoanthropology: A research model for interpreting ancient human remains, *Anthropologie, Brno* **13**(2):35–46.

Dutta, P. C., 1981, The aspect of origin of the Harappa civilisation and the ancestry of its authors, *Indian Museum Bulletin,* Calcutta **17**:19–24.

Dutta, P. C., 1983a, *The Bronze Age Harappans,* Anthropol. Surv. of India, Calcutta.

Dutta, P. C., 1983b, An odontometric study of molar crown characters of the Bronze Age Harappans, *Anth. Anz.* **41**:67–72.

Dutta, P. C., 1983c, A study of the molar teeth of the Bronze Age Harappans in the context of evolutionary biology, *Anthropologie, Brno.* **21**(2).

Dutta, P. C., Pal, A., and Biswas, J. N., 1972, Late stone age human remains from Sarai Nahar Rai: The earliest skeletal evidence of man in India, *Bull. Anthropol. Surv. India* **21**:114–138.

Ghosh, A. K., and Sen, A. K., 1981, Fresh light on phylo-taxonomy of Siwalik hominoids, in: *Proc. Field Conf. Neogene–Quaternary Boundary, India* (M. V. A. Sástry, T. K. Kurien, A. K. Dutta, and S. Biswas, eds.), Geological Survey of India, Calcutta, pp. 55–62.

Gupta, P., Dutta, P. C., and Basu, A., 1962, *Human Remains from Harappa,* Anthropol. Surv. of India, Calcutta.

Gupta, H. P., 1976, Holocene palynology from Meander Lake in the Ganga Valley, District Pratapgarh, U. P., *Palaeobotanist* **25**:109–119.

Hiernaux, J., 1965, Une nouvelle mesure de distance anthropologique entre populations, utilisant simultanément des frequences géniques, des pourcentage de traits descriptifs et des moyennes metriques, *C. r. hebd. Séanc. Acad. Sci., Paris* **260**:1748–1750.

Huizinga, J., 1962, From *DD* to D^2 and back, the quantitative expression of resemblance, *Proc. Kon. ned. Akad. Wet.,* Series C **65**:1–12.

Kennedy, K. A. R., 1975, Biological adaptations of prehistoric South Asian populations to different and changing ecological settings, in: *Biosocial Interrelations in Population Adaptation,* (E. S. Watts, F. E. Johnston, and G. W. Lasker, eds.), Mouton Publishers, The Hague, pp. 65–90.

Khan, F. A., 1965, Excavations at Kot Diji, *Pakistan Archaeol.* **2**:13–85.

Mahalanobis, P. C., 1936, On the generalized distance in statistics, *Proc. Nat. Inst. Sci. India* **2**:49–55.

Marshall, Sir John, 1931, *Mohenjo-daro and the Indus Civilization,* 2 volumes Arthur Probasthan, London.

Martin, R., and Saller, K., 1956, *Lehrbuch der Anthropologie,* 3 Lief, Gustav Fischer, Jena.

Mughal, M. R., 1979, The present state of research on the Indus Valley civilization, in: *Ancient Cities of the Indus* (G. L. Passehl, ed.), Vikas Publishing, New Delhi, pp. 90–98.

Pearson, K., 1926, On the coefficient of racial likeness, *Biometrika* **18**:105–117.

Penrose, L. S., 1954, Distance, size and shape, *Ann. Eugen., Lond.* **18**:337–343.

Pilbeam, D. R., Meyer, G. E., Rose, M. D., Pickford, M. H. L., Behrensmeyer, A. K., and Shah, S. M. J., 1977, New hominoid primates from the Siwaliks of Pakistan and their bearing on hominoid evolution, *Nature* **270**:689–695.

Ralph, E. K., Michael, H. N., and Han, M. A., 1973, Radiocarbon and reality, *MASCA Newsletter* **9**(1):1–20.

Rao, C. R., 1952, *Advanced Statistical Methods in Biometric Research,* John Wiley, New York.

Talbot, P. A., and Mulhall, H., 1962, *The Physical Anthropology of Southern Nigeria: A Biometrical Study in Statistical Method,* Cambridge University Press, bridge.

Vats, M. S., 1940, *Excavations at Harappa,* 2 volumes, Govt. India Press, Delhi.

Wheeler, R. E. M., 1947, Harappa 1946: The defences and cemetery R 37, *Anc. India* **3**:58–130.

CHAPTER 4

The Indo-Aryan Invasions: Cultural Myth and Archaeological Reality

JIM G. SHAFFER

1. Introduction

The concept of an Indo-European or Indo-Aryan group of peoples has played a prominent role in interpretative studies of Old World history and archaeology. For almost 200 years, scholars and quasi scholars have attributed the linguistic, cultural, and racial affiliations of very disparate groups to a common Indo-Aryan heritage. In such widely seperated areas as Europe and India, many significant cultural changes recorded for the first and second millennia B.C. are attributed to an influx, or invasion, of Indo-Aryan peoples who shared a common cultural base and who were responsible for important socioeconomic and linguistic changes in the areas they invaded. In the framework of European prehistory, the analytical importance of these Indo-European or Indo-Aryan intrusions has been replaced somewhat by the current emphasis on ecological reconstruction and indigenous cultural development, although invasion or migration explanations are still found (e.g., Gimbutas, 1973).

However, in South Asian studies the concept of an Indo-Aryan invasion continues to be the main explanation for the cultural history of that region. The importance of these invasions is linked to the persistent opinion that the Indo-Aryan invaders were the authors of early Vedic (Sanskrit) literature, which is viewed as the foundation for all subsequent "Indian civilization." To understand better the importance that the Indo-Aryan invasion concept has within the context

JIM G. SHAFFER • Department of Anthropology, Case Western Reserve University, Cleveland, Ohio 44106.

of South Asian studies, some attention must be given the concept's historical development and interpretive use in Europe and India.

2. Indo-Aryan Invasions: The Concept

According to Poliakov (1974), the concept of an Indo-Aryan invading group can be traced to the 18th century, and is associated with attempts by Western scholars to free themselves from the confines of Judeo-Christian thought, while at the same time maintaining biblical revelations. These early interpretations paid special attention to the concept of "the Flood" and the importance of mountains in the early origin myths of the ancient world (e.g., Noah's ark was grounded on the heights of Mount Ararat). Many scholars, such as Buffon, found suggestions within the Bible itself that the origins of mankind and the "arts of civilization" were to be found in a human group located east of the Caspian Sea and that this knowledge was preserved by the Brahmans of India. The location of seashells in all latitudes was interpreted by Enlightenment scholars as confirming the existence of the Flood and also suggesting that it was in mountainous areas that people and the arts of civilization had survived the Flood. Since the highest mountains were found in India and China, it was thought that, in those regions, civilization had developed and was preserved.

> Now it was know that the highest mountains in the world towered over India and China. But the fact remains that tradition, perhaps influenced by the reluctance of the Whites to admit affiliation to the Yellow races, focused attention on the near side of the Himalayas and of Kashmir, not beyond them. (Poliakov, 1974, p. 184)

Concomitant with the development of these ideas was the fact that during the 18th century, European scholars were becoming increasingly aware of the complexities of Indian culture, due to their countries' colonial expansions in Asia. Many scholars, such as Kant and Herder, began to draw analogies between the myths and philosophies of ancient India and the West. In their attempt to separate Western European culture from its Judaic heritage, many scholars were convinced that the origin of Western culture was to be found in India rather than in the ancient Near East. Even Voltaire was "convinced that everything has come down to us from the banks of the Ganges, astronomy, astrology, metempsychosis, etc." (Voltaire, quoted in Poliakov, 1974, p. 185). These 18th-century developments are summarized by Poliakov:

> Thus we see that a wide variety of authors and schools located the birthplace of the entire human race between the Indus and the Ganges. It only remained for linguistics to make its contribution, in a decisive though ambiguous manner, by dispelling with one certain truth a fog of adventurous suppositions, and at the same time advancing a new hypothesis as fragile as any of those which preceded it. According to this new theory it was not the whole human race but one particular race—a white race which

> subsequently became Christian—which had descended from the mountains of Asia to colonize and populate the West. It seemed as if the Europeans of the scientific age, having freed themselves from the conventional Noachian genealogy and rejected Adam as a common father, were looking around for new ancestors but were unable to break with the tradition which placed their origin in the fabulous Orient. It was the science of linguistics which was to give a name to these ancestors by opposing the Aryans to the Hamites, the Mongols—and the Jews. (Poliakov, 1974, p. 188).

The developing discipline of linguistics provided a comprehensive and acceptable structure for these 18th-century ideas, which in turn helped legitimize historical linguistics as a field of "scientific" study.

Sir William Jones, a justice of the High Court of Bengal, is usually accepted as the first to recognize the affinities of Sanskrit with Greek and Latin.

> The Sanscrit language, whatever may be its antiquity, is of a wounderful structure; more perfect than the Greek; more copious than the Latin, and more exquisitely refined than either yet bearing to both of them a stronger affinity, both in the roots of verbs and in the forms of grammar, than could possibly have been produced by accident; so strong, indeed, that no philosopher could examine them all three without believing them to have sprung from some common source which, perhaps, no longer exists; there is a similar reason, though not quite so forcible, for supposing that both the Gothick and the Celtick, though blended with a very different idiom, had the same origin with the Sanscrit. (Jones, 1788, quoted in Poliakov, 1974, p. 190)

Jones's analysis established at once both the concept of a family of Indo-European languages and provided the historical, and presumed scientific, link between Indian and European cultures that scholars were seeking. Although Jones's analysis was quickly accepted among Orientalists, it was Friedrick Schlegel who developed the Indo-Aryan concept in its final form. Schlegel provided an anthropological twist to the concept by correlating a relationship of language with that of biological race. Despite the early misgivings of some scholars about such a correlation between language and race (Tylor [1881], also 1960, p. 55) and the circular nature of many of the arguments (Reinach, 1893), the concept of a common linguistic, cultural, biological, and historical heritage linking European and Indian peoples became internationally accepted as more fact than theory. Based on linguistic reconstructions, the prehistoric to historic chronologies of Europe and India were interpreted as reflecting various invasions of Indo-European or Indo-Aryan peoples who possessed a common cultural heritage, albeit remote. For Europe, this concept ultimately resulted in the disaster of the Third Reich, whereas in South Asia, the concept of Indo-Aryan peoples played a quite different cultural role.

The 19th century saw the development of modern historical studies concerned with India (R. Thapar, 1978, pp. 1–25). Initially, many of the historical syntheses were written by Europeans—Christen Larssen and Vincent Smith—who imposed a Western framework on the data. Indian history was presented as a series of three major periods—Hindu, Muslim, and Christian (British). At the same time, Indian scholars such as R. G. Bhandarkar also began to write on ancient Indian history. These early Indian scholars adopted the prevailing perspectives of European Orientalists, concentrating on political histories and analyses of Vedic literature. The focus on the early Vedic literature was very appropriate because it constituted the earliest written records for this area. Two important developments emerged from this period of Indian historiography. First, the development of the concept of a common cultural heritage linking Europe with ancient India via the Indo-Aryan peoples gave studies of ancient India a unique position in the general study of ancient non-European history. No other Asian or African cultural group undergoing colonization could define a common cultural heritage, no matter how remote, with Europe. Therefore, the Indo-Aryan concept became an important aspect of cultural identity within the framework of Indian history. Secondly, the fact that the last two major periods of Indian history—Muslim and Christian—were the result of invasions from the west made plausible the acceptance of an earlier Indo-Aryan invasion into India, with its introduction of Hindu culture. Such an invasion theory, used as a means to explain Indian cultural origins, was enhanced by the fact that a similar invasion theory was used to define cultural development in the West. Together, the two developments gave a degree of historical reality not usually associated with such origin myths to early Vedic literature.

Indian historians in the first half of the 20th century were greatly influenced by the subcontinent's national movement. Such writers tended to glorify ancient Indian society, stressing that it was equal in cultural achievement to the ancient societies of Europe. Such an argument seemed very rational because the peoples of India and Europe shared a common cultural, linguistic, and biological heritage, that is, Indo-European or Indo-Aryan. Ancient Indian society was viewed by these historians as "a comparatively unchanging society over the period from 1000 B.C. to A.D. 1000 with a uniformly high quality of achievement; the basis of this stability was the ancient Aryan culture" (R. Thapar, 1978, p. 12).

At the same time, there was an attempt to push the antiquity of the Vedic literature as far back in time as possible, thereby emphasizing the distinctiveness of Indian achievements as well as their equality with those defined for the West. There was also an attempt to stress the cultural and political unity of Indian peoples from earliest times, at the expense of regional diversity.

> Thus the rise of the Mauryan empire in the third century B.C. and its extension over almost the entire sub-continent was seen as an expression of an all-India consciousness. (R. Thapar, 1978, p. 12).

By the time of national independence, the concept of Indo-Aryans and the historical validity of the Vedic literature had become an important aspect of the cultural and political identities of the subcontinent.

This brief historical discussion indicates that the Indo-European or Indo-Aryan concept was intimately connected with other social, cultural, and political movements from the 18th to the 20th centuries. In Europe, it was tied to the attempt to distinguish a Christian heritage from that of the Jews. Once formulated, it underwent social and political changes climaxing in what was Nazi Germany. In India, the concept provided a distinct cultural identity and still linked Indian culture to European culture. At the same time in India during the 20th century, the validity of an Indo-Aryan affiliation was tied to cultural and political movements leading to national independence. In both instances, the Indo-Aryan concept was never subjected to rigorous validation beyond the field of historical linguistics. Linguistic reconstructions were used to interpret archaeological materials, which in turn were used to substantiate the original cultural reconstructions. It was not until the mid-20th century that archaeological data were independently used to examine the validity of the Indo-Aryan concept. It is these data, within a South Asian context, that will be the focus of discussion.

3. The Archaeological Data

Excavations conducted in the 1930s at Mohenjo-Daro and Harappa initiated a comprehensive attempt to reconstruct South Asia's pre- and protohistoric past. These excavations clearly established the presence of a literate urban civilization dating from the Bronze Age that was comparable to those in Mesopotamia. The potential antiquity of these sites, together with the presumed antiquity of the Vedic literature, almost immediately prompted speculation about the possible Aryan authorship of this impressive Harappan cultural complex. Moreover, the failure of the early excavations to define an ancestral pre-Harappan period of cultural development indicated to many scholars that the Harappan culture represented yet another Western intrusion into South Asia, further strengthening the idea that it was the product of Indo-Aryan invasions. Based on an analysis of the material culture of the Harappans, Sir John Marshall, the original excavator, argued that the Mature phase of the Harappan culture was pre-Aryan in date and cultural affiliation—a view that was supported by later scholars (Piggott, 1950). However, the idea of an Aryan origin for the Harappan culture has continued to persist. Some, like Sastri (1965), argue for an Aryan origin on the basis of similarities in the material culture found at these sites and material described in the Vedic literature. Others argue that parts of the Vedic literature, such as the *Mahabharata,* have a much greater antiquity, dating to 3100 B.C. (see Gupta and Ramachandran, 1976, for discussion), which would make the literature contemporary with and possibly part of the Harappan culture. On the other hand, some scholars (e.g., Agrawal and Kusumgar, 1974) advocate a "short chronology" for the Harappan culture based on material-culture correlations with Mesopotamia. This chronology places the date for the Mature Harappan culture between 2300 and 2000 B.C. Acceptance of this chronology by some scholars has perpetuated the hypothesis of an Indo-Aryan origin for the Harappan culture.

> If, as we have seen, the Harappan civilization with its remarkable cultural unity, came into existence only around 2150 B.C., it is necessary to admit that not only the end of the cities, but even their initial impetus may have been due to Indo-European speaking peoples. (Allchin and Allchin, 1968, p. 144).

The archaeological data gathered throughout the last two decades, however, consistantly indicate that the Harappan culture is *non-Aryan*. The more important aspects of these recent data are the following.

1. The discovery of extensive nonceramic occupations associated with early domesticates at Mehrgarh, dated to pre-6000 B.C. (Jarrige and Meadow, 1980). This site clearly establishes the antiquity of humans in the Greater Indus Valley and, therefore, provides the chronological depth, making plausible the hypothesis that the domestication of plants and animals and the rise of civilization in the Indus Valley was an indigenous cultural process.
2. There is a growing awareness among scholars (Mughal, 1973) that such so-called "pre-Harappan" sites as Kot Diji, Amri, Sothi, and Gumla may actual constitute an early developmental phase of the Harappan culture. (See Dutta, this volume).
3. Recalibrated C-14 dates indicate that the Harappan culture existed between 2500 and 1700 B.C. (Dales, 1973), or well before the post-1500 B.C. date accepted by most scholars for the Indo-Aryan invasions.
4. The widespread reference to iron tools in the Vedic literature and their apparent absence in the Harappan culture (for the possibility of an "iron awareness" in Harappan culture see Shaffer, 1983).
5. The absence of archaeological evidence for hereditary social elites in the Harappan culture versus the prominent role such elites played in the early Vedic literature (Shaffer, 1982a).
6. The increasing evidence suggesting that the Painted Grey Ware (hereafter PGW) culture was the predominant culture in the Ganga-Yamuna region during the post-1500 B.C. period, the generally accepted data for the Indo-Aryan incursions (Tripathi, 1976).

If there is some reluctance in attributing Aryan responsibility for the Harappan culture, there is little hesitation in defining Indo-Aryan invasion(s) as the main cause for the culture's disappearance. Several factors add to the ready acceptance of this interpretation, the most important being the location of several skeletons found in the streets and buildings of a late occupation at Mohenjo-Daro. The context of these skeletons suggests that they were massacred, and earlier scholars quickly assumed that the Aryans were responsible for the massacre (Childe, 1934; Wheeler, 1947). Another reason for accepting this interpretation was the earlier correlation of Harappa with Hariyupiya—the location of a battle in the Vedic literature (no evidence suggesting a massacre was uncovered in the excavations at this site). A critical reexamination of the evidence, however, does not support such an interpretation:

> The contemporaneity of the skeletal remains is anything but certain. Whereas a couple of them definitely seem to represent a slaughter, *in situ,* the bulk of the bones were found in contexts suggesting burials of the sloppiest and most irreverent nature. There is no destruction level covering the latest period of the city, no sign of extensive burning, no bodies of warriors clad in armor and surrounded by the weapons of war. The citadel, the only fortified part of the city, yeilded no evidence of a final defense. (Dales, 1964, p. 43).

Despite the absence of archaeological evidence for an Aryan massacre of the people at Mohenjo-Daro and the accumulating evidence of alternative explanations for the abandonment of the site itself (Dales, 1966), this interpretation of an Aryan invasion is still found in literature on South Asian protohistory (Wheeler, 1968, pp. 129–133).

Attempts have also been made to correlate the various post-Mature Harappan cultures in the Greater Indus Valley (Jhukar, Cemetery H., Ochre Colored Pottery, Black-and-Red Ware, copper hoards, etc.) and Chalcolithic Deccan cultures with the Aryans. Initially, their post-Mature Harappan stratigraphic position and their seemingly different cultural traits reinforced such interpretations. Indeed, some very specific correlations with various aspects of the Vedic literature (Sankalia, 1964; R. Thapar, 1975) have been made, based on the material culture traits and geographic distribution of these cultures. Ultimately, these interpretations depend on the validity of the Iranian affinities of these groups. That is, if they represent Indo-Aryans, they would have had to pass through Iran to arrive in India. Although Sankalia (1973, 1974, pp. 550–559) no longer designates these groups as Aryans, his continued emphasis on their Iranian origins implies a continued Aryan identity. However, these Iranian affinities are not convincing and have been severely criticized.

> First, this hypothesis of a population movement from Iran and elsewhere to Peninsular India does not conform to the geographic framework suggested earlier in the present paper on the basis of documented political and economic records. . . . Second, almost all the suggested analogies are too general to be of any use in a valid and meaningful archaeological comparison. . . . Third, some of the analogies cited are positively misleading. . . . Fourth, the suggested West Asiatic analogies do not belong to any single cultural assemblage or even different assemblages of any specific period. . . . Finally, it should be pointed out that not a single demonstrably West Asiatic type fossil occurs in the cited Indian assemblages. . . . Moreover, the basic character of these Indian assemblages is very different from that of their supposedly parent [in Sankalia's hypothesis they are parent sites] West Asiatic sites, a difference which

> should be obvious to anybody who studies these assemblages without primarily looking for similarities. (Chakrabarti, 1977, pp. 33–34).

In light of these criticisms it is difficult to attach any validity to an Aryan, or even West Asiatic, origin for these post-Mature Harappan cultural developments.

Currently, the archaeological culture for which the most convincing argument may be made for an Indo-Aryan parentage is that of the PGW. Extensive researches of B. B. Lal (1954–1955) and others (see Tripathi, 1976, for discussion) have yielded an archaeological reconstruction of this culture that corresponds well with accepted beliefs about Indo-Aryan culture. The major characteristics of PGW that suggest its Indo-Aryan origin are the following.

1. Stratigraphically and chronologically, PGW culture corresponds to the generally accepted date of the Indo-Aryan invasions (middle of the second millennium B.C.). There seems to be a stratigraphic gap between occupations of the last protohistoric cultures (post-Mature Harappan) and the PGW. Carbon-14 dates place the absolute date of PGW at between 1100 and 300 B.C.
2. The geographic distribution of PGW sites appears confined to the Ganga-Yamuna region—the same region emphasized in the early Vedic literature.
3. PGW was the initial occupation at several sites that were thought to be associated historically with the literature—such as Hastinapur in the *Mahabharata*.
4. PGW stratigraphically overlapped with the historically known culture of the Northern Black Polished Ware.
5. PGW is the earliest culture associated with a variety of iron artifacts—and widespread use of iron is indicated in the Vedic literature.
6. The domestic horse, an important animal in the Vedic literature, is found at PGW sites.
7. The absence of mud-brick architecture and the distinctive painted and plain gray pottery associated with PGW seem to represent a sharp break with previous protohistoric cultures. Moreover, many similarities exist between the gray ware vessel forms and those of later historic periods, much more so than exist between PGW vessel forms and those of earlier protohistoric cultures. These archaeological considerations have led many scholars to make a definitive association of PGW with at least a later Aryan invasion.

> Whether the Aryans should be regarded as the authors of the Painted Grey Ware or not has been a matter of dispute. While most Indian scholars have held that they were, others have doubted it. It is not necessary to reconsider the matter here in detail, and it would suffice to emphasize that the geographical horizon of the later Aryans is coterminous with that of the Ware; there is also a remarkable chronological proximity between the dates of the beginning of the Ware and the later Vedic

> age, which no critical scholar would place before the start of the first millennium B.C. There can, therefore, be no reasonable doubt in ascribing the Ware to the later Aryans. (Ghosh, 1973, pp. 5–6).

Although scholars generally have accepted the correlation of PGW with Indo-Aryans in northern India, a few have been critical of this hypothesis. If PGW represents the Indo-Aryans, then, according to accepted theories, similar or antecedent types of pottery should be located west of the Ganga-Yamuna region on the Iranian Plateau. B. K. Thapar (1970) has noted the absence of any PGW antecedent types of pottery anywhere along the route supposedly taken by the Aryans, and he has outlined the chronological problems associated with existing accounts. Chakrabarti, on the other hand, has proposed an eastern, rather than western, origin for the PGW, thereby negating the PGW–Aryan correlation.

> The Painted Grey Ware culture, thus, with its traits of rice cultivation and the use of domestic pig and buffalo seems to suggest a culture distinctly eastern in bias and not a western one as its suggested Aryan authorship would indicate. (Chakrabarti, 1968, p. 353)

Recent archaeological research in Eastern Punjab (Shaffer, 1981) substantiates objections to the PGW = Aryan correlation.

J. P. Joshi's excavations (1976, 1977, 1978a, 1978b; Joshi and Madhu, 1982) at Bhagwanpura, Dadheri, Nagar, and Katpalon have significantly altered the perspective of the archaeological sequence in the Punjab, particularly that regarding the PGW culture. At these sites, Joshi found PGW pottery and structures associated in the same stratigraphic unit with material belonging to the indigenous protohistoric culture of this region—Siswal. Moreover, Joshi was able, for the first time, to associate substantial mud-brick architecture units with PGW, and to define overlapping ceramic attributes between the Siswal and PGW cultures. At the same time, Chakrabarti (1974, 1977) and I (Shaffer, 1983) argue for an indigenous development of iron technology within the Indian subcontinent. At present, the archaeological record indicates no cultural discontinuities separating PGW from the indigenous protohistoric culture. That is, PGW culture represents an indigenous cultural development and does not reflect any cultural intrusion from the West, that is, an Indo-Aryan invasion. Therefore, there is no archaeological evidence corroborating the fact of an Indo-Aryan invasion.

Two conclusions may be drawn from the archaeological data. First, there is no connection between PGW culture and that of the Aryans. Second, if the "Aryan" concept is to have any cultural meaning, then such a culture (PGW) had an *indigenous* South Asian origin within the protohistoric cultures of the Ganga-Yamuna region. There was no invasion from the West. The current archaeological evidence suggests that the original reconstruction indicating the occurrence of an Indo-Aryan invasion mistakenly associated linguistic change with the migration of peoples. Linguistic changes and affiliations are brought about by a complex series of cultural processes, many of which do not involve the physical movements of social groups (Barth, 1972). Yet, the Vedic literature does exist, and few would deny that it totally lacks historical and cultural significance. If these myths do not reflect a factual human invasion, what do they reflect?

4. Indo-Aryan Invasions: A Reconsideration

Anthropologists and others have long recognized that myths, in part, reflect a coding of social information and an attempt to explain relationships between phenomena that are both cultural and natural. As Middleton (1967, p. x) has noted: "Myths are ways of explaining paradoxes, the paradoxes of social order within extra-social chaos, of the relationship of authority to power and the like." If this interpretation is applied to the early Vedic literature, correlating it with the emerging South Asian archaeological data, a different explanation of these myths is possible.

Recent reevaluations (Fentress, 1976; Shaffer, 1982a) of the protohistoric cultural developments in South Asia, especially that of the Harappan culture, highlight many unproved assumptions about this culture, while indicating its uniqueness when contrasted to contemporary cultures in the West. Of particular note is that despite the technological sophistication associated with the Harappan urban, literature culture, it appears to lack precisely those cultural patterns usually associated with the development of well-defined hereditary sociopolitical elites (palaces, temples, high-status burials, etc.), which were crucial to development of comparable cultures in Mesopotamia. In other words,

> In the Indus Valley, a technically advanced, urban, literate culture was achieved without the usually associated social organization based on hereditary elites, centralized political government (states, empires) and warfare. (Shaffer, 1982a, p. 47).

If this interpretation can be substantiated, it presents a striking contrast to the culture depicted in the Vedic literature that is described as having hereditary elites and centralized political, religious, and economic organizations. The Vedic literature reflects then, not a foreign human invasion, but a radical alteration in the social, political, and economic organizations of the indigenous culture. That a dominant social group is depicted as a conquering invader in this social reorganization may reflect a cultural rationalization, or justification, for the ascendancy of one social group over others.

However, if the Vedic literature reflects an indigenous cultural phenomenon, how can the linguistic similarities between Sanskrit and Western languages be accounted for; they have long been isolated as proof of an Indo-

Aryan invasion. There are at present two possible interpretations that can account for these similarities. First, these linguistic relationships are seen as having much greater antiquity than the mid-second millennium B.C. To some extent, such relationships may reflect the existence of a Zagrosian family of language linking Elamite and Dravidian on the Iranian Plateau, as proposed by McAlpin (1974, 1975). The existence of a Zagrosian family would provide a basic linguistic similarity linking northern South Asia with the Iranian Plateau in the remote prehistoric past. Such linguistic similarities may have diffused west from the plateau as a result of the extensive trading networks linking cultures in the plateau with those in Mesopotamia and beyond. Kohl's (1978) analysis of "international" trade during the third millennium B.C. indicates that not only by that time were there extensive trading networks linking the plateau with Mesopotamia, but also that such trade was crucial in the development of sociopolitical elites and early states in those regions. Likewise, Tosi (1974) defines the existence of a contemporary turquoise trade, linking groups on the plateau with the Kelteminar culture of central Asia. It is doubtful that such an extensive and important trading system could have existed for apparently millennia without some degree of linguistic diffusion among the affected regions. However, at present, it does not appear that the Harappan culture was involved to any great extent with this "international" trade of the third millennium B.C. (Shaffer, 1982b). Indeed, Harappan economic organization had developed an intensive, internal trading network within the Greater Indus Valley that supplied most commodities, though limited contact with western areas may be documented. Therefore, membership in a basic linguistic family—Zagrosian—may account for some of the linguistic similarities of later periods. Furthermore, it may be proposed that this different economic organization of the Harappans fostered development of a sociopolitical organization that did not emphasize hereditary social elites. Along with developing linguistic differences, this combined to reinforce a distinctive ethnic identity among the Harappans vis-à-vis western groups who had different sociopolitical organizations. The appearance of hereditary social and political elites and the associated restructuring of social and economic organization during the mid-second millennium B.C., similar to that found among western groups, may have reemphasized those linguistic traits linking hereditary social elites in both regions.

A second possible interpretation is that such linguistic similarities are a result of post-second millennium B.C. contacts with the West. The Vedic literature represents an oral tradition that was codified during several different periods (Gupta and Ramachandran, 1976). The language used to record these myths in writing reflects the language used at the time of documentation that, given the extensive interaction with the West in later periods, may or may not accurately reflect linguistic traditions of the more remote past. Therefore, these linguistic similarities may reflect later, not original cultural interactions. Once codified, it was advantageous for the emerging hereditary social elites to stabilize such linguistic traits with the validity of the explanations offered in the literature enhancing their social positions.

5. Conclusions

It is argued that current archaeological data do not support the existence of an Indo-Aryan or European invasion into South Asia at any time in the pre- or protohistoric periods. Instead, it is possible to document archaeologically a series of cultural changes reflecting indigenous cultural development from prehistoric to historic periods. The early Vedic literature describes not a human invasion into the area, but a fundamental restructuring of indigenous society that saw the rise of hereditary social elites. It has also been suggested that the linguistic similarities that are cited as proof of these human invasions have alternative explanations.

The Indo-Aryan invasion(s) as an academic concept in 18th- and 19th-century Europe reflected the cultural milieu of that period. Linguistic data were used to validate the concept that in turn was used to interpret archaeological and anthropological data. What was theory became unquestioned fact that was used to interpret and organize all subsequent data. It is time to end the ''linguistic tyranny'' that has prescribed interpretative frameworks of pre- and protohistoric cultural development in South Asia. Linguistic reconstructions have a reputation of scientific validity based on the study of existing languages (written and non-written). However, linguistic reconstructions based upon supposed rates of linguistic change are the archaeological equivalents of estimating absolute chronology from the depth of deposits. There are simply too many intervening cultural and historical variables to permit any great degree of cross-cultural accuracy. In archaeology, such methods were replaced when better aids to cultural identification, such as radiocarbon dating, became available. Linguistic reconstructions for the area are no longer independently supported by the archaeological data, and even if one is reluctant to disregard these reconstructions completely, the present data nonetheless suggest critical reevaluation of earlier interpretations.

References

Agrawal, D. P., and Kusumgar, S. 1974, *Prehistoric Chronology and Radiocarbon Dating in India,* Munshiram Manoharlal, New Delhi.

Allchin, B., and Allchin, R., 1968, *The Birth of Indian Civilization,* Penguin Books, Baltimore.

Barth, F., 1972, Ethnic processes on the Pathan-Baluch boundary, in: *Directions in Sociolinguistics* (J. J. Gumperz and D. Hymes, eds.), Holt, Rinehart & Winston, New York, pp. 454–464.

Chakrabarti, D. K., 1968, The Aryan hypothesis in Indian archaeology, in: *Indian Studies Past and Present* **4**:333–358.
Chakrabarti, D. K., 1974, Beginning of iron in India: Problem reconsidered, in: *Perspectives in Palaeoanthropology,* (A. K. Ghosh, ed.), Firma K. L. Mukhopadhyay, Calcutta, pp. 345–356.
Chakrabarti, D. K., 1977, India and West Asia—An alternative approach, *Man and Environment* **1**:25–38.
Childe, V. G., 1934, *New Light on the Most Ancient East,* Routledge and Kegan Paul, London.
Dales, G. F., 1964, The mythical massacre at Mohenjo-Daro, *Expedition* **6**:36–43.
Dales, G. F., 1966, The decline of the Harappans, *Sci. Am.* **241**:92–100.
Dales, G. F., 1973, Archaeological and radiocarbon chronologies for protohistoric South Asia, in: *South Asian Archaeology* (N. Hammond, ed.), Duckworth, London, pp. 157–170.
Fentress, M. A., 1976, Resource Access, Exchange Systems, and Regional Interaction in the Indus Valley: An Investigation of Archaeological Variability at Harappa and Mohenjodaro, Ph.D. Thesis, Department of Anthropology, University of Pennsylvania, Philadelphia.
Ghosh, A., 1973, *The City in Early Historical India,* Indian Institute of Advanced Study, Simla.
Gimbutas, M., 1973, The beginning of the Bronze Age in Europe and the Indo-Europeans: 3500–2500 B.C., *The J. Indo-European Stud.* **3**:163–214.
Gupta, S. P., and Ramachandran, K. S. (eds.), 1976, *Mahabharata: Myth and Reality—Differing Views,* Agam Prakashan, Delhi.
Jarrige, J. F., and Meadow, R. H., 1980, The antecedents of civilization in the Indus Valley, *Sci. Am.* **243**:122–133.
Joshi, J. P., 1976, Excavations at Bhagwanpura, in: *Mahabharata: Myth and Reality—Differing Views* (S. P. Gupta and K. S. Ramachandran, eds.), Agam Prakashan, Delhi, pp. 239–240.
Joshi, J. P., 1977, Overlap of Late Harappan Culture and Painted Grey Ware Culture in Light of Recent Excavations in Haryana, Punjab, and Jammu, Paper presented at a seminar, Indus Civilization: Problems and Issues, Indian Institute of Advanced Study, Simla.
Joshi, J. P., 1978a, Interlocking of late Harappan culture and Painted Grey Ware culture in light of recent excavations, *Man and Environment* **2**:98–100.
Joshi, J. P., 1978b, A note on the excavations at Bhagwanpura, *Puratattva* **8**:178–180.
Joshi, J. P., and Madhu, B. 1982, Manda: A Harappan site in Jammu and Kashmir, in: *Harappan Civilization: A Contemporary Perspective* (G. L. Possehl, ed.), American Institute of Indian Studies, Oxford, and I. B. H. Publishers, New Delhi, pp. 185–195.
Kohl, P. L., 1978, The balance of trade in southwestern Asia in the mid-third millennium B.C., *Curr. Anthropol.* **19**:463–492.
Lal, B. B., 1954–55, Excavations at Hastinapur and other explorations in the upper Ganga and Sutlej basins, 1950–52 in *Anc. India* **10–11**:5–152.
McAlpin, D., 1974, Towards proto-Elamo-Dravidian, *Language* **50**:89–101.
McAlpin, D., 1975, Elamite and Dravidian: Further evidence of relationship, *Curr. Anthropol.* **16**:93–104.
Middleton, J., 1967, Introduction, in: *Myth and Cosmos* (J. Middleton, ed.), Natural History Press, Garden City, Long Island, pp. ix–xi.
Mughal, M. R., 1973, *Present State of Research on the Indus Valley Civilization,* Department of Archaeology and Museums, Ministry of Education and Culture, Government of Pakistan, Karachi.
Piggott, S., 1950, *Prehistoric India,* Penguin Books, Middlesex.
Poliakov, L., 1974, *The Aryan Myth,* Basic Books, New York.
Reinach, J., 1893, Le mirage oriental, *L'Anthropologie* **4**:540–555.
Sankalia, H. D., 1964, Traditional Indian chronology and C-14 dates of excavated sites, *J. Indian Hist.* **13**:635–650.
Sankalia, H. D., 1973, Prehistoric colonization in India, *World Archaeol.* **5**:86–91.

Sankalia, H. D., 1974, *Prehistory and Protohistory of India and Pakistan,* Deccan College Postgraduate and Research Institute, Pune.

Sastri, K. N., 1965, *New Light on the Indus Civilization,* Vol. II, Atma Ram & Sons, Delhi.

Shaffer, J. G., 1981, The protohistoric period in the eastern Punjab: A preliminary assessment, in: *Indus Civilization—New Perspectives* (A. H. Dani, ed.), Centre for the Study of the Civilization of Central Asia, Quaid-i-Azam University, Islamabad, pp. 65–102.

Shaffer, J. G., 1982a, Harappan culture: A reconsideration, in: *Harappan Civilization: A Contemporary Perspective* (G. L. Possehl, ed.), American Institute of Indian Studies, Oxford and I. B. H. Publishers, New Delhi, pp. 41–50.

Shaffer, J. G., 1982b, Harappan commerce: An alternative perspective, in: *Anthropology in Pakistan: Recent Socio-Cultural and Archaeological Perspectives* (S. Pastner and L. Flam, eds.), South Asia Occasional Papers and Theses No. 8, South Asia Program, Cornell University, Ithaca, pp. 166–210.

Shaffer, J. G., 1983, Bronze Age iron from Afghanistan: Its implications for South Asian protohistory, in: *Studies in the Archaeology and Paleoanthropology of South Asia,* (K. A. R. Kennedy and G. L. Possehl, eds.), Oxford and I. B. H. Publishers, New Delhi, pp. 65–102.

Thapar, B. K., 1970, The Aryans: A reappraisal of the problem, in: *India's Contribution to World Thought and Culture* (L. Chandra, S. P. Gupta, D. Swarup, and S. Goel, eds.), Vivikananda Rock Memorial Committee, Madras, pp. 147–164.

Thapar, R., 1975, Puranic lineages and archaeological cultures in *Puratattva* **8**:86–98.

Thapar, R., 1978, *Ancient Indian Social History,* Orient Longman, Delhi.

Tosi, M., 1974, The problem of turquoise in protohistoric trade on the Iranian Plateau, *Studi di Palentologia, Paleoantropologia, Paleonologia e Geologia del Quaternario* **2**:147–162.

Tripathi, V., 1976, *The Painted Grey Ware: An Iron Age Culture of Northern India,* Concept Publishing Co., Delhi.

Tylor, E. B., 1960, *Anthropology,* 2nd ed., University of Michigan Press, Ann Arbor (first published in 1881).

Wheeler, M., 1947, Harappa 1946: The defences and cemetery R37, *Anc. India* **3**:58–130.

Wheeler, M., 1968, *The Indus Civilization,* Cambridge University Press, Cambridge.

CHAPTER 5

Excavations at the Early Farming Village of Inamgaon 1968–1982

H. D. SANKALIA, Z. D. ANSARI, AND M. K. DHAVALIKAR

1. Introduction

Though archaeological excavations in India are over 120 years old, no complete plan of a town or village has been exposed. Hence, it was impossible to determine the antiquity of village planning practices despite the fact that India is still largely a country of villages.

This lacuna was recently filled for the area of western Maharashtra near Pune by the excavations that Deccan College conducted at Inamgaon. Since 1968, support from the University Grants Commission, through the University of Pune, has permitted annual excavations at Inamgaon. The excavations were deliberately planned and carefully executed because the conditions at this site were ideal. There were no deposits of the historic period, as is shown by several C-14 dates of the charred remains from the latest phases of occupation (*ca.* 1000–700 B.C.).

From the beginning, data recovery at Inamgaon was contextual, so that detailed information regarding the life of the inhabitants could be gathered. We wished to determine the size of the family, food habits, craft specializations, religious practices, and methods for disposal of the dead. These objectives have been largely fulfilled because an expert interdisciplinary team of excavators and laboratory specialists have been involved in the work at Inamgaon. The 11 years

---

H. D. SANKALIA, Z. D. ANSARI, AND M. K. DHAVALIKAR • Department of Archaeology, Deccan College, Pune 411 006 India. Generous financial support from the University Grants Commission made the excavations at Inamgaon possible.

of excavation and analysis have not only given a fairly good idea of village life 3500 years ago, but they have shown how village life changed in response to new cultural forces and climatic alterations.

A recent survey of the modern villages of Inamgaon and Wangdari, across the Ghod River from prehistoric Inamgaon, showed that many important features in the layout of these villages (such as methods of house construction and grain storage) were quite similar to those revealed in the excavated village. Thus, the modern village of Inamgaon provides a good opportunity for detailed investigation of problems in ethnoarchaeology. These similarities between prehistoric and modern villages illustrate that India is a country where ancient traditions still survive to modern times.

Brief reports of the earlier excavations have appeared in *Expedition* and *Asian Perspectives* (Sankalia, Ansari, and Dhavalikar, 1973; Sankalia, Ansari, and Dhavalikar, 1975). This chapter summarizes the main discoveries and interpretations made at Inamgaon during the past 5 years (1977–1982).

Inamgaon is situated on the right bank of the Ghod River, 85 km east of Pune. The ancient site is nearly 1m east–west and 1m north–south. This area was erosionally dissected into five separate mounds; Mound I is the largest (Figure 1). During the past 5 years over 70 houses and more than 150 burials

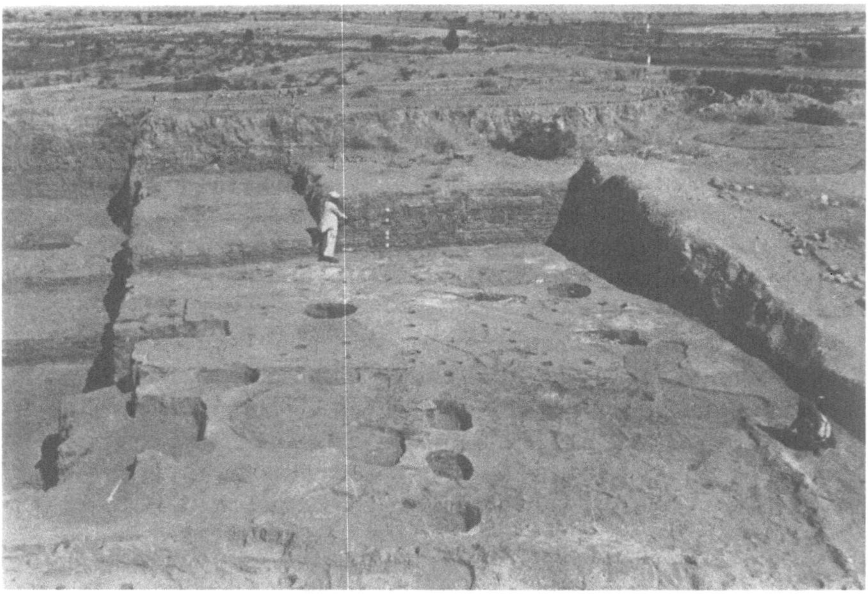

Figure 1. House 51, Period II, showing round mud floor and silo.

have been carefully excavated. The contents of each house were meticulously recorded so that analysis could be done in house-by-house fashion.

2. Settlement Pattern

2.1. House Construction

Houses and burials were found throughout the entire site, and they belong stratigraphically to three main periods: Period I (Malwa, *ca.* 1600–1400 B.C.); Period II (Early Jorwe, 1400–1000 B.C.); and Period III (Late Jorwe, 1000–700 B.C.). The earliest inhabitants lived on the black soil in houses that were circular or rectangular; house floors were well pounded after the black soil was covered with a thin layer of river gravel and yellow silt. This was the most common and practical method of preparing the living floor, as is attested to by our excavations at Navdatoli and Nevasa (Sankalia, Deo, and Ansari, 1960; Sankalia, Deo, Ansari, and Ehrhardt, 1971). However, this practice was not uniformly followed either in Period I or in subsequent periods. The variations in the mode of floor construction give us some idea about the varying social and economic conditions (or temperament) of the inhabitants of a particular house. For example, House 108 has a well-rammed floor, whereas in House 109 the floor was plastered as well. Houses 111 and 112 had the distinction of well-demarcated boundaries and lime-plastered floors, whereas House 113 had neither floor nor postholes. The oval shape of House 113 reminds us of the present-day temporary grass huts commonly found in rural India. From the earliest levels the houses at Inamgaon were built close to each other. House 90 was very well made. It was rectangular (4.15 m × 2.90 m) and had a well-constructed floor with raised edges, so that rain water could not enter. House 87 was originally large and rectangular (6.50 m × 3.35 m). Still later, there were rectangular houses, a circular house, and two courtyards in the same area.

Typical houses of Period II (Early Jorwe) are well represented by houses 63 and 65. In the latter, the floor was remade six times. In addition, it had a low mud wall with postholes, and contained a three-armed *chulah* (fireplace). The *chulah* does not appear to be a normal feature for cooking at Inamgaon.

An idea of town planning in this early village is indicated by the fact that between Early Jorwe houses 66–68, 62–63, and 70–71, there was a passage about 4.90 m wide running on a north–south axis. Further, what has been interpreted as a lane is seen adjacent to House 72.

House 112 of the Late Jorwe period, exhibits well-demarcated boundaries, a lime-plastered floor, and two courtyards. One courtyard contains a number of postholes; these were probably used to tether domestic animals. A large rectangular house, 105, was the scene of a tragedy. It was found completely burned. Its wooden posts and grain were charred, and in one corner a partially burned skeleton of a child was found.

3. House Structures and Implements

These houses contained abundant utilitarian pottery for eating, drinking, storing food grains, and water, and usually one or two burial urns were found. Less common domestic artifacts and house structures include the three-armed *chulah,* grain storage structures (silos, clay jars, and bins), saddle querns and grinding stones, microliths, and figurines.

3.1. Chulas

While fire pits were found in a number of houses in all three occupation periods, the three-armed *chulah* (fireplace), occurs in only two houses. *Chulas* are of two types: One has a semicircular clay border with an opening for inserting thin firewood; the other type is made by placing three stones in a roughly semicircular position, with the front open.

3.2. Grain Storage Structures

Silos occur frequently at Inamgaon and are lined with a thin layer of lime plaster. In several instances large and small storage jars made of unbaked clay were found. Typical cases (cited later) give an idea of the varied life-styles of the inhabitants of Inamgaon.

Silos were found in four houses; each had a notable feature. Two large silos were located in the courtyard of House 86; along their periphery there were a number of postholes indicating that these silos had roofs. These are very similar to the earliest silo found in Bihar. The two silos in House 74 were also located in a courtyard and had postholes along the periphery.

The occurrence of a poorly baked female figure with a punch decoration round her neck was found between three silos in House 69. The figurine may symbolize fertility, and it possibly functioned to protect the grain stored in the silos. The grain stored in House 74 has been identified as barley. Barley is usually stored in a silo today, but not wheat. Storage jars occur in all the three periods. The earliest occurrence was noticed in a rectangular house (4.15 m × 2.90 m) of the Early Jorwe period. Two large storage jars were made of unbaked clay with a beveled body. The storage jar in House 93 had a flat base, but the two found in the Late Lorwe period were four legged. One of these was found empty, but an adult was buried in a sitting posture in the other. These large unbaked clay jars must have been used for storing dry things.

These were not the only methods of grain storage at Inamgaon; bins were also used. Grain storage bins were round or oval mud platforms about 15 cm in height upon which a large cane basket was placed; the basket was then plastered with clay.

4. Evidence of Craft Specialization

4.1. Saddle Querns

Until recently, saddle querns were a common item in households. However, of all the houses excavated at Inamgaon, only three contained saddle querns (houses 75, 93, and 107). In addition to two saddle querns, House 93 contained a storage jar and a fire pit. The house itself was large, rectangular, and of the Malwa-Jorwe period. These features indicate that the occupants of House 93 perhaps were of high socioeconomic status or they may have had a large family.

A saddle quern is normally associated with one flat, or planoconvex, grinding stone. However, in House 75, four grinding stones were found, but there was no saddle quern. The significance of this is unclear, but perhaps the resident of this house was either a producer or distributor of grinding stones.

Throughout the three periods at Inamgaon cotton was spun on spindle whorls. These were either specially made or produced from broken pottery by boring holes in the shreds. In the past we found many spindle whorls, but during the last 5 years only one, made of pottery, was found in House 84 (Period I, Malwa). However, we are certain that many more spindle whorls must have been in use and that every family probably spun its own yarn.

Similarly, every family must have had at least one experienced hunter who could shoot with a sling ball. But only one sling ball, of stone, was found, in House 79-80.

4.2. Microlithic Implements

Microlithic blades, flakes, and cores are found in varying numbers in all houses, suggesting that making stone tools was practiced by every family. In House 102, however, a resident of the Late Jorwe period seems to have specialized in making lunates only (see Figure 2). In a section of this house a stone (quern) was placed on the floor to serve as an anvil. More than 1000 lunates were found around the quern—among masses of flakes and chips. By any standard this is an impressive number of lunates, and it can only be interpreted as evidence of

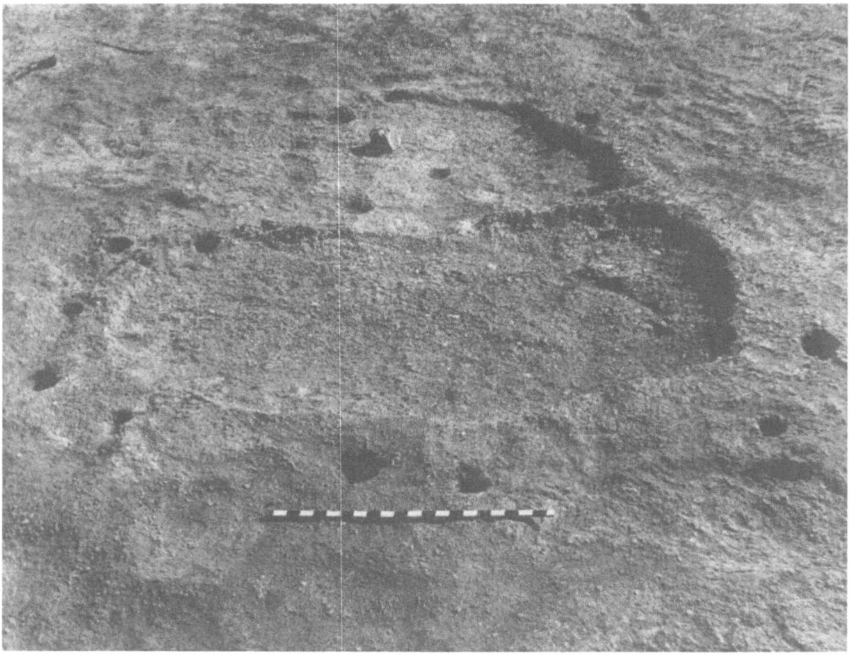

Figure 2. Lunate-makers' house, Period III.

craft specialization at Inamgaon. Similar evidence of craft specialization was discovered at the site of Shahr-i-Sokhta. A sandstone quern was found on a specially made floor in a semicircular area of House 109, and in House 13 a cruciblelike object was found that might have been used by a goldsmith.

In addition to these household crafts we have discussed, evidence of pot making and lime making was discovered. Two complete potter's kilns, a small one from Period I and a larger one from Period II, have been found.

In 1968 we noticed that lime was occasionally used as a thin coating in the construction of a silo. However, its regular use seems to have begun gradually. That it was used extensively and perhaps traded during the last phase was indicated by a number of lime balls found on the surface of Period I. Raw material in the shape of *kankar* (lime nodules) is abundantly available on the left bank of the Ghod River about a mile upstream from Inamgaon.

4.3. Figurines

Two nude female figurines made of clay were found in a clay box during the 1973 excavation season, and they may represent a Mother Goddess. Male and

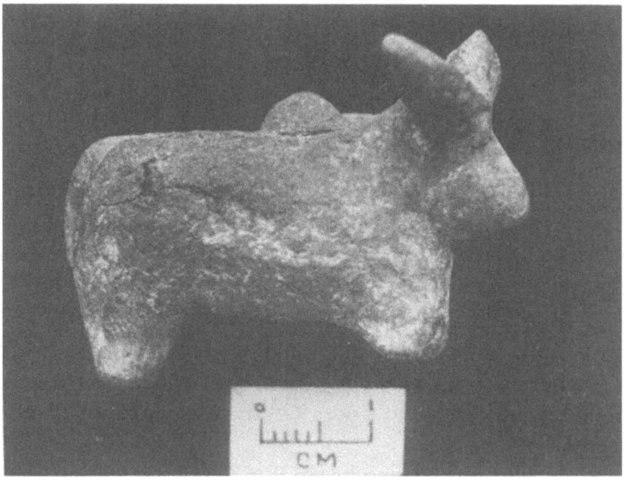

Figure 3. Clay figurine of a bull.

female terracotta figurines were also found, but not in a definite cultural context. However, in one case that was mentioned previously, a terracotta figurine with a punctured decoration round the neck was found between three silos. This suggests that both males and females may have been worshipped. Animal figurines have also been found (see Figure 3).

5. Human Burials

5.1. Features of a Typical Burial

Evidence regarding belief in an afterlife is found in 223 burials uncovered at Inamgaon. The deceased were invariably buried within the house under the living floor. The remains of children were placed in two or three pots with one or two bowls and a spouted jar. Adults were placed in an extended position in a specially dug pit that was sometimes lined with grass. The head usually was placed toward the north and the feet toward the south. Bowls and spouted pots were often placed in the burial pit. Food and drink may have been placed in the vessels at the time of the burial, but from the position of the pots and the absence of organic remains in them, it would appear that this was not done.

Though house burials are a normal feature at Inamgaon, many interesting departures from this practice were recorded. These variations in burial practices perhaps indicate variations in social conditions. Burial 129 is a typical child burial. The skeleton was placed in two Grey Ware urns with their mouths oriented in a north-south direction. Grave goods associated with this burial consisted of a bowl and a spouted pot of Jorwe Ware.

5.2. Examples of Atypical Burials

In Burial 127, the northern jar was made of the painted Malwa fabric and the southern pot was a typical Grey Ware. The rim of the painted pot was cut to the neck. A unique example is provided by Burial 128 in which a large red storage jar contained two Grey Ware burial urns. This unusual burial contained no grave goods at all. Among the grave goods found in Burial 132 were two bowls of Malwa fabric with vertical sides and two bowls of Grey Ware. In Burial 130, a child was buried in a single Grey Ware urn, which was placed vertically. This child might have belonged to a poor family that could not afford the normal burial equipment.

Three persons were buried together in Burial 125, which may be regarded as a very unique burial from the Early Jorwe period. This multiple burial might be due to a calamity, an accident, disease, or simple poverty. Burial 91 consisted of an isolated skull found in the burial pit, and only a single urn and a bowl were associated with Burial 99. These burials (91, 99, 125) were probably those of poor persons, or of individuals whose deaths were due to disease or accident. Burial 89 was a fairly tall person (1.65 m or 5 ft 6 inches) who was buried with his knees flexed toward the right. Normally, in adult burials the legs are fully extended, but in this case, the person either died in this posture or perhaps was accorded this unique posture because of an elite social status. This burial also provided definite evidence that when deceased individuals were buried under the house floor the family continued to occupy the house, but only after covering the burial pot and relaying the floor.

Frequently, when an adult was buried in an extended position the legs were removed. However Burial 160, an adolescent, was found buried in an extended position, but the legs had not been removed. This departure from the normal burial custom might be due to the person's young age and short stature that would have required minimal burial space. Other social or economic reasons are also possible for this departure from the norm.

Burial 152 lacked human skeletal remains, but it contained an atypical spouted jar with vertical neck. Spouted jars normally have a flaring neck. Burial 152 could be a symbolic burial, or it may represent an example of how preparations were made for burying the dead, but the burial place, for some reason, was not utilized.

Twin burial 83 is notable because both urns are of equal size and the spouted pot found in one of the urns has an unusual flaring mouth. A wide-mouthed pot

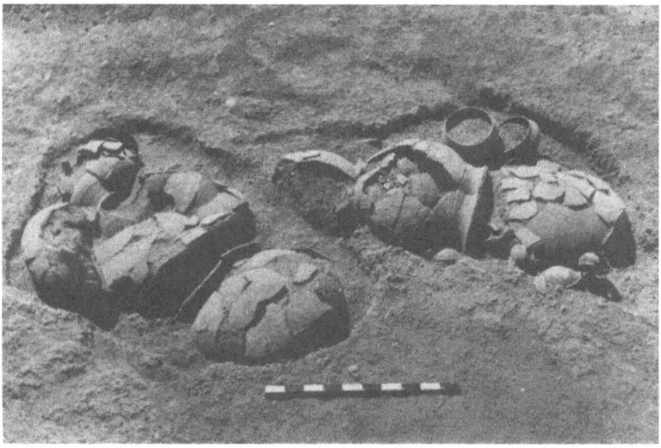

Figure 4. Three- and four-urn burial, Period III.

was used in this case because a smaller pot was placed within it with its mouth toward the northeast. In addition, the deceased child's body was covered with grass. This twin-urn burial was different in several respects from normal twin-urn burials.

In the Late Jorwe period we find abnormal burial practices. In the courtyard of House 106, a double adult burial was discovered (Burial No. 146), whereas in House 113, a child burial was found without the skull. Also, a rare three-urn burial (163) was found (see Figure 4) in which each urn was made differently. Although the central urn was a handmade storage jar, the southern urn, which was the smallest of the three, was a coarse, red-and-gray pot. The skull of the individual in Burial 163 was present, but it was badly crushed. All this evidence might indicate a hasty burial, but the fact that there were seven funerary pots in the burial pit—one of which was made of Late Jorwe fabric and the rest were Black-and-Red-Ware pots—is significant. This suggests that these people were among the latest inhabitants of Inamgaon and either were not well acquainted with, or equipped for using Early Jorwe burial customs. An alternative interpretation is that they were affluent and could easily afford to place seven pots in the burial pit.

A still more striking example indicating either higher social rank or specialized status of the buried individual is Burial 113. In this instance, a four-legged clay jar was used to bury a person in sitting posture. A similar jar was found during the course of earlier excavations (1977–1978), but it was empty. This burial posture is used today by the Lingayats—a sect that dates to the 13th century in Karnatak.

6. Cultural Contacts beyond the Deccan Plateau

6.1. Malwa (Central Indian) Contacts

The Chalcolithic settlement at Inamgaon, located, as it appears today, off the main roads in a perpetually semiarid region of India, shows contact with Malwa (Central India) to the north and Andhra-Karnatak to the south. Though revealing some evidence of outside contact, Inamgaon maintained its individuality and gradually lost its Malwa influence. This is best seen in the tableware, ordinary household pottery, and the disposal of the dead. In houses of the earliest period, dated *ca.* 1600 B.C., we find the typical Malwa style of pottery in use. Its fabric or surface treatment is distinctive as are the few pottery shapes including *lotas* (water vessels) and bowls. But for some unknown reason, other characteristic shapes—dishes, dishes on stands, and goblets (bowls on stands) with their rich naturalistic paintings—were totally absent. Instead, the Inamgaon inhabitants had large and small spouted pots with flaring mouths and bowls with carinated bellies. What we call *thalis* (dishes) are totally absent. If they used such flat-based dishes, they might have used Grey-Ware basins.

Later, in Period II, this limited Malwa influence is practically absent, and it disappears completely in Period III. These conclusions, summarized so briefly here, are based on a very thorough analysis of complete pots and numerous potsherds that give an idea of the shape of each vessel from each excavated house.

6.2. Andhra-Karnataka (South India)

During Period III, the typical pottery, which had a smooth, red surface with simple geometric designs painted in black, began to lose its fineness and the surface became coarser. However, at this time another type of pottery, bowls of Black-and-Red ware, makes an appearance (see Figure 5). The presence of this Black-and-Red Ware suggests cultural contact with South India. These bowls had definitely entered the kitchen because they were found among the grave goods.

The exact date of introduction of the typical Black-and-Red Ware is not known, but at present we regard it as being of South Indian origin. In fact, such influence can also be postulated as the source of Grey Ware pots with flaring mouths, which were for burying children and for other purposes in the kitchen (see Figure 6). The large number of these pots in every house attests to their usefulness.

Again, spouted vessels in Grey Ware with an almost teapotlike recurved spout occurred in the Neolithic settlements at Tekkalkota in Karnataka and in Tamil Nadu.

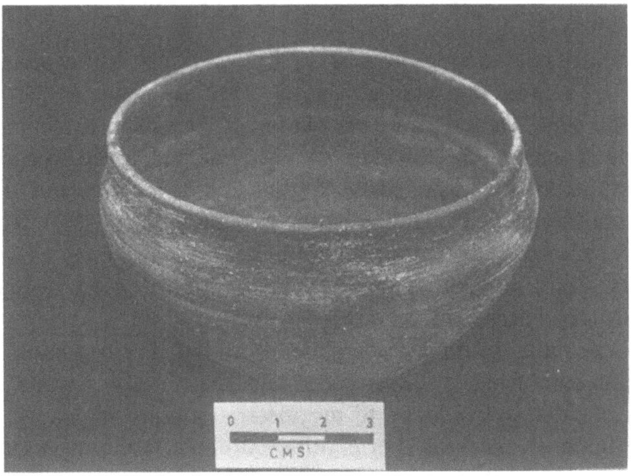

Figure 5. Bowl: Black-and-Red Ware, Period III.

The people of Maharashtra, as shown by the excavations at Nevasa, Daimabad, and now Inamgaon, did not fully borrow these South Indian fabrics or forms, nor did they borrow the polished axe. Thus far, only a few polished axes have been found at Inamgaon and Nevasa. At Inamgaon, the individuality

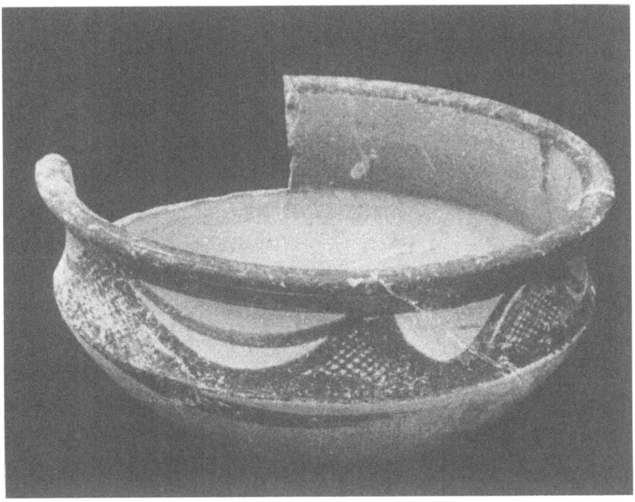

Figure 6. Concave-sided bowl, Period III.

of the Jorwe culture as a typical Maharashtrian Chalcolithic culture is once again a striking feature.

Contact with coastal areas is indicated by a necklace of tiny sea shells found on the neck of a child in a twin-urn burial (176) excavated in the 1981–1982 season. At this time, we are aware of how important such ornaments were to the Jorwe people at Inamgaon. However, the materials employed—copper beads at Nevasa and Chandoli but paste, sea shells, and copper at Inamgaon—indicate the economic conditions of the families at the two sites.

Earlier, heavy anklets or "wristlets" of copper were found as well as a few other objects. Thus, although copper was known to the people of Inamgaon, its use was restricted because of its rarity.

This Chalcolithic settlement depended from the very beginning on hunting and the cultivation of barley. Later sheep and goats, wheat, lentils, and two or three kinds of pulse were added to the material culture inventory. Increasing dependence upon a vegetarian diet is reflected in the preliminary studies of the adult skeletal remains (Lukacs and Badam, 1976–1977).

One of the most important results of these 5 years' work, aided by scientific studies in paleobotany and paleoanthropology, is that we now know that the latest inhabitants of Inamgaon were not economically impoverished—either in the size of their houses and food resources or in their general health (Lukacs, Bogorad, R., Walimbe, and Dunbar, 1983).

Further ethnographic studies of villages around the site, such as Wagdari and Inamgaon, show that although the prehistoric settlement faded out, possibly

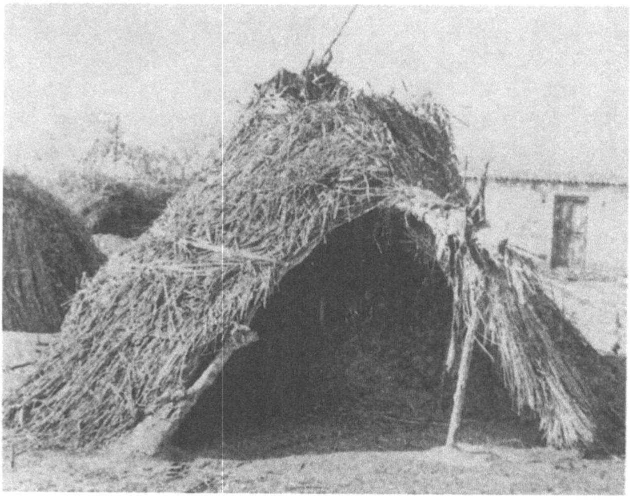

Figure 7. Present hut at Inamgaon.

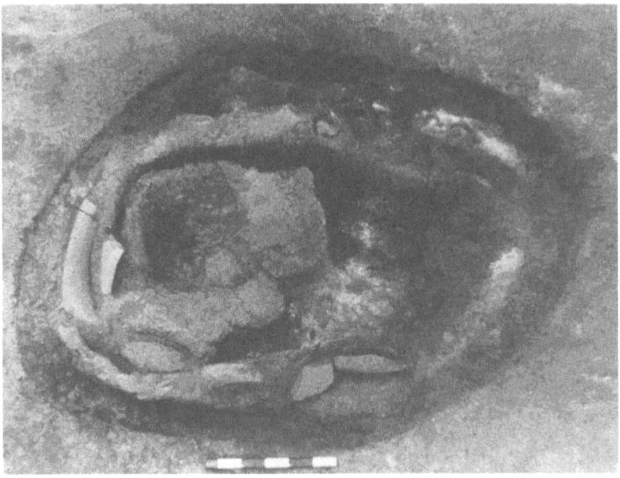

Figure 8. Clay-lined fire pit, Period I.

because of climatic changes, it left its legacy. The best evidence is found in modern villages where the methods of building hatched huts (see Figures 7 and 8), and mud-platform storage bins are similar to those of the archaeological culture.

ACKNOWLEDGMENTS

We wish to thank the Physical Research Laboratory (Ahmedabad) and the Birbal Sahni Institute (Lucknow) for promptly providing radiocarbon dates.

References

Lukacs, J. R., and Badam, G. L., 1976–1977, Biological Anthropology of Human Skeletal Remains from Chalcolithic Inamgaon, western India, *Bull. Deccan Coll. Res. Instit.* **36:**73–83.

Lukacs, J. R., Bogorad, R., Walimbe, S. R., and Dunbar, D. C., (1983) Paleopathology at Inamgaon (1600–700 B.C.), A prehistoric agrarian village in western India, *Am. J. Phys. Anthropol.*

Sankalia, H. D., Deo, S. B., Anasari, Z. D., and Ehrhardt, S., 1960, *From History to Prehistory at Nevasa (1954–1956).* Pune: Deccan College.

Sankalia, H. D., Deo, S. B., and Ansari, Z. D., 1971, *Chalcolithic Navdatoli,* Pune.

Sankalia, H. D., Ansari, Z. D., and Dhavalikar, M. K., 1975, An early farmer's village in central India, *Expedition* **17**(2):2–11.

Sankalia, H. D., Ansari, Z. D., and Dhavalikar, M. K., 1973, Inamgaon: A Chalcolithic settlement in western India, *Asian Perspectives* **14:**139–146.

CHAPTER 6

Paleodemography at Inamgaon: An Early Farming Village in Western India

JOHN R. LUKACS AND SUBHASH R. WALIMBE

1. Introduction

The human skeletal remains from the early farming village of Inamgaon are of major anthropological significance because (1) infant and juvenile skeletons have been systematically and thoroughly analyzed, and (2) a paleodemographic perspective has been adopted in analyzing all human skeletal elements from the site. In these respects this study is the first of its kind in South Asian paleoanthropology and provides valuable insights into the biological adaptations of these early occupants of the Deccan Plateau.

Inamgaon is not unique among the late Chalcolithic settlements of western India in yielding abundant, and often well-preserved, skeletal remains of infants and juveniles. Though more than 90 burials of immature individuals were recovered in three excavation seasons at Nevasa, the value of an anthropological analysis of these specimens was overlooked. Consequently, the descriptive and comparative anthropometric study of the Nevasa skeletal series focused primarily on the four adult specimens from that site (Kennedy and Malhotra, 1966). A similar situation is found at Chandoli where 24 burials were excavated and only one was an adult (Deo and Ansari, 1965). The remaining 23 burials were never subjected to anthropological description (Malhotra, 1965).

JOHN R. LUKACS • Department of Anthropology, University of Oregon, Eugene, Oregon 97403 and *SUBHASH W. WALIMBE* • Department of Archaeology, Deccan College Postgraduate and Research Institute, Pune 411 006. This research was made possible by grants from the American Institute of Indian Studies (NSF, INT-8106982-A01) and the Smithsonian Institution (Grant No. 10832700). The support of these agencies is deeply appreciated.

In South Asian paleoanthropology, descriptive and comparative osteometric analyses frequently include only the better preserved adult crania from a more extensive collection of fragmentary and immature specimens (Gupta, Dutta, and Basu, 1962; Bernhard 1967, 1969, 1981; Basu and Pal, 1980). This practice is attributable to the investigator's objective of establishing the "racial" or "ethnic" indentity of the skeletal sample, and in this endeavor only complete adult crania provide relevant data. A demographic perspective in South Asian paleoanthropology has been slow to develop because numerous investigators adhere to racial paradigms in their analyses of human skeletal series. The unfortunate result is that numerous immature and fragmentary skeletal specimens, having great potential anthropological value, are routinely disregarded. When a demographic perspective is adopted as the primary research orientation, every piece of human bone—cranial or postcranial, fragmentary or complete—must be scrutinized because it may yield valuable information regarding the health, status, occupation, age, and sex of the individual.

A paleodemographic perspective was adopted from the beginning in our analysis of the human skeletons from Inamgaon, but initial descriptive and comparative studies were limited by the small number of specimens available (Lukacs and Badam 1975, 1976–1977). A full paleodemographic analysis of 53 human skeletons from Early and Late Jorwe phases at Inamgaon was conducted by Lukacs and Badam (1981). This study emphasized the importance of a paleodemographic orientation in South Asian paleoanthropology, described the demographic structure of the Inamgaon skeletal sample, and found the people of Inamgaon relatively free from skeletal and dental diseases (Lukacs and Badam, 1981).

Official excavations at Inamgaon were concluded at the close of the 1981–1982 field excavations. Between January and August, 1982, we described and analyzed all new human skeletal remains recovered from Inamgaon since 1979, and completed a reanalysis of those skeletal remains excavated prior to 1979. This chapter summarizes the major research conclusions derived from a paleodemographic analysis of the entire collection of human skeletons from Inamgaon.* The main topics discussed here include the structure of the Inamgaon skeletal sample, phenotypic features of healthy adults and infants, and a preliminary description of paleopathological lesions. Specialized studies on various aspects of the Inamgaon skeletal series will be published separately.

*Preparation of the final report on the human skeletal remains from Inamgaon is currently in progress (Lukacs and Walimbe, 1983) and will ultimately be published by Deccan College.

A detailed description and interpretation of the paleopathological lesions in the Inamgaon series is in preparation and will be published separately (Lukacs, Bogorad, Walimbe, and Dunbar, 1983). Analytic and comparative studies of the size and morphology of the deciduous (Lukacs, Joshi, and Makhija, 1983) and permanent (Lukacs, 1983) teeth from Inamgaon are in progress and will be published in the near future.

Table I
Distribution of Human Skeletons from Inamgaon by Age, Sex, and Cultural Phase

Age category	Malwa			Early Jorwe			Late Jorwe			Subtotal			Grand total
Infant (0–1 yr)		15			27			61			103 (72.0)		
Early child (2–6 yr)		1			11			12			24 (16.8)		
Late child (7–11 yr)		—			4			12			16 (11.2)		
Subtotal		16 (11.2)			42 (29.4)			85 (59.4)					143 (81.25)
	Sex			Sex			Sex			Sex			
	M	F	?	M	F	?	M	F	?	M	F	?	
Adolescent (12–16 yr)				—	—	1	1	2	4	1	2	5	8 (24.2)
Young adult (17–31 yr)				—	1	1	4	1	2	4	2	3	9 (27.3)
Middle-aged adult (32–46 yr)				—	3	3	4	2	4	4	5	7	16 (48.5)
Old adult (47)				—	—	—	—	—	—	—	—	—	0 (0.0)
Subtotal (by sex)				—	4	5	9	5	10	9(27.3)	9(27.3)	15(45.5)	33 (18.75)
Subtotal (sexes pooled)		0 (0.0)			9 (27.3)			24 (72.7)			33 (18.75)		
Grand Total		16 (9.1)			51 (29.0)			109 (61.9)					176

2. Materials and Methods

2.1. Sample and Definition of Terms

A total of 228 burials were exposed during the course of 12 years of excavation at Inamgaon. Many of these burials are "symbolic" and are devoid of any human bone; others are so poorly preserved that no human skeletal remains survived the processes of exposure, excavation, and transport to the laboratory. The minimum number of individuals from Inamgaon is 176. The distribution of these individuals by age, sex, and cultural phase is given in Table I. The term *individual* is employed here in the paleontological sense; a particular individual may be represented by a complete and well-preserved skeleton, or by a single tooth or a few fragmentary cranial or postcranial bones.

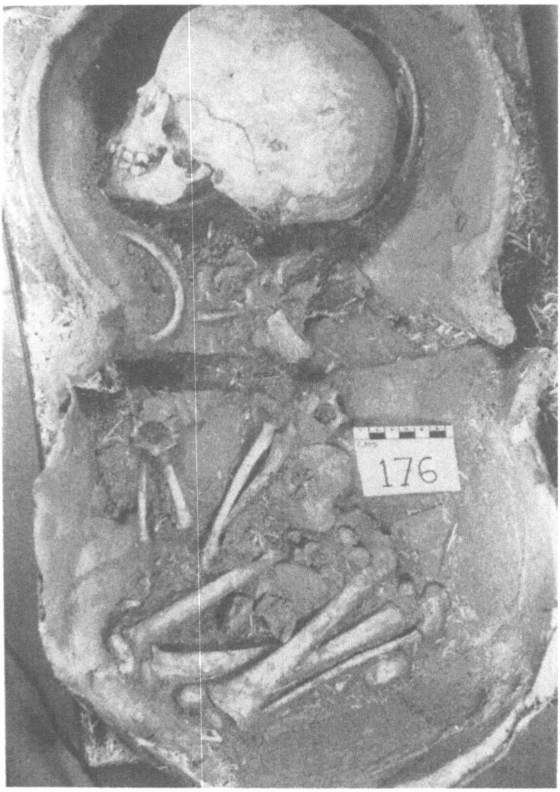

(a)

Figure 1. Inamgaon burials (a) typical twin-urn burial (INM 176) and (b) atypical mud-sarcophagus burial (INM 198).

In addition, the term *burial* cannot be equated with *individual,* although in many instances one burial has yielded one individual. In such instances where more than one individual is derived from one burial, they are denoted by letters (INM 206-A, 206-B, etc.).

2.2. Preservation of Skeletal Remains

The state of preservation of the Inamgaon skeletons varies greatly. Some specimens consist of nearly complete and well-preserved infant skeletons; others consist of very fragmentary bone chips and isolated teeth. Local differences in soil chemistry appear to play a major role in preservation; some bones are bleached white and have a chalky texture, whereas those from other burials appear partially mineralized. The integrity of the single or twin burial urns in

(b)
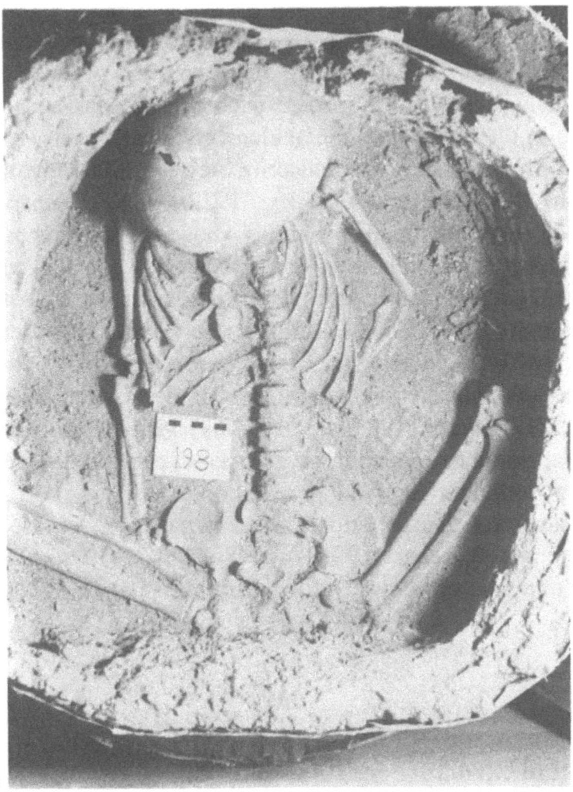

Figure 1. (*continued*)

which an infant is interred also plays a role in preserving skeletal and dental elements in good condition (see Figure 1). Specimens derived from broken burial urns are less complete and less well preserved.

When the likelihood of preservation of different skeletal parts is considered, teeth and bones of the cranial base (basi-occipital, condylar portion of occipital and petrous portion of temporal) are the most frequently preserved elements in fragmentary infant burials. In fragmentary adult burials, dental and gnathic structures and portions of the occipital and temporal bones are most frequently preserved. A more complete discussion of the state of preservation of each specimen and a quantitative evaluation of differential preservation of skeletal parts will be included in the final report (Lukacs and Walimbe, 1983).

2.3. Methods of Analysis

Age and sex of the adult segment of the sample was determined by the standardized criteria described in Brothwell (1972) and Stewart (1979). Sex determination for the preadolescent portion of the sample was not attempted. Age estimates for preadolescent individuals are based on dental eruption sequences (Olivier, 1969; Stewart, 1979), or the progress of dental calcification if only isolated dental crowns are present (Schour and Massler 1940; Hunt and Gleiser 1959). In the absence of dental elements, long bones were employed in age estimation using the charts provided by Stewart (1979), the tabular data for Arikara Indians (Merchant and Ubelaker, 1977), or by comparison with long bones of individuals in the Inamgaon series whose age was determined dentally.

The problem of differences in chronological-, dental-, and skeletal-age estimates in paleodemographic and paleopathological research is discussed by Buikstra and Cook (1980). The use of European standards for dental eruption is justifiable because differences in the timing of tooth eruption between European and Indian populations are not significant (Banerjee and Mukherjee, 1967; Mukherjee, 1973; Prakash, 1974, Rami Reddy, 1981). European standards for dental calcification are employed in the absence of published standards for dental crown and root formation in Indian populations.

The diagnosis and interpretation of skeletal pathology is based on Brothwell (1972), Ortner and Putschar (1981), and Steinbock (1976). Description and interpretation of dental pathology follows Brothwell (1963, 1972) and Glickman (1964).

3. Results

3.1. Population Structure and Sample Bias

Reference to Table 1 shows that the Inamgaon skeletal sample is composed predominantly of preadolescent individuals (81.25%). The adult segment of the series consists of 33 individuals (18.75%), nearly half of which are of indeterminate sex. More than half the skeletal series (61.9%; 109/176) is derived from the Late Jorwe cultural phase. The Early Jorwe cultural phase yielded 51 individuals (29%), and the Malwa phase only 16 (9.1%).

This distribution of individuals by age, sex, and cultural phase is clearly biased; that is, in the overrepresentation of preadolescents and the underrepresentation of individuals from earlier cultural phases. These points require clarification. The abundance of immature individuals (81.25%; 143/176) is primarily due to differential preservation; burial urns afforded protection to the skeletal elements from the destructive pressure of the superincumbant earth. The paucity of adolescent and adult individuals (18.75%; 33/176) in the Inamgaon skeletal series is best attributed to exposure, disposal, and possibly cremation as alternatives to the practice of burial beneath the house floor (see Figure 2). Burial of the deceased in a cemetery located outside the habitation area is another possible explanation for the paucity of adult specimens in the Inamgaon skeletal series. However, archaeological exploration has failed to locate such a burial ground. The proximity of the Ghod River to the occupation mound may have facilitated the disposal of the decomposed, osseous, or ashen remains of individuals who were exposed or cremated.

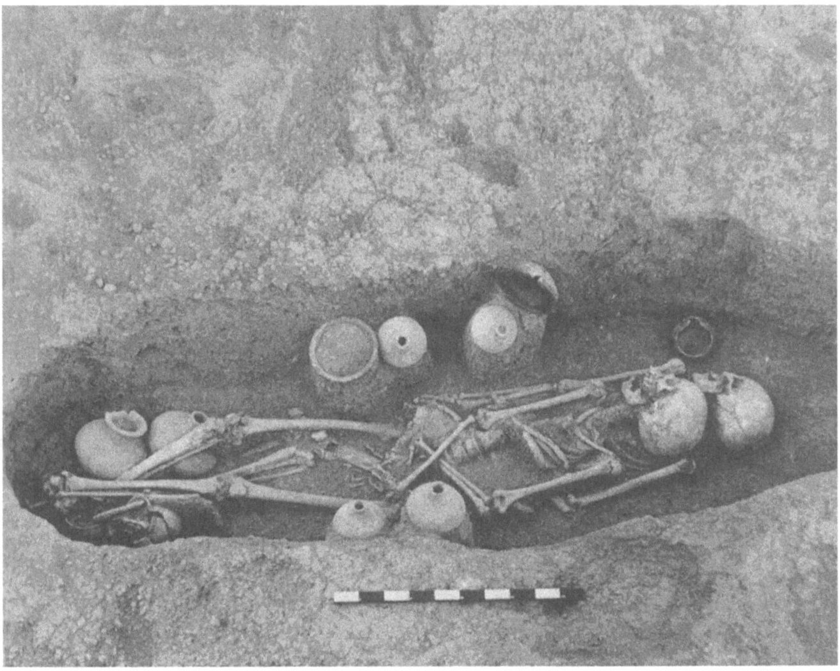

Figure 2. Atypical extended double burial (No. 146) from Late Jorwe period. The female (INM 146-A) is located stratigraphically above the male (INM 146-B).

The differential representation of human skeletal remains by cultural phase (Late Jorwe, 61.9%; Early Jorwe, 29.4%; Malwa 9.1%) is primarily due to the more extensive excavation of later cultural phases. Thirteen of the 16 specimens from the Malwa phase were recovered during the 1979–1980 excavation season when this horizon was intensively excavated.

3.2. Biological Characteristics of the Inamgaon People

3.2.1. The adult phenotypic pattern. This description of the biological characteristics of the Inamgaon people is based on a small sample of well-preserved specimens (Figures 3 and 4). Because adult individuals are few in number at Inamgaon, as they are at all late Chalcolithic sites in the Deccan Plateau, this assessment of cranial and postcranial skeletal variation must be regarded as tentative.

Craniometric data for three adults from Late Jorwe levels at Inamgaon are presented in Table II. A comparative framework for interpreting the Inamgaon data is provided by the inclusion of craniometric data for selected prehistoric skeletal series and living inhabitants of Maharashtra.

The similarity in craniometric characters between Inamgaon and the skeletal series from Nevasa is striking. Values for the Cranial Index of the Inamgaon specimens fall near the dolicho-mesocranial border, and the male specimen from Nevasa is clearly dolichocranial. The only other important difference between the two series is the hyperacrocranic skull of INM 146-B. In all other facial and cranial features, the Inamgaon and Nevasa series exhibit close similarity. This is not surprising, in view of the close geographic, temporal, and cultural associations between these two sites.

When compared with the Harappan sample, the Inamgaon crania are most similar in length, breadth, and Cranial Index to specimens from Cemetery R-37. Crania from Cemetery H (Stratum II) at Harappan are longer and broader than the Inamgaon specimens, but they exhibit similar cranial indexes. In facial structure, both Harappan samples are considerably broader across the zygoma than are the Inamgaon specimens. This fact is also true for Burzahom and is reflected in the lower valves for the Upper Facial Index of males at these sites. Nasal height and breadth are also greater among Harappan males than at Inamgaon. In nasal structure the Burzahom series is more similar to the Harappan samples than it is to the Inamgaon specimens.

A multivariate analysis of the Inamgaon skulls is currently in progress with the collaboration of Dr. Wolfram Bernhard (Universität Mainz). This investigation will provide a clearer picture of the biological affinities of the Inamgaon skeletal series.

Mandibular measurements for two male and three female specimens from Inamgaon are presented in Table III. Male and female specimens show consider-

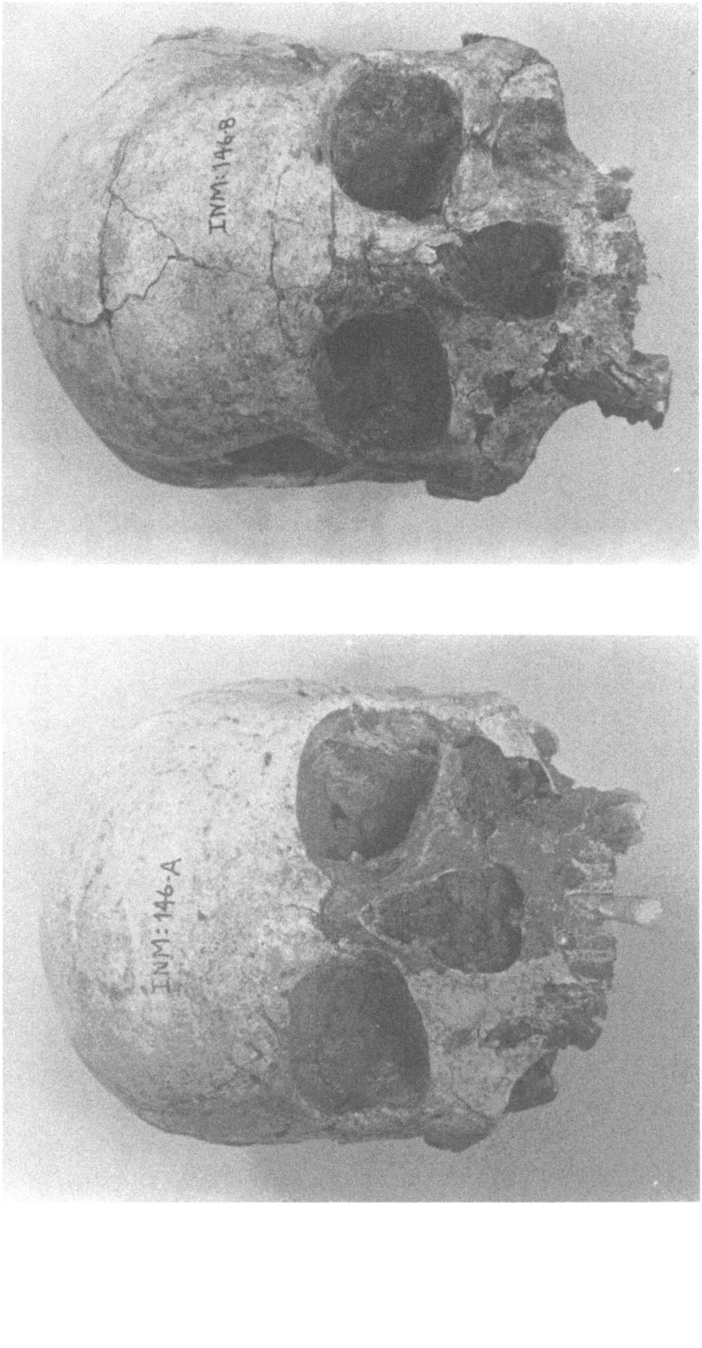

Figure 3. Crania of INM 146, *Norma Frontalis* (a left; b right).

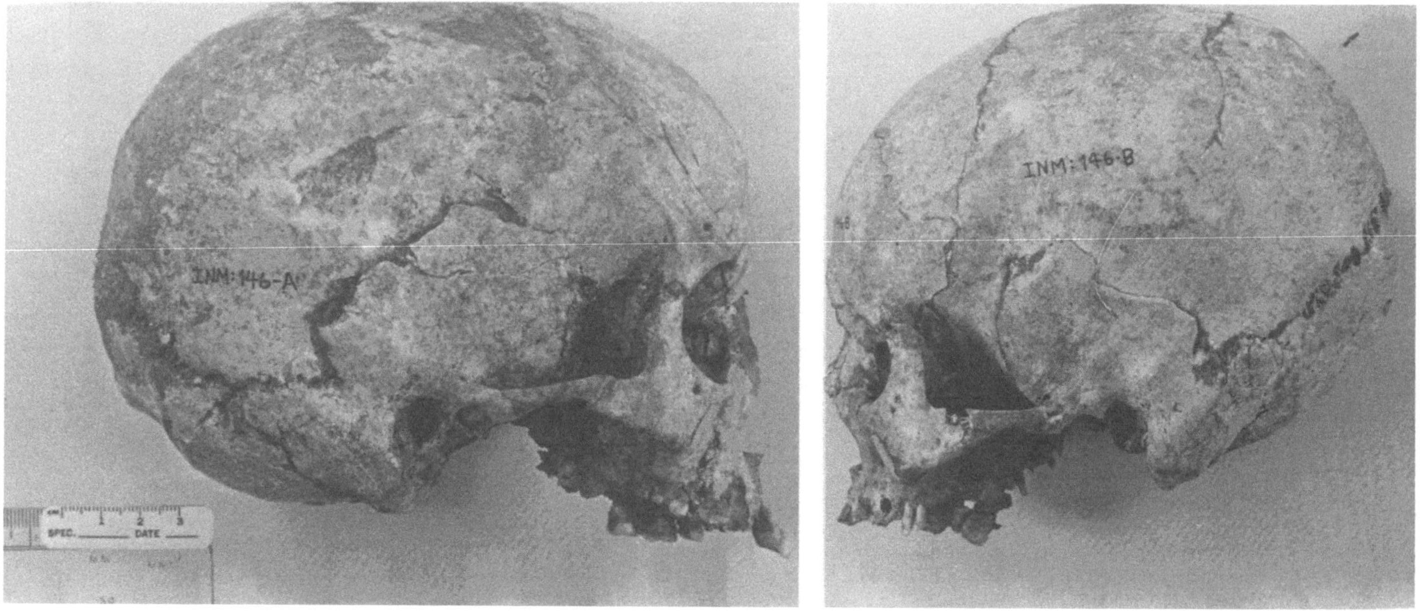

Figure 4. Crania of INM 146, *Norma Lateralis* (left, 146-A; right, 146-B).

Table II
Comparative Craniometric Data for Inamgaon and Selected Prehistoric and Living South Asian Populations (in mm)

	Prehistoric Indians											Living Indians	
	Inamgaon			Nevasa[a]		Harappa—R-37[b]		Harappa H-II[b]		Burzahom[c]		Bhils[d]	Marathas[e]
	Male		Female	Male	Female	Male	Female	Male	Female	Male	Female	Male	Male
	59	146-B	146-A	(n = 1)	(n = 2)	(n = 7)	(n = 3)	(n = 7)	(n = 6)	(n = 2)	(n = 2)		
Measurements													
Cranial length (1)	176	181	183	186	180	180	174	189	181	188.5	187.5	179.50	183.93
Cranial breadth (8)	137	138	137	125	133	138	125	144	133	136.5	128.0	135.96	144.23
Basion-bregma height (17)		137	136		134	133	123	134	134	140.0	—		
Auricular-vertex height (21)	111	121	115	115						122.5	119.5	114.70	130.12
Auricular-bregma height (20)	109	119	113	110	114	115	111	119	109	—	—		
Minimum frontal diameter (9)	101	87	100	89	111	95	93	95	93	97.0	92.5	99.38	104.87
Bizygmatic diameter (45)	(128)	122	(118)	122	125	131	124	136	117	142.0	(125.5)	132.40	134.87
Prosthion-nasion height (48)		(65)	(65)	64	64	70	65	70	66	(74.0)	(69.0)		
Basion-nasion (5)		101	102							110.0			
Basion-prosthion (40)		102	(95)							100.0			
Nasal height (55)		46	46	46	46	51	47	52	45	(52.5)	(51.5)	43.36	49.39
Nasal breadth (54)		22	24	24	24	26	24	25	24	(30.5)	(27.0)	37.56	36.33
Orbital height (52)		31	32	32	32	34	33	33	33	37.0	34.0		
Orbital breadth (51)		36	41	35	40	42	40	41	40	44.0	—		

(continued)

Table II *(Continued)*

	Prehistoric Indians											Living Indians	
	Inamgaon			Nevasa[a]		Harappa—R-37[b]		Harappa H-II[b]		Burzahom[c]		Bhils[d]	Marathas[e]
	Male		Female	Male	Female	Male	Female	Male	Female	Male	Female	Male	Male
	59	146-B	146-A	(n = 1)	(n = 2)	(n = 7)	(n = 3)	(n = 7)	(n = 6)	(n = 2)	(n = 2)		
Indexes													
Cranial index	77.86	76.24	74.86	67.20	74.10	76.40	74.40	76.70	76.00	72.45	68.30	74.94	78.58
Cranial module		152.00	152.00		149.00	150.30	140.70	155.70	149.30	155.00	—		
Cranial capacity	1318.64	1444.26	1358.78	1301.31	1316.53					1481.09	1383.12		
Upper facial index		53.28	55.10		53.60	52.60		50.00		52.30	55.11	46.72	49.10
Zygo-frontal index	78.91	71.31	84.75	72.95	88.89	72.50	75.00	69.90	79.50	68.30	73.70		77.96
Height (Ba-Br) length		75.69	74.32		72.40			70.90	74.00	73.70	—		
Height (Ba-Br) breadth		99.28	99.27		100.00			93.10	100.80	105.30	—		
Height (Au-Br) length		65.75	61.75	59.10	61.60	61.30	61.90	62.10	62.60	—	—		
Height (Au-Br) breadth		86.23	82.48	88.00	85.00	86.20	85.40	85.60	82.30	—	—		
Height (Au-Vx) length		66.85	62.84	61.80						64.95	63.75	64.15	71.14
Height (Au-Vx) breadth		87.68	83.94	92.00						89.85	93.35	85.74	90.62
Nasal index		47.83	52.17	52.10	51.00	51.00	51.90	47.60	53.30	59.45	52.40	86.79	74.15
Orbital index	76.19	86.11	78.05	91.40	80.00	80.80	83.20	79.20	82.70	81.40	—		

[a]Kennedy, K. A. R. and K. C. Malhotra (1966)
[b]Gupta, P., P. C. Dutta, and A. Basu (1962)
[c]Basu, A. and A. Pal (1980)
[d]Srinivasan, S. and R. K. Gulati (1973)
[e]Karve (1948)

Table III
Comparative Mandibular Measurements (in mm)

	Prehistoric Indians												
	Inamgaon					Nevasa[a]		Harappa R-37[b]		Harappa H,St II[b]		Burzahom[c]	
	Male		Female			Male	Female	Male	Female	Male	Female	Male	Female
	59	146-B	146-A	106	68	(n = 2)	(n = 2)						
Measurements													
Bicondylar breadth (65)	114	(130)	109	118	94	112.0	102.0	103.9	108.3	(112.5)	111.5	117.0	118.5
Bigonial breadth (66)	99	(90)	82	98	77	94.5	102.0	89.1	81.0	79.0	83.6	89.3	86.5
Symphyseal height (69)	35	(34)	31	25	22	33.5	31.5	33.5	30.0	30.3	30.0	34.0	30.0
Height of corpus (69[1]) M_2	28	31	25	25	23	—	—	—	—	—	—	32.2	30.0
Ascending ramus height (71)	—	58	44	53	—	63.0	55.0	68.4	59.0	62.0	57.8	64.8	56.5
Min. breadth of ascending ramus (71)	35	37	32	31	32	30.0	33.0	34.3	31.5	35.0	31.7	32.8	32.5
Condylo-symphyseal length	(98)	103	106	99	92	105.0	105.5	81.9	75.0	87.0	74.7	76.5	68.5
Mandibular angle	124°	121°	124°	120°	116°	116.3°	129.5°	120.2°	118.7°	110.5°	122.6°	117.0°	120.0°

[a]Kennedy, K. A. R. and K. C. Malhotra (1966)
[b]Gupta, P., P. C. Dutta, and A. Basu (1962)
[c]Basu, A. and A. Pal (1980)

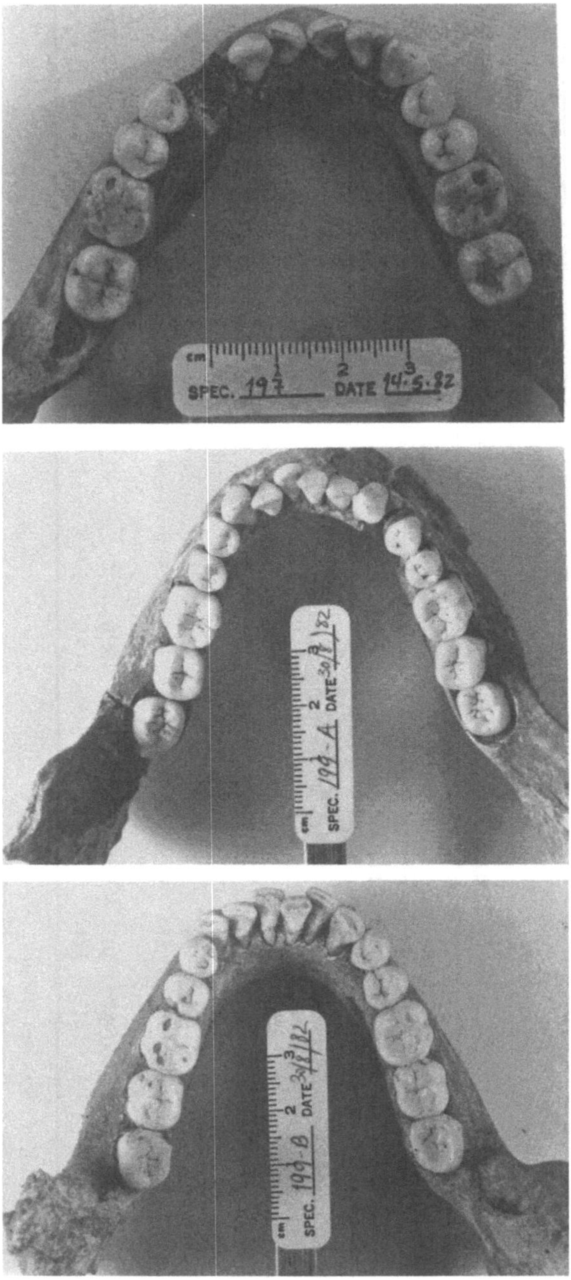

Figure 5. Adult mandibles, superior view of dental arcade (top, INM 197; middle, 199-A; bottom, 199-B).

able overlap in measurements of mandibular length and breadth (Figure 5). Sexual dimorphism is detectable in the height of the symphysis and corpus, and the height of the ascending ramus. Male values for the mandibular angle fall within the range of female values. The pattern of sexual dimorphism in mandibular structure observed in the Inamgaon specimens is found to be generally characteristic of other skeletal series from South Asia (see Table III). The high variability of mandibular measurements in the Inamgaon series precludes any statement regarding its biological affinities with other Indian skeletal series.

The best clues to the genetic affinities of the Inamgaon skeletal series will derive from detailed morphometric analyses of the deciduous and permanent teeth from this site. These investigations are currently in progress and will be published separately (Lukacs, 1983; Lukacs *et al.*, 1983).

Though postcranial skeletal elements of adults were frequently damaged, stature estimates could be made for eight individuals whose long bones were well preserved. These estimates were computed from formulas of Athawale (1963)

Table IV
Individual and Mean Stature Estimates for Males and Females

Specimen Number	Athawale (1963)	Calculations Based On	Trotter (1970)
		Males	
INM-59	162.70 ± 3.62	Ulna	168.40 ± 4.23
INM-146-B		Femur	164.23 ± 3.27
		Humerus	166.24 ± 4.05
INM-157		Tibia	177.29 ± 3.37
INM-199-A		Humerus	152.69 ± 4.05
	155.16 ± 3.84	Ulna	165.07 ± 4.23
INM-200		Humerus	172.09 ± 4.05
	175.86 ± 3.84	Ulna	185.05 ± 4.23
Mean Stature 1	164.57 (n = 3)		169.76 (n = 5)
2	169.28 (n = 2)		172.48 (n = 4)
		Females	
INM-68		Ulna	155.97 ± 4.30
INM-106		Humerus	155.75 ± 4.45
		Radius	166.32 ± 4.24
		Ulna	167.50 ± 4.30
INM-146-A		Radius	171.06 ± 4.24
Mean Stature 1			163.41 (n = 3)
2			167.13 (n = 2)

and Trotter (1970) for males, and Trotter (1970) for females. The two late-adolescent individuals (INM 199-A, INM-68) are omitted from the calculation of average stature because they apparently have not attained full adult stature. The mean stature for males is 172.48 cm ($n = 4$) and for females, 167.13 cm ($n = 2$); both these averages are derived from Trotter's formulas for "whites." The individual stature estimates, the bone whose length this estimate was calculated from, and the mean stature figures for each sex are presented in Table IV. Comparative data for stature and selected postcranial indexes of other prehistoric skeletal series are presented in Table V. The average stature for Inamgaon males falls in the middle of the range of mean stature for four other skeletal series. The average stature of Inamgaon females, however, is considerably above the mean stature of the four other series with which it is compared. It is interesting to note that sex dimorphism in stature is less for Inamgaon (difference between male and female means [5.35 cm]) and Nevasa (6.06 cm), and greater at Burzahom (15.55 cm) and Harappa: R-37 (15.83) and Cemetery H, Stratum II (12.68). The significance of this finding is presently unclear, but it may be related to differences in diet, subsistence, and occupational activities between the people of the Deccan Plateau (Inamgaon and Nevasa) and those from Harappa and Burzahom. Mean values for the platymeric and platycnemic indexes for Inamgaon and four other South Asian skeletal series are also presented in Table V. Male and female tibiae from Inamgaon are eurymeric and femora are platymeric.

In skeletal morphology, females tend to be robust and males somewhat gracile in both cranial and postcranial features. Estimation of sex on cranial and postcranial criteria other than pelvic features tends to be very risky in this series. The adult skeletal sample from Inamgaon described previously undoubtedly represents a biased sample and may be derived from the higher socioeconomic strata of the society. In many instances, manual labor may be unacceptable for a person of high sociopolitical and religious standing, but traditional chores of carrying water, infants, and other burdens fall on the female regardless of her

Table V
Comparison of Mean Stature Estimate and Postcranial Indexes

	Stature (in cm)		Platymeric Index		Platycnemic Index	
Site	Male (*n*)	Female (*n*)	Male (*n*)	Female (*n*)	Male (*n*)	Female (*n*)
Inamgaon	172.48(4)	167.13(2)	84.48(1)	76.45(3)	82.54(1)	70.43(2)
Nevasa	170.70(2)	164.64(2)	91.15(2)	92.78(2)	89.29(1)	70.97(1)
Harappa R-37	173.24(2)	157.41(1)	82.24(7)	90.91(1)		
Harappa H. (St. II)	170.24(8)	157.56(5)	77.05(4)	85.71(5)		
Burzahom	175.35(4)	159.88(2)	70.70(3)	71.10(2)	66.50(4)	63.60(1)

Table VI
Mean Long-bone Length of Inamgaon Infants (0–6 mos.)

Bone	Mean length (n)	Minimum	Maximum	SD
Humerus	73.03 (9)	63.5	91.5	8.29
Radius	55.98 (10)	51.3	74.0	7.50
Ulna	71.62 (5)	65.0	81.0	7.48
Femur	83.80 (5)	70.6	109.3	15.37
Tibia	66.30 (3)	61.2	70.0	4.57
Fibula	65.70 (3)	62.1	68.0	3.16

status or affiliation. This may account for the lack of a clear pattern of sex dimorphism in the skeletal anatomy of the Inamgaon adults.

3.2.2. Osteometry of the newborn. All infant long bones that were complete and well preserved were measured with a Helios dial caliper. Due to the incomplete representation of all long bones of individuals from all age groups, detailed analysis of skeletal growth is not possible for the Inamgaon series. However, the age group from 0 to 6 months of age contained enough specimens to give an approximate mean long-bone length. The mean diaphyseal length of the six primary long bones for Inamgaon infants (0–6 months) are given in Table VI with minimum and maximum values and standard deviation. Because data for skeletal growth of long bones for South Asian populations is unknown to me, the Inamgaon data are compared with figures for Arikara new-

Table VII
Comparison of Mean Long-bone Lengths of Inamgaon Infants and Arikara Indians

	Inamgaon[a] (0–6 mo)		Arikara[b] newborn		Arikara[c] (0–6 mo)	
Bone	$\bar{X}$	(n)	$\bar{X}$	Range	$\bar{X}$	(n)
Humerus	73.0	(9)	66.0	63.5–71.5	70.5	(49)
Radius	56.0	(10)	55.0	50.5–60.0	57.4	(47)
Ulna	71.6	(5)	63.0	60.5–70.0	66.1	(47)
Femur	83.8	(5)	75.0	73.5–81.5	82.2	(51)
Tibia	66.3	(3)	67.0	63.0–74.5	71.6	(47)
Fibula	65.7	(3)	63.0	60.0–69.5	68.9	(37)

[a]This study.
[b]Stewart (1979).
[c]Merchant and Ubelaker (1977).

Table VIII
Occurrence of Superficial Porotic Hyperostosis

Specimen number	Age in months	Layer	Cultural phase	Bones affected
86	12–18 mo	8	Early Jorwe	Two fragmentary long bones: (1) ?femur (2) ?tibia
96	4–5 mo	5	Late Jorwe	Two long bones: (1) distal tibia (2) unidentifiable fragment
133	24 mo	15	Malwa	One long bone: (1) tibia
145	24–36 mo	4	Late Jorwe	Three ribs and four long bones: (1) two humeri (2) tibia (3) fibula
147	6–12 mo	2	Late Jorwe	One long bone: (1) tibia
156	12–14 mo	4	Late Jorwe	Two long bones: (1) tibia (2) unidentifiable fragment

born (Stewart, 1979) and the 0–6-month age group (Merchant and Ubelaker, 1977). The length of Inamgaon long bones compare favorably with both newborn and the 0–6-month age group of the Arikara (see Table VIII). Comparable data for Indian populations would be very desirable, but they are unavailable at present.*

3.3. Paleopathology

A recent review of the literature on South Asian paleopathology is provided by Kennedy (1983); his valuable interpretations and summary provide a context for this discussion of paleopathology at Inamgaon. In the preliminary report on paleodemography at Inamgaon, Lukacs and Badam (1981) noted the absence of skeletal and dental lesions in the 46 immature specimens recovered prior to 1979. Pathological lesions were also reported as rare in the adult segment of this Inamgaon skeletal sample. Thorough macroscopic examination of the 123 skeletons recovered from Inamgaon since 1979 yields evidence of several new congenital and nutritional deficiency diseases. All of the pathological lesions described here are previously unreported for prehistoric South Asian skeletal series.

3.3.1. Skeletal and dental lesions of immature individuals. The most prevalent pathological lesion found in the subadult portion of the Inamgaon skeletal series is the superficial porotic hyperostosis (SPH). Six individuals be-

*Mr. Simons, a graduate student in the Department of Anatomy at B. J. Medical College, Pune, is analyzing long-bone lengths of stillbirths and neonatal deaths as part of his dissertation research project.

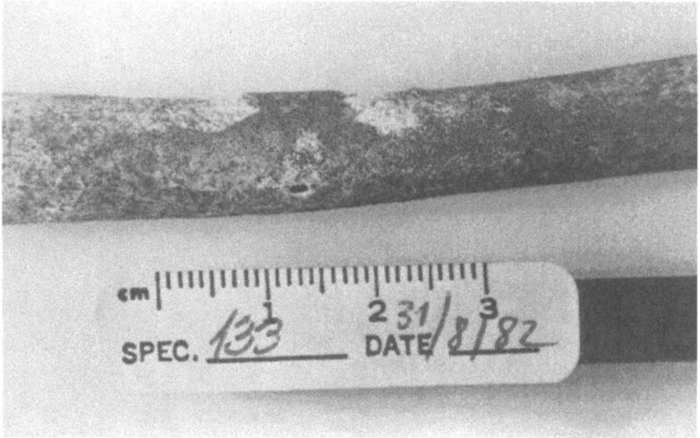

Figure 6. Superficial porotic hyperostosis on the diaphysis of the right tibia of INM 133.

tween the ages of 4 months and 3 years exhibit ossified SPH on one or more of their long bones (Figure 6). Details regarding afflicted specimens are provided in Table VIII, which shows that individuals with ossified SPH are found in all three cultural phases, and that the tibia is the most frequently affected bone. The frequency of occurrence of SPH among infants for all cultural phases combined is 4.85% (n = 5/103), whereas the incidence of these lesions in each cultural phase is primarily a function of differences in sample size (Malwa = 6.7%, n = 1/15; Early Jorwe = 3.7%, n = 1/27; Late Jorwe = 4.29%, n = 3/61).

Interpreting the etiology of these lesions is difficult because several different causes may be responsible. Infantile scurvy, or Barlow's disease, produces ossified SPH. These lesions commonly occur in individuals between 6 months and 1 year of age, and severe cases are frequently fatal (Steinbock, 1976). Paleobotanical evidence from Inamgaon confirms that sources of ascorbic acid (vitamin C) were not abundant locally (Kajale, 1977). These data suggest infantile scurvy as a probable cause for the SPH lesions observed in the Inamgaon infants. Two additional diseases, infantile cortical hyperostosis (Caffey's disease) and hypervitaminosis A, cannot be excluded as causal agents because both produce similar lesions in immature individuals (Saul, personal communication).

Two subadolescent individuals from Late Jorwe levels at Inamgaon exhibit pathological lesions that have tentatively been identified as cranial yaws and trigonocephaly. The external surface of the occipital bone of specimen 196, a 7- or 8-year-old child, exhibits an elliptical depression 13 mm long and 9 mm wide, with a slightly raised rim of smooth compact bone (Figure 7). Coarsely textured porous bone lines the floor of this depression, and the internal surface of the occipital bone is unaffected and appears normal. Though this lesion compares favorably with photographs and descriptions of cranial yaws, two points make

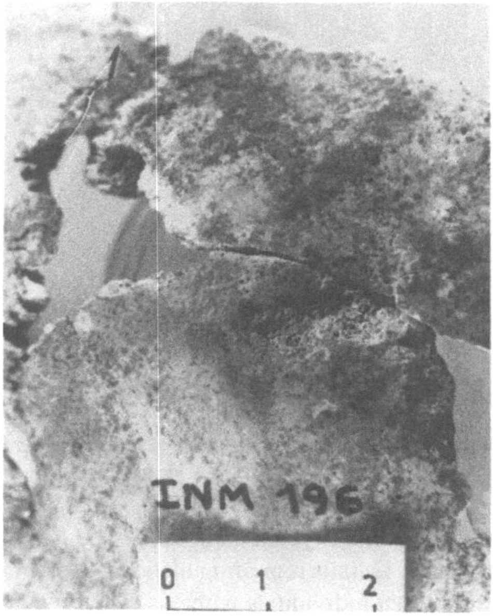

Figure 7. Osteolytic lesion on the occipital bone of INM 196.

this attribution uncertain: (1) cranial yaws most frequently affect the frontal bone and the frontal of specimen 196 is unaffected; and (2) in severe cases of yaws, phalanges and long bones may also be affected and in specimen 196 they are not. If confirmed, the presence of this highly contagious treponemal infection at Inamgaon would not be surprising because it occurs in high frequency today in tropical and predominantly agricultural countries like India and Africa.

Prominent midsagittal keeling of the frontal bone is present in specimen H-105, a child of 5 or 6 years of age at death (Figure 8). Above each orbit, the frontal bone is flatter than normal and is angulated toward a conspicuous elevated ridge between glabella and bregma. Keeling is absent from the partial bones of this individual, though this is a more common site for midsagittal elevation of the cranial vault in some fossil hominids and modern human populations. Premature closure of the metopic suture is the most likely cause of frontal keeling in this specimen. It imparts a very narrow appearance to the frontal bone and to the upper facial region of this individual. This is the only instance of trigonocephaly known to me from the Indian subcontinent.

The frontal bone of specimen H-105 is undamaged in the supraglabellar region; consequently, the observed flexure of the frontal bone cannot be attributed to imprecise reconstruction. This specimen has been exposed to fire, and many of the cranial, dental, and postcranial elements are blackened. The smooth, uncracked, and unwarped surface of all blackened bones indicates that once

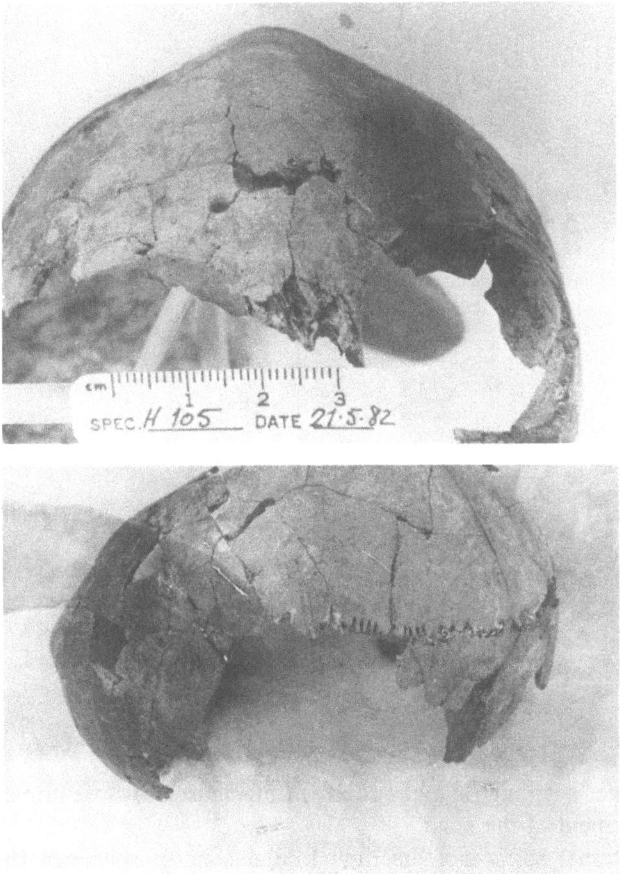

Figure 8. Sagittal keeling of the frontal bone of specimen H 105; (a) inferior frontal view; (b) *Norma Superioris*.

defleshed, dry bone was exposed to a fire of low heat, probably unintentionally. Exposure to fire can confidently be excluded as a possible cause for midsagittal keeling of the frontal bone of specimen H-105.

Additional skeletal anomalies occur in the immature segment of the Inamgaon series, but these will only be briefly described here because a more complete description and interpretation will be published separately, as mentioned previously. The cranial base of specimen INM-198 (5–6 years of age at death) exhibits a prominent tuberosity (10–11 mm in diameter) at the posteriolateral margin of the left occipital condyle (Figure 9). The *rectus capitis lateralis* muscle inserts in this region on the jugular process of the occipital bone. The prominence of this tuberosity on the left side, and its complete absence on the

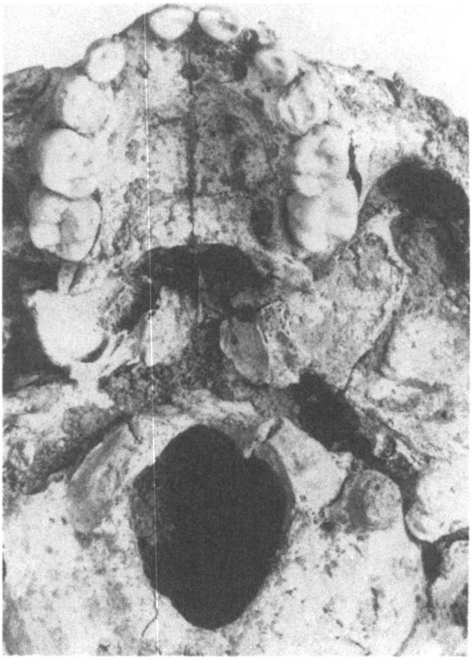

Figure 9. Juxta-condylar tuberosity of INM 198.

right, indicates asymmetric hypertrophy of this muscle, whose prime function is lateral movement of the head.

The internal surface of the right frontal bone of specimen INM-226, an infant, exhibits hyperostosis of cancellous bone. The areas affected include the anterior and lateral portions of the endocranial surface of the frontal. This lesion is not due to hyperostosis of the diplöe, but to sub-periosteal ossification on the surface of the inner table of the frontal bone. The significance of this lesion is undetermined, though it may have resulted from a hereditary hemolytic anemia, such as thalassemia or sickle-cell anemia, trauma, or an ossified hemorrhage.

The dental health of the immature individuals from Inamgaon is very good. The frequency of dental caries and gross enamel hypoplasias in the deciduous dentition is very low. An unusual anomaly that occurs with low frequency in the Inamgaon primary teeth is best described as a congenital/developmental enamel deficiency. These lesions are characterized by incomplete formation of enamel in certain areas of the tooth crown resulting in a circular depression in the enamel. These depressions are several millimeters in diameter, of varying depth, and primarily occur in the occlusal surface of the deciduous first molar teeth and on the labial surface of deciduous canine teeth (Figure 10). In some individuals,

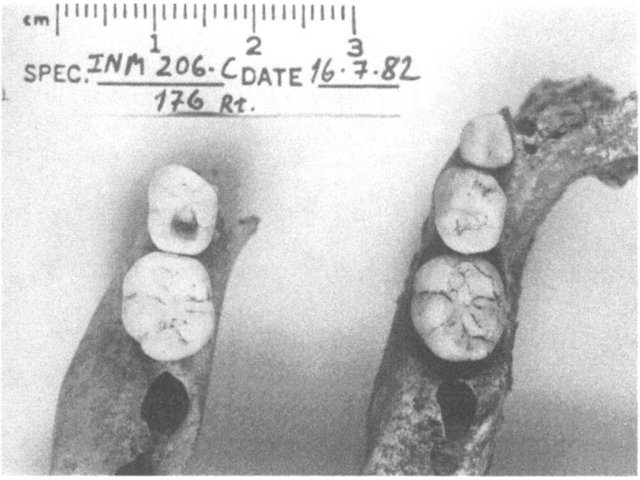

Figure 10. Enamel deficiency defect on occlusal surface of ldm_1 of INM 206-C. The normal ldm_1 of INM 176 is provided for comparison.

these lesions are bilaterally present, and lesions may occur on both deciduous canine and deciduous first molar teeth of the same individual. These lesions were also found in the maxillary and mandibular permanent molar teeth of specimens from Inamgaon and from other prehistoric sites in western and southern India (Lukacs, 1983). Histological analyses of these lesions will be conducted in order to determine the precise mode of their formation and their etiology.

3.3.2. Paleopathology of adult specimens. Pathological lesions were less frequent in the adult segment of the Inamgaon skeletal series. The most common affliction is thickening of the parietal and occipital bones in association with varying degrees of osteoporosis. One specimen, INM-168-A, exhibits very thick parietal bones (max. 13.0 mm) and cribra orbitalia of the right lacrimal fossa (Figure 11). Though these two lesions often appear together in individuals with severe iron-deficiency anemia, it is possible that the cribra orbitalia in this individual may be caused by irritation of the lacrimal gland (Steinbock, 1976, p. 243). The location of these hyperostosis lesions on the cranial vault suggests that iron-deficiency anemia is a more likely causal agent than hereditary hemolytic anemias.

Osteophytic lipping occurs on lumbar vertebrae of several individuals in this series. The size of osteophytes are usually small to medium in most individuals. However, specimen INM-200 (male, 35–40 years) exhibits large "parrots-beak" osteophytic projections in the lumbar region, bony ankylosis of two thoracic vertebrate, and ankylosis of a third thoracic vertebra is imminent.

Spina bifida occulta is present in the sacrum of specimen INM-146-A

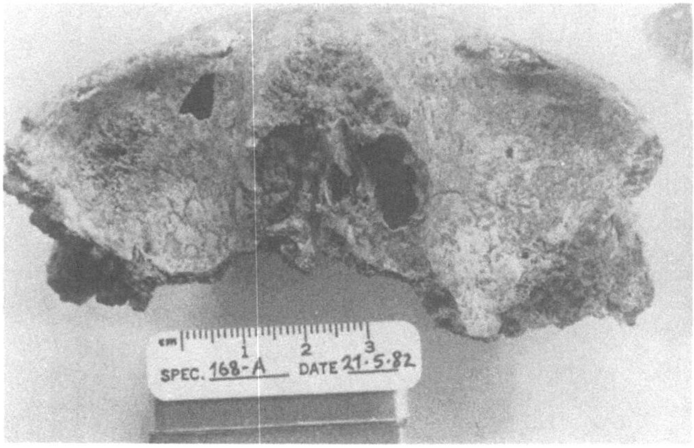

Figure 11. Unilateral *cribra orbitalia* of the right orbit of INM 168-A.

(female, 30–40 years); the neural arches failed to form on part of the third, fourth, and fifth sacral vertebrae.

Dental health of the adult individuals at Inamgaon is good; dental caries and gross enamel hypoplasia are low in frequency. The most common dental problem is antemorten tooth loss, a condition found in nearly all individuals over about 35 years of age. Adolescents and young adults appear to have very healthy dental arcades, but the stress of heavy mastication and the associated severe dental attrition (rather than caries) appears to be the primary cause of early tooth loss. Generally, only one or two teeth were lost antemortem, as in specimens INM-59 and INM-106, each having lost one lower molar tooth, and INM-116, which lost two lower molars. A higher incidence of antemortem tooth loss afflicted specimens INM 146-A and 146-B; the former lost four teeth, the latter, eight teeth antemortem. Upper and lower jaws were affected in both individuals, and the most frequently affected tooth class was the molar (Figure 12).

Conclusions

The major conclusions derived from this analysis of 176 individuals from the early farming village of Inamgaon are the following.

1. Biases in the representation of different age groups at Inamgaon is due to different burial practices for infants and children as opposed to adults.
2. The distribution of specimens by cultural phase is biased primarily by the more extensive excavation of later cultural horizons. These biases preclude any meaningful analysis of the Inamgaon skeletal series from the perspective of survivorship or mortality rates.

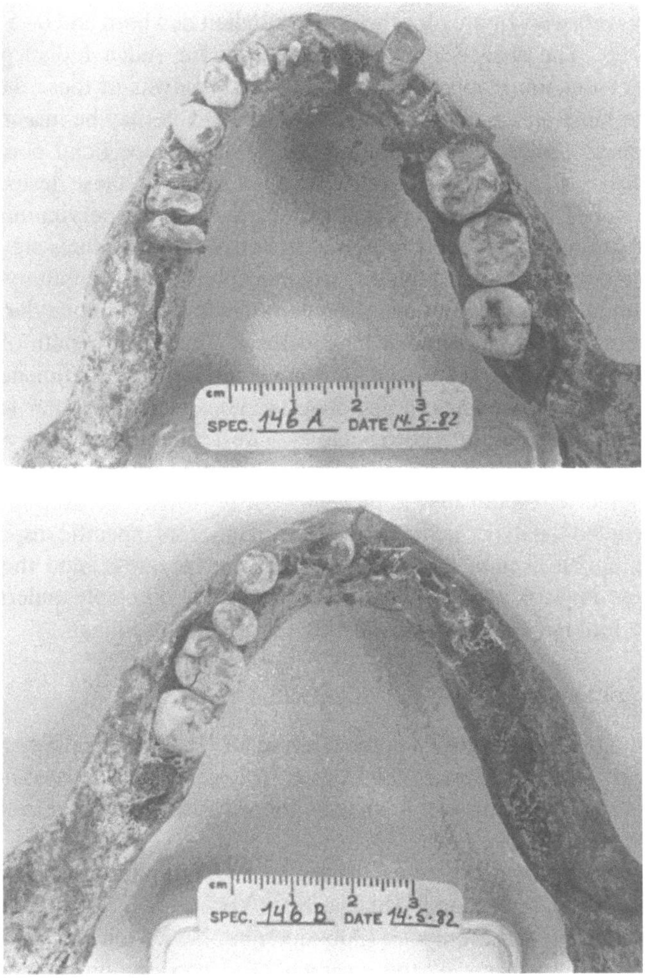

Figure 12. Superior view of mandibles of INM 146-A and B, showing tooth loss and alveolar resorption.

3. The adult phenotype of the Inamgaon skeletal series exhibits close similarity to other Chalcolithic populations of the Deccan Plateau—Nevasa in particular. Although sexual dimorphism can be noted in certain cranial and mandibular measurements and in stature, in general it is small. Males tend to be somewhat gracile in skeletal structure, and females exhibit robusticity, especially in the postcranial skeleton but also in the skull.
4. The mean length of long bones of Inamgaon infants compares reasona-

bly well with figures for the Arikara Indian newborn and 0–6 month age group. The absence of comparable data for Asian Indian populations precludes more appropriate comparative analysis of these data.
5. The most prevalent infant disease at Inamgaon may be infantile scurvy, with six individuals exhibiting one or more superficial porotic hyperostosis. Caution is necessary because some of these lesions may be produced by infantile cortical hyperostosis and hypervitaminosis A.
6. Additional skeletal lesions found in immature individuals are interpreted as evidence of cranial yaws, trigonocephaly, and hereditary hemolytic anemia. Anomalous bone growths include a juxta-condylar tuberosity and a case of endocranial hyperostosis. The dental health of immature individuals was very good, but congenital enamel deficiencies appear with low frequencies in deciduous canines and first molar teeth.
7. Skeletal lesions in adult specimens are less common, but evidence of iron-deficiency anemia, osteophytosis, spina bifida occulta, and early antemortem tooth loss is present.
8. Detailed analytic and comparative studies of specific aspects of the Inamgaon skeletal series are currently in progress, and the results of these investigations will contribute to a more complete understanding of the biological adaptations of this early farming village.

ACKNOWLEDGMENTS

The authors express their appreciation to Dr. H. D. Sankalia (past director) and Dr. S. B. Deo (director) of the Deccan College Post-Graduate and Research Institute (Pune) for permission to analyze the valuable human skeletal collection from Inamgaon.

The senior author expresses thanks to Dr. William Alexander (Eugene, Oregon) Dr. K. A. R. Kennedy (Ithaca, New York), Dr. Frank P. Saul (Toledo, Ohio), and Dr. R. Ted Steinbock (Albuquerque, New Mexico), with whom he discussed specific aspects of the research. The cooperation of these scholars contributed to the improvement of this final draft.

The authors wish to thank Dr. Donald C. Dunbar and Miss Rebecca Kimbrell for assistance in the preparation and analysis of skeletal remains during part of the 1982 field season. The senior author appreciates the patient assistance and encouragement of his wife, Shirley—a valuable source of inspiration.

References

Athawale, M. C., 1963, Estimation of height from lengths of forearm bones: A study of one hundred Maharashtrian male adults of ages between twenty-five and thirty years. *Am. J. Phys. Anthropol.* **21**:105–112.

Banherjee, P., and Mukherjee, S., 1967, Eruption of deciduous teeth among Bengalee children. *Am. J. Phys. Anthropol.* **26**:357.

Basu, A., and A. Pal, 1980, Human remains from Burzahom, *Mem. Anthropol. Surv. India* **56**:1–90.

Bernhard, W., 1967, Human skeletal remains from the cemetery of Timargarha, *Anc. Pakistan* **3**:291–407.

Bernhard, W., 1969, Human skeletal remains from the prehistoric cemetery of Sarai Khola, *Pakistan Archaeol.* **6**:100–116.

Bernhard, W., 1981, Ethnic and morphological affinities of the Iron Age cemetery of Sarai Khola near Taxila (Pakistan), *J. Mediterranean Anthropol. and Archaeol.* **1**:180–210.

Brothwell, D. R., 1963, The macroscopic dental pathology of some earlier human populations, in: *Den. Anthropol.* (D. R. Brothwell, ed.), Pergamon Press, London, pp. 271–288.

Brothwell, D., 1972, *Digging up Bones,* 2d ed., British Museum (Natural History), London.

Buikstra, J., and Cook, D. C., 1980, Paleopathology: An American account. *Annu. Rev. Anthropol.* **9**:433–470.

Deo, S. B., and Ansari, Z. D., 1965, *Chalcolithic Chandoli,* Deccan Coll. Post-graduate and Research Institute, Pune.

Glickman, I., 1964, *Clinical Periodontology,* W. B. Saunders, Philadelphia.

Gupta, P., Dutta, P. C., and Basu, A., 1962, Human Remains from Harappa. Mem. Anthropol. Surv. of India **9**:3–186.

Hunt, E. E., and Gleiser, E., 1959, The estimation of age and sex of preadolescent children from their bones and teeth, *Am. J. Phys. Anthropol.* **13**:479–487.

Kajale, M. D., 1977, Plant Economy at Inamgaon, *Man and Environment* **1**:54–56.

Karve, I., 1948, Anthropometric Measurements of the Marathas. Deccan College Monog. Ser. No. 2, Pune, pp. 1–71.

Kennedy, K. A. R., 1983, Growth, nutrition and pathology in changing paleodemographic settings in South Asia, in: *Paleopathology and Socio-economic change at the origins of agriculture* (M. Cohen and G. Armelagos, eds.), (in press).

Kennedy, K. A. R., and Malhotra, K. C., 1966, Human skeletal remains from Chalcolithic and Indo-Roman levels from Nevasa: An anthropometric and comparative analysis, *Deccan Coll. Build., Centen. and Silver Jubilee Ser.* **55**:1–135.

Lukacs, J. R., and Badam, G. L., 1975, Bio-anthropology of human skeletal remains from Inamgaon, West India, *Curr. Anthropol.* **16**(4):667–668.

Lukacs, J. R., and Badam, G. L., 1976–1977, Biological anthropology of human skeletal remains from Chalcolithic Inamgaon, western India, *Bull. Deccan Coll. Res. Inst.,* **36**:73–83.

Lukacs, J. R., and Badam, G. L., 1981, Paleodemography of post-Harappan Inamgaon: A preliminary report, *J. Indian Anthropol. Soc.* **16**:59–74.

Lukacs, J. R., 1983, Dental morphology and the biological affinities of the people of Inamgaon. Paper presented at a conference, Recent Advances in Indian Archaeology, Pune, India, December 9–12, 1983.

Lukacs, J. R., and Walimbe, S. R., 1983, *Physical anthropology of human skeletal remains from prehistoric Inamgaon: An osteobiographic analysis,* Deccan Coll. Post-Graduate and Research Institute, Pune. (In prep.)

Lukacs, J. R., Joshi, M. R., and Makhija, P. G., 1983, Deciduous tooth crown dimensions in living and prehistoric populations of western India. *Am. J. Phys. Anthropol.* **61**(3):383–387.

Lukacs, J. R., Bogorad, R., Walimbe, S. R., and Dunbar, D. C., 1983, Paleopathology at Inamgaon: an early farming village in western India. *Am. J. Phys. Anthropol.* (in press).

Malhotra, K. C., 1965, Human skeletal remains from Chandoli, in: *Chalcolithic Chandoli* (S. B. Deo and Z. D. Ansari, eds.), Deccan Coll. Pune, pp. 143–184.

Merchant, V. L., and Ubelaker, D. H., 1977, Skeletal growth of the protohistoric Arikara, *Am. J. Phys. Anthropol.* **46**:61–72.

Mukherjee, D. K., 1973, Deciduous dental eruption in low income group Bengali Hindu children. *J. Trop. Pediatr. Env. Child Hlth.* **19**:207–210.

Olivier, G., 1969, *Practical Anthropology*, Charles C Thomas Publishers, Springfield, Illinois.

Ortner, D. J., and Putschar, W. G. J., 1981, Identification of pathological conditions in human skeletal remains, *Smithsonian Contrib. to Anthropol.* **28,** Smithsonian Institution Press, Washington, D.C.,

Prakash, S., 1974, A note on the estimation of age from deciduous teeth. *Eastern Anthropol.* **27**(3):263–265.

Rami Reddy, V., 1981, Eruption of deciduous teeth among the children of Gulbarga, South India, *Indian J. Med. Res.* **73**:772–781.

Schour, I., and Massler, M., 1940, Studies in tooth development: The growth pattern of human teeth, *J. Amer. Dent. Assoc.* **27**:1778–1793, 1918–1931.

Srinivasan, S., and Gulati, R. K., 1973, The Bhils of west Khandesh (Maharashtra), *Bull. Deccan Coll. Res. Inst. C.* **31/32**:301–316.

Steinbock, R. T., 1976, *Paleopathological Diagnosis and Interpretation: Bone Disease in Ancient Human Populations*, Charles C Thomas Publisher, Springfield, Illinois.

Stewart, T. D., 1979, *The Essentials of Forensic Anthropology*, Charles C Thomas Publisher, Springfield, Ill.

Trotter, M., 1970, Estimation of stature from intact limb bones, in: *Personal Identification in Mass Disasters* (T. D. Stewart, ed.), National Museum of Natural History, Washington, D.C., pp. 71–83.

CHAPTER 7

Dental Anthropology of South Asian Populations: A Review

JOHN R. LUKACS

1. Introduction

Morphological and metrical variations of the human dentition have not been utilized to their full potential by anthropologists concerned with patterns of human biological variation in South Asia. While dental anthropology has contributed major insights into the evolution and migration of many of the world's populations, physical anthropology in South Asia consists primarily of traditional descriptions of the anthropometric, dermatoglyphic, and immunogenetic characteristics of the subcontinent's diverse populations.

The recent appearance of numerous publications on the dental variation of Indian populations prompts one to ask several questions: (1) why has evidence of the human dentition been disregarded by both Indian and Western scholars in the anthropological study of South Asian people; (2) what factors contributed to the recent emergence of dental anthropology as a viable and promising research orientation in South Asian anthropology; and (3) what conclusions can be drawn from existing data on dental morphology and tooth size regarding the biological relationships and evolutionary trends in South Asian populations?

These queries are best answered by tracing the origin, historical development, and recent rapid growth of dental anthropology in South Asia. This histor-

---

JOHN R. LUKACS • Department of Anthropology, University of Oregon, Eugene, Oregon 97403. The fieldwork and library research on which this paper is based was supported by grants from the American Institute of Indian Studies (1974–1975, 1982); Fulbright-Hays Program (1981–1982); Indo-American Fellowship Program (1979) and Smithsonian Institution (1982). The author is indebted to these institutions for their continued research support.

ical literature review provides a summary overview of the development of dental anthropology as a research orientation in South Asian anthropology. The literature cited was selected to document major landmarks and trends in the history of the discipline and is not intended to be an exhaustive reference bibliography.

2. Dental Variation in Living South Asians

2.1. Early Studies of Dental Variation

The first discussions of South Asian dental variation encountered in the anthropological literature are by European anthropologists employing dental traits as racial markers. These early works are of two broad types: population descriptions and comparative surveys. In the first approach, evidence of the dentition is systematically collected and analyzed as one part of a general anthropometric and serological description of a specific population. The Andaman Islanders figure prominently in this early descriptive literature, and the studies of Flower (1880, 1885a) and Owen (1863) are characteristic of this approach. Both writers include basic observations on tooth size, attrition, and dental health in their osteological investigations, the primary objective of which was to ascertain the racial stock to which the Andamanese were most closely related.

In the second approach, data on tooth size and morphology of South Asian populations were presented as part of a comparative survey of dental variation in the races of the world. Flower's (1885b) use of 42 crania of "low caste natives of Central and Southern India (mostly male)" in formulating the Dental Index as a racial characteristic is a classic example. The world's races were grouped into microdont, mesodont, and megadont categories for this index, which was calculated by dividing the dental length (from the mesial surface of P^3 to the distal surface of M^3) by basion–nasion length. European, British, and Asian Indian populations were found to be microdont, while African, American Indian, and Asian groups were classified as mesodont. Megadont races included Melanesians, Anadamanese, Australians, and Tasmanians.

Two decades later, De Terra (1905) included seven Tamil and five Singhalese skulls in his monograph on the odontography of human races. This work is organized geographically (by continent) and presents data on length and breadth of the dental crown, cusp number, and groove pattern of molar teeth, premolar shape, and root variations. Maximum and minimum figures are reported for crown dimensions, rather than mean values that are commonly used today. De Terra found that Tamil and Singhalese samples were in the mesodont range for Flower's Dental Index.

In these comparative surveys of dental variation, data from South Asia was not the prime focus of study but was presented in the context of worldwide patterns of dental variation. Early studies of this kind provided useful baseline data on tooth size and morphology for many populations, but because the proveniences, ages, and sexes of the skeletal remains from non-European countries were not reported, the anthropological value of the South Asian data is limited. Though some European populations in De Terra's survey are represented by adequate numbers of specimens, the small sample size of many non-European populations, including the Tamil and Singhalese, make one believe that sampling error is involved. It is with these publications that the discipline of dental anthropology began to develop in South Asia. Unfortunately, these valuable contributions to the anthropology of South Asia were not followed by more intensive and systematic study of the dentitions of larger and more carefully selected samples.

The early 20th century witnessed rapid growth in the field of dental anthropology and evolution, which was attributable in part to the discovery of fossil hominid remains and the need for a comparative framework of dental variation in modern human populations. At this time, the human dentition was analyzed in considerable detail from phylogenetic (Gregory, 1916, 1922; Gregory and Hellman, 1926), ontogenetic (Bolk, 1914), and racial perspectives (Hellman, 1928). The voluminous literature on population variation in the size and morphology of teeth cannot be documented here for lack of space. However, a cursory review of major contributions to the literature of dental anthropology during the second and third decades of the 20th century reveals that South Asian populations were *not* a focus of investigation. During this period, Campbell (1925) reported on the dentition and palate of the Australian aboriginals; Drennan (1929) described dental variation of African Bushmen; Leigh (1925 a,b, 1929, 1930) investigated the dental pathology and morphology of American Indians, Eskimos, and the prehistoric inhabitants of Guam; and Shaw (1931) analyzed the teeth, bony palates and mandibles of the Bantu of equatorial and southern Africa. Though monographic publications on the dentition of many of the world's populations clearly begins at this time, reports on South Asian populations are conspicuous by their absence. More recently, thorough descriptive analyses of the dentition of East Greenland Eskimo (Pedersen, 1949), Norwegian Lapps (Selmer-Olsen, 1949), American Indians (Dahlberg, 1951), Aleuts (Moorrees, 1957), Arctic peoples (Turner, 1967), and South African blacks (Jacobson, 1982) have been published. Comprehensive and systematic analysis of the dentition of South Asian populations has not yet been conducted.

Considerable progress was made during the 1920s in documenting variation in the frequency of occurrence of specific dental traits among the world's populations. The classical investigations of Hrdlička (1920) on shovel-shaped incisor teeth and Hellman (1928) on lower molar cusp number and groove pattern do not contain data for South Asian populations. In addition to American whites and black samples, Hrdlička's study included Chinese, Hawaiian, and Japanese groups. Hellman presents data for American white and blacks, Chinese, Eskimo, European, and Mongol (the Buriat of Central Asia) groups, but not South Asians. It is interesting to note that Hellman depicts the mandible of a "Hindu male" to illustrate changes in cusp number and groove pattern in the first and second molar teeth (Hellman 1928, p. 163, Fig. 5), but no data are provided for Hindu samples.

Recent surveys of the worldwide variation in the tooth-crown morphology of living populations include as *Asian* primarily people of eastern Asia and the New World (Cadien, 1972). Data for South Asian populations are frequently *not* included in such surveys. Surprisingly, a recent review of current knowledge on variation in expression of Carabelli's trait and the canine distal accessory ridge throughout the world *does* include data for "Asiatic Indians" (Scott, 1977, 1980). However, this sample is an immigrant Indian community in South Africa, and the precise geographic, social, and religious roots of the people in India are not well known (Scott and Morris, personal communication). Immigrant Indian settlements are often ethnically, socially, and religiously heterogeneous groups, and it is likely that this sample includes members of more than one endogamous group (Schwartz, 1967).

Following the pattern of Flower and Owen, Bowles (1943) included observations on dental variation in conjunction with anthropometric and linguistic evidence in reaching conclusions on the racial affinities of the Munda of India. The frequency of shovel-shaped incisor teeth among the Bhotia, Kanawri, Khasi, and Manchati were reported by Bowles (1943).

Comprehensive data on the physical anthropology of Ceylonese populations was collected by Marett between 1937 and 1939 as one phase of the Ethnological Survey of Ceylon. Serving as an assistant in ethnology at the Colombo National Museum, Marett gathered data on tooth eruption, dental crowding, tooth size, and caries, along with standard anthropometric observations. Unfortunately, the dental data were very crudely assembled with no meaningful standardization or quantitative assessment of dental variations. All observations were anthroposcopic and grouped into two or three categories; tooth eruption was judged as complete or incomplete; tooth size as large, medium, or small. Traditional anthrometric methods in which Marett had been instructed by Hooton at Harvard were rigorously applied, and the resulting data were later statistically summarized and interpreted by Stoudt (1961). The absence of high standards in the collection of dental data is lamentable, because this survey had the potential to be the earliest thorough analysis of South Asian dental variation.

Unquestionably, the first substantive investigations of dental morphology in South Asia were conducted by Tratman (1938, 1950). A practicing dentist at the dental school and clinic of King Edward VII Medical College, Singapore, Tratman amassed considerable data on tooth crown and root variations of his patients. The extracted teeth of a variety of immigrant populations, including South Indian (mostly Tamil), Malay, and Chinese, formed the basis for his investigations. His research is the first to describe and compare the dental features of South Asians with those of other populations on the basis of large samples of known provenience. Turner (1971) recognizes Tratman (1938) as the first scholar to discover the "racial" significance of three-rooted mandibular first molars, a trait that he found in high frequency in Asiatic populations. Unfortunately, dental trait frequencies are not reported in Tratman's (1950) classic study that characterized the main differences between the Indo-European and the Mongoloid dental patterns. Nevertheless, this publication became a landmark in anthropological research because it emphasized the patterned distribution of multiple dental traits and demonstrated the uniqueness of the Mongoloid dentition. Tratman (1950) found that the Mongoloid dentition exhibited high frequencies of shovel-shaped incisor teeth, shortness of roots, crowns situated at an angle on the roots, three-rooted mandibular molar teeth, wrinkled occlusal surface of molar teeth, enamel extensions and pearls, and a low frequency of Carabelli's trait. Observations and comparative studies were also conducted on the congenital absence of teeth and supernumerary teeth (Tratman and Chiam, 1941).

Tratman's contributions to the dental anthropology of South Asian populations are historically significant, but a few limitations should not be overlooked. His perception of the Indian phenotypic pattern as uniform overlooks small-scale dental differences that may characterize regional populations of the subcontinent. Though these have yet to be defined, anthropologists today would dispute the practice of lumping Tamil, Sikh, Telugu, and Malabari populations into one pool for anthropological investigation.

The research was conducted as a by-product of his dental practice rather than as an exclusively anthropological research project. While it can be disputed whether the consequent sampling bias had an effect on the results of the investigation, it is apparent that much of the meager data for tooth size and morphology published on South Asian populations during the 1960s and 1970s is similarly derived from studies conducted in dental hospitals and clinics. The research was usually done by clinically oriented dental practitioners, sometimes on patients, but often on dental students with healthy teeth (Babbar, 1963; Biviji, Shourie, Baldev Singh, and Menezes, 1967; Biviji and Bhatt, 1971; Joshi *et al.*, 1972). The primary focus of these later studies was to generate data that would clarify the relationship between tooth size, crowding, and malocclusion. The ethnic composition of all the samples is heterogeneous, severely limiting the anthropological value of the data. Frequently, these publications report only mesiodistal dimensions of the dental crown.

2.2. Recent Anthropological Analyses of Dental Variation

The description and comparative analysis of dental morphology and tooth size in living and skeletal South Asian populations by trained anthropologists commenced in the 1960s and is characterized more by studies of dental morphology than by studies of dental crown dimensions. The Anthropological Survey of India (Calcutta) and Calcutta University figure prominently in early studies of dental variation in living and recent skeletal populations of India. Ganguly (1960), an officer of the Anthropological Survey, investigated shovel-shaped incisors and the frequency of missing incisors in the Nicobarese. His observations were made intraorally in living subjects. Anadi Pal (1964), a colleague of Ganguly's at the survey, reported the frequency of shovel-shaped incisors, tuberculum dentale, supernumerary teeth, missing teeth, attrition, and caries of the people of eastern India. Cusp number and groove pattern in a series of modern Hindu crania were reported by Pal (1967), but the provenience of the series, now housed with the Anthropological Survey, is not stated. This research was followed by an investigation of incisor shoveling among the Andaman Islanders (Pal, 1972) in which both skeletal remains and intraoral observations were used.

Banerjee (1963, 1964, 1967) reported the incidence of congenitally missing teeth and root number of premolars and molars in a collection of 93 crania and 87 mandibles from Midnapur District, West Bengal. Joshi *et al.* (1972) employed plaster casts in their analysis of variation in Carabelli's trait among Gujarati Hindu children in Ahmedabad.

Though anthropological in orientation and subscribing to accepted standards of dental analysis (Hrdlička, 1920; Hellman, 1928; Dahlberg, 1951, 1963; Kraus, 1951), these studies suffered from sampling problems. When living populations were investigated, no attempt was made to analyze endogamous groups separately. In addition, the skeletal series employed in these studies originated either through the collection of unclaimed bodies from Calcutta or corpses collected following a famine or drought in rural areas surrounding Calcutta. Consequently, the endogamous group or religious affiliation of individuals in these skeletal series are not known with any certainty, thus limiting the anthropological value of these data.

Since 1972, studies of dental morphology in living South Asians have been based on the analysis of plaster dental casts. Series of dental casts become valuable research tools because they may be referred to repeatedly for data verification, and they can provide data not only for dental morphologists but for studies of crown dimensions, arch shape, and occlusion.

While Prakash and Sharma (1972) described and compared dental arch shapes of the Jats, Sharma and Kaul (1977) reported on morphological features of the Punjabi dentition based on a sample of 80 individuals. Odontometry, morphological features of anterior and posterior teeth, and occlusal variation were also reported for Punjabis by Sharma and Kaul (1977). Subsequently, comparative studies of the dental features of Bhutanese (Prakash, Kaul, and Kanta, 1978) and Jats (Bhasin, Sharma, and Singh, 1979; Kaul and Prakash, 1981) were conducted. This was the first time that dental features of deciduous teeth were reported for an Indian population (Kaul and Prakash, 1981).

Morphological variations in Bengali and Maharashtrian dentitions were described by Lukacs (1977) who also presented data on dental crown dimensions. The joint Indo-Soviet anthropological expedition of 1971 included in its final report a detailed analysis of the dental morphology of five endogamous groups from Delhi (Zubov, 1980). These studies were based on dental casts made in India and subsequently analyzed in the United States and in Russia.

The incidence of shovel-shaped incisors, Carabelli's trait, cingulum variations, third-molar agenesis and diastema were reported for the Pattusalis (Rami Reddy *et al.*, 1982a) and Muslims (Rami Reddy *et al.*, 1982b) of Andhra Pradesh. The frequencies of incisor shoveling in deciduous and permanent teeth of the people of Gulbarga (Karnataka) were analyzed by Rami Reddy (MS I, MS II). These studies of the dental morphology of Dravidian-speaking people are based on intraoral observation and are the only recent studies of South Indian dental variation known. A small sample of dental casts has been made of Ladaki children of Leh (Jammu-Kashmir) by N. Ohnu. Though his research is in progress, the specific nature of his analysis remains unknown (R. Mengi, personal communication).

Anthropological studies of South Asian dental crown dimensions in addition to those cited previously are relatively rare. Benyon (1971) reported on molar crown dimensions of male Afghan Tajik; and Sakai, Hanamura and Ohno (1971) give dental crown dimensions and indexes of the Pushtun and Tajik of Afghanistan. The occlusal surface index of molar teeth of Indians was found to be smaller than the indexes of both Australian and Japanese samples by Ozaki, Ohnuki, and Tsuruoka (1977).

2.3. A Comparative Review of Morphological and Metrical Data for South Asian Dentitions

Current knowledge of dental variation among living South Asians is presented in this section. A brief comparative analysis of dental morphology and crown dimensions is concluded with suggestions for further research. Close study of all the sources cited previously reveals that very few are useful in a comparative analysis of South Asian dental morphology. Factors that limit the value and hamper the comparability of these data include the following: (1) small sample sizes, (2) pooling the sexes, (3) combining different endogamous groups, and (4) using different standards for the evaluation of dental trait variation. In addition, results are often reported differently; some investigators use the tooth count method, whereas others use the more widely accepted individual count technique (Scott, 1980). Dental trait frequencies reported according to one method are not strictly comparable with data reported by the other method.

Some of these limitations may be overcome if data sets are carefully scrutinized for the following: (1) for consistency in trait-scoring standards (or carefully determining correspondences between different systems); (2) to be sure observations are limited to a single endogamous group; and (3) to be certain results are reported by the same method. These precautions were taken in preparing Table I, which contains frequency data for selected morphological traits in living South Asians. It is noteworthy that these data are almost exclusively for North Indian populations, and data for South Indian and tribal populations are unavailable.

Nine different studies are summarized in Table I. All are based on the individual count method, and the same standards were employed by most investigators. Where discrepancies occurred between trait evaluation standards, synonymies were established to enhance comparability of data sets. Most investigators followed traditional sources in their evaluation of dental trait expression: shovel shape (Hrdlička, 1920); Carabelli's trait (Kraus, 1951); hypocone (Dahlberg, 1951); cusp number and groove pattern (Hellman, 1928; Jørgensen, 1955). Variation in cusp 7 (metaconulid), deflecting wrinkle, and distal trigonid crest in the first mandibular molar teeth are reported only by Zubov who records as present only full expressions of these traits (Turner, personal communication). Trait-scoring methods of Zubov are further explained in his textbook on odontology (Zubov, 1968).

The analysis by Zubov (1980) is particularly valuable because of the following: (1) a single observer has collected data on five endogamous groups (Ahirs, Chamar, Gujar, Jat, and Rajput); (2) sample sizes are adequate; and (3) several less common but biologically significant traits (metaconulid, deflecting wrinkle, and trigonid crest) are reported. Zubov draws several important conclusions from these data. The groups studied exhibit an overall similarity to people of the "western odontological type"; this is reflected in the low frequency of shovel-shaped incisors and metaconulid, and the high incidence of four-cusped lower molar teeth. Signs of admixture from eastern (Asian) populations are indicated by increased frequency of the deflecting wrinkle, distal trigonid crest, and a corresponding decrease in incidence of Carabelli's trait. The Chamar dentition exhibits the most evidence of eastern influence of the five groups studied, particularly in showing the highest frequencies for the deflecting wrinkle and distal trigonid crest. The most western of the five groups is the Ahirs, who exhibit the highest frequency for Carabelli's trait and the lowest incidence of incisor shoveling. Though Chamars exhibit slight evidence of eastern admixture and Ahirs show some indication of western admixture, Zubov concludes that in their overall dental pattern the five groups studied are quite homogeneous.

Incisor shoveling, Carabelli's trait, and lower molar cusp and groove patterns have been independently reported for Jats by Bhasin *et al.* (1979), Kaul and Prakash (1981), and Zubov (1980). Striking differences occur between Zubov and the other two studies in the frequency of incisor shoveling and the expression of Carabelli's trait. In both instances, Zubov reports a much lower incidence for these dental features than Bhasin *et al.* or Kaul and Prakash. If Zubov's grade 1

Table I
Dental Trait Frequencies for Living South Asians (in percentages)

Morphological Trait	Ahir[a]	Chamar[a]	Gujar[a]	Rajput[a]	Jat[a]	Jat[b]	Jat[c]	Nicobar[d]	Asian Indian[e]	Tajik[f]	Bengali[g]	Bhutani[h]	Pushtun[i]	Tajik[i]	Eastern Indian[i]	Northern Indian[i]	Sherpa[i]
Shovel-shape (I¹)[1]																	
Absent	80.0	64.1	56.5	72.6	66.0	18.0	8.3	38 8	—	85.0	—	12.8	61.8	76 2	63.9	64.4	9.4
Trace	17.6	28.3	37.3	17.8	23.0	36.8	19.4	25.8		—	—	25.7	26.5	23.8	16.5	22.1	59.4
Semi	2.3	7.5	5.5	9.5	11.0	26.5	63.3	22.2		15.0	—	12.8	10.3	—	15.6	10.6	21.9
Marked						18.7	8.3	13.2		—		48.7	1.4	—	4.5	2.9	9.4
Carabelli's trait (M¹)[2]																	
Absent	43.6	61.5	62.3	60.9	50.6	34 2	38.8	—	37.8	59.0	—		40.9	63.6	—	20.2	53.1
Pit	28.2	21.9	14.8	22.8	28 2	26.0	41.6		31.6	—			23.9	9.1		40.4	21.9
Groove	21.8	9.8	11.8	14.1	16.5	17.8			21.5	41.0							
Small cusp	3.8	4.3	4.9	0.0	4.7	11.5	15.2		5.6	—			21.1	18.2		22.2	21.9
Large cusp	2.5	2.1	5.8	2.2	0.0	10.5	4.4		3.6	—			14.1	9.1		17.2	3.1
Hypocone (M¹)																	
4	94.5	96.2	100 0	89.0	96.2	82.1	—	—	—	—	97.5	—	7.2	82.6	—	100.0	100.0
4−	3.3	3.8	—	10.0	3.8	11.3				—	2.5		11.4	13.0		—	—
3+	1.1	—	—	—	—	6.6				—	—		1.4	—		—	—
3	1.1	—	—	1.0	—	—				—	—		—	4.4		—	—
Cusp number (M_1)																	
6	—	0.9	3.9	1.0	1.0	3.7	—	—	—	—	—	—	—	—	—	—	—
5	85.5	83.0	86.2	86.5	88.6	80.9	76.4			95.0	68 0	—	79.3	79.0		85.1	96.8
4	14.4	16.0	10.8	12.4	10.3	14.6	23.5			5.0	32.0	—	20 7	21.0		14.9	3.2
3	—	—	—	—	—	—	—			—	—	—	—	—		—	—
Groove pattern (M_1)																	
Y	59.0	67.9	56.9	69.0	58.7	60.7	58.5	—	—	—	—	—	83.2	66.7	—	80.5	64.5
+	33.7	30.1	41.1	26.8	36.0	29.9	33.8						16 8	33.3		19.5	35.5
X	7.2	1.9	2.9	4.1	5.2	9 4	7.3						—	—		—	—
Metaconulid (C-7, M_1)	3.4	1.0	3.9	2.9	1.1	—	—	—		—	—	—					
Deflecting wrinkle (M_1)	10.6	11.2	10.4	2.0	9.7	—	—			—	—	—					
Distal trigonid crest (M_1)	9.1	19.0	5 9	12.5	11.5	—	—			—	—	—					

[a]Zubov, 1980
[b]Kaul and Prakash, 1981
[c]Bhasin, Sharma, and Singh, 1979
[d]Ganguly, 1960
[e]Scott, 1980
[f]Benyon, 1971
[g]Banerjee, 1967
[h]Prakash, Kaul, and Kanta, 1979
[i]Ohnu, 1981

[1]Figures include semi and marked grades
[2]Figures include pit and groove grades

for shovel shape is taken as equivalent to Dahlberg's or Hrdlička's grade 0 (= absent), as Turner suggests, then the differences are even more striking (Turner, personal communication). Explaining these frequency differences is difficult. They may reflect sampling error, differences in trait gradation and scoring, or interobserver error. That such major differences in trait frequencies may accurately reflect the biological diversity of a single *jati* seems unlikely. In groove pattern and cusp number, a much greater level of agreement is attained. Bhasin *et al.* (1979) and Kaul and Prakash (1981) note a higher frequency of four-cusped lower first molar teeth than does Zubov (1980). They also report slightly higher frequencies for the X-groove pattern. These discrepancies are much less divergent than those mentioned previously for shovel-shaped incisors and Carabelli's trait.

In incisor shoveling, the Bhutanese exhibit the highest frequency (48.7%) of marked shovel (equivalent to the shovel category of Hrdlička, 1920). The only other groups for which similar high frequencies of marked (pronounced) shovel are reported include the Bhotia (44%) of the western Himalayas and the Khasi (32%) of Assam (Bowles, 1943). The Tajik of Afghanistan exhibit a low frequency of shoveling, with 85% (n = 30) of this small sample lacking any trace of marginal ridges (Benyon, 1971).

Similar levels of expression of Carabelli's trait are exhibited by Ahirs, Jats (Bhasin *et al.* [1979] and Kaul and Prakash's samples [1981]), and Scott's (1980) Asiatic Indian sample. By contrast, the small cusp form and the groove form of this polymorphic trait are reported in lower frequencies for Chamars, Gujars, and Rajputs (Zubov, 1980). The greatest frequency of Carabelli's cusp is recorded for Jats by Kaul and Prakash (1981) in which group the total frequency of small and large cusps together is 22%.

In lower first molar cusp number, Bengalis (Banerjee, 1967), like the Jats (Bhasin *et al.*, 1979; Kaul and Prakash, 1981), show the greatest reduction, exhibiting high frequencies of four-cusped teeth.

The dental morphology of eastern Indians from Calcutta, northern Indians from Lucknow, Sherpas of eastern Nepal, and Pushtun and Tajik of Afghanistan were recently reported by some Japanese odontologists (Sakai, Hanamura and Ohnu, 1969, 1970; Ohnu, 1981). They report dental trait frequencies based on the individual count method, and their results help broaden the data base for comparative study of North Indian dental morphology.

Among Afghans, the Tajik (Benyon, 1971; Sakai, Hanamura, and Ohnu, 1969, 1971) show greater affinity to western populations than do the Pushtun. This is indicated by the lower incidence of central incisor shoveling and by the high frequency of the plus (+) groove pattern in lower first-molar teeth. The Pushtun exhibit higher frequencies of the semi- and marked expressions of central incisor shoveling in conjunction with a higher incidence of Carabelli's trait than either Tajik sample.

The northern Indian sample of Ohnu (1981), consisting of 211 male and female subjects, compares favorably with Zubov's (1980) results for north Indians from Delhi in expressions of shovel shape, hypocone variation, and lower molar cusp number, but significant differences exist in the frequencies reported for Carabelli's trait and lower molar groove pattern. In the expression of Carabelli's trait, Ohnu's (1981) northern Indian sample shows similarities to figures reported for Jats by Bhasin *et al.* (1979) and Kaul and Prakash (1981).

Ohnu (1981) also presents dental trait frequencies for the Sherpa dentition that can be characterized by a very high incidence of the trace grade of shoveling, moderate frequency of Carabelli's trait, no reduction in hypocone size, little reduction in lower molar cusp number and a high incidence of the plus (+) groove pattern. The Sherpa pattern of incisor shoveling contrasts dramatically with figures reported for the Bhutanese (Prakash, Kaul, and Kanta, 1979) and emphasizes the importance of close adherence to accepted standards of trait variation. Unfortunately, further comparison of the Sherpa and Bhutanese samples is precluded by different reporting methods. Further studies of cis- and trans-Himalayan populations will help to clarify clinal variation in dental morphology across the great Himalayan barrier. This preliminary review of dental morphology in living South Asians reveals some very important areas for further investigation.

The range of variation exhibited by a polymorphic dental trait in a single *jati* needs to be precisely defined, taking into account sampling error, observer error, and related phenomenon. In addition to traditional observations of mandibular molar cusp number and groove pattern, the presence of extra cusps (C-6, entoconulid, and C-7, metaconulid), deflecting wrinkles, and distal trigonid crests must be recorded. Finally, data must be gathered for central and southern Indian populations if clinal variation in dental morphology is to be discerned.

Dental crown dimensions of living South Asians are reported much less frequently than morphological features and often specific teeth or dimensions are omitted from the analysis. This practice does not allow the computation of summed molar crown areas, a commonly used index of tooth size comparison. Sharma and Kaul (1977) do not record buccolingual dimensions of lower incisor and canine teeth. Prakash *et al.* (1979) omit buccolingual dimensions of lower incisors but include them for lower canines, and omit third-molar teeth from the analysis completely.

Data for molar crown size, as indicated by cross-sectional crown area, is presented in Table II. These data must be regarded as very preliminary and may serve as a base for comparative evaluation of new dental data. It should be noted that the "Indian" sample of Biviji and Bhatt (1971) is undoubtedly biased in that teeth requiring extraction (the basis of their study) may be larger in size than nonextracted teeth. In addition, the ethnic composition of their sample is not mentioned but probably includes many diverse endogamous groups. The

Table II
Cross-sectional Areas of Molar Teeth of Living South Asians (in mm²)

	Afghan Tajik[a]	Punjabi[b]	Indian[c]
Maxillary			
M1	—	112.14 (67)	115.50 (77)
M2	—	108.68 (67)	115.83 (141)
M3	—	96.27 (28)	103.40 (112)
Subtotal	—	317.09	334.73
Mandible			
M1	113.36 (40)	115.88 (66)	121.90 (121)
M2	103.00 (35)	102.90 (69)	114.40 (94)
M3	104.94 (20)	105.22 (29)	124.20 (97)
Subtotal	321.30	324.00	360.50
Total molar crown area	—	641.09	695.23

[a]Benyon, 1971
[b]Sharma and Kaul, 1977
[c]Biviji and Bhatt, 1971

summed molar crown area of their "Indian" sample is 695 mm^2, a figure that compares favorably with certain prehistoric samples with Neolithic and Mesolithic cultural associations. Deciduous tooth crown dimensions were reported by Lukacs, Joshi, and Makhija (1983) for Gujarati Hindus from Ahmedabad. Crown size, as reflected by cross-sectional area, was found to be smaller in living Gujaratis than in a prehistoric population from Inamgaon, an early farming village in western India. Obviously, much more data on dental crown dimensions is required from all areas of the Indian subcontinent. This is a much neglected area of research in South Asian anthropology.

3. Dental Variation in Prehistoric South Asians

3.1. The Early Development of Paleodontology in South Asia

The discovery of human skeletal remains in South Asia during the second half of the 19th century included few comments of any value on the dentition. Taylor (1873) illustrated the skull and dentition of a specimen from Jewurge, and Branfill (1881), like others, made notes on the degree of dental attrition. No systematic analysis of dental morphology, size, attrition, or disease occurred until the 1920s when human skeletal remains were recovered from Nal and the Indus Valley sites of Harappa and Mohenjo-Daro.

Sewell and Guha (1929, 1931a, 1931b) described and compared the human skeletal remains collected by Stein in Makran, those excavated by Marshall

(1931) at Mohenjo-Daro and by Hargreaves (1929) at Nal. Their studies are noteworthy because of the systematic treatment they gave the dentition. Observations on the preservation of teeth, their state of health, and degree of attrition are consistently made. Morphological details of dental variations are not recorded, probably due to the moderate-to-heavy attrition in most specimens. Though metrical data for crown length and breadth are consistently reported, and although one may question the anthropological significance of reporting crown dimensions of worn teeth, it is significant that these investigators recognized the utility of dental data in their research. Reports on the Mohenjo-Daro and Nal specimens include attempts to evaluate the dental dimensions of prehistoric South Asians comparatively with data for living and prehistoric populations from outside the subcontinent.

The attention Sewell and Guha gave to descriptive and comparative analysis of the teeth may possibly derive from Sewell's education in medicine. He graduated from Saint Bartholomew's Hospital in London and subsequently served in the Indian medical services from 1908–1935. It was as director of the Zoological Survey of India (1925–1933) that he and B. S. Guha conducted their osteological and dental investigations. Unfortunately, the example they set in systematic dental descriptions was not followed by other physical anthropologists working on prehistoric South Asian skeletal collections.

A large number of osteological reports describing human skeletal remains from prehistoric contexts in South Asia either lack any mention of teeth or provide only casual and incomplete analysis. Frequently, photographic plates or excavation reports indicate that dental remains were recovered from a site, but descriptive or comparative analyses of the teeth are not contained in the osteological report. This situation pertains to the skeletal remains from Chanhu-Daro (Krogman and Sussman, 1943), Harappa (Chatterjee and Kumar, 1963a, 1970), Lothal (Chatterjee and Kumar, 1963b), Piklihal (Ayer, 1960) and Yelleswaram (Gupta and Dutta, 1962).

Many publications list the teeth preserved and describe their states of preservation. A most common occurrence is the partial or incomplete analysis of prehistoric dental remains, with an emphasis upon the description, in very qualitative terms, of dental attrition. The use of standards is lacking in these evaluations of dental attrition. Teeth from Bhramagiri (Sarkar, 1960) and Harappa (Gupta, Dutta, and Basu, 1962) are variously described as being "completely worn out," "very much eroded," or "badly worn down."

Morphological features of the dentition are very infrequently reported in these osteological studies, and measurements of the tooth crown, if reported, are for the molar teeth only. Occasional descriptions of dental pathology occur, but they are limited to comments on dental caries, alveolar resorption, and dental abscesses, and the observations appear not to have been systematically conducted.

3.2. Current Research in South Asian Paleodontology

The systematic and thorough anthropological analysis of prehistoric dental remains from archaeological sites in South Asia began in the mid-1960s with the work of Kennedy. His analyses of the Balangoda skeletons from Bellan Bandi Palassa, Sri Lanka (Kennedy, 1965), and skeletal series from Langhnaj (Ehrhardt and Kennedy, 1965) and Nevasa (Kennedy and Malhotra, 1966) in India show detailed attention to the description and comparative analysis of the dentition. Kennedy routinely and systematically described dental attrition, pathology, and morphology, and he included dental crown measurements as part of his osteological research on these skeletal collections. Because the sample size of well-preserved dental arcades was often small, conclusions regarding the biological affinities of these populations were sometimes difficult to draw from comparative surveys of dental features alone (Kennedy, 1979).

Kennedy's interest in human dental variation in South Asia stimulated his Indian colleagues and students to begin research in this area of physical anthropology. A reanalysis of the human skeletons from Neolithic Piklihal was conducted by Malhotra (1967) who focused on the systematic description and comparative analysis of the dentition. Lukacs (1977) analyzed the dental crown dimensions, morphology, and pathology of specific prehistoric populations of northern India. The recent growth and development of paleodontology in South Asia may be partly attributable to Kennedy's research and influence.

The following review of recently completed research and research in progress on the dental anthropology of prehistoric South Asians is a necessary prerequisite to a discussion of major research conclusions. The dental anthropology of Iron Age skeletal series from Pomparippu, Sri Lanka, was described by Lukacs (1976) and Lukacs and Kennedy (1981). The problems of sample bias in deciphering the relationship between ecology, subsistence, and the pattern of dental disease in Neolithic/Chalcolithic populations of India was reviewed by Lukacs (1978). More recently, the dental pathology of the Iron Age megalith builders of central India (Lukacs, 1981a) and the Harappans (Lukacs, 1982a) has been described and interpreted. Macroscopic and histological studies of dental pathology in the Sarai Khola skeletal sample are in the analytic stage (Schultz and Lukacs, 1983; Lukacs and Schultz, 1983), and analysis of the macroscopic dental pathology of the Timargarha skeletal remains is in progress.

Descriptive and comparative studies of the morphological variations and dimensions of the permanent dental crown have recently been completed for prehistoric skeletal series from Apegaon (Lukacs, 1980), Bagor (Lukacs, 1982b), Bhimbetka (Lukacs, 1983a), and Mahurjhari (Lukacs, 1983e) in India, and Mehrgarh (Lukacs, 1983c), Sarai Khola, and Timargarha (Lukacs, 1983d) in Pakistan. A preliminary study of the crown size of deciduous teeth from prehistoric Inamgaon (Lukacs, 1981b) is currently being supplemented by morphological and metrical analyses of a larger sample of deciduous teeth from this early farming village (Lukacs, Joshi, and Makhija, 1983). Similar studies are currently being completed on the permanent teeth from Inamgaon.

Officers of the Anthropological Survey of India have traditionally given little attention to the description and comparative study of dental morphology and crown dimensions. As recently as 1970, in their description of the human remains from Kumar Tekri, the dental evidence was incompletely described and not all tooth classes were measured (Gupta, Basu, and Dutta, 1970).

However, the survey's recent report on the human skeletal remains from Burzahom, an important Neolithic site in the Kashmir Valley, provides a thorough description of the dentition and indicates a new research orientation at that institution (Basu and Pal, 1980). In a series of publications, Dutta (1980, 1983a) conducted a reanalysis of molar crown size of the Bronze Age Harappans and interpreted the results in a selective evolutionary context. Independently and with different data sets, Dutta (1983b) and Lukacs (1983b) reached similar conclusions about the reduced crown size of the Bronze Age Harappans. Dental anthropology has been included in the research program of the Anthropological Survey of India since 1960, but until very recently, the focus was entirely upon living populations or recent skeletal collections (Ganguly, 1960). What conclusions about the spatiotemporal pattern of dental variation in South Asia can be drawn from the available data?

3.3. Comparative and Interpretive Analysis of Tooth Crown Size

The literature reviewed in the preceding paragraphs indicates that dental data for prehistoric South Asians is unevenly distributed in space and time, thereby limiting the conclusions that can be drawn in particular chronological periods or in specific geographic areas. Though many researchers include observations on dental attrition, pathology, morphology, and crown dimensions in their reports, a chronic lack of standardization prohibits precise comparison of these results between different populations, especially when different investigators are involved. Another problem that precludes the detection of trends in dental variation for South Asia is the small size of many skeletal series. This limitation severely hampers morphological investigations because the effects of sampling error are great, especially for rarely occurring morphological variants. Consequently, this discussion of dental variation in prehistoric South Asia focuses on the pattern of variation in tooth size as is reflected by the crown area. With these limitations in mind, the major conclusions regarding dental variation in prehistoric South Asians will be outlined in the following paragraphs.

According to Brace (1980, p. 143), "The best indicator of tooth size—and hence the actual trait on which natural selection operates—is the cross-sectional area, a product of the mesial-distal and buccal-lingual (MD × BL) crown measurements." The mean crown areas presented later were obtained by averaging the crown areas of a given tooth for all specimens in the series. In instances where individual dental crown data were unavailable, mean MD diameter was multiplied by mean BL diameter to obtain an estimate of the mean cross-sectional crown area for that series. Variations in the method of computing the mean cross-sectional area of a tooth result in minor differences in crown area, but they do not substantially change the summed molar crown area (or the total crown area) for a given skeletal sample.

Lukacs, Joshi, and Makhija (1983) recently reported the crown diameters and crown areas of deciduous teeth from prehistoric and living populations in western India. Table III presents individual tooth crown areas and summed crown areas for the maxilla, mandible, and total dentition for prehistoric skeletal series from Inamgaon (1600–700 B.C.), Timargarha (1400–850 B.C.) and Pomparippu (300 B.C.). Also included in Table III are crown areas for a living sample of Gujarati schoolchildren with normal occlusion. Since sex is indeterminate in the skeletal remains of prepubescent children, all data presented in Table III, including the Gujarati sample, are based on pooled samples of males and females.

Table III shows that the Inamgaon sample exhibits a larger total cross-sectional area than either the Timargarha or the Gujarati sample. The total cross-

Table III
Crown Areas for Deciduous Teeth of Prehistoric and Living South Asians

	Prehistoric samples						Living sample	
	Inamgaon		Timargarha		Pomparippu		Gujarati Hindu	
Tooth	x̄ (n)	SD	x̄ (n)	SD	x̄ (n)	SD	x̄ (n)	SD
Maxilla								
di1	36.13 (19)	3.89	34.21 (4)	3.39	—		34.20 (100)	3.93
di2	27.99 (20)	3.64	26.45 (6)	3.66	—		26.11 (100)	3.35
dc	40.26 (27)	5.45	40.06 (9)	5.37	40.44 (2)	5.07	40.72 (100)	4.89
dm1	67.68 (32)	5.89	68.95 (8)	7.41	66.51 (6)	10.42	64.57 (100)	7.11
dm2	95.13 (32)	11.00	87.86 (8)	5.74	86.29 (5)	10.56	91.15 (100)	9.69
total	267.19		257.53				256.75	
Mandible								
di1	17.74 (20)	1.90	14.88 (4)	2.67	—		15.84 (100)	1.81
di2	21.81 (22)	2.62	20.61 (6)	3.20	—		20.32 (100)	2.41
dc	31.62 (22)	3.83	32.51 (9)	3.62	30.60 (1)	0.0	32.24 (100)	3.52
dm1	62.21 (36)	6.37	58.10 (13)	5.95	63.10 (2)	7.50	59.80 (100)	6.86
dm2	97.34 (36)	10.16	90.44 (13)	7.36	89.26 (5)	3.80	91.13 (100)	9.59
total	230.72		216.54				219.33	
Total crown area	497.91		474.07				476.08	

sectional area for the Pomparippu sample cannot be computed because labiolingual diameters of anterior teeth were not reported (Lukacs, 1976).

If the summed molar crown area is compared across groups, Inamgaon (332 mm^2) exhibits larger molar teeth than the other three groups. Timargarha (305 mm^2), Pomparippu (305 mm^2), and the living Gujarati sample (307 mm^2) are all similar to one another in having small molar crown areas that average 16 mm^2 less than the figure reported for Inamgaon.

Lukacs, Joshi, and Makhija (1983) have suggested that these differences in deciduous tooth crown areas may be partially attributable to differences in the levels of technology, diet, and subsistence among the groups studied. Inamgaon is an early farming village in western India whose inhabitants possessed a typical late Chalcolithic culture and practiced a subsistence pattern that included hunting. The occupants of Timargarha (Iron Age), Pomparippu (Iron Age), and Gujarat (modern) all possess more developed technologies than Inamgaon, and agricultural subsistence has a greater antiquity among these groups. These variations in culture and subsistence may partly explain the observed differences in tooth size between the groups studied.

The first systematic discussion of variation in permanent tooth crown size in South Asia was limited to an analysis of the cross-sectional molar crown areas of prehistoric skeletal series (Lukacs, 1983b). Table IV is a revised version of the table that accompanied that presentation. Mean summed molar crown areas (SMCAs) of prehistoric South Asian skeletal series are arranged in order of decreasing size. Also given in Table IV are the site names, approximate antiquity, and the sources from which the data were derived.

In most instances, the SMCA is derived from a single skeletal series and represents the sample mean of a biological (breeding) population. In a few instances, data from several small skeletal series were pooled into larger groups; these are identified as *Mesolithic pooled, late Neolithic pooled,* and *Chalcolithic pooled* in Table IV. The Mesolithic pooled sample includes data from the sites of Lekhahia and Sarai-Nahar-Rai in the Ganga Plains (Sharma, 1973, 1975) and from Bagor (Rajasthan) and Langhnaj (Gujarat) in western India. The late Neolithic pooled sample is derived from the sites of Piklihal and Tekklakota in peninsular India, and specimens from Chandoli, Inamgaon, and Nevasa provided data for the Chalcolithic pooled sample. The conclusions originally were derived from a close study of these data, and they are still valid and are reiterated as follows:

1. Skeletal samples with the largest tooth sizes have Mesolithic or early Neolithic cultural associations.
2. Early Neolithic, prepottery farming cultures of the northwestern borderlands also exhibit large tooth sizes.
3. Tooth sizes among early Neolithic farmers of South Asia and southwestern Asia are very similar.

4. Late Neolithic samples from peninsular India have smaller molar teeth than early Neolithic groups of the northwestern borderlands.
5. Early urban centers of the second and third millennia B.C. (civilizations of the Bronze Age) exhibit the smallest tooth size figures.
6. Early farming Chalcolithic cultures of peninsular India have smaller molar teeth than Mesolithic inhabitants of central and western India.

Table IV
Summed Molar Crown Areas of Prehistoric South and Southwest Asian Skeletal Series (in mm²)

Cultural association	Archaeological site	Summed molar crown area	Approximate antiquity	Source of data
South Asia				
Mesolithic	Bellan Bandi Palassa	713	4650 B.C.	Kennedy (1965)
Mesolithic	Mahadaha	692	—	Kennedy (ms.)
Early Neolithic	Mehrgarh	680	6500 B.C.	Lukacs (1983c)
Mesolithic	Bhimbetka	678	—	Lukacs (1983a)
Iron Age	Mahurjhari	677	800 B.C.	Lukacs (1983e)
Mesolithic (pooled)	Northern India	674	8100–1600 B.C.	Lukacs (1977)
Late Neolithic (pooled)	Peninsular India	658	1600 B.C.	Lukacs (1977)
Chalcolithic	Inamgaon	653	1600–700 B.C.	Lukacs (1983a)
Iron Age	Timargarha	642	1400–850 B.C.	Lukacs (1983d)
Chalcolithic (pooled)	Peninsular India	635	1200 B.C.	Lukacs (1977)
Iron Age	Pomparippu	626	300 B.C.	Lukacs (1976)
Iron Age	Sarai Khola	614	300 B.C.	Lukacs (1983d)
Bronze Age	Mohenjo-Daro	607	2000 B.C.	Sewell and Guha (1931a)
Bronze Age	Harappa	606	2000 B.C.	Dutta (1983)
Bronze Age	Harappa	595	2000 B.C.	Gupta *et al.* (1962)
Late Neolithic	Burzahom	560	2400–1800 B.C.	Basu and Pal (1980)
Early Historic	Kumhar Tekri	493	200 B.C.	Gupta and Basu (1970)
Southwestern Asia				
Mesolithic	Natufian	720	—	Dahlberg (1960)
Neolithic	Abou Gosh	685	6500 B.C.	Arensburg *et al.* (1978)
Neolithic	Jarmo	680	6750 B.C.	Dahlberg (1960)
Bronze Age	Kish	614	2500–600 B.C.	Rathbun (1975)
Bronze Age	Umm an-Nar	609	2500 B.C.	Højgaard (1980)
Bronze Age	Hasanlu IV	605		Rathbun (1972)

7. Skeletal series with Iron Age cultural associations are derived from geographically, temporally, and ecologically diverse settings, and, correspondingly, they exhibit a wide range of molar tooth sizes.
8. The most recent skeletal series for which dental crown dimensions are available is the collection from Kumhar Tekri near Ujjain, which yields a SMCA of 493 mm^2 (Gupta and Basu, 1970).

These points are explained in much greater detail in Lukacs's (1983b) discussion of cultural variation and dental reduction in South Asia.

The addition of three new data points (Abou Gosh, Burzahom, and Timargarha) to Table IV permits further insight into the patterning of tooth size variation in South Asia. In this regard, several important points need to be emphasized: (1) a given cultural level yields a range of tooth sizes; (2) average tooth sizes for a given cultural level are similar despite geographical remoteness of the groups; and (3) "primitive" cultures are associated with large teeth and "developed" cultures are associated with small teeth.

Iron Age cultures of South Asia vary in molar tooth size from a large SMCA of 677 mm^2 for Mahurjhari (central India) to a small figure of 614 mm^2 at Sarai Khola (northern Pakistan), yielding a range of 63 mm^2. Tooth sizes among Mesolithic and early Neolithic cultures vary from a large figure of 713 mm^2 for Bellan Bandi Palassa (Sri Lanka) to a small size of 678 mm^2 for Bhimbetka (central India). Similar ranges in SMCA are found to characterize southwestern Asian prehistoric people. These variations in tooth size occur among people of a crudely similar level of cultural development because subtle differences in diet, methods of food preparation, and genetic composition exist between them.

If an average SMCA is computed for all Mesolithic/early Neolithic samples, the similarities in tooth size between South and southwestern Asians is striking: 691 mm^2 for four South Asian sites and 695 mm^2 for three southwestern Asian sites. If the average SMCA is computed for Bronze Age people of South and southwestern Asia, the results are similarly impressive: 602 mm^2 for two sites in South Asia and 609 mm^2 for three sites in southwestern Asia. Cruder technologies and coarser diets are correlated with larger molar teeth in geographically diverse regions. On the other hand, more efficient technologies and softer foods are associated with smaller molar teeth.

Parallel differences are found in SMCA between Mesolithic/early Neolithic cultures on the one hand, and Bronze Age cultures on the other, in both South and southwestern Asia. Molar teeth of Bronze Age inhabitants of northwestern India are 89 mm^2 (12.9%) smaller than the molar teeth of people associated with the Mesolithic/early Neolithic cultures of South Asia. In southwestern Asia, people with Bronze Age cultural associations have molar teeth that are 84 mm^2 (12.1%) smaller than the molar teeth of Mesolithic/early Neolithic people in that region of the world. These cultural and molar-tooth-size variations in different regions of southern Asia have important implications for the causative role of culture in influencing the pattern of dental variation in crown sizes. Cultural variation makes natural selective processes of dental reduction much more plausible mechanisms for dental evolution than the process of accumulating random mutations.

Absence of SMCAs for early historic and living populations of South Asia precludes continuation of this analysis through to its logical conclusion: Documentation of clinal variation in SMCAs of living South Asians and correlating the observed tooth-size clines with differing levels of cultural development. The paucity of data for SMCAs exists despite several recent publications on dental crown dimensions of living Indian peoples.

Limitations of this approach to dental reduction are undoubtedly evident to the reader, but they should be explicitly and clearly stated. First, the obvious limitation of the data: Many skeletal series contain only a few fragmentary specimens and some consist only of isolated teeth. The number of skeletal samples for which SMCAs are available is small, and firm documentation of these trends and correlations requires more data points derived from larger skeletal series.

Second, the low but positive correlation between tooth size and body size may introduce a source of error into the analysis. Dental size differences that are attributed here to changes in technology or subsistence strategy may in some instances simply reflect a change in average body size. Third, the chronological position of many archaeological sites yielding human skeletal remains is uncertain or controversial. This limitation is less crucial than the previous two because cultural association is of greater import than temporal position in interpreting patterns of tooth size variation.

ACKNOWLEDGMENTS

Dr. H. D. Sankalia and Dr. S. B. Deo (Deccal College, Post-Graduate and Research Institute, Pune), Dr. W. Bernhard (Anthropologisches Institut, Universitat Mainz), and Dr. Jean-Francois Jarrige (Musée Guimet, Paris) graciously provided access to skeletal and dental remains under their curatorial care. Their cooperation is appreciated.

Translation from Russian was done by Fruim Yurevich (University of Oregon, Eugene) and C. K. Thapar (Ranade Institute, Pune); and from Japanese by Osamu Kataoka and Hiroshi Inoue. The author appreciates their willingness to assist in this project.

References

Arensburg, B., Smith, P., and Yakar, R., 1978, The human remains from Abou Gosh, in: *Abou Gosh at Beisamoun: deux gisements du VIIe millenaire avant L'ere chretienne en Israel* (M. Lechavellier, ed.), Association Paleorient, Paris, pp. 95–106.

Ayer, A. A., 1960, Report on the human skeletal remains excavated at Piklihal near Mudgal, in: *Piklihal Excavations* (F. R. Allchin, ed.), Andhra Pradesh Govt. Archaeol. Ser. **1**, Hyderabad.

Babbar, A. C., 1963, Arch form and tooth size in Indian male adults with neutrocclusion, *J. All India Dent. Assoc.* **35**:87–105.

Banerjee, P., 1963, Missing teeth in Bengalee Skulls, *Science and Culture* **29**:407.

Banerjee, P., 1964, Weight of Bengalee skulls, mandibles and teeth, *Science and Culture* **30**:207.

Banerjee, P., 1967, Some evolutionary aspects in dental morphology of Benaglese skulls, *Man in India* **147**:103–112.

Basu, A., and Pal, A., 1980, *Human Remains from Burzahom,* Anthropological Survey of India, Calcutta.

Benyon, A. D. G., 1971, Dentition of the Afghan Tajik, in: *Dental Morphology and Evolution* (A. A. Dahlberg, ed.), University of Chicago Press, Chicago, pp. 271–282.

Bhasin, M. K., Sharma, A., and Singh, I. P., 1979, A study on dental traits among Jats of Haryana, North India, *Indian J. Phys. Anthropol. Hum. Genet.* **5**(1):7–18.

Biviji, A. T., and Bhatt, A. P., 1971, Odontometric data of Indian teeth: II. Posterior teeth, *J. Indian Dent. Assoc.* **43**:250–252.

Biviji, A. T., Shourie, K. L., Baldev Singh, and Menezes, C. J., 1967, Odontometric data of Indian teeth, I. Anterior teeth, *J. Indian Dent. Assoc.* **39**(5):27–31.

Bolk, L., 1914, Supernumerary teeth in the molar region in man, *Dental Cosmos* **56**:154–167.

Bolk, L., 1916, Problems of the human dentition, *Am. J. Anat.* **19**:91–148.

Bowles, G. T., 1943, Linguistic and racial aspects of the Munda problem, *Harvard Univ., Peabody Mus. Pap.* **20**:81–101.

Brace, C. L., 1980, Australian tooth-size clines and the death of a stereotype, *Curr. Anthropol.* **21**(2):141–164.

Branfill, B. R., 1881, On the Savandurga rude stone cemetery, central Maisur, *Indian Antiquary* **10**:1–12.

Cadien, J. D., 1972, Dental variation in man, in: *Perspectives on Human Evolution,* Volume 2 (S. L. Washburn and P. Dolhinow, eds.), Holt, Rinehart & Winston, New York, pp. 199–222.

Campbell, T. D., 1925, Dentition and Palate of the Australian Aboriginal, *University of Adelaide Publications* **1.**

Chatterjee, B. K., and Kumar, G. D., 1963a, *Comparative Study and Racial Analysis of the Human Remains of Indus Valley Civilization with Particular Reference to Harappa,* W. Newman, Calcutta.

Chatterjee, B. K., and Kumar, G. D., 1963b, Racial elements in post-Harappan skeletal remains at Lothal, in: *Anthropology on the March* (Bala Ratnam, ed.), Social Sciences Assn., Madras, pp. 104–110.

Chatterjee, B. K., and Kumar, G. D., 1970, Ethnogenesis of ancient inhabitants of Indo-Pakistan, central and western Asia, *Bull. Indian Mus. (Calcutta)* **5**:126–141.

Dahlberg, A. A., 1951, The dentition of the American Indian, in: *Papers on the Physical Anthropology of the American Indian* (W. S. Laughlin, ed.), Fourth Viking Fund Summer Seminar in Physical Anthropology (1949), Viking Fund, New York, pp. 138–176.

Dahlberg, A. A., 1960, The dentition of the first agriculturalists (Jarmo, Iraq), *Am. J. Phys. Anthropol.* **18**:243–256.

Dahlberg, A. A., 1963, Analysis of the American Indian dentition, in: *Dental Anthropology* (D. R. Brothwell, ed.), Pergamon Press, New York, pp. 149–177.

Drennan, M. R., 1929, The dentition of a Bushman tribe, *Ann. South Africa Mus.* **24**:61–88.

Dutta, P. C., 1980, Molar crown characteristics of the Bronze Age Harappans and natural selection, *Proc. of the Symp. on Three Decades of Development in Paleontol. Strat. in India, Hyderabad (10–12 September 1980).*

Dutta, P. C., 1983a, A study of the molar teeth of the Bronze Age Harappans in the context of evolutionary biology, *Anthropologie* (in press).

Dutta, P. C., 1983b, An odontometric study of the molar crown characters of the Bronze Age Harappans. *Anthropologischer Anzeiger.* **41**(1):1–19.

Ehrhardt, S., and Kennedy, K. A. R., 1965, Excavations at Langhnaj: 1944–1963. Part III: The human remains, *Deccan Coll. Build. Centen. Silver Jubilee Ser.* **27.**

Flower, W. H., 1880, On the osteology and affinities of the natives of the Andaman Islands, *J. R. Anthropol. Inst. Gr. Br. Ir.* **9:**108–135.

Flower, W. H., 1885a, Additional observations on the osteology of the natives of the Andaman Islands, *J. R. Anthropol. Inst. Gr. Br. Ir.* **14:**115–120.

Flower, W. H., 1885b, On the size of teeth as a character of race, *J. R. Anthropol. Inst. Gr. Br. Ir.* **14:**183–186.

Ganguly, P., 1960, Observations on the Teeth of Nicobar Islanders, *Bull. Anthropol. Surv. India* **9:**43–50.

Gregory, W. K., 1916, Studies on the evolution of the primates, *Bull. Am. Mus. Nat. Hist.* **35:**239–356.

Gregory, W. K., 1922, *The Origin and Evolution of the Human Dentition,* Williams and Wilkins, Baltimore.

Gregory, W. K., and Hellman, M., 1926, The dentition of *Dryopithecus* and the origin of man, *Anthropol. Pap. Am. Mus. Nat. Hist.* **28**(1):1–123.

Gupta, P., and Basu, A., 1970, Early historic crania from Kumhar Tekri, Ujjain, in: *Ancient Human Remains* (P. Gupta, A. Basu, and P. C. Dutta, eds.), Anthropol. Surv. India, Calcutta, pp. 35–74.

Gupta, P., and Dutta, P. C., 1962, Human remains excavated from megaliths at Yelleswaram (Andhra Pradesh), *Man in India* **42**(1):19–34.

Gupta, P., Basu, A., and Dutta, P. C., 1970, Ancient human remains, *Mem. Anthropol. Surv. India (Calcutta)* **20:**1–74.

Gupta, P., Dutta, P. C., and Basu, A., 1962, *Human skeletal remains from Harappa, Mem. Anthropol. Surv. India (Calcutta)* **9:**3–186.

Hargreaves, H., 1929, Excavations in Baluchistan 1925, Sampur Mound, Mastung and Sohr Damb, Nal, *Mem. Archeol. Surv. India (New Dehli)* **35.**

Hellman, M., 1928, Racial characters in the human dentition, *Proc. Am. Philos. Soc.* **67:**157–174.

Højgaard, K., 1980, Dentition on Umm and an-Nar (Trucial Oman), *Scand. J. Dent. Res.* **88:**355–364.

Hrdlička, A., 1920, Shovel shaped teeth, *Am. J. Phys. Anthropol.* **3:**429–465.

Jacobsen, A.,1982, *The Dentition of the South African Negro,* Higginbotham, Inc., Anniston.

Jørgensen, K. D., 1955, The *Dryopithecus* pattern in recent Danes and Dutchmen, *J. Dent. Res.* **34:**195–208.

Joshi, M. R., Gondiawala, R. N., and Dutia, A., 1972, Carabelli's trait in Hindu children from Gujarat, *J. Dent. Res.* **50**(3):706–711.

Kaul, V., and Prakash, S., 1981, Morphological features of Jat dentition, *Am. J. of Phys. Anthropol.* **54:**123–127.

Kennedy, K. A. R., 1965, Human skeletal material from Ceylon, with an analysis of the island's prehistoric and contemporary populations, *Bull. Brit. Mus. Nat. Hist.* (Geology) **11:**137–213.

Kennedy, K. A. R., 1979, Implications of dental anthropology in the study of biological continua: Balangodese and Veddas, *Spolia Zeylan.* **35:**319–322.

Kennedy, K. A. R., and Malhotra, K. C., 1966, Human skeletal remains from Chalcolithic and Indo-Roman levels from Nevasa: An anthropometric and comparative analysis, *Deccan Coll. Building Centen. Silver Jubilee Ser.* **55:**1–135.

Kraus, B. S., 1951, Carabelli's anomaly of the maxillary molar teeth. Observations on Mexicans and Papago Indians and an interpretation of the inheritance, *Am. J. Hum. Genet.* **3:**348–355.

Krogman, W. M., and Sassman, W. H., 1943, Skull found at Chanhudaro, in: *Chanhudaro Excava-*

tions 1935–1936 (E. J. H. MacKay, ed.), American Oriental Society, New Haven, pp. 253–263.

Leigh, R. W., 1925a, Dental pathology of Indian tribes of varied environmental and food conditions, *Am. J. Phys. Anthropol.* **8:**179–199.

Leigh, R. W., 1925b, Dental pathology of the Eskimo, *Dent. Cosmos* **67:**884–898.

Leigh, R. W., 1929, Dental morphology and pathology of prehistoric Guam, *Mem. Bernice P. Bishop Mus.* **11:**255–273.

Leigh, R. W., 1930, Dental morphology and pathology of prehistoric Guam, *J. Dent. Res.* **10:**451–479.

Lukacs, J. R., 1976, Dental anthropology and the biological affinities of an Iron Age population from Pomparippu, Sri Lanka, in: *Ecological Backgrounds of South Asian Prehistory* (K. A. R. Kennedy and G. L. Possehl, eds.), Occasional Paper No. 4, Cornell University, South Asia Program, Ithaca, pp. 197–215.

Lukacs, J. R., 1977, Anthropological Aspects of Dental Variation in North India: A Morphometric Analysis, Unpublished Ph.D. thesis, Cornell University, Ithaca, New York.

Lukacs, J. R., 1978, Biocultural interaction in prehistoric India: Culture, ecology and the pattern of dental disease in Neolithic-Chalcolithic populations, in: *American Studies in the Anthropology of India* (S. Vatuk, ed.), Manohar, Delhi, pp. 425–444.

Lukacs, J. R., 1980, The Apegaon mandible: Morphology and pathology, *Bull. Deccan Coll. Res. Inst.* **39:**88–95.

Lukacs, J. R., 1981a, Dental pathology and nutritional patterns of South Asian megalith builders: The evidence from Iron Age Mahurjhari, *Proc. Am. Philos. Soc.* **125:**220–237.

Lukacs, J. R., 1981b, Crown dimensions of deciduous teeth from Prehistoric India, *Am. J. Phys. Anthropol.* **55:**261–266.

Lukacs, J. R., and Kennedy, K. A. R., 1981, Biological Anthropology of human remains from Pomparippu, in: *Excavations of Iron Age Burials at Pomparippu* (V. Begley, ed.), 1970, *Ancient Ceylon* **4:**97–142.

Lukacs, J. R., 1982a, Dental disease, dietary patterns and subsistence at Harappa and Mohenjo-daro, in: *Harappan Civilization: A Contemporary Perspective* (G. L. Posseh, ed.), Oxford and IBH Publishing Co., New Delhi, pp. 301–307.

Lukacs, J. R., 1982b, Biological anthropology of human skeletal remains from Bagor: The dentition, in: *Bagor and Tilwara, Late Mesolithic Cultures of Northwest India: Volume I. The Human Skeletal Remains* (J. R. Lukacs, V. N. Misra, and K. A. R. Kennedy, eds.), Deccan Coll., Pune, pp. 61–85.

Lukacs, J. R., 1983a, Human skeletal remains from Bhimbetka: A comparative analysis of the Susan Haas Collection, *Deccan Coll. Monogr. Ser.*, Pune (in press).

Lukacs, J. R., 1983b, Cultural Variation and Dental Reduction: Evolutionary Mechanisms and the Evidence from South Asia, Paper Presented at the Indian Statistical Institute Conference on Human Genetics and Adaptation, Calcutta (February 1–5, 1982), pp. 1–18.

Lukacs, J. R., 1983c, Human dental remains from early Neolithic levels at Mehrgarh, Baluchistan, *Curr. Anthropol.* **24**(3):390–392.

Lukacs, J. R., 1983d, Dental anthropology and the origins of two Iron Age populations from Northern Pakistan, *Homo* (W. Germany) **34:**1–15.

Lukacs, J. R., 1983e, Dental anthropology of human skeletal remains from Iron Age Mahurjhari, in: *Excavations at Mahurjhari* (S. B. Deo, ed.), Deccan College, Pune.

Lukacs, J. R., and Schultz, M., 1983, Macroscopic dental pathology of the human skeletal remains from Sarai Khola, northern Pakistan. *Am. J. Phys. Anthropol.*, in press.

Lukacs, J. R., Joshi, M. R., and Makhija, P. G., 1983, Deciduous tooth crown dimensions of living and prehistoric populations in western India, *Am. J. Phys. Anthropol.* **61**(3):383–387.

Malhotra, K. C., 1967, Further observations on the human skeletal remains from Neolithic Piklihal, *Anthropologist* **14:**99–111.

Marshall, Sir J., 1931, *Mohenjo-daro and the Indus Civilization,* Arthur Probsthain, London.

Moorrees, C. F. A., 1957, *The Aleut Dentition,* Harvard University Press, Cambridge.

Ohnu, N., 1981, Observations on the dentition of northern Indians and the North-east Sherpas, *Aichi-Gakuin J. of Dent. Sci.* **19**(3):84–97.

Owen, R., 1863, On the osteology and dentition of the aborigines of the Andaman Islands, and the relations thereby indicated to other races of mankind, *Trans. Ethnol. Soc. Lond.* **1**:34–39.

Ozaki, T., Ohnuki, E., and Tsuruoka, M., 1977, Occlusal surface index of the molars of Indians, *J. Anthropol. Soc. Nippon* **85**:237–243.

Pal, A., 1964, Observations on the dentition of the crania from eastern India, *Anthropol. Surv. India* **13**:9–18.

Pal, A., 1967, Observations on groove configurations and cusp numbers on the occlusal surface of the human molars, *Anthropol. Surv. India* **16**:219–254.

Pal, A., 1972, Shovel-shaped incisors among the Negritos of Andaman Island, *Man in India* **52**(3):239–251.

Pedersen, P. O., 1949, The East Greenland Eskimo dentition, numerical variations and anatomy, *Med. om Gronland* **142**:1–244.

Prakash, S., and Sharma, K. K., 1972, Shape of dental arch in the Jats of Harayana. *Anthropologist* **19**(1/2):53–57.

Prakash, S., Kaul, V., and Kanta, S., 1979, Observations on Bhutanese dentitions, *Hum. Biol.* **51**:23–30.

Rami Reddy, V., Ramakrishna, K., Naidu, G. P., and Reddy, B. K. C., 1982, Dental morphology and pathology among the Pattusalis of Chittoor District, Andhra Pradesh. *Indian Anthropologist* **12**(1).

Rami Reddy, V., Vijayalakshmi, P. B., and Reddy, B. K. C., 1982, Some dental features among the Muslims of southeastern Andhra Pradesh. *Man in India* **62**(4):395–404.

Rami Reddy, V., MS I, Shovel-shaped Deciduous Incisors among the Children of Gulbarga, Karnataka.

Rami Reddy, V., MS II, Shovel-shaped Permanent Incisors among the People of Gulbarga, Karnataka.

Rathbun, T. A., 1972, A Study of the Physical Characteristics of the Ancient Inhabitants of Hasanlu, Iran, Field Research Projects, Miami (180 pages).

Rathbun, T. A., 1975, A Study of the Physical Characteristics of the Ancient Inhabitants of Kisk, Iraq, Field Research Projects, Miami (255 pages).

Sakai, T., Hanamura, H., and Ohnu, N., 1969, The dentition of the Pushtun and Tajik in Afghanistan, *Aichi-Gakuin J. Dent. Sci.* **7**:106–137.

Sakai, T., Hanamura, H., and Ohnu, N., 1970, The dentition of the Pushtun and Tajik in Afghanistan, *Aichi-Gakuin J. Dent. Sci.* **7**:265–314.

Sakai, T., Hanamura, H., and Ohnu, N., 1971, Tooth size of the Pushtun and Tajik in Afghanistan, *J. Anthropol. Soc. Nippon* **79**(2):159–177.

Sarkar, S. S., 1960, Human skeletal remains from Brhmagiri, *Bull. Anthropol. Surv. India,* **9**(1):2–25.

Schultz, M., and Lukacs, J. R., 1983, Microscopic analysis of dental pathology in the human skeletal series from Sarai Khola, northern Pakistan.

Schwartz, B. M., 1967, *Caste in Overseas Indian Communities,* Chandler Publishing Corp., San Francisco.

Scott, G. R., 1977, Classification of sex dimorphism, association, and population variation of the canine distal accessory ridge, *Hum. Biol.* **49**:453–469.

Scott, G. R., 1980, Population variation of Carabelli's trait, *Hum. Biol.* **52**(1):63–78.

Selmer-Olsen, R., 1949, An odontometrical study on Norwegian Lapps, *Skrifter utgitt av det Norke Videnskaps-Akademis Oslo, I Math. Naturv. Klasse* **3,** pp. 1–167.

Sewell, R. B. S., and Guha, B. S., 1929, Report on the bones excavated at Nal, *Mem. Archaeol. Surv. India* **35**:56–89.

Sewell, R. B. S., and Guha, B. S., 1931a, Human remains in: *Mohenjo-Daro and the Indus Civilization,* Volume 2 (J. Marshall, ed.), Arthur Probsthan, London, pp. 599–648.

Sewell, R. B. S., and Guha, B. S., 1931b, Report on a collection of bones made by Sir Aurel Stein in Makran, *Mem. Archaeol. Surv. India* **43**:191–200.

Sharma, G. R., 1973, Mesolithic lake cultures in the Ganga Valley, India, *Proc. of the Prehist. Soc.* **39**:129–144.

Sharma, G. R., 1975, Season Migrations and Mesolithic Lake Cultures of the Ganga Valley, *Indian Prehist. Soc. (Delhi), Presidential Address,* pp. 1–20.

Sharma, J. C., and Kaul, V., 1977, Dental morphology and odontometry in Panjabis, *Indian Anthropol.* **12**:213–226.

Shaw, J. C. M., 1931, *The teeth, the bony palate and the mandible in Bantu races of South Africa,* John Bale and Sons and Danielson, London.

Stoudt, H. W., 1961, The physical anthropology of Ceylon, *Ceylon Natl. Mus. Ethnogr. Ser. Publ.* **2,** Colombo Museum, Colombo.

Taylor, P. M., 1873, Descriptions of carins, cromlechs, kistvaens and other Celtic, Druidical or Scythian monuments in the Dekhan, *Trans. R. Ir. Acad.* **24**:329–362.

de Terra, M., 1905, *Beitrage zu einer Odontographie der Menschenrassen,* Berlinische Verlagsanstalt, Berlin.

Tratman, E. K., 1938, Three-rooted lower molars in man and their racial distribution, *Brit. Dent. J.* **64**:264–274.

Tratman, E. K., 1950, A comparison of the teeth of people: Indo-European racial stock with the mongoloid racial stock, *Dental Record* **70**(2/3):31–53, 63–88.

Tratman, E. K., and Chiam, K. N., 1941, On supernumerary teeth, *Malayan Branch, Br. Med. Assoc. J.* **5**:31.

Turner, C. G. II, 1967, The Dentition of Arctic Peoples, Unpublished Ph.D. Dissertation, University of Wisconsin, Madison.

Turner, C. G. II, 1971, Three-rooted mandibular first permanent molars and the question of American Indian origins, *Am. J. Phys. Anthropol.* **34**:229–242.

Zubov, A. A., 1968, *Odontology: Methodology for Anthropological Research,* Nauka Publishing Company, Moscow. (In Russian)

Zubov, A. A., 1980, Anthropological characteristics of the union territory of Delhi on the basis of odontological features, in: *New Anthropological Data for Northern India: Results of the Joint Indo-Soviet Expedition 1971* (M. G. Abdushalishvili and K. C. Malhotra, eds.), Academy of Sciences of U.S.S.R., Moscow, pp. 218–240. (In Russian)

CHAPTER 8

South Asian Prehistoric Human Skeletal Remains and Burial Practices

KENNETH A. R. KENNEDY AND PEGGY C. CALDWELL

1. Introduction

South Asia is assuming a frontier position with respect to recent advances in human paleontology, skeletal biology, paleodemography, and paleoecology. For many years the exclusive preserve of archaeological investigation, the Indian subcontinent is now yielding a prehistoric skeletal record that promises to answer many questions of a biological and demographic nature that the study of the artifactual and stratigraphical record does not supply. Not only have the numbers of prehistoric skeletal specimens increased through recent excavations, but many skeletal specimens and series collected in earlier times are being reinvestigated. Furthermore, the information derived from modern morphometric analyses of skeletal remains extends far beyond a preoccupation with racial identification and discernment of biological affinities. Reorientation of research designs means a closer association of anatomical and statistical analyses of skeletal materials to specific archaeological issues as well as the application of these data to the broader spectrum of world prehistory and human evolution. In his or her search for comparative skeletal data, the biological anthropologist is discovering the

---

KENNETH A. R. KENNEDY • Ecology and Systematics, Division of Biological Sciences, Cornell University, Ithaca, New York 14853 and *PEGGY C. CALDWELL* • Department of Anthropology, National Museum of Natural History, Washington, D.C. 20560. Appreciation is expressed to the National Science Foundation, the Smithsonian Institution, the Howard Foundation, the American Institute of Indian Studies, the American Institute of Pakistan Studies, the South Asia Program at Cornell University, and the Faculty Research Grants Committee at Cornell University.

richness of research materials available in South Asia, a skeletal record that has a considerable, if discontinuous, antiquity of some 9 to 15 million years for hominoids.

This chapter provides biological anthropologists and prehistorians with a short catalog of human skeletal remains collected from ancient sites in South Asia. As a summary, it includes those skeletal specimens and series that are currently available for study and for which some anatomical description has been published. Along with information about names of discoverers and dates of discovery, size of the collection, dating, archaeological context, anatomical references, and place of last reported repository, the catalog includes descriptions of burial practices and circumstances of deposition. This section is organized by temporal, geographical, and cultural criteria for skeletal specimens of (1) Pleistocene or uncertain antiquity; (2) Holocene hunter–gatherer communities; (3) farming and nomadic populations of the northwestern sector of the subcontinent (the Harappan civilization and the Gandharan Grave culture); (4) early farming and herding communities of central and southern India; and (5) the megalith builders and their Iron Age collaterals. This makes a total of 63 sites.

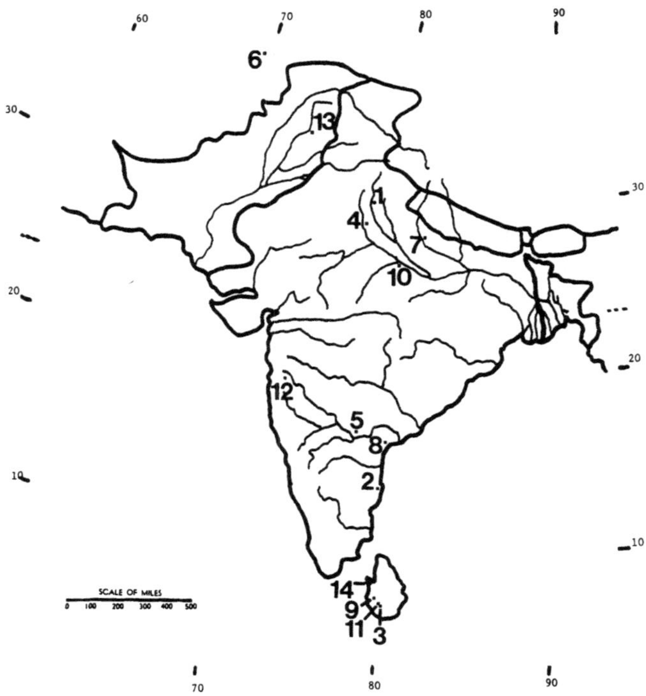

Figure 1. Location of sites yielding anatomically described human skeletal specimens of Pleistocene or uncertain antiquity in India, Pakistan, and Sri Lanka (see Table I-A).

A list of 108 sites that have yielded currently available but, as of yet, anatomically undescribed or unpublished studies of skeletons follows the catalog section. Further information about these collections may be obtained by writing to the authors, but permission to examine any of the collections rests, of course, with the institution presently curating the specimens. Lost specimens for which anatomical descriptions may have been published are not included in the catalog section or in the list of undescribed materials. The map figures indicate the geographical locations of the sites of described specimens.

Readers seeking summary sources about the biological anthropology of prehistoric man in South Asia will find these in the writings of Büchi (1968), P. Gupta (1975), S. P. Gupta (1979), Kennedy (1973, 1980), Murty (1974a), M. R. Sahni (1956), and Sarkar (1964, 1972). Summary studies of South Asian burial practices are by Bose (1966), Buxton and Rice (1931), Codrington (1930), Durrani (1978), P. Gupta (1976), Leshnik (1967), and Singh (1970). This chapter does not include discussion of the Neogene hominoids of the Siwalik Hills of India and Pakistan, but the senior author has written a brief summary of this record in a separate publication (Kennedy 1980, pp. 391–396).

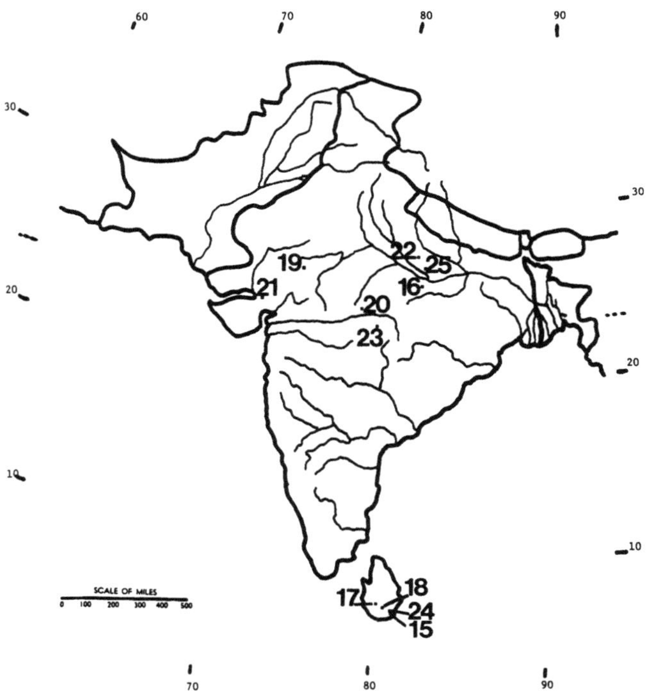

Figure 2. Location of sites yielding anatomically described human skeletal specimens of early Holocene and later hunter–gatherer communities (see Table I-B).

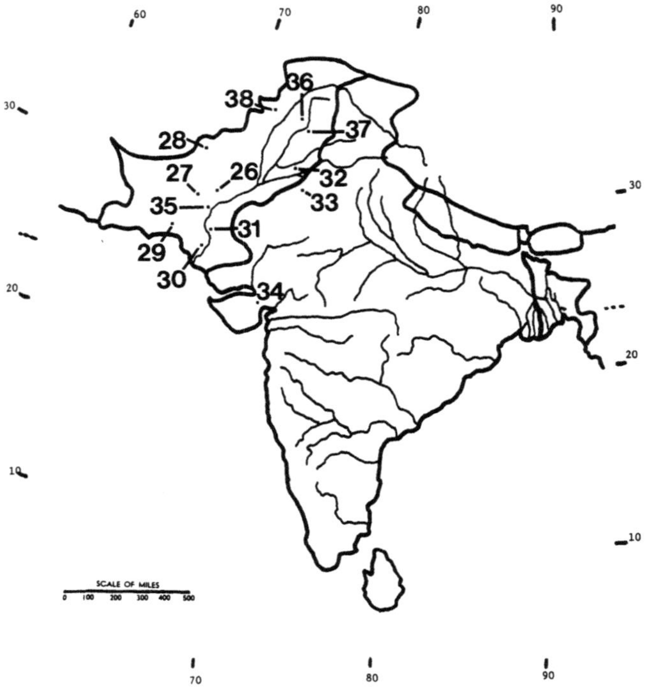

Figure 3. Location of sites yielding anatomically described prehistoric human skeletal specimens from farming and nomadic populations of the northwestern sector of the subcontinent (see Table I-C).

Key to Abbreviations

A summary of burial information accompanies each entry of the catalog and appears as the base line(s). There are 10 categories of information that appear in the following order, but in cases where an item of information is unknown or is irrelevant, the number of categories may be reduced. The 10 categories are as follows:

1. Intentional or unintentional (depositional) burial.
2. Condition or state of preservation of the human remains.
3. Bone(s) present.
4. Age and sex distribution of the human remains.
5. Type(s) of burial(s) present.
6. Location of the burial(s) in relation to other site features; presence or absence of a surface burial marker.
7. Position of the body at time of burial and/or excavation.
8. Orientation of the body at time of burial and/or excavation.

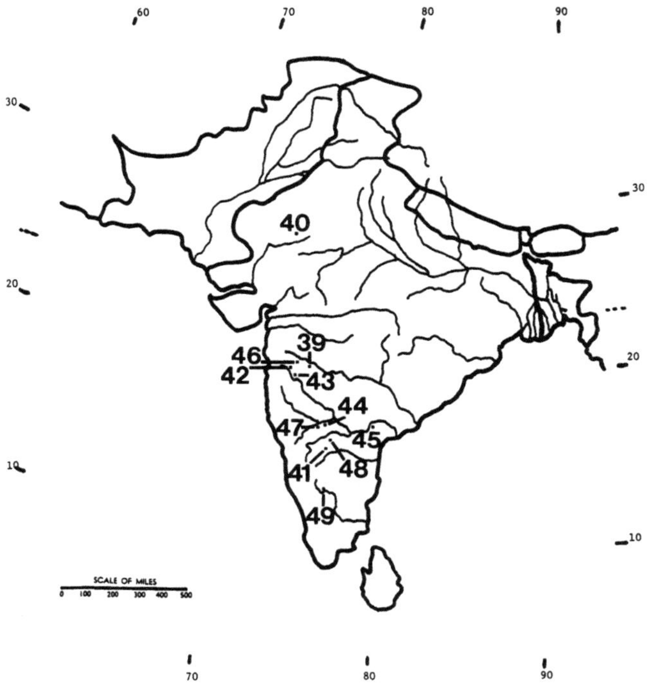

Figure 4. Location of sites in Central and South India yielding anatomically described human skeletal specimens of early farming and herding communities of Central and South India (see Table I-D).

9. Type of deposit.
10. Grave goods, direct associations of artifacts with human remains.

The abbreviations found in each of the preceding categories are the following:

1. BP (burial practices); BP (gen) (burial practices in general); BC (burial circumstances).
2. BaP (badly preserved); PP (poorly preserved); WP (well preserved); ExP (excellently preserved); Fos (fossilized); SFos (semifossilized).
3. Skeles (complete or incomplete skeletons); Frags (fragments); other information detailed.
4. Ad (adult); Ch (child); Juv (juvenile); Inf (infant); M (male); F (female).
5. PB (primary burial); SB (secondary burial); CC (complete cremation); PC (partial cremation); Fr (fractional or excarnated remains); other information detailed.
6. BIH (burial in the habitation); BCC (burial in a cemetery context);

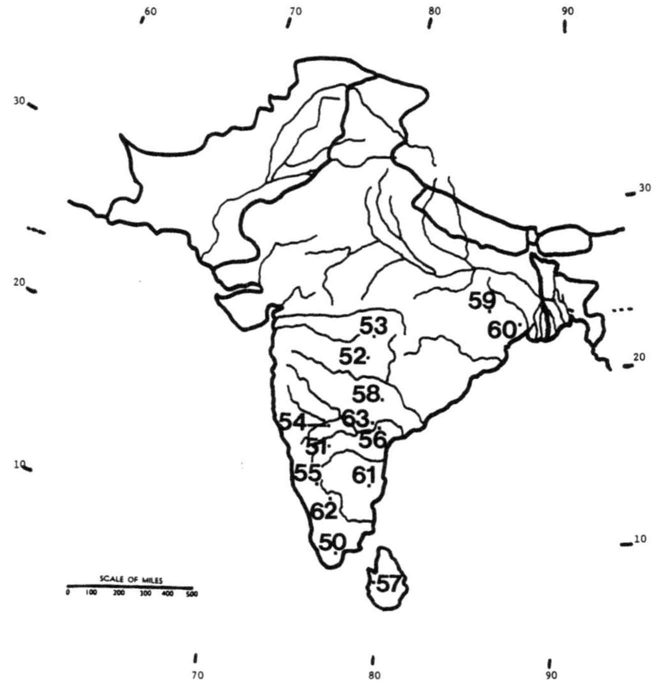

Figure 5. Location of sites yielding anatomically described human skeletal specimens of the Megalith Builders and their Iron Age collaterals (see Table I-E).

CAH (cemetery associated with habitation, compass directions used to indicate location of cemetery); BSM+ (burial surface monument present and described).

7. TFl (tightly flexed); Fl (flexed); Ext (extended); R (right side of body in contact with the burial surface); L (left side of body in contact with the burial surface); Var (no pattern discernable among burials).
8. N (north); S (south); E (east); W (west). Direction of head placement given first.
9. LF (living floor); other information detailed.
10. GG (grave goods); As (associations that are unintentional but that are located directly with the skeletal specimens); As w/i dep (associations in the deposit that are unintentional and not in direct association with the human remains); = (sign to indicate types of following artifacts); AgObjs (silver objects); AT (antler tools); AuObjs (gold objects); Bds (beads); BT (bone tools); CuObjs (copper objects); CuSnObjs (bronze objects); FeObjs (iron objects); FMB (fossil mammal bones); FRB (fossil reptile bones); IObjs (ivory objects); LF (living floor); MB

(*Continued on p. 185.*)

Table I
Catalog of Human Skeletal Remains at South Asian Sites

Map number	Place name and locality	Discoverer, date of discovery	Number of specimens	Dating references	Primary archaeological references	Primary anatomical references	Repository last reported
A. Specimens of Pleistocene or uncertain antiquity							
1.	AHIRPURA Gorakhpur, Uttar Pradesh	Carlleyle, 1875–1876	5	Holocene: Kennedy, 1973	Carlleyle, 1879	Carlleyle, 1879	Government Museum, Madras
BC: Skeles, Ad (2M, 1F, 2?), PB (intrusive?), Ext/?, 4N-S, 1SW-NE, within foundations of a small temple—1 lying across doorway, 2 on either side of an outer wall and 2(1M, 1F) side by side at rear end of temple. As w/i dep = FMB, IObj, TObj, Pt, BT							
2.	ATIRAMPAKAM Chingleput, Madras	Foote & King, 1863	1	Pleistocene(?): Sahni, 1956	Foote, 1914, 1916; Lydekker, 1880	Lydekker, 1880	Government Museum, Madras
BC: Tibia, in dry streambed; As w/i dep: ST.							
3.	BALAHAPUVA (KARANGODA) Ratnapura, Sabaragamuva	Piyasena, 1959	1	Terminal Middle Pleistocene(?): Deraniyagala, 1955a, 1960b, 1963a,d	Deraniyagala, 1959, 1960b	Deraniyagala, 1963a	Ratnapura Museum
BC: WP upper L. central incisor w/o root, 18 ft deep in gem sand dep.; As: ST, FMB.							
4.	BAYANA Agra, Uttar Pradesh	Wolff, 1910	1	Upper Pleistocene or Holocene: Keith, 1929; Vredenburg, 1919	Keith, 1919; Kirtikar, 1912	Keith, 1919; Kirtikar, 1912	Anthropological Survey of India, Calcutta
BC: fos skull, Ad(F), 35 ft below riverbed level in alluvial dep; As: none.							

(continued)

Table I *(Continued)*

Map number	Place name and locality	Discoverer, date of discovery	Number of specimens	Dating references	Primary archaeological references	Primary anatomical references	Repository last reported
5.	BILLA SURGAM Kurnool, Andhra Pradesh	Newbold, 1844; Foote, 1883 & 1884	2	Pleistocene: Lydekker, 1886; Murty, 1974b, 1979	Cammiade, 1926; Foote 1884a,b, 1885, 1916; Khatri, 1963; Murty 1974b, 1979; Newbold, 1884	Lydekker, 1886	Government Museum, Madras
BC: Chapter House Cave: Lg molar, 4 ft below surface of cave interior; As: none. Charnel House Cave: Frags, close to N wall of cave interior just under surface and broken limestone blocks, on disturbed dep; As w/i dep: MB, BT, AT.							
6.	DARRA-I-KUR Wakhan, Kataghan-Badakhshan	Dupree, 1966	1	Upper Pleistocene: Dupree, 1972	Dupree, 1972	Angel, 1972	Smithsonian Institution, Washington, D.C.
BC: Fos broken R temporal bone; As w/i/dep: Mousterian artifacts.							
7.	GORAKHPUR (UMHUT) Gorakhpur, Uttar Pradesh	Tucker, 1847	app 2	Pleistocene (?): P. Mitra, 1923; Theobald, 1881	Anderson, 1883; Blanford, 1864; P. Mitra, 1923; Theobald, 1881; Tucker, 1847	P. Mitra, 1927	Anthropological Survey of India, Calcutta
BC: Frags of app 2 skeles in a pit 12–15 ft deep; As: Shls, AT, FMB.							
8.	GUNDLAKAMMA Guntur, Andhra Pradesh	Foote, 1880	4	Holocene (?): Foote, 1916	Foote, 1880, 1916	Foote, 1916	Geological Survey of India, Calcutta
BC: Frags, 16–20 ft deep in alluvial sand cliffs; As w/i dep: Shls.							

9.	JAHINGE ANGILIYA (RATNAPURA) Ratnapura, Sabaragamuva	Mudiyanse, 1954	1	Middle Pleistocene (?): Deraniyagala, 1957, 1963a	Deraniyagala, 1958b, 1960b, 1963 a,d	Deraniyagala, 1957, 1963a	Ratnapura Museum
BC: Fos L. supraorbital ridge, 12.5 ft deep in black sand; As w/i dep: FMB							
10.	KARIMKHAN Hamirpur, Uttar Pradesh	Smith & Dean, 1833; Burt, 1833	"several"	Pleistocene or Holocene: Anonymous, 1833; Dean, 1835; Kennedy, 1973; Smith, 1833	Prinsep, 1833a,b, 1835a,b	Falconer, 1865, Prinsep, 1835a,b	Museum of the Asiatic Society, Calcutta
BC: Bones & Frags, 2.5–18 in. deep in clay shoal of river channel; As w/i dep: FMB, FRB, Shls.							
11.	LINDAGAVA Ratnapura, Sabaragamuva	Workmen, 1960–1963(?)	1	Pleistocene (?): Deraniyagala 1955a, 1963a	Deraniyagala, 1963a, 1965	Deraniyagala, 1963a	Ratnapura Museum
BC: WP upper L. premolar, 15 ft deep in gem pit; As: lion's carnassial tooth.							
12.	PUNE Pune, Maharashtra	Sankalia & Rajaguru, 1962	2	Holocene (?): Rajaguru & Kennedy, 1964	Rajaguru & Kennedy, 1964	Rajaguru & Kennedy, 1964	Deccan College, Pune
BC: SFos mandibles, Ad(M,F), in a talus dep below a vertical cliff; As w/i dep: sheep mandible.							
13.	SIALKOT Lahore, West Punjab	Hingston, 1912	1	Upper Pleistocene or Holocene: Keith, 1929; Vredenburg, 1919	Hingston, 1912; Keith, 1919; Kirtikar, 1912	Keith, 1919; Kirtikar, 1912	Anthropological Survey of India, Calcutta
BP: Skele, Ad(M), PB, TF1/R side, 6 ft below surface, protruding from a stream bank; As: none.							

(continued)

Table I (*Continued*)

Map number	Place name and locality	Discoverer, date of discovery	Number of specimens	Dating references	Primary archaeological references	Primary anatomical references	Repository last reported
14.	TIRUKKE-TISWARAM Manar, North Central Province	Shanmuganathan, 1950	1	Holocene: Chanmugam & Jayawardena, 1954	Begley, 1976; Chanmugam & Jayawardena, 1954	Chanmugam & Jayawardena, 1954	National Museum, Colombo
BP: WP Skele, Ad(F), PB, F1/Supine, W-E facing S, 4′8″ below surface in sandy soil/clay; GG = Bds; As w/i dep: Pt.							
B. Specimens of early Holocene and later hunter–gatherer communities							
15.	ALU GALGE (TELULLA) Badulla, Uva	Caldera & Sarannelis, 1954	1	Deraniyagala, 1955a	Deraniyagala, 1955a, 1963c	Deraniyagala, 1955b, 1957	National Museum, Colombo
BP: BaP Skele, Ad(M), PB, BIH, F1/L side facing E, covered w/ST, in rockshelter dep; GG = ST, Shls, BT; As w/i dep: ST, BT, Pt, MB, RB, Shls.							
16.	BAGHAI KHOR Mirzapur, Uttar Pradesh	Varma, 1964	1	Varma, 1964, 1965	Varma, 1964, 1965	Kennedy, unpublished	Allahabad University
BP: PP Skele, Ad(F), PB, BIH, Ext/Supine, W-E, lying on dressed bedrock platform w/raised platforms for head & feet, covered w/ST, in a rockshelter dep; As w/i dep: Pt, ST.							
17.	BATADOMBA LENA Ratnapura, Sabaragamuva	Deraniyagala, 1939	"several"	Deraniyagala, 1943a	Deraniyagala 1940, 1942, 1943a,b, 1953, 1957	Deraniyagala, 1953, 1957	National Museum, Colombo
BP: PP Bones & Frags, Ad/Ch-(teeth), PB, BIH, in rockshelter dep; As w/i dep: ST, BT, Pt.							
18.	BELLAN BANDI PALASSA Balangoda, Sabaragamuva	Delgoda, 1956; P. Deraniyagala; Dela & Hart, 1961; S. Deraniyagala & Kennedy, 1970	15	Deraniyagala, 1958a, 1971; Wintle & Oakley, 1972	Deraniyagala, 1956a,b,c,d, 1957, 1958a,b, 1959, 1960a,c, 1962, 1963d; S. Deraniyagala & Kennedy, 1972	Deraniyagala, 1957, 1958a,b, 1962, 1963a,b,c; Kennedy, 1965	National Museum, Colombo, and American Museum of Natural History, New York

BP (Gen): PP Skeles, Ad(M,F), PB, BIH, TF1/Var, W-E most facing E or SE, on limestone bedrock or limestone slab, head/thorax often covered w/another slab, skull often resting on hands, M/F pairs common, skull bones often damaged or found in isolation; in 4 ft thick midden dep; GG = ST, BT, AT, MB; As w/i dep: ST, BT, AT, MB, Pt.							
19.	BAGOR Bhilwara, Rajasthan	Misra, 1967–1970	1	IAR, 1956–1957	Misra, 1971a,b, 1972, 1973a	Lukacs, Misra, & Kennedy, 1982	Deccan College, Pune
BP: PP Skele, Ad(F), PB, BIH, Ext/Supine, NW–SE on LF in sand dune dep; GG = ST; As w/i dep: ST, MB, LFs.							
20.	BHIMBETKA Raisen, Madhya Pradesh	Wakankar, 1957; Bajpai & Pandey, 1971; Wakankar, 1972–1978; Misra, 1973	"Several"	Misra, 1973b	IAR 1975–1976, 1976–77; Misra, 1973b, 1974, 1976, 1978; Misra *et al.*, 1977; Wakankar, 1973, 1975	Tiwari & Banerjee, 1980	Vikram University, Ujjain, and Deccan College, Pune
BP (Gen): PP Skeles, Ad(M,F)/Ch, PB, BIH, F1 or Ext/Var, Var 0, usually resting on stone(s) in rockshelter dep; GG = ST, Pt, AT, BT, Ochre nodules, Bds, MB.							
21.	LANGHNAJ Mehsana, Gujarat	Sankalia & Karve, 1941–1942, 1944–1945; Sankalia, 1947; Subbarao, 1959; Kennedy & Karve-Corvinus, 1963	14	Agrawal & Kusumgar, 1969; Sankalia, 1965; Zeuner, 1952	Clutton-Brock, 1965; Karve-Corvinus & Kennedy, 1964; Sankalia, 1943a,b, 1946, 1949, 1955, 1956, 1965; Sankalia & Karve, 1944, 1945; Zeuner, 1950, 1951, 1952, 1963	Ehrhardt, 1960, 1963; Ehrhardt & Kennedy, 1965; Karve & Kurulkar, 1945; Khan & Karve, 1946; Sankalia & Karve, 1949	Deccan College, Pune
BP (Gen): PP Skeles, Ad(M,F)/Ch, PB & ?SB (indications of violence), BIH, TF1/R side, E-W; Var: 1 Ext/Supine, W-E; 2–6 ft deep in sand dune dep; GG = None; As w/i dep: ST, Pt, MB, Bds, CuObjs.							

(continued)

Table I *(Continued)*

Map number	Place name and locality	Discoverer, date of discovery	Number of specimens	Dating references	Primary archaeological references	Primary anatomical references	Repository last reported
22.	MAHADAHA Pratapgarh, Uttar Pradesh	Sharma, 1977–1979	26	Sharma *et al.*, 1980	IAR, 1977–1978, Sharma *et al.*, 1980	Kennedy 1983	Allahabad University
BP: SFos Skeles, Ad(M,F)/Ch, PB, BIH (often disturbed by hearths), Ext/Supine, W-E facing N; Var: 2 E-W, 2 double burials—1 w/ F laid over M, 1 w/ F to N of M; in shallow oblong pits sloping gently W-E, some graves w/soil cushion for head made of diff. soil from that of grave pit; GG = Bone Objs, Charred MB, ST, BT, Shls							
23.	PACHMARHI (DOROTHY DEEP) Hoshangabad, Madhya Pradesh	Hunter, 1932, 1933–1935	4	Hunter, 1935	Hunter, 1935, 1936	Buxton, 1935; Morant, 1936; Penniman, 1935	University Museum, Oxford
BP: BaP Skele & Frags, 1 Ad(M?)/Ch, PB, BIH, 1 burial (Ad) in situ—Ext/Supine, E-W, 18–21 in. below surface in rockshelter dep; rest = clustered frags on surface and in fill; GG = ST.							
24.	RAVAN ALLE Badulla, Uva	Caldera, 1945	1	Deraniyagala, 1953	Deraniyagala, 1945a,b,c, 1953, 1955a, 1957, 1958a	Deraniyagala, 1953; Oakley, 1983	National Museum, Colombo
BC: WP Frontal bone, Upper L Third Molar } Ad(M), PB, near cave wall, 16 ft from entrance { 1 ft 7 in. below surface covered by 3 rock slabs; 2 ft 6 in. below surface. As.w/i.dep.: ST, BT, Pt.							
25.	SARAI NAHAR RAI Pratapgarh, Uttar Pradesh	Dutta, 1968, 1970	35	Agrawal, 1971; Agrawal & Kusumgar, 1974; Dutta *et al.*, 1971	Dutta, 1971; Dutta *et al.*, 1971; Sharma, G. R., 1973, 1975	Dutta & Pal, 1972; Kennedy, 1983a,b; Sharma, G. R., 1975	Allahabad University

BP (Gen): SFos Skeles, Ad(M,F)/ PB, BIH (hearths distinct from burials), Ext/Supine, W-E, in compact, hard silt; GG = Pt, ST, Shls; As w/i dep: TObjs, charred MB							
C. Specimens from farming and nomadic populations of the northwestern sector of the subcontinent							
The Harappan civilization and the Gandharan grave culture							
26.	DAMB BUTHI Larkana, Sind	Majumdar, 1930–1931	"Several"	Majumdar, 1934	Majumdar, 1934	Guha, 1934	Anthropological Survey of India, Calcutta
BP: PP Frags, Ad(M,F)/ Misc, SB/Fr, BIH; bones scattered on LF of doorless small rooms; GG = Pt, ST, TObjs, ShlObjs, MB, Bds, Shl w/ RO							
27.	NAL (SOHR DAMB) Jhalawan, Kalat	Marshall, 1904–05 Jacobs, 1908 Hargreaves, 1925–26	18+	Hargreaves, 1929	Hargreaves, 1929	Sewell & Guha, 1929	Anthropological Survey of India, Calcutta
BP: 1: PP Skeles, 1 Ad(M)/4Ch, PB, BIH, Ad = Fl/L side, E-W facing S, Ad & 2Ch in mud-brick-lined graves; 2 other Ch in undefined graves; GG = Bds 2: PP Skulls & Frags, Ad(M,F)/Ch, SB/Fr, BCC/CAH, Frags scattered on grave floors; GG = Pt, MB, Bds, ST, CuObjs, BT, RO							
28.	QUETTA	Fairservis, 1949–1951	2	Fairservis, 1956	Fairservis, 1956	Cappieri, 1970; Riesenfeld, 1956	Uncertain
BP: PP Skull & Skele, Ad(M)-Skull/Ch-Skele, Ch = PB?, Ad = SB?/sacrifice, BIH, Ad Skull = face up in stone cavity in center of stone cairn under the main wall of a massive public building; BP of Ch Skele = ?; GG = none.							
29.	SHAHI-TUMP Turbat, Makran	Stein, 1926–1928	3	Stein, 1931	Stein, 1931	Sewell & Guha, 1931a	Anthropological Survey of India, Calcutta
BP: 1: WP Skeles, 2 Ad(M), PB, BIH, Fl/L side or supine, E-W; GG = Pt 2: PP Frags, SB/PC-CC, BIH; GG = Pt, MB							
30.	ALLAHDINO (NAL BAZAAR) Tatta, Sind	Fairservis, 1973–1974, 1973–74	1	Shaffer, 1974	Hoffman, 1974a,b; Hoffman & Shaffer, 1976; Khan, 1968; Shaffer, 1974	Lukacs, unpublished	American Museum of Natural History, New York
BC: WP Skull found near the surface in the fill of an alleyway; As w/i dep: none.							

(continued)

Table I (*Continued*)

Map number	Place name and locality	Discoverer, date of discovery	Number of specimens	Dating references	Primary archaeological references	Primary anatomical references	Repository last reported
31.	CHANDU-DARO Nawabshah, Sind	Majumdar, 1927–1931; Mackay, 1935–1936	1	Majumdar, 1934	Mackay, 1943; Majumdar, 1934	Krogman & Sassman, 1943	Indian Museum, Calcutta
BP: WP skull w/o mandible, Ad(F), SB/Fr, BIH, placed in a lg storage jar; GG = Shl, CuObjs, CuSnObjs, also in jar							
32.	HARAPPA Montgomery, Sind	Mason, 1826; Burnes, 1831; Cunningham, 1853–1856; Sahni, 1920–21; Vats, 1923–25, 1926–34; Sastri, 1937; Wheeler, 1946; Mughal, 1966	265	Sahni, 1926; Wheeler, 1947	Khan, 1968; Marshall, 1931; Sahni, 1926, 1927; Sarkar, 1954; Vats, 1940; Wheeler, 1947	Bartel, 1979; Chatterjee & Kumar, 1962, 1963a; Dutta, 1972; Gupta, Dutta & Basu, 1962; Kennedy, 1983d	Anthropological Survey of India, Calcutta

Cemetery H (Sahni, 1921–1925; Vats, 1926–1927, 1929–1930, 1933–1934; Wheeler, 1946).

BP: Stratum I: Ads & Ch: PP Skulls & Frags, Ad(M,F)/Ch, SB/Fr, BCC (S of city, but not contemporary with habitation); all remains in Pts, often commingled, skull(s) generally placed in center of Pt; Infs: PP Skeles, PB, BCC (see notes above), wrapped and placed in distinct Pt; several Pts had Infs & Ad(F—SB/Fr or PC) deposited together.

Stratum II: PP Skeles & Frags, Ad(M,F)/Ch, PB (some SB?/Fr?), BCC/CAH, Ext/Var, E-W (or NE-SW) in pits, GG = Pt MB.

Cemetery R37 (Sastri & Bose, 1937–41; Wheeler, 1946).

BP: Skeles & Frags, Ad(M,F)/Ch, PB, BCC (S of city)/CAH, Ext (1F1)/R or L side, N-S (1 S-N) facing W, in grave pits;

Var: 1 w/pile of mud bricks over it; 1 in wooden coffin; 2 in brick-lined cists; 1 w/pile of 5 skulls only; GG = (mostly around head) Pt (2–40 per burial), ShlObjs, CuObjs, AuObjs, Bds, MB, ST.

Area G (Vats, 1926–1927, 1929–1930, 1933–1934).

BP: PP Skulls & Frags, Ad(M,F)/Ch, SB/Fr, dumped in a single midden grave; As w/i dep: Pt, MB

Mound AB. (Vats, 1926–1927, 1929–1930, 1933–1934).

BP: PP Skulls & Frags, Ad(M,F)/Ch, SB/Fr?, BIH, in Pt.

Mound F. (Sarkar, 1930–1931—under Vats).

BP: PP Skeles. Ad(?), PB, BIH, Ext/R side, W-E, under LF; GG = Pt (reburied).

33.	KALIBANGAN Ganganagar, Rajasthan	Lal & Thapar, 1961–1969	11	IAR, 1962–1963	IAR, 1962–1963, Lal, 1979; Lal & Thapar, 1967; Thapar, 1973, 1975	Sharma, A. K., 1969–1970, 1972, 1979	Anthropological Survey of India, Calcutta

BP: 3 types—No. 1 and No. 2 distinct from each other in location; No. 3 scattered but predominantly in area of No. 1

1. PP Skeles, Ad(M,F)/Ch, PB, BCC (WSW of city)/CAH, Ext/Supine, N-S (1 = Fl/Prone, S-N), in oblong pits on brownish clay "carpet" of pit floor; Var: 1 grave lined w/mud bricks covered w/plaster & w/body lying on top of some 70+ Pts instead of grave floor, 1 reused grave of type 1 superimposed on type 2, 1 grave of 3 skulls & frag long bones only; GG = (placed around head mostly) Pt, CuObjs, Bds, ShlObjs, BT.
2. No bones, oval or circular pits w/Pt, ShlObjs, Bds.
3. No bones, rectangular or oval pits on N-S axis w/Pt, ShlObjs, Bds; pits not filled w/earth—left open

34.	LOTHAL Ahmedabad, Gujarat	Rao, 1954–1960	21	Rao, 1956–1957	Rao, 1956–1957, 1973	Chatterjee & Kumar, 1963b; Possehl & Kennedy, 1979; Sarkar, 1972	Anthropological Survey of India, Calcutta

BP: PP Skeles & Frags, Ad(M mostly, F)/Ch, PB, BCC (NW of city)/CAH, Ext/Supine predominently, N-S facing E, in rectangular pits covered by a low tumulus; Var: 1 grave lined w/mud brick, 3 examples of double burial (2 M,F—1 M,M), 3 examples of Pt urn burial of frags in circular pits, but there is no distinction in the cemetery of location of Ext vs urn burials; GG = Pt (1–2 near head), MB, CuObjs, ShlObjs.

35.	MOHENJO-DARO Larkana, Sind	Banerjee, 1920; Banerjee, Vats; Dikshit, Hargreaves under Marshall, 1922–1927; Mackay, 1927–1931; Wheeler, 1950; Dales, 1964–1965	46	Marshall, 1931	Dales, 1964, 1965; Hasan, 1975; Khan, 1968; MacKay, 1938; Marshall, 1931	Cappieri, 1970; Guha & Basu, 1938; Kennedy, 1983d; Sewell & Guha, 1931b	Anthropological Survey of India, Calcutta

(*continued*)

Table I (*Continued*)

Map number	Place name and locality	Discoverer, date of discovery	Number of specimens	Dating references	Primary archaeological references	Primary anatomical references	Repository last reported
BC: PP Skeles & Frags, Ad(M,F)/Ch, primary deposition, BIH (all in lower town, none in citadel), but may not be contemporary w/habitiation; positions and orientations var; Indications of tragic death suggested by body positions, locations, and injuries; As w/i dep: (scattered) Pt, IObjs, Bds, CuObjs							
BP?: 4 PP Skeles, Ad(M,F), PB, BIH, Ext/L side, N-S facing E w/head on L hand; located below LF or in courtyard; GG = none.							
Gandharan grave culture							
36.	BUTKARA II Swat, N.W. Frontier	Tucci & Khan, 1955; Tucci, 1960–1962; Taddei, 1961–1962	50	Stacul, 1966; Tucci, 1963	Antonini, 1963, 1969; Tucci, 1958	Alciati, 1967; Alciati & Fedeli, 1965; Genna, 1965	Italian Archaeological Mission, Saidu Sharif, & Institute of Archaeology, University of Rome
BP (Gen): WP Skeles & Frags, Ad(M,F)/, PB, and SB/PC= PB = Fl/R or L side, S-N w/head toward hill facing E or W, lying in center of tomb's lower cavity. GG mainly at feet (N); Var: 2 examples of double burial; SB/PC= Frags in Pt urn, covered w/lid; BCC (on side of hill), in distinctive tombs having 2 cavities: upper cavity = rectangular w/rounded corners, earth fill(?) (the upper cavity contained remains of the crematory process in the case of the SB/PC—bone frags, ashes, charcoal); lower cavity = circular and narrower than upper cavity, contained PB or SB/PC human remains; slabs of stone and a lining of schist separated the cavities w/smaller stones filling in gaps; GG = Pt ($\bar{x}$ = 10 per burial, placed around urn exterior), TObjs, CuObjs, Bds mixed in w/frags.							
37.	SARAI KHOLA Taxilla, N.W. Frontier	Sharif, 1967; Khan, 1968–1971; Halim, 1968–1969	122	Halim 1970–1971, 1972	Halim, 1970–1971, 1972; Khan, 1968; Mughal, 1972	Bernhard, 1969	Department of Archaeology, Karachi, and University of Mainz
BP: PP-WP Skeles, Ad(M,F)/Ch, PB, BCC (on high portion of mound to N), BSM+ (Early Cemetery: one stone each at head (E) and feet (W) ends of grave on top of fill; graves also shallow; Late Cemetery: large to medium pebbles scattered over top of fill; graves also deeper than those of Early Cemetery);							

Ext/Supine—Age/Sex Vars =
Ad(M) = arms parallel to body; young M = arms parallel to body, 1 leg bent so foot touched opposite ankle;
Ad(F) = 1 hand over pelvic region, other hand over ribs or parallel to body; young F = 1 hand over pelvic region, other hand over abdomen or ribs; 1 leg bent so foot touched opposite ankle;
Ch = arms parallel; 1 leg bent so foot touched opposite leg, or both legs bent so feet touched; E-W (1 = N-S) facing N or S or skyward; Skeles lying on prepared (hardened) floors of rectangular grave pits, laid out in parallel rows; generally, M, F burials occurred in distinct rows, but later burials were added in between existing graves w/o regard for the ''sex'' of a particular given row; GG = FeObjs, Bds, ShlObjs.

38.	TIMARGARHA Dir, N.W. Frontier	Dani, 1964–1965	137	Alciati, 1967; Dani, 1967	Dani, 1967, 1968; Dani & Durrani, 1964	Bernhard, 1967, 1968	Anthropological Institute, University of Mainz & Museum, Department of Archaeology, Peshawar University

BP: *Period I:* PP Skeles, Ad(M,F)/Ch, PB, BCC (on side of hills), BSM+ (circle of stones above fill), TFL/R or L side w/hands together below face, SW-NE, in deep rectangular pits lined (at their lower extremes) w/stone masonry and covered over by stone rubble above more fill; GG = Pt (to sides of skeles), TObjs, CuSnObjs IObjs.
Period II: (Burials of Period I persist): PP Frags, Ad(M,F)/Ch, SB/PC in Pt urns, BCC (on sides of hills, often above Period I burials), BSM+ & grave construction are same as in Period I, but SB/PC urn present in pit instead of TF1 Skele; urn usually covered; ashes/bone frags not always present; GG = Pt, CuSnObjs, Bds, ShlObjs, Bone Objs, IObjs, AuObj.
Period III: (Burials of Periods I and II persist): PP Frags, Ad(M,F)/Ch, SB/Fr in Pt urns, BCC (on sides of hills, often above Periods I & II burials), BSM+ & grave construction are same as in Period I, but SB/Fr urn now replaces position of TF1 Skele or SB/PC urn; GG = Pt, FeObjs, TObjs, CuSnObjs, Bds.

D. Specimens from early farming and herding communities of central and southern India

39.	APEGAON Aurangabad, Maharashtra	Deo, 1976	1	Deo *et al.*, 1979	Deo *et al.*, 1979	Lukacs, 1980	Deccan College, Pune

BC: Mandibular frag w/3 molars found in ''Layer 3'' of site; As w/i dep = None.

40.	BAGOR Bhilwara, Rajasthan	Misra, 1967–1970	3	IAR, 1956–1957	IAR, 1956–1957; Leshnik, 1968; Misra, 1970a,b, 1972	Lukacs, Misra & Kennedy, 1982	Deccan College, Pune

(*continued*)

Table I (*Continued*)

Map number	Place name and locality	Discoverer, date of discovery	Number of specimens	Dating references	Primary archaeological references	Primary anatomical references	Repository last reported
BP: BaP Skeles, Ad(M,F), PB, BIH, BSM+ (in 1 case only—circular enclosure of stones overlying burial), TF1/R side, E-W facing N or S, placed on a LF of stone slabs and covered by a new LF; GG = CuObjs, Pt (near head and/or feet), MB, Bds, TObjs.							
41.	BRAHMAGIRI Chitaldrug, Karnataka	Krishna, 1942; Wheeler, 1947	20	Wheeler, 1947–1948	Wheeler, 1947–1948	Sarkar, 1960, 1972	Anthropological Survey of India, Calcutta
BP: PP Skeles, Ad(1 partially uncovered)/Ch-1 Juv & 18 Ch & Infs, PB, BIH, Age var = Ad & Juv (N = 2) = Ext/Supine, E-W facing N; GG = Pt near pelvis and head; Ch & Infs (N = 18) = TF1 in globular Pt urns placed in small pits; Frags only remain; urns covered; GG = Pt, CuSnObj.							
42.	CHANDOLI Pune, Maharashtra	Deo & Ansari, 1957, 1961	24	Deo & Ansari, 1965	Deo & Ansari, 1965	Malhotra, 1963, 1965a	Deccan College, Pune
BP: BaP Skeles, Ad(M)/Ch-1 Juv & Infs, PB, BIH, Age Var: Ad & Juv (N = 2) = Ext/Supine, N-S, lying on LF of burnt clods covered by interconnecting Pt; Feet removed (possibly) prior to burial; N bones of the Ad charred (accidental?); GG = Pt; Ch & Infs (N = 22) = in 2 globular Pt urns placed mouth to mouth horizontally on N-S axis; no pit—lying on LF; N urn generally contained bones of thorax up—S urn generally contained pelvic & leg bones, or was empty; Var: 3 examples of deposition in 1 Pt urn placed vertically; 1 example of deposition in 3 urns; GG = Pt, CuObjs, Bds, ShlObj.							
43.	INAMGAON Pune, Maharashtra	Sankalia, 1967, 1968–1975	70	Agrawal, 1969; Sankalia, Ansari & Dhavalikar, 1971	IAR 1974–1975; IAR 1977–1978; Sankalia, 1977; Sankalia, Ansari & Dhavalikar, 1971, 1975	Badam, 1977; Lukacs, 1981a; Lukacs & Badam, 1975, 1977	Deccan College, Pune
BP: WP Skeles, Ad(M,F)/Ch, PB (some Ch = SB/Fr), BIH, Age Var= Ad = Ext/Supine, N-S, in pits inside house floors or in courtyards, feet removed before burial; Var.: 1 example of M placed in 4-legged unbaked Pt urn in a sitting posture (TF1) w/feet present; 1 example of 2 4-legged urns placed mouth to mouth on N-S axis in a pit, but no bones (symbolic burial?) and in same area as burial described previously; GG = Pt; Ch = in 2 Pt globular urns placed mouth to mouth horizontally on N-S axis in small pits w/i house floors; N urn contained head, S urn contained rest of body; Var: several examples of single urn burial; GG = Pt, Bds, CuObjs; evidence that both Ad & Ch were wrapped in grass before burial.							

44.	MASKI Raichur, Karnataka	Yazdani, 1935–1937; Thapar, 1954	329	Thapar, 1957	Gordon & Gordon, 1943; Richards, 1939; Thapar, 1957; Yazdani, 1938, 1939	Sarkar, 1972	Anthropological Survey of India, Calcutta
BP: None described (see Iron Age), but Yazdani briefly mentions some urn and extended burials.							
45.	NAGARJUNA-KONDA Guntur, Andhra, Pradesh	Saraswati, 1926; Soundara Rajan, 1954–1957; Sinha, Subrahmanyan *et al.*, 1957–1958, 1958–1959, 1959–1960	13	IAR, 1957–1958; Soundara Rajan, 1958	IAR, 1957–1958; Sarkar & Mishra, 1966; Soundara Rajan, 1958	Gupta, Basu & Dutta, 1970	Anthropological Survey of India, Calcutta
BP: PP Skeles & Frags, Ad(M,F)/Ch, PB and SB/Fr, BIH, and BCC (2000 m to W of habitation site)/CAH—Var = BIH = 1 Ad(M)/2 Ch; Ad = PB, Ext/Supine, N-S, w/feet missing, compressed into a circular (hearth) pit, covered by a cairn heap; 2 Ch = SB/Fr, inside Pt urns; GG = none. *BCC:* Ad(6M,3F,1?); PB(5 graves yielding M individuals except 1 with a F) and SB/Fr (3 graves yielding 2 M-F double burials and 1 single burial of ? sex), Ext/Supine, N-S (in the SB/Fr examples, the disarticulated, incomplete skeles were laid out in app. anatomical order on a N-S axis); SB/Fr double burials had 1M-1F side by side; GG = Pt (near feet), MB.							
46.	NEVASA Ahmednagar, Maharashtra	Sankalia, 1954–1956; Deo & Ansari, 1959–1960, 1960–1961	130	Sankalia, Deo, Ansari & Ehrhardt, 1960	Sankalia, Deo, Ansari & Ehrhardt, 1960	Kennedy & Malhotra, 1966	Deccan College, Pune
BP: WP Skeles, Ad(M,F)/Ch, PB = Ads & Infs, SB/Fr = Ch, BIH, Age Var = Ad = Ext/Supine (some F1), N-S, in pits lined w/lime or in horizontally placed Pt urns, under LF, feet removed before burial; GG = Pt, Bds; Ch = SB/Fr, (PB, TF1 of Infs), in 2 Pt globular urns placed horizontally mouth to mouth primarily on N-S axis under LF in pits or on LF covered over with soil; Var: some instances of covered single-urn burial, vertically placed double-urn burial (urns still placed mouth to mouth), and triple-urn burial horizontally; 2 examples of double burial w/i 2 urns (1 Ch in each urn); In all horizontal urn burials, N urn contained bones from the thorax up—S urn contained pelvic and leg bones; somne burial urns devoid of remains (symbolic burial?); GG = Pt, Bds, CuObjs							
47.	PIKLIHAL Raichur, Karnataka	Allchin, 1952	4	Allchin, 1960	Allchin, 1960	Ayer, 1960; Malhotra, 1967; Sarkar, 1972	Archaeological Survey, Hyderabad

(*continued*)

Table I *(Continued)*

Map number	Place name and locality	Discoverer, date of discovery	Number of specimens	Dating references	Primary archaeological references	Primary anatomical references	Repository last reported
BP: PP Skeles & 1 Frag, Ad(1M,1F)/1Ch, PB, BIH, BSM+ (boulder for Ad M), Ext/Supine (Ads), R side (Ch), SE-NW (Ch), N-S (F), S-N (M), in shallow pits; GG = none w/Ch, Pt, ST near head, pelvis and/or feet of Ads.							
48.	TEKKALAKOTA Bellary, Karnataka	Rao, 1963–1965	9+	Rao, 1967; Rao & Malhotra, 1965	Rao, 1967; Rao & Malhotra, 1965	Malhotra, 1965b	Deccan College, Pune
BP: *Phase I:* WP Skeles, Ad(M,F)/Ch, mainly SB/Fr, BIH, BSM+ (boulders above grave fill), Age Var = Ad = SB/Fr but laid out in approx. anatomical order in Ext/Supine burial, S-N, in shallow pit; Var: 1 grave w/3 individuals, 1 grave = PB, Ext/R side, W-E facing S, in a shallow pit between 4 rocks outside a house—bones below upper legs removed to make body fit in grave area; GG = Pt near head (on abdomen in case of PB just described); Ch = SB/Fr outside house to N; 1 in a covered urn w/ST, 1 in debris from house; Inf (*N* = 1): PB under LF on a rock, TF1 but not in an urn; *Phase II:* WP Skeles, Ad(M,F)/Ch, PB = ads, SB/Fr = Ch, BIH, Age Var= Ad = Ext/Supine or R side, N-S facing W, in oval pits; Var: 1 SB/Fr but laid out in approx. anatomical position buried under interconnecting Pts.; GG = Pt near feet; Ch = SB/Fr in urns under LF.							
49.	T. NARASIPUR Mysore, Karnataka	Foote (ca. 1865), Seshadri, 1959–1960, 1962–1963, 1965	1	Seshadri, 1971	Seshadri, 1971	Malhotra, 1971	Archaeological Survey, Mysore
Baseline: PP Skele, Ad(F), PB, BIH, Ext/Supine, E-W facing S, with hands crossed over abdomen, in an oblong pit with a posthole on either side (function?); GG = Pt (near head), TObj ("headrest").							
E. Specimens of the megalith builders and their Iron Age collaterals							
50.	ADITTANALLUR (ADICHANAL-LUR)	Jägor, 1876; Rea, 1899–1905, 1908; Lapique,	16+	Rea, 1902–1903	Grunwedel, 1914; Rea, 1902–1903a,b, 1903–	Chatterjee & Gupta, 1963; Kennedy, 1983c;	Anthropological Survey of India, Calcutta

	Tinnevelly, Madras	1903–1905			1904, 1915	Sarkar, 1965, 1972; Smith, 1927; Thurston, 1909; Zuckerman, 1930	
BP:	PP Skeles & Frags, Ad(M,F)/Ch, ?PB & SB/Fr—possible age var?, BCC (to S of habituation)/CAH, PB = TF1 vertically in sitting posture, PB & SB/Fr all in large, 1-legged, globular urns w/lids; some urns w/complete Skeles, others w/Frags, and still others devoid of remains; GG = Pt, AuObjs, CuObjs, CuSnObjs, FeObjs, Bds, PR, some inside and some outside of urn; weapons found point down.						
51.	BRAHMAGIRI Chitraldrug, Karnataka	Krishna, 1942; Wheeler, 1947	20	Wheeler, 1947–1948	Wheeler, 1947–1948	Sarkar, 1960, 1972	Anthropological Survey of India, Calcutta
BP:	WP Bones, Ad(M,F)/Ch, SB/Fr, BCC (surrounding town site on NE & SE)/CAH, BSM+ of 2 types (not distinct in location). 1. Cist circles = burial pit lined w/granite slabs resting on a floor slab and covered by a capstone; E wall had a sealed port-hole; ramp leading to porthole on E side w/lined walls that then extended all the way around the cist; low cairn covered the cist on surface; inside cist, GG lay on the floor slab, covered by ca. 6 in. of earth with remains (and sometimes more GG-secondary offerings) on top of this. More earth added and port-hole sealed; bones lay in center of cist, or to W of center, commingled and scattered in all 6 excavated examples. 2. Pit circles = single or double stone circle enclosing a circular or oval (E-W axis) pit "sealed" by nonfunctional doors, w/shallow ramp approaching pit from the E; Floor of pit had 4 stone slabs overlaid with earth fill; GG in earth fill and bones (only in 2 of the 4 excavated examples) above earth fill—Possible that these were excarnation pits rather than intentional burials; GG in Cist Circles = Pt (6–62 per megalith), FeObjs, Bds, TObjs; GG in pit circles = Pt, FeObjs, Bds, CuObjs, Shl.						
52.	KHAPA Nagpur, Maharashtra	Deo, 1968–1969	5	Deo, 1970; IAR, 1967–1968	Deo, 1970, 1978	V. V. Rao, 1970	Deccan College, Pune
BP:	PP Frags, Ad(M,F), SB/Fr, BCC (W side of river; town site is on E side of river)/CAH, BSM+ = single stone circle placed on surface and filled w/earth; bones and GG in earth fill (5 of 9 excavated megaliths contained frags or teeth); remains clustered in one or more quadrants of circle w/GG; Var = 2 examples of remains being found in center of circle—1 group in a Pt, other group in a Cu dish; GG = Pt, MB (*Equus* often), Bds, FeObjs, CuObjs.						
53.	MAHURJHARI Nagpur, Maharashtra	Deo, 1970–1972, 1979	28	Deo, 1973a	Deo, 1973b	Lukacs, 1981b; Rao, 1973	Deccan College, Pune

(*continued*)

Table I *(Continued)*

Map number	Place name and locality	Discoverer, date of discovery	Number of specimens	Dating references	Primary archaeological references	Primary anatomical references	Repository last reported
BP:	WP Skeles & Frags, Ad(M,?F), PB & SB/Fr, BCC, BSM+ (single and double stone circles occur, but all human remains were recovered from megaliths with only a single circle); PB = Ext/Supine, E-W, lying on natural surface under earth fill inside stone circle, feet missing in all examples; Var: 1 Skele lying on thin bed of earth, 2 double burials—1 w/skeles lying one above the other over a series of Pts, 1 w/skeles laid side by side; SB/Fr = Frags clustered in quadrants of circle; PB & SB/Fr = no distinction in quadrants where remains occur, but only a few of the excavated circles contained remains in the NE quadrant. Virtually all excavated circles contained remains of more than 1 individual; GG = Pt, Bds, MB (*Equus* often), CuObjs, Cu & Fe Objs, FeObjs, AuObjs.						
54.	MASKI Raichur, Karnataka	Yazdani, 1935–1937; Thapar, 1954	9+	Thapar, 1957	Thapar, 1957	Sarkar, 1972	Anthropological Survey of India, Calcutta
BP:	None described from excavation of Chalcolithic and Iron Age burials by Yazdani. B.P. information on Iron Age burials excavated by Thapar: WP Skeles & Frags, Ad(M,F)/Ch, 5 types distinguished (located in different parts of the site); 1. PB, BIH, Ext/Supine, N-S facing W, in the center of an elliptical pit (N-S axis) lying on ash layer on bottom of pit, w/ash spread over body too; Var: 1 w/lime instead of ash over body, 1 w/7 slabs instead of ash over body, 1 lying directly on pit floor—Fl/L side, S-N facing E, w/o GG; GG = Pt, FeObjs, MB; 2. SB/Fr, BCC/CAH, in an elliptical pit (E-W) axis), ash on pit floor covered by stacked Pt, bones scattered over the Pt in the center of the pit and covered by more ash; GG = Pt, FeObj, MB; 3. SB/Fr, BCC/CAH in a Pt urn w/lid, in shallow pit just deep enough to cover urn; GG = Pt inside and outside of urn; 4. PB, BIH, BSM+ (circle of boulders with rubble packing), Ext/Supine, N-S facing W, in an oblong pit, lying on stone slabs and covered w/stone slabs upon which GG were placed; GG = Pt (& 2 stone balls found w/Ch skele); 5. SB/Fr, BCC/CAH, BSM+ (low cairn within a circle of boulders), remains located in pit under the center of the low cairn w/shallow ramp on E side; 7 in. of ash fill in bottom of pit over which remains scattered w/GG; GG = Pt, FeObjs.						
55.	MYSORE Mysore, Karnataka	Bain, 1890?	1	Bain, 1890	Bain, 1890	Bain, 1890	Not collected
BP:	WP Skele, Ad(M), BCC? (only 1 megalith excavated), BSM+ (3 concentric stone circles), Ext/Supine?, lying on floor slab of a ''dolmen'' (w/roof, walls and floor slab(s)) located 4 ft under surface below BSM+; GG = Pt, PR, FeObjs, AuObj, CuObj						

56.	NAGARJUNA-KONDA Guntur, Andhra Pradesh	Saraswati, 1926; Soundara Rajan, 1954–1957; Sinha, Subrahmanyan, *et al.*, 1957–1958, 1958–1959, 1959–1960	19	IAR, 1957–1958; Soundara Rajan, 1958	IAR, 1957–1958; Sarkar & Mishra, 1966; Soundara Rajan, 1958	Gupta, Basu & Dutta, 1970	Anthropological Survey of India, Calcutta
BP:	PP Skeles & Frags, Ad(M,F)/Ch, SB/Fr (primarily) and PB, BCC (WNW of habitation)/CAH, BSM+ (single stone circle) 2 types: 1. Cist Circles (2 examples excavated): E-W chamber of 4 orthostats, covered by 2 slabs, w/o a porthole, under BSM+; SB/Fr (1 contained remains of 3 Ads, the other contained 2 Ad femora); GG = CuObj, Pt, FeObjs, MB 2. Pit circles (12 examples excavated): Unlined rectangular pits (oriented E-W or N-S, no distinction in burials) under BSM+ w/ ash layer on pit floor; PB (2 graves), SB/Fr (7 graves), 1 w/ no human bones, 1 with splinters only, and 1 w/ a few frags in NE corner; PB = Ad (1F,1?), Ext/left side, 1 facing E(F), the other facing S (Sex?); SB/Fr = Ad(M,F)/Ch laid out in app. anatomical order N-S (Var: 1 E-W oriented triple burial group of 2 Ads and 1 Ch); Four double burials of Ads (1M-M,1M-F,2?-?); 1 Ch burial w/ 2 animals located one above the other in fill over burial; GG = Pt, FeObjs, TObjs, Bds, MB.						
57.	POMPARIPPU North Central Province	Hocart, 1916; DeSilva, 1956–1957; Bronson, Begley & Kennedy, 1970	27	Begley, Kennedy, & Lukacs, 1981	Begley, 1976; Begley, Lukacs, & Kennedy, 1981	Lukacs, 1976; Lukacs & Kennedy, 1981	University of Pennsylvania, Philadelphia
BP:	PP Skulls & Frags, Ad(M,F)/Ch, SB/Fr & possible PC for Ch, BCC, BSM+ (large limestone boulders or tumulus/cairn—1 under possible brick floor); bones and GG placed in bottom of a large Pt urn (bones often placed w/i GG Pt) and urns then buried in pits singly or (more frequently) in groups below BSM+; commingling of bones common; GG = Pt, Bds, FeObjs, CuObjs, ST, MB.						
58.	RAIGIR Hyderabad, Andhra Pradesh	Hunt, 1920s	24 burials (6 calvariae remaining)	Hunt, 1916, 1924	Hunt, 1916, 1924	Kennedy, 1965[a]	British Museum (Natural History), London

(*continued*)

Table I *(Continued)*

Map number	Place name and locality	Discoverer, date of discovery	Number of specimens	Dating references	Primary archaeological references	Primary anatomical references	Repository last reported
BP: BaP Skeles & Frags, Ad(M,F)/Ch, PB & SB/Fr & a few PC (Sacrificial?), BCC, BSM+ (cairn circles), PB = TF1/? (3 Ext/Supine), N-S; SB/Fr = bones found in piles near PBs—sacrificial victims?; SB/PC urn burial of Ch rare but present, some SB/Fr of Ch too; all burials found in cists under BSM+; commingling and multiple burials very common; GG = Pt (lying on top of stones on floor of cist), Bds, FeObjs, CuObjs, Au/AgObj							
59.	RANCHI Ranchi, Bihar	Basu, 1935?	3	Mitra, 1936	Mitra, 1936	Mitra, 1936	Anthropological Survey of India, Calcutta
BP: WP Skulls (& Skeles ?), Ad(M,F), found in a "dolmenic grave"; GG = FeObjs, ST, Pt.							
60.	RUAMGARH Dhalbhum, Bihar	Murray, 1926	2	Murray, 1940	Guha, 1935; Murray, 1940	Kennedy, 1972	British Museum (Natural History), London
BC/BP: WP Skulls, Ad(M), found on surface debris near the N entrance to the ruins of a brick-built, circular watchtower; 2 monoliths noted protruding from the foundations of tower to S of location of skulls; neither the skulls nor the monoliths were noted by Murray when he examined the site 2 years prior to the discovery of the human remains.							
61.	SANUR Chingleput, Madras	Banerjee & Soundara Rajan, 1950, 1952	3+	Banerjee, 1956	Banerjee, 1956; Banerjee & Soundara Rajan, 1959	Bose, 1959	Government Museum, Madras
BP: BaP Skulls & Frags, Ad(M,F), SB/, BCC, BSM+ (cairn w/i large stone circle); 2 types found: 1. Pit burial under BSM+; pit was oblong (E-W axis) w/ E and W upper sides lined w/rubble packing; bones lying in central space w/GG along sides of pit surrounding remains; bones had been laid out on an E-W alignment in an organized pattern, but not in anatomical order; GG = Pt, MB, FeObjs (some in fill).							

2. Dolmenoid cists enclosing sarcophagi below BSM+; cists composed of 7 orthostatic boulders and oriented on an E-W axis; E side of cists had porthole sealed by slab(s); 1 cist w/5 sarcophagi (E-W, 1 N-S) of which 1 contained frags w/GG inside and outside of sarcophagus; other cist had 3 sarcophagi (E-W, 1 NE-SW) of which 2 contained skulls and skele remains heaped inside; some bones also in Pt around sarcophagi and scattered on cist floor; GG located outside of sarcophagi; GG = Pt, FeObjs, ST.

62.	SAVANKURGA Bangalore, Karnataka	Branfill, 1879	ca. 6	Branfill, 1881	Branfill, 1881	Branfill, 1881	Uncertain

BP: BaP Skele & Frags, Ad(?)/Ch?, SB/PC, BCC, BSM+ (oblong dolmens on E-W axis, above ground surrounded by stone circle(s); 4 orthostats of sides dressed, capstone natural); SB/PC frags found in 3 megaliths: each contained 2 bowls w/remains, usually placed near sides of dolmen; 1 megalith contained SB/PC frags in fill and a skele lying on a prepared platform on the floor of the dolmen—TF1/R side, E-W facing N (Ad F?); GG = Pt, FeObjs, CuObjs, MB.

63.	YELLESWARAM Nalgonda, Andhra Pradesh	Sreenvivasacher, 1955–1956, Khan, 1960–1962	16	Khan, 1963	Khan, 1963	Gupta & Dutta, 1962; Sarkar, 1972	Department of Archaeology, Hyderabad

BP: WP Skeles & Frags, Ad(M,F)/Ch, BCC (all under Buddhist Temple), BSM+ (but not exposed to surface); 5 Types:

1. PB, in a pit; 1 Skele. Ext/Supine, N-S looking up; GG = Pt, FeObjs.
2. PB, under a cairn circle in an elliptical pit (N-S axis); 2 skeles (one above the other) lying on thin ash layer covered w/Pt; Ext/Supine, N-S facing up; GG = Pt, FeObjs, MB (*Equus*)—MB (*Equus*) also found in Pt dish in fill.
3. SB/Fr, of 1 Ch & 1 Ad in a Pt urn covered w/ a lid and a BSM+ (capstone) above it; GG = Pt, FeObjs (inside urn).
4. SB/PC, frags in Pt inside a dolmenoid cist (N-S axis) w/sealed porthole in N orthostat; GG = Pt, FeObjs, smaller cist to W side.
5. SB/Fr, skulls & frags inside a dolmenoid cist (N-S axis) w/o a porthole; cist was partitioned by a rough slab w/2 skulls & bones in E compartment, and 1 skull & bones in W compartment; GG = Pt.

Table II
List of Prehistoric South Asian Sites at Which Skeletal Specimens Have Been Found (Descriptions Unpublished or Unavailable)

Specimens of uncertain or Pleistocene antiquity	
Antichak, Bihar	Chandravalli, Karnataka
Barlagondi Hill, Karnataka	Sijua, Uttar Pradesh
Bhimbetka, Madhya Pradesh	Urumutta, Sri Lanka
Specimens of early Holocene and later hunter–gatherer communities	
Beli-Lena Athula, Sri Lanka	Lekhahia Rock Shelter, Uttar Pradesh
Jalampura, Gujarat	Morhana Pahar, Uttar Pradesh
Kuruvita, Sri Lanka	
Specimens from farming and nomadic populations of the northwestern sector	
Abdul-But, Baluchistan	Mehi, Baluchistan
Dabar-Kot, Baluchistan	Nokjo Shah-Dinzai, Baluchistan
Kaudani, Baluchistan	Periano Ghundai, Baluchistan
Kulli, Baluchistan	Suktagen-Dor, Baluchistan
Las Bela, Baluchistan	Sur-Jangal, Baluchistan
Mundigak, Kandahar, Afghanistan	
Harappan civilization	
Burzahom, Kashmir[a]	Mehrgarh, Baluchistan
Chandigarh, Punjab	Rampara II, Gujarat
Gumla, Gomel Valley	Randal Dadwa, Saurashtra
Hathala, Gomel Valley	Rupar, Punjab
Ispelinji, Baluchistan	Tarkanwala Dera, Rajasthan
Mahra Sharif, Gomel Valley	Uchali, Punjab
Gandharan Grave culture	
Bakamak, Chitral	Loebanr I, Swat
Bala Hisar, Chitral	Panchpir, Dir
Balambat, Dir Panjkora Valley	Pulanr, Buner
Bros (Tamunak), Chitral	Rashnel, Chitral
Chakdara, Dir	"Stone Enclosed Cemetery," Baluchistan
Charpat, Dir	Tarika, Buner
Dolmutse, Chitral	Tashneb, Chitral
Gogdara, Swat	Thana, Swat
Katelai I, Swat	Ushoram, Chitral
Kherai, Kohistan	Zarif Karuna, Peshawar Plain
Labbatai, Buner	Ziarat, Dir
Specimens from early farming and herding communities of central and southern India	
Amreli, Gujarat	Moghul-Ghundai, Baluchistan
Chaperkai Hill, Baluchistan	Nasirabad, Baluchistan
Daimabad, Maharashtra	Pandu Rajar Dhibi, West Bengal
Damba-Koh, Baluchistan	Sonpur, Bihar
Gatti, Baluchistan	Take-Dap, Baluchistan
Gevarjak, Baluchistan	Tekwada, Maharashtra

Table II (*Continued*)

Hallur, Karnataka	Tor-Dherai, Baluchistan
Jhangar, Sind	Zangian, Baluchistan
Jiwanri, Baluchistan	
Specimens of the megalith builders and their Iron Age collaterals	
Agiripalli, Andhra Pradesh	Montapalam, Tamil Nadu
Amirthamangalam, Tamil Nadu[b]	Nilgiris Hills, Karnataka
"Asura Graves," Bihar	Noghormuri, Chitral
Chandravalli, Karnataka	Paikara, Karnataka
Damloti Water Works, Sind	Palni Hills, Tamil Nadu
Gulsohankanatte, Sri Lanka	Paryampalli, Tamil Nadu
Gurugal Hinna, Sri Lanka	Perambour, Andhra Pradesh
Halingali, Karnataka	Perimbe, Tamil Nadu
Jewurji, Maharashtra	Pochampad, Andhra Pradesh
Junapani, Madhya Pradesh	Porkalam, Kerala
Kadambapur, Andhra Pradesh	T. Kallupatti, Tamil Nadu
Kathiraveli, Sri Lanka	Tennar, Andhra Pradesh
Kokebe, Sri Lanka	Tiruvicar, Tamil Nadu
Kot Allah-Dad, Gomel Valley	Twenty-first Mile Post on the Puttalam-Pomparippu Road, Sri Lanka
Kunnattur, Tamil Nadu	Uppalapadu, Andhra Pradesh
Makewita, Sri Lanka	Veerabyina Kinta, Andhra Pradesh
Maski, Karnataka	
Maula Ali, Hyderabad	

[a]Basu and Pal, 1980.
[b]Bose, 1966; Gupta, Dutta, and Dutta, 1967.

(mammal bones); PR (plant remains); Pt (pottery); RB (reptile bones); RO (red ochre); Shls (shells); ShlObjs (shell objects); TObjs (terracotta objects).

Other abbreviations that are used are the following: Var (variations in burial customs); w/ (with); w/i (within); w/o (without); & (and); ? (questionable or maybe); *N* (number or sample size); O (orientation); App (approximately).

Burial practices represented in South Asian sites yielding human skeletal remains present two remarkable features. First, burial practices within a given period illustrate striking similarities to each other in body position and/or orientation, location of the burial(s), occurrence of grave-good types, burial type, and so on. Second, burial practices of a given time period (aside from the early Holocene and later hunter–gatherer communities complex) in the southern reaches of the subcontinent tend to mirror the burial practices of the preceding time period in the northern reaches of the subcontinent, with minor variations. This tendency strongly suggests a north to south pattern of cultural diffusion in the later phases of South Asian prehistory.

ACKNOWLEDGMENTS

This summary of the current record of human skeletal remains from prehistoric deposits in South Asia represents for the senior author a synthesis of research programs conducted since 1960 under the sponsorship of several funding institutions. It would be impossible to list the many colleagues who have contributed to the realization of this continuing research effort concerning the skeletal biology and evolution of prehistoric man in South Asia, but the three persons who were crucial to the initiation of this study were Dr. Theodore D. McCown of the University of California at Berkeley, Dr. Kenneth P. Oakley of the British Museum of Natural History at London, and Dr. H. D. Sankalia of Deccan College, Pune, India. The junior author wishes to thank Dr. Charles F. Merbs of Arizona State University for initiating her interest in cross-cultural burial practices through time and space and Dr. J. Lawrence Angel and other staff members of the Department of Anthropology, Smithsonian Institution, for allowing her the opportunity to conduct professional projects.

References

Agrawal, D. P., 1969, *C-14 Date List, June 1969,* Tata Institute of Fundamental Research, Bombay.

Agrawal, D. P., 1971, *C-14 Date List, March 1971,* Tata Institute of Fundamental Research, Bombay.

Agrawal, D. P., and Kusumgar, S., 1969, Tata Institute radiocarbon date list VI, *Radiocarbon* **11:**188–193.

Agrawal, D. P., and Kusumgar, S., 1974, *Prehistoric Chronology and Radiocarbon Dating in India,* Munshiram Manoharlal, New Delhi.

Alciati, G., 1967, I resti ossei umani necropoli dello Swat (W. Pakistan), *Rep. Mem. Ital. Medio.* **8:**1–66.

Alciati, G., and Fedeli, M., 1965, On some traumatic lesions in human bone remains of the necropolis of Butkara II (Swat, West Pakistan), *East & West* **15:**168–173.

Allchin, F. R. (ed.), 1960, Piklihal excavations, *Andhra Pradesh Gov. Archaeol. Ser.* **1.**

Anderson, J., 1883, *Handbook of the Indian Museum: General Archaeology,* Government Press, Calcutta.

Angel, J. L., 1972, A Middle Palaeolithic temporal bone from Darra-I-Kur, Afghanistan, in: *Prehistoric Research in Afghanistan (1959–1966)* (L. Dupree, ed.), *Trans. Am. Philos. Soc.* **62**(4)**:**54–56.

Anonymous, 1833, Proceedings, *J. Asiat. Soc. Bengal* **2:**648.

Antonini, C. S., 1963, Preliminary notes on the excavation of the necropolises found in western Pakistan, *East & West* **14:**13–25.

Antonini, C. S., 1969, Swat and central Asia, *East & West* **19**(1–2)**:**100–115.

Ayer, A. A., 1960, Report on human remains excavated at Piklihal near Mudgal, in: *Piklihal Excavations* (F. R. Allchin, ed.), *Andhra Pradesh Gov. Archaeol. Ser.* **1**:143–154.
Badam, G. L., 1977, Inamgaon: Human skeletal remains, in: Inamgaon seminar, (H. D. Sankalia, ed.), *Man & Environ.* **1**:56–58.
Bain, D. S. E., 1890, Antiquities of Southern India, *J. Anthropol. Soc. Bombay* **2**:229–231.
Banerjee, N. R., 1956, The Megalithic problem of Chingleput in the light of recent exploration, *Anc. India* **12**:21–34.
Banerjee, N. R., and Soundara Rajan, K. V. (eds.), 1959, Sanur 1950 and 1952: A megalithic site in district Chingleput, *Anc. India* **15**:4–42.
Bartel, B., 1979, A discriminant analysis of Harappan civilization human populations, *J. Archaeol. Sci.* **6**:49–61.
Basu, A., and Pal, A., 1980, *Human Remains from Burzahom*, Anthropological Survey of India, Calcutta.
Begley, V., 1976, Proto-historic material from Sri Lanka (Ceylon) and Indian contacts, in: *Ecological Backgrounds of South Asian Prehistory* (K. A. R. Kennedy and G. L. Possehl, eds.), South Asian Occasional Papers and Theses, Cornell University, pp. 191–196.
Begley, V., Lukacs, J. R., and Kennedy, K. A. R. (eds.), 1981, Excavations of Iron Age burials at Pomparippu: 1970, *Anc. Ceylon* **4**:51–131.
Bernhard, W., 1967, Human skeletal remains from the cemetery of Timargarha, in: *Timargarha and the Gandhara Grave Culture* (A. H. Dani, ed.), *Anc. Pakistan* **3**:289–407.
Bernhard, W., 1968, Human skeletal remains from the Bronze and early Iron Age cemetery of Timargarha (Dir State, West Pakistan), *Proc. 8th Int. Congr. Anthropol. Ethnol. Sci., Tokyo* **2**:144–154.
Bernhard, W., 1969, Preliminary report on the human skeletal remains from the prehistoric cemetery of Sarai Khola, *Pak. Archaeol.* **6**:100–116.
Blanford, H. F., 1864, Proceedings, *J. Asiat. Soc. Bengal* **33**:575–576.
Bose, H. K., 1959, Preliminary report on skeletal remains, in: *Sanur 1950 and 1952: A Megalithic Site in District Chingleput* (N. R. Banerjee and K. V. Soundara Rajan, eds.), *Anc. India* **15**:40–42.
Bose, H. K., 1966, Preliminary report on the skeletal and cranial remains from Amirthamangalam, in: *Amirthamangalam 1955: A Megalithic Urn Burial Site in District Chingleput, Tamilnadu, Ancient India* (N. R. Banerjee, K. S. Ramachandran, eds.) *Bull. Archaeol. Surv. India* **22**:1–36.
Branfill, B. R., 1881, On the Savandurga rude stone cemetery, Central Maisur, *Indian Antiquary* **10**:1–12.
Büchi, E. C., 1968, *Rassengeschichte der Menschheit*, Volume 1 (K. Saller, ed.), Olderbourg, Munich, pp. 109–184.
Buxton, L. H. D., 1935, Report, in: *Interim Report on an Excavation* (G. R. Hunter, ed.), *Nagpur Univ. J.* **1**:51–52.
Buxton, L. H. D., and Rice, D. T., 1931, Report on the human remains found at Kish, *J. R. Anthropol. Inst. G. B. Irel*, **61**:57–119.
Cammiade, L. A., 1926, Notes on the exploration of the Kurnool bone caves, *Man in India* **16**:174–181.
Cappieri, M., 1970, The population of the Indus civilization, *Field Res. Proj. Occas. Pap.* **11**:1–46.
Carlleyle, A. C. L., 1879, Reports of tours in the Central Doab and Gorakhpur in 1874–75 and 1875–76, *Rep. Archaeol. Surv. India* **12**:1–230.
Chanmugam, P. K., and Jayawardena, F. L. W., 1954, Skeletal remains from Tirukketiswaram, *Ceylon J. Sci. Sect. G.* **5**(2):65–68.
Chatterjee, B. K., and Gupta, P., 1963, *Report on the Adittanalur Skulls*, Anthropological Survey of India, Calcutta.

Chatterjee, B. K., and Kumar, G. D., 1962, Etude comparee et analyse racial des restes humains de Harappa, Pakistan Occidental, *Anthropologie* **66**:335–337.

Chatterjee, B. K., and Kumar, G. D., 1963a, *Comparative Study and Racial Analysis of the Human Remains of the Indus Valley Civilization with Particular Reference to Harappa,* Newman, Calcutta.

Chatterjee, B. K., and Kumar, G. D., 1963b, Racial elements in post-Harappan skeletal remains at Lothal, in: *Anthropology on the March* (B. Ratnam, ed.), Social Sciences Association, Madras, pp. 104–110.

Clutton-Brock, J., 1965, Excavations at Langhnaj 1944–63: Part II: The fauna, *Deccan Coll. Build. Centen. Silver Jubilee Ser.* **28.**

Codrington, K. de B., 1930, Indian cairn and urn burials, *Man* **30:**190–196.

Dales, G. F., 1964, The mythical massacre at Mohenjodaro, *Expedition* **6**(3):37–43.

Dales, G. F., 1965, New investigations at Mohenjodaro, *Archaeology* **18**(2):145–150.

Dani, A. H. (ed.), 1967, Timargarha and the Gandhara Grave Culture, *Anc. Pakistan* **3:**1–407.

Dani, A. H., 1968, Gandhara Grave Complex in West Pakistan, *Asian Perspect.* **11:**99–110.

Dani, A. H., and Durrani, F. A., 1964, A new grave complex in West Pakistan, *Asian Perspect.* **8**(1):164–165.

Dean, E., 1835, On the fossil bones of the Jamna river: Extract from a letter dated 2nd April, 1834, accompanying the first dispatch of specimens. *J. Asiat. Soc. Bengal* **4:**495–500.

Deo, S. B. (ed.), 1970, *Excavations at Takalghat and Khapa (1968–1969),* Nagpur University, Nagpur.

Deo, S. B., 1973a, The dating of megaliths in Maharashtra: Evaluation and some new evidence, in: *Radiocarbon and Indian Archaeology* (D. P. Agrawal and A. Ghosh, eds.), Tata Institute of Fundamental Research, Bombay, pp. 131–137.

Deo, S. B. (ed.), 1973b, *Mahurjhari Excavations 1970–1972,* Nagpur University, Nagpur.

Deo, S. B., 1978, The Megalithic Problem: A Review, Paper presented at the Symposium on Recent Advances in Indo-Pacific Prehistory, Pune.

Deo, S. B., and Ansari, Z. D. (eds.), 1965, *Chalcolithic Chandoli, Deccan Coll. Build. Centen. Silver Jubilee Ser.* **39.**

Deo, S. B., Dhavalikar, M. K., and Ansari, Z. D., 1979, *Apegaon Excavations,* Deccan College, Pune.

Deraniyagala, P. E. P., 1940, The Stone Age and cave men of Ceylon: Part I, *J. R. Asiat. Soc. Ceylon* **34**(92):351–373.

Deraniyagala, P. E. P., 1942, Ground and polished prehistoric artifacts from Ceylon, *Nature* **149**(3779):384–385.

Deraniyagala, P. E. P., 1943a, Some aspects of the prehistory of Ceylon: Part I, *Spolia Zeylan.* **23**(2):93–115.

Deraniyagala, P. E. P., 1943b, The Stone Age and cave men of Ceylon: Part II, *J. R. Asiat. Soc. Ceylon* **35**(4)(96):159–162.

Deraniyagala, P. E. P., 1945a, Balangoda culture phase: Collections at the museum, *Ceylon Times,* March 8, 1945.

Deraniyagala, P. E. P., 1945b, A Neolithic culture phase of Ceylon and South India, *Proc. 32d Indian Sci. Congr.* (Part 3, Sect. 6) **10:**52.

Deraniyagala, P. E. P., 1945c, Some aspects of the prehistory of Ceylon, Part II, *Spolia Zeylan.* **24**(2):121–144.

Deraniyagala, P. E. P., 1953, Some aspects of the prehistory of Ceylon: Part III: The Balangoda culture, *Spolia Zeylan.* **27:**125–131.

Deraniyagala, P. E. P., 1955a, Ceylon's Stone Ages, *New Lanka* **6:**39–41.

Deraniyagala, P. E. P., 1955b, Some aspects of the prehistory of Ceylon: Part IV: Some skeletal remains, implements, and food of Balangoda man, *Spolia Zeylan.* **27**(2):295–303.

Deraniyagala, P. E. P., 1956a, Land oscillation to the northwest of Ceylon, *J. R. Asiat. Soc. Ceylon* **4**(2):127–142.

Deraniyagala, P. E. P., 1956b, A Mesolithic burial tumulus from Ceylon, *Nature* **178**(4548): 1481–1482.

Deraniyagala, P. E. P., 1956c, Some aspects of the prehistory of Ceylon: Part V: The Balangoda culture, *Spolia Zeylan.* **28**(1):117–120.

Deraniyagala, P. E. P., 1956d, Some early human races of Ceylon, *Ceylon Today* **5**(10):15–16.

Deraniyagala, P. E. P., 1957, Races of the Stone Age and the Ferrolithic of Ceylon, *J. R. Asiat. Soc. Ceylon* **5**:1–23.

Deraniyagala, P. E. P., 1958a, An open-air habitation site of *Homo sapiens balangodensis:* Part I, *Spolia Zeylan.* **28**:223–261.

Deraniyagala, P. E. P., 1958b, The Pleistocene of Ceylon, *Ceylon Mus. Nat. Hist. Ser.* **1958**:1–164.

Deraniyagala, P. E. P., 1959, The persistence of Paleolithic types among the stone artifacts of Ceylon, *Proc. 46th Indian Sci. Congr.* **38**:432.

Deraniyagala, P. E. P., 1960a, An open-air habitation site of *Homo sapiens balangodensis: Part II, Spolia Zeylan.* **29**(1):95–109.

Deraniyagala, P. E. P., 1960b, Some mammals of the extinct Ratnapura fauna of Ceylon: *Part IV, Spolia Zeylan.* **29**(1):1–14.

Deraniyagala, P. E. P., 1960c, Stone Age man in Ceylon, in: *The Concise Encyclopaedia of Archaeology* (L. Cottrell, ed.), Hutchinson and Company, London, pp. 128.

Deraniyagala, P. E. P., 1962, The extinct Hominoidae of Ceylon, *Anthropol. Ann. Vidyodaya Univ. Ceylon* **1962**:52–62.

Deraniyagala, P. E. P., 1963a, Further descriptions of the three extinct hominoids of Ceylon, *Spolia Zeylan.* **30**:27–34.

Deraniyagala, P. E. P., 1963b, The hybridization of the Veddas with the Sinhalese, *Spolia Zeylan.* **30**:111–147.

Deraniyagala, P. E. P., 1963c, An open-air habitation site of *Homo sapiens balangodensis: Part III, Spolia Zeylan.* **30**:87–110.

Deraniyagala, P. E. P., 1963d, Prehistoric archaeology in Ceylon, *Asian Perspect.* **7**:189–192.

Deraniyagala, P. E. P., 1965, Some extinct hominoids and other Mammalia of Ceylon, in: *Dr. D. N. Wadia Commemorative Volume,* (A. G. Jhingran, ed.), Mining and Metallurgical Institute of India, Calcutta, pp. 290–300.

Deraniyagala, P. E. P., 1971, The age of Ceylon's extinct human, Balangoda man, *Loris* **12**:212.

Deraniyagala, S., and Kennedy, K. A. R., 1972, Bellan-Bandi Palassa 1970: A Mesolithic burial site in Ceylon, *Anc. Ceylon* **2**:18–47.

Dupree, L. (ed.), 1972, Prehistoric research in Afghanistan (1959–1966), *Trans. Am. Philos. Soc.* **62**(4):1–84.

Durrani, F. A., 1978, Ethnographical facts and archaeological theory through ancient burials, *J. Soc. Sci.* (Peshawar Univ.) **1**:22–38.

Dutta, P. C., 1971, Earliest Indian human remains found in a late Stone Age site, *Nature* **233**(5320):500–501.

Dutta, P. C., 1972, The Bronze Age Harappans: A re-examination of the skulls in the context of the population concept, *Am. J. Phys. Anthropol.* **36**:391–396.

Dutta, P. C., and Pal, A., 1972, The earliest Indian human skeletal find and the estimation of stature, *Curr. Sci.* **41**(9):334–335.

Dutta, P. C., Pal, A., and Dutta, B. C., 1971, Sarai Nahar Rai: A Late Stone Age site in the plain of the Ganga, *J. Indian Anthropol. Soc.* **6**:15–28.

Ehrhardt, S., 1960, Schlagspüren, Brüche und Sprunge an den Skeletten von Langhnaj im Nordlichen Gujarat, Vorderindien, *Anthropol. Anz.* **24**:178–183.

Ehrhardt, S., 1963, Frühmenschliche Skelette aus Langhnaj in Gujarat, Vörderindien, *Z. Morphol. Anthropol.* **54**:151–162.

Ehrhardt, S., and Kennedy, K. A. R., 1965, Excavations at Langhnaj: 1944–1963: Part III: The Human Remains, *Deccan Coll. Build. Centen. Silver Jubilee Ser.* **27.**

Fairservis, W. A. (ed.), 1956, Excavations in the Quetta Valley, West Pakistan, *Anthropol. Pap. Am. Mus. Nat. Hist.* **45**(2):169–402.

Falconer, H., 1865, On the asserted occurrence of human bones in the ancient fluviatile deposits of the Nile and Ganges, *Proc. Q. J. Geolog. Soc. London* **21**:372–389.

Foote, R. B., 1880, On the geological structure of the eastern coast from Latitude 15° northward to Masulipatam, *Mem. Geol. Surv. India* **16:**1–107.

Foote, R. B., 1884a, Rough notes on Billa Surgam and other caves in the Kurnool district, *Rec. Geol. Surv. India* **17**:27–34.

Foote, R. B., 1884b, Mr. H. B. Foote's work at the Billa Surgam caves, *Rec. Geol. Surv. India* **17**:200–208.

Foote, R. B., 1885, Notes on the results of Mr. H. B. Foote's further excavations in the Billa Surgam caves, *Rec. Geol. Surv. India* **18**:227–235.

Foote, R. B., 1914, *The Foote Collection of Indian Prehistoric and Protohistoric Antiquities: Catalogue Raisonne,* Government Press, Madras.

Foote, R. B., 1916, *The Foote Collection of Indian Prehistoric and Protohistoric Antiquities: Notes on Their Ages and Distribution,* Madras Government Museum, Madras.

Genna, G., 1965, First anthropological investigations of the skeletal remains of the necropolis of Butkara II (Swat, West Pakistan), *East & West* **15:**161–167.

Gordon, D. H., and Gordon, M. E., 1943, The cultures of Maski and Madhavpur, *J. R. Asiat. Soc. Bengal* **9**(1):83–97.

Grunwedel, A., 1914, *Aus Fedor Jagor's Nachlass Mit Unterstutzung der Jagor Staftung herausgegeben von der Berliner Gesellshaft fur Anthropologie, Ethnologie und Urgeschichte,* Band 1: *Sudindische Volksstamme,* Dietrich Reimer (Ernst Vohsen), Berlin.

Guha, B. S., 1934, Human remains, in: *Explorations in Sind, Being a Report of the Exploratory Survey Carried Out during the Years 1927–28, 1929–30, and 1930–31* (N. C. Majumdar, ed.), *Mem. Archaeol. Surv. India* **48:**157–158.

Guha, B. S., 1935, The racial affinities of the peoples of India, *Census of India 1931* Vol. 1, Part III: *Ethnographical,* Sec. A, Government of India, Simla.

Guha, B. S., and Basu, P. C., 1938, Report on the human remains excavated at Mohenjo-daro in 1928–29, in: *Further Excavations at Mohenjo-daro* (E. J. H. Mackay, ed.), Government of India, New Delhi, pp. 613–638.

Gupta, P., 1975, Human remains in the Indian subcontinent during pre- and protohistoric periods, *Bio-anthropological Research in India: Proceedings of the Seminar in Physical Anthropology and Allied Sciences* (H. K. Rakshit, ed.), Anthropological Survey of India, Calcutta, pp. 9–19.

Gupta, P., 1976, Antiquity of man in India, in: *Anthropology in India: Physical Anthropology* (H. K. Rakshit, ed.), Anthropological Survey of India, Calcutta, pp. 96–106.

Gupta, P., and Dutta, P. C., 1962, Human remains excavated from megaliths at Yelleswaram (Andhra Pradesh), *Man in India* **42:**19–34.

Gupta, P., Dutta, P. C., and Basu, A., 1962, Human skeletal remains from Harappa, *Mem. Anthropol. Surv. India* **9:**13–188.

Gupta, P., Basu, A., and Dutta, P. C., 1970, Ancient human remains: Part I: A study of the Nagarjunakonda skeletons, *Mem. Anthropol. Surv. India* **20:**1–33.

Gupta, P., Dutta, P. C., and Dutta, B. C., 1967, Report of the human skeletal remains discovered from urn burials at Amirthamangalam, District Chingleput, Madras, *Bull. Anthropol. Surv. India,* Calcutta, **16:**77–82.

Gupta, S. P., 1979, *Disposal of the Dead and Physical Types of Ancient India,* Oriental Publishers, Delhi.

Halim, M. A., 1970–1971, Excavations at Sarai Khola: Part I, *Pak. Archaeol.* **7**:23–89.

Halim, M. A., 1972, Excavations at Sarai Khola: Part II, *Pak. Archaeol.* **8:**1–112.
Hargreaves, H., 1929, Excavations in Baluchistan 1925: Sampur Mound, Mastung, and Sohr Damb, Nal, *Mem. Archaeol. Surv. India* **35.**
Hasan, K., 1975, The burial practices among the people of the Indus Valley civilization, in: *Proc. Int. Symp. Mohenjo-daro 1973* (A. N. Khan, ed.), National Book Foundation, Karachi, pp. 94–99.
Hingston, R. W. G., 1912, Letter to Mr. W. S. Millard, Honorary Secretary, Bombay Natural History Society, dated 8th August 1912, in: *Notes on two skulls (Homo sapiens) from upper India* (K. R. Kirtikar, ed.), *J. Anthropol. Soc. Bombay* **9:**527–529.
Hoffman, M. A., 1974a, *An Analysis of the Lithic Material from the 1973 Excavations at Allahdino,* University of Virginia, Charlottesville.
Hoffman, M. A., 1974b, *An Analysis of the Occupational Features at Allahdino,* University of Virginia, Charlottesville.
Hoffman, M. A., and Shaffer, J. G., 1976, The Harappan settlement of Allahdino: Analyzing the sociology of an archaeological site, in: *Ecological Backgrounds of South Asian Prehistory* (K. A. R. Kennedy and G. L. Possehl, eds.), South Asian Occasional Papers and Theses, Cornell University, pp. 94–117.
Hunt, E. H., 1916, Hyderabad cairns: Their problems, *J. Hyderabad Archaeol. Soc.* **10:**180–224.
Hunt, E. H., 1924, Hyderabad cairn burials and their significance, *J. R. Anthropol. Inst. G. B. Irel.* **54:**140–156.
Hunter, G. R. (ed.), 1935, Interim report on an excavation, *Nagpur Univ. J.* **1:**28–57.
Hunter, G. R. (ed.), 1936, Final report on the excavation in the Mahadeo Hills, *Nagpur Univ. J.* **2:**127–144.
Indian Archaeology: A Review, 1956–1957, Archaeol. Surv. India, Delhi.
Indian Archaeology: A Review, 1957–1958, Archaeol. Surv. India, Delhi.
Indian Archaeology: A Review, 1962–1963, Archaeol. Surv. India, Delhi.
Indian Archaeology: A Review, 1967–1968, Archaeol. Surv. India, Delhi.
Indian Archaeology: A Review, 1974–1975, Archaeol. Surv. India, Delhi.
Indian Archaeology: A Review, 1975–1976, Archaeol. Surv. India, Delhi.
Indian Archaeology: A Review, 1976–1977, Archaeol. Surv. India, Delhi.
Indian Archaeology: A Review, 1977–1978, Archaeol. Surv. India, Delhi.
Karve, I., and Kurulkar, G. M., 1945, *A Preliminary Report on the Human Remains Found at Langhnaj in February and December 1944,* Times of India Press, Pune.
Karve-Corvinus, G., and Kennedy, K. A. R., 1964, Preliminary report on Langhnaj, *Bull. Deccan Coll. Res. Inst.* **24:**44–57.
Keith, A., 1919, Report on two human crania of considerable antiquity, *J. Anthropol. Soc. Bombay* **11:**663–672.
Keith, A., 1929, *The Antiquity of Man,* 2nd ed., Williams and Norgate, London.
Kennedy, K. A. R., 1965a, Megalithic calvariae from Raigir, Andhra Pradesh, *Anthropologist* **11:**1–24.
Kennedy, K. A. R., 1965b, Human skeletal material from Ceylon with an analysis of the island's prehistoric and contemporary populations, *Brit. Mus. Geol. Palaeontol. Ser.* **2**(4).
Kennedy, K. A. R., 1972, Anatomical description of two crania from Ruamgarh: An ancient site in Dhalbhum, Bihar, *J. Indian Anthropol. Soc.* **7:**129–141.
Kennedy, K. A. R., 1973, The search for fossil man in India, in: *Physical Anthropology and Its Extending Horizons,* S. S. Sarkar Memorial Volume (A. Basu *et al.*, eds.), Orient Longman, Calcutta, pp. 25–44.
Kennedy, K. A. R., 1980, Prehistoric skeletal record of man in South Asia, *Ann. Rev. Anthropol.* **9:**391–432.
Kennedy, K. A. R., 1983a, Palaeo-ecological factors in the isolation of populations in the Indian

Mesolithic, Paper read at the *Symposium on Quarternary Environments and Cultural Succession in South Asia,* Vancouver, B.C., August 22, 1983.

Kennedy, K. A. R., 1983b, Preliminary report of the Mesolithic human skeletal remains from Sarai Nahar Rai: Their skeletal biology and evolutionary significance, in: *History and Archaeology,* Volume 2 (G. R. Sharma, ed.), Centre of Advanced Study and the Department of Ancient History, Culture, and Archaeology, Allahabad.

Kennedy, K. A. R., 1983c, Hauntings at Aditanallur: An anthropological ghost story, in: *Recent Research of American Anthropologists in India* (J. Jacobson, ed.), American Institute of Indian Studies, Chicago.

Kennedy, K. A. R., 1983d, Trauma and disease in the ancient Harappans: Recent reassessments of the skeletal record, in: *Aspects of Harappan Culture: Sir Mortimer Wheeler Commemorative Volume* (S. P. Gupta and B. B. Lal, eds.), Indian History and Culture Society, New Delhi.

Kennedy, K. A. R., and Malhotra, K. C., 1966, Human skeletal remains from Chalcolithic and Indo-Roman levels from Nevasa: An anthropometric and comparative analysis, *Deccan Coll. Postgrad. Res. Inst. Build. Centen. Silver Jubilee Ser.* **55.**

Kennedy, K. A. R., Misra, V. N., and Burrow, C. B., 1981, Dental mutilations from prehistoric India, *Curr. Anthropol.* **22**(3):285–286.

Khan, A. H., and Karve, I., 1946, Identification of a few bone remains from Langhnaj, in: *Investigations into Prehistoric Archaeology of Gujarat, Being the Official Report of the First Gujarat Prehistoric Expedition 1941–42* (H. D. Sankalia, ed.), Sri-Pratapasimha Maharaja Rajyabhisheka Grantha-male Memoir 4, Baroda State Press, Baroda, pp. 313–314.

Khan, A. R., 1968, Ancient settlements in the Karachi region, *Dawn, Sunday Magazine Sect.,* July 21 and 28, p. 12.

Khan, A. W., 1963, A Monograph on Yeleswaram excavations, *Andhra Pradesh Gov. Archaeol. Ser.* **14.**

Khan, F. A., 1968, Exploration in Pakistan; excavations; conservation, *Pak. Archaeol.* **5:**1–249.

Khatri, A. P., 1963, Recent exploration for the remains of early man in India, *Asian Perspect.* **7:**160–182.

Kirtikar, K. R. (ed.), 1912, Notes on two skulls (*Homo sapiens*) from upper India, *J. Anthropol. Soc. Bombay* **9:**524–530.

Krogman, W. M., and Sassman, W. H., 1943, Skull found at Chanhu-daro, in: *Chanhu-daro Excavations 1935–1936,* (E. J. H. Mackay, ed.), American Oriental Society, New Haven, pp. 252–263.

Lal, B. B., 1979, Kalibangan and the Indus civilization, in: *Essays in Indian Protohistory* (D. P. Agrawal and D. K. Chakrabarti, eds.), B. R. Publishing Corporation, Delhi, pp. 65–97.

Lal, B. B., and Thapar, B. K., 1967, Excavations at Kalibangan: New light on the Indus civilization, *Cult. Forum* **9:**86–96.

Leshnik, L. S., 1967, Archaeological interpretation of burials in the light of central Indian ethnography, *Z. Ethnol.* **92:**23–32.

Leshnik, L. S., 1968, Prehistoric exploration in North Gujarat and parts of Rajasthan, *East & West* **18**(3–4)**:**295–310.

Lukacs, J. R., 1976, Dental anthropology and the biological affinities of an Iron Age population from Pomparippu, Sri Lanka, in: *Ecological Backgrounds of South Asian Prehistory,* (K. A. R. Kennedy and G. L. Possehl, eds.), South Asian Occasional Papers and Theses, Cornell University, pp. 197–215.

Lukacs, J. R., 1980, The Apegaon mandible: Morphology and pathology, *Bull. Deccan Coll. Res. Inst.* **39**(1–4)**:**88–95a.

Lukacs, J. R., 1981a, Crown dimensions of deciduous teeth from prehistoric India, *Am. J. Phys. Anthropol.* **55:**261–266.

Lukacs, J. R., 1981b, Dental pathology and nutritional patterns of South Asian megalith builders: The evidence from Iron Age Mahurjhari, *Proc. Am. Philos. Soc.* **125**(3):220–237.

Lukacs, J. R., and Badam, G. L., 1975, Bioanthropology of human skeletal remains from Inamgaon, West India, *Curr. Anthropol.* **16**:667–668.

Lukacs, J. R., and Badam, G. L., 1977, Biological anthropology of human skeletal remains from Chalcolithic Inamgaon, western India, *Bull. Deccan Coll. Res. Inst.* **36**:78–83.

Lukacs, J. R., and Kennedy, K. A. R., 1981, Biological anthropology of human remains from Pomparippu, in: *Excavations of Iron Age burials at Pomparippu,* 1970 (V. Begley, J. R. Lukacs, and K. A. R. Kennedy, eds.), *Anc. Ceylon* **4**:97–130.

Lukacs, J. R., Misra, V. N., and Kennedy, K. A. R., 1982, Bagor and Tilwari: Late Mesolithic cultures of Northwest India, Volume 1: The human skeletal remains, *Bull. Deccan Coll. Res. Inst.*

Lydekker, R., 1880, A sketch of the history of the fossil vertebrata of India, *J. Asiat. Soc. Bengal* **49**:8–40.

Lydekker, R., 1886, The fauna of the Karnul caves, *Palaeontol. Indica, Mem. Geol. Surv. India* **4**:23–58.

MacKay, E. J. H. (ed.), 1938, *Further Excavations at Mohenjo-daro,* Government of India, New Delhi.

MacKay, E. J. H. (ed.), 1943, *Chanhu-daro Excavations 1935–36,* American Oriental Society, New Haven.

Majumdar, N. G. (ed.), 1934, Explorations in Sind, being a report of the exploratory survey carried out during the years 1927–28, 1929–30, and 1930–31, *Mem. Archaeol. Surv. India* **48.**

Malhotra, K. C., 1963, The Chandoli skull, *Link* **November 24:**41.

Malhotra, K. C., 1965a, Human skeletal remains from Chandoli, in: *Chalcolithic Chandoli,* (S. B. Deo and Z. D. Ansari, eds.), *Deccan Coll. Build. Centen. Silver Jubilee Ser.* **39**:69–80.

Malhotra, K. C., 1965b, Human skeletal remains from Neolithic Tekkalakota, in: *The Stone Age Hill Dwellers of Tekkalakota: Preliminary Report of the Excavations at Tekkalakota* (M. S. N. Rao and K. C. Malhotra, eds.), *Deccan Coll. Build. Centen. Silver Jubilee Ser.* **31**:109–162.

Malhotra, K. C., 1967, Further observations on the human skeletal remains from Neolithic Piklihal, *Anthropologist* **14**:99–111.

Malhotra, K. C., 1971, Report on the human skeleton from the burial, in: *Report on the Excavations at T. Narsipur,* (M. Seshadri, ed.), Government of India, Bangalore, pp. 79–104.

Marshall, J. (ed.), 1931, *Mohenjo-daro and the Indus Civilization,* Probsthain, London.

Misra, V. N., 1970a, Cultural significance of three copper arrowheads from Rajasthan, India, *J. Near Eastern Stud.* **29**(4):221–232.

Misra, V. N., 1970b, Evidence for a Chalcolithic culture in South Rajasthan, *Indian Antiquary* **4**(1–4):85–95.

Misra, V. N., 1971a, Two late Mesolithic settlements in Rajasthan: A brief review of investigations, *J. Univ. Pune* **35**:59–77.

Misra, V. N., 1971b, Two microlithic sites in Rajasthan: A preliminary investigation, *East. Anthropol.* **24**:237–288.

Misra, V. N., 1972, Burials from prehistoric Bagor, Rajasthan, in: *Archaeological Congress and Seminar Papers* (S. B. Deo, ed.), University of Nagpur, Nagpur, pp. 58–65.

Misra, V. N., 1973a, Bagor: A late Mesolithic settlement in Northwest India, *World Archaeol.* **5**:92–110.

Misra, V. N., 1973b, Bhimbaithka ki Guphao ke Rahasya [The secrets of the Bhimbetka caves], *Dharamyug* **September 30:**17–23.

Misra, V. N., 1974, The Acheulian Industry of Rockshelter IIF-23 at Bhimbetka, Central India: A Preliminary Analysis, Paper presented at the Seminar on Indian Prehistory, Pune.

Misra, V. N., 1976, Ecological adaptations during the terminal Stone Age in western and central India, in: *Ecological Backgrounds of South Asian Prehistory,* (K. A. R. Kennedy and G. L. Possehl, eds.), South Asian Occasional Papers and Theses, Cornell University, pp. 28–51.

Misra, V. N., 1978, Acheulian Succession at Bhimbetka, Central India, Paper presented at the Symposium for Recent Advances in Indo-Pakistan Prehistory, Pune.

Misra, V. N., Mathpal, Y., and Nagar, M., 1977, *Bhimbetka: Prehistoric Man and His Art in Central India,* Sakal, Pune.

Mitra, P., 1923, *Prehistoric India: Its Place in the World's Culture,* 1st ed., University of Calcutta, Calcutta.

Mitra, P., 1927, *Prehistoric India: Its Place in the World's Culture,* 2nd ed., University of Calcutta, Calcutta.

Mitra, P., 1936, The early Chalcolithic races of India, *16th Congr. Int. Anthropol. Archaeol. Prehist.,* Brussels **1:**135–146.

Morant, G. M., 1936, Report of human skeletal remains excavated in a rockshelter near Pachmarhi, Central Province, in: *Final Report on the Excavation in the Mahadeo Hills* (G. R. Hunter, ed.), *Nagpur Univ. J.* **2:**144.

Mughal, M. R., 1972, A summary of excavations and explorations in Pakistan (1971 and 1972), *Pak. Archaeol.* **8:**113–158.

Murray, E. F. O., 1940, The ancient workers of western Dhalbhum, *J. R. Asiat. Soc. Bengal* **6:**79–104.

Murty, M. L. K., 1974a, Twenty-five years of research on human osteological remains from prehistoric sites in India, *Bull. Deccan Coll. Res. Inst.* **34:**116–133.

Murty, M. L. K., 1974b, A late Pleistocene cave site in southern India, *Proc. Am. Philos. Soc.* **118:**196–230.

Murty, M. L. K., 1979, Recent research on the Upper Palaeolithic phase in India, *J. Field Archaeol.* **6**(3):301–320.

Newbold, T., 1884, Note on the osseous breccia and deposits in the caves of Billa Surgam, Lat. 15° 25′ and Long. 78° 15′ southern India, *J. Asiat. Soc. Bengal* **13:**610–611.

Oakley, K. P., 1983, Two essays written in commemoration of Paul Edward Pieris Deraniyagala: (a) Some problems of Balangoda man; (b) Fossils as *materia medica* in Sri Lanka, in: *Dr. P. E. P. Deraniyagala Commemorative Volume* (W. T. P. Gunawardana, ed.), Colombo, Lake House Investments, Ltd.

Penniman, T. K., 1935, Letter, in: *Interim Report on an Excavation* (G. R. Hunter, ed.), *Nagpur Univ. J.* **1:**51–52.

Possehl, G. L., and Kennedy, K. A. R., 1979, Hunter–gatherer/agriculturalist exchange in prehistory: An Indian example, *Curr. Anthropol.* **20:**592–593.

Prinsep, J., 1833a, Notes on the specimens of the Kankar formation and the fossil bones collected on the Jamna, *J. Asiat. Soc. Bengal* **2:**622–635.

Prinsep, J., 1833b, Proceedings, *J. Asiat. Soc. Bengal* **2:**648.

Prinsep, J., 1835a, On the fossil bones of the Jamna river, *J. Asiat. Soc. Bengal* **4:**495–500.

Prinsep, J., 1835b, Note, *J. Asiat. Soc. Bengal* **4:**500–506.

Rajaguru, S. N., and Kennedy, K. A. R., 1964, The skeletal evidence for Pleistocene man in India, *Bull. Deccan Coll. Res. Inst.* **24:**71–76.

Rao, M. S. N., 1967, New evidence for Neolithic life in India: Excavations in the southern Deccan, *Archaeology* **20**(1):28–35.

Rao, M. S. N., and Malhotra, K. C. (eds.), 1965, The Stone Age hill dwellers of Tekkalakota: Preliminary report of the excavations at Tekkalakota, *Deccan Coll. Build. Centen. Silver Jubilee Ser.* **31.**

Rao, S. R., 1956–1957, The excavations at Lothal, *Lalit Kala* **3,4:**82–89.

Rao, S. R., 1973, *Lothal and the Indus Civilization,* Asia Publishing House, New York.

Rao, V. V., 1970, Skeletal remains from Takalghat and Khapa excavation, in: *Excavations at Takalghat and Khapa (1968–1969)* (S. B. Deo, ed.), Nagpur University, Nagpur, pp. 60–77.

Rao, V. V., 1973, Skeletal remains from Mahurjhari, in: *Mahurjhari Excavations 1970–1972,* (S. B. Deo, ed.), Nagpur University, Nagpur, pp. 63–76.

Rea, A., 1902–1903a, Adichanallur excavations, *Ann. Rep. Archaeol. Surv. Madras and Coorg,* **1902–03:**9–14.

Rea, A., 1902–1903b, Prehistoric antiquities in Tinnevelly, *Ann. Rep. Archaeol. Surv. India* **1:**111–140.

Rea, A., 1903–1904, Prehistoric pottery from Tinnevelly, *Ann. Rep. Archaeol. Surv. India* **1903–04,** Calcutta, India.

Rea, A., 1915, *Catalogue of the Prehistoric Antiquities from Adichanallur and Perumbair,* Madras Government Museum, Madras.

Richards, F. J., 1939, Review of annual report of the archaeological department of H. E. H. the Nizam's dominions: 1934–5, 1935–6, *Antiquity* **13:**468–469.

Riesenfeld, A., 1956, Human skeletal remains, in: *Excavations in the Quetta Valley, West Pakistan* (W. A. Fairservis, ed.), *Anthropol. Pap. Am. Mus. Nat. Hist.* **45**(2):378–381.

Sahni, D. R., 1926, Northern circle: Harappa, *Ann. Rep. Archaeol. Surv. India* **1923–24:**52–54.

Sahni, D. R., 1927, Northern circle: Harappa, *Ann. Rep. Archaeol. Surv. India* **1924–25:**73–80.

Sahni, M. R., 1956, A century of palaeontology, palaeobotany and prehistory in India and adjacent countries, *J. Palaeontol. Soc. India* **1:**7–51.

Sankalia, H. D., 1943a, In search of early man along the Sabarmati, *J. Gujarat Res. Soc.* **1943:** 75–86.

Sankalia, H. D., 1943b, Pre- and proto-history of Gujarat, in: *The Glory That Was Gurjaradesa,* Part I, Ch. 2, Mularaja Solanki Millenial Celebration Volume, Bharatiya Vidya Bhavan, Bombay, pp. 13–26, 34–40.

Sankalia, H. D. (ed.), 1946, Investigations into prehistoric archaeology of Gujarat, being the Official Report of the First Gujarat Prehistoric Expedition 1941–42, *Mem. Sri Pratapasimha Maharaja Raiyabisheka Grnathamala* **4,** Baroda State Press, Baroda.

Sankalia, H. D., 1949, Studies in the historical and cultural geography of Gujarat (Places and peoples in inscriptions of Gujarat: 300 B.C. to 1300 A.D.), *Deccan Coll. Monograph Ser.* **3.**

Sankalia, H. D., 1955, Excavations at Langhnaj, Gujarat, *Man* **55**(33):26.

Sankalia, H. D., 1956, The microlithic industry of Langhnaj, Gujarat, *J. Gujarat Res. Soc.* **18**(4):275–284.

Sankalia, H. D., 1965, Excavations at Langhnaj: 1944–1963: Part I: Archaeology, *Deccan Coll. Build. Centen. Silver Jubilee Ser.* **29.**

Sankalia, H. D. (ed.), 1977, Inamgaon Seminar, *Man and Environment* **1:**44–60.

Sankalia, H. D., and Karve, I., 1944, The Second Gujarat Prehistoric Expedition: A preliminary account of the search for microlithic man in Gujarat, *New Indian Antiquary* **7**(1):1–6.

Sankalia, H. D., and Karve, I., 1945, *Preliminary Report on the Third Gujarat Prehistoric Expedition,* Times of India Press, Bombay.

Sankalia, H. D., and Karve, I., 1949, Early primitive microlithic culture and people of Gujarat, *Am. Anthropologist* **51:**28–34.

Sankalia, H. D., Deo, S. B., Ansari, Z. D., and Ehrhardt, S., 1960, Chronology, in: *From History to Prehistory at Nevasa: Report on the Excavations and Explorations in and around Nevasa 1954–56,* Department of Archaeology and Ancient Indian History, Deccan College, University of Pune, Publication **1,** pp. 64–70.

Sankalia, H. D., Ansari, Z. D., and Dhavalikar, M. K., 1971, Inamgaon: A Chalcolithic settlement in western India, *Asian Perspect.* **14:**139–146.

Sankalia, H. D., Ansari, Z. D., and Dhavalikar, M. K., 1975, An early farmer's village in central India, *Expedition* **47**(2):2–11.
Sarkar, S. S., 1954, *The Aboriginal Races of India,* Appendix I: *Disposal of the Dead at Harappa,* Bookland Limited,Calcutta, pp. 141–145.
Sarkar, S. S., 1960, Human skeletal remains from Brahmagiri, *Bull. Dept. Anthropol., Gov. India* **9**:5–26.
Sarkar, S. S., 1964, *Ancient Races of Baluchistan, Punjab, and Sind,* Bookland Limited, Calcutta.
Sarkar, S. S., 1965, Review of Chatterjee and Gupta's report on the Adittanalur skulls, *Sci. and Cult.* **31**:136–137.
Sarkar, S. S., 1972, *Ancient Races of the Deccan,* Munshiram Manoharlal, New Delhi.
Sarkar, S. S., and Mishra, B. N., 1966, *Nagarjunakonda,* New Delhi.
Seshadri, M. (ed.), 1971, *Report on the Excavations at T. Narsipur,* Government of India, Bangalore.
Sewell, R. B. S. and Guha, B. S., 1929, Report on the bones excavated at Nal, *Mem. Archaeol. Surv. India* **35**:56–86.
Sewell, R. B. S., and Guha, B. S., 1931a, Report on a collection of bones made by Sir Aurel Stein in Makran, *Mem. Archaeol. Surv. India* **43**:191–200.
Sewell, R. B. S., and Guha, B. S., 1931b, Human remains, in: *Mohenjodaro and the Indus Civilization* (J. Marshall, ed.), Volume 2, Probsthain, London, pp. 599–648.
Shaffer, J. G., 1974, *Allahdino and the Mature Harappan: A Preliminary Report on the Cultural Stratigraphy,* Case Western Reserve University, Cleveland.
Sharma, A. K., 1969–1970, Kalibangan human skeletal remains: An osteoarchaeological approach, *J. Orient. Inst. Baroda* **19**:109–113.
Sharma, A. K., 1972, Harappan cemetery at Kalibangan: A demographic survey, *Proc. 4th Indian Archaeol. Congr., Nagpur,* pp. 113–116.
Sharma, A. K., 1979, Harappan Cemetery at Kalibangan: A Study, Paper presented at the Conference on Harappan Civilization, Srinigar.
Sharma, G. R., 1973, Mesolithic lake culture in the Ganga Valley, *Proc. Prehistoric Soc.* **39**: 129–146.
Sharma, G. R., 1975, Seasonal migrations and Mesolithic lake cultures of the Ganga Valley, in: *K.C. Chattopadhyaya Memorial Volume* (G. R. Sharma, ed.), Dubey, Allahabad, pp. 1–20.
Sharma, G. R., Mishra, V. D., Mandal, D., Mishra, B. B., and Pal, J. N., 1980, *Beginnings of Agriculture: Epi-Palaeolithic to Neolithic Excavations at Chopani-Mando, Mahadaha, and Mahagara,* Abinash Prakashan, Allahabad.
Singh, P., 1970, *Burial Practices in Ancient India,* Prithivi Prakshan, Varanasi.
Soundara Rajan, K. V., 1958, Studies in the Stone Age of Nagarjunakonda and its neighborhood, *Anc. India* **14**:49–113.
Smith, E., 1833, Notes on the specimens of the Kankar formation and the fossil bones collected on the Jamna, *J. Asiat. Soc. Bengal* **2**:622–635.
Smith, G. E., 1927, *The Evolution of Man: Essays,* 2d ed., Oxford University Press, London.
Stacul, G., 1966, Notes on the discovery of a necropolis near Kherai in the Gorband Valley (Swat, West Pakistan), *East and West* **17**:185–219.
Stein, A., 1931, An archaeological tour in Gedrosia, *Mem. Archaeol. Surv. India* **43.**
Thapar, B. K., 1957, Maski 1954: A Chalcolithic site of the southern Deccan, *Anc. India* **13**:4–142.
Thapar, B. K., 1973, New traits of the Indus civilization at Kalibangan: An appraisal, in: *South Asian Archaeology* (N. Hammond, ed.), Noyes Press, Park Ridge, pp. 85–104.
Thapar, B. K., 1975, Kalibangan: A Harappan metropolis beyond the Indus Valley, *Expedition* **47**(2):19–32.
Theobald, W., 1881, The Siwalik group of the sub-Himalayan region, *Rec. Geol. Surv. India* **14**:66–125.

Thurston, E., 1909, *Castes and Tribes of Southern India,* Government of India, Madras.
Tiwari, S. C., and Banerjee, S., 1980, A preliminary appraisal of Mesolithic racial elements from India, *Indian Anthropol.* **10**(2):131–144.
Tucci, G., 1958, Preliminary report on an archaeological survey in Swat, *East and West* **9**:279–328.
Tucci, G., 1963, The tombs of the Asvakayana—Assakenoi, *East and West* **14**:27–28.
Tucker, H.C., 1847, Letter to the Secretary of the Asiatic Society of Bengal, Calcutta, *J. Asiat. Soc. Bengal* **16**:376–377.
Varma, R. K., 1964, *The Stone Age Cultures of Mizapur,* Ph.D. thesis, Allahabad University, India.
Varma, R. K., 1965, Comment on the Mesolithic phase in the prehistory of India, in: *Indian Prehistory 1964* (V. N. Misra and M.S. Mate, eds.), *Deccan Coll. Build. Centen. Silver Jubilee Ser.* **32**:73–76.
Vats, M. S., 1940, *Excavations at Harappa,* Government of India, Calcutta.
Vredenburg, E., 1919, Note, *J. Anthropol. Soc. Bombay* **11**:673–674.
Wakankar, V. S., 1973, Bhim-Betka excavations, *J. Indian Hist.* **51**:23–32.
Wakankar, V. S., 1975, Bhimbetka: The prehistoric paradise, *Prachya Pratibha* **3**:7–29.
Wheeler, R. E. M., 1947, Harappa 1946: The defences and cemetery R37, *Anc. India* **3**:58–130.
Wheeler, R. E. M., 1947–1948, Brahmagiri and Chandravalli 1947: Megalithic and other cultures in Mysore State, *Anc. India* **4**:180–311.
Wintle, A. G., and Oakley, K. P., 1972, Thermoluminescent dating of fired rock crystal from Bellan Bandi Palassa, Ceylon, *Archaeometry* **14**:277–279.
Yazdani, G., 1938, Note on the excavations at Maski, Appendix B, *Ann. Rep. Archaeol. Dept. H.E.H. Nizam's Domin. 1935–36* **13**:22–24, 28–31.
Yazdani, G., 1939, Excavations: Kadkal and Maski, *Ann. Rep. Archaeol. Dept. H.E.H. Nizam's Domin. 1936–37* **8**:14–16.
Zeuner, F. E., 1950, Stone Age and Pleistocene chronology in Gujarat, *Deccan College Monograph Series* **6**, pp. 1–46.
Zeuner, F. E., 1951, Prehistory in India: Four broadcast talks on early man, *Deccan College Handbook Series* **1.**
Zeuner, F. E., 1952, The microlithic industry of Langhnaj, Gujarat, *Man* **52**(182):129–131.
Zeuner, F. E., 1963, Environment as inferred from fauna and flora, in: *Environment of Early Man with Special Reference to the Tropical Regions,* The Maharafa Sayajirao Memorial Lectures 1960–1961, Lecture 3, University of Baroda Press, Baroda, pp. 19–28.
Zuckerman, S., 1930, The Adichanallur skulls, *Bull. Madras Gov. Mus.* **2**:1–24.

PART II

Biological Anthropology of the Living

CHAPTER 9

The Epidemiological Transition in Dental Occlusion in a North Indian Population

SAMVIT S. KAUL and ***ROBERT S. CORRUCCINI***

1. Introduction

One factor of interest in the epidemiology of malocclusion is the repeated finding that persons living in the rural areas of developed countries show better dental occlusion. Goose *et al.* showed in 1957 that West Midlands country youths had a lower prevalence of malocclusion. They suggested respiratory infections, early deciduous tooth loss, sucking habits, and age changes as possible mechanisms. Lavelle (1973) confirmed this trend among youths and their parents in central England. He also showed that the younger (presumably more urbanized) English were characterized by narrower maxillary arches. In Australia, Barnard (1956) reported that country dwellers were better occluded. Finally, Corruccini and Whitley (1981) showed that the middle-aged adults in a rural Kentucky community were very much better occluded than the youths and young adults, and that this was not merely a result of age differences. The younger subjects had been raised in a more urbanized environment, insofar as commercially purchased (rather than coarser home-produced) food was concerned.

This general finding is surely important for tracing the etiology of malocclusion, and therefore occlusal surveys contrasting rural and urban youths in new ethnic groups would be valuable. The Punjabi population of Chandigarh, India,

---

SAMVIT S. KAUL • Department of Anthropology, Punjab University, Chandigarh 160014 and ***ROBERT S. CORRUCCINI*** • Department of Anthropology, Southern Illinois University, Carbondale, Illinois 62901. We are grateful to the Smithsonian Foreign Currency Program (Grant #10832900) for full financial support.

shows several special social characteristics of value to an epidemiological study of occlusal variation. Within a short geographic distance, Punjabi communities cover the entire spectrum of persons from completely urban, modern, sedentary, professional, and social levels to immigrant laborers and farmers, usually living just outside the city in reduced circumstances that are typical of long-standing isolation in the countryside. In fact, the city of Chandigarh was started only 35 years ago as a capital for the new Indian state, Punjab, and to rehabilitate the immense displaced population from West Punjab (now Pakistan) after the partition of 1947. The entire urbanization phenomenon has taken place in the relatively short intervening time. Chandigarh has a relatively high per capita income, and the higher socioeconomic stratum includes children that have always known a cosmopolitan urban environment, including many who have been abroad. The lowest stratum, on the other hand, is composed largely of laborers and recent immigrants from rural circumstances who tend to retain their original dietary and residence habits. Neither group has had access to significant amounts of orthodontic care (less than 2% of the upper middle class), and this circumvents the inevitable problems that arise in occlusal surveys of industrialized countries where large segments have had the natural phenotype changed completely through orthodontistry.

Furthermore, whereas the city dwellers appear to have the typical high caries and malocclusion incidence of Western societies, we have frequently noticed instances in which the elderly populations of villages retained all 32 permanent teeth, without caries. The jaws of these persons were capable of stripping raw sugar cane. We determined, therefore, to survey occlusal variation in Chandigarh youths in relation to various environmental and social characteristics.

2. Materials and Methods

The subjects were drawn from and examined at seven schools located inside or within 2 km of Chandigarh. The schools were selected to provide a representative cross-sectional sample (Kaul *et al.*, 1975) of roughly 1% of the school-going population between ages 12–16. This age range ensured that eruption of the full permanent dentition through the second molar and minimal effects from tooth loss or caries would be found. Youths missing more than one tooth or retaining more than one deciduous premolar were excluded.

To conform to the earlier study of permanent-tooth emergence in this population (Kaul, 1975; Kaul *et al.*, 1975), the sample was divided into high-, middle-, and low-socioeconomic groups (SEG), because this division closely predicts social behavioral characteristics and geographic family background. The resulting samples are the following.

1. Seventy-eight high-SEG youths (41 male and 37 female), classified according to family income over 1000 rupees/month. This criterion almost always connoted postgraduate education, professional employment, and fairly distant urban birth of parents.
2. One hundred sixteen middle-SEG youths (58 of each sex) of family income of 450–1000 rupees/month. Most of these youths had been born in Chandigarh of parents who were usually longtime area residents who were employed as assistants or tradesmen.
3. Seventy-one low-SEG youths (46 male and 25 female) of rural birth, whose parents (frequently from birthplaces now in Pakistan) made no more than 400 rupees/month as agriculturalists, servants, and workers.

When the subjects had been selected at each school, Indian team members interviewed each to ascertain their ages and places of birth and their parents' birthplaces, education, occupation, and income. They then conducted oral examinations of tooth emergence and number, anomalies, periodontal disease (gingivitis scored from absent to advanced following the World Health Organization [WHO, 1971] criteria), and the number of carious (decayed or filled) teeth. Then the subjects went to a location where the occlusion (in terms of Angle Class I, II, or III) and dental crowding were noted, and a soft wax bite impression (Aluwax denture forms) was taken of the mouth in centric occlusion. From the oral examination and the wax impression, one of us assessed the following occlusal variables (see also details in Corruccini and Whitley, 1981):

1. *Overjet (horizontal incisor relation):* Scored as normal (maxillary central incisor is 2–4 mm anterior to mandibular central incisor); slight positive (5–7 mm) or extreme positive (more than 7 mm) maxillary overjet; and slight negative (0–2 mm) or extreme negative (mandibular overjet more than 1 mm).
2. *Vertical over bite:* Scored as normal (when the maxillary central incisor overlaps the mandibular antagonist by 0 to about 2/3 of the cervical height of the latter); slightly positive (overlap of 2/3 to the full height of the mandibular central incisor); extreme positive (the mandibular incisal edge contacts the gingivae posterior to the maxillary incisor); slight negative (open bite of around 1 mm); and extreme negative (open bite 2 mm or more).
3. *Posterior cross-bite:* Scored as normal (maxillary molar mesiolingual cusp occludes with the mandibular molar central fossa); slight positive (buccal cross-bite; a mandibular molar is buccally displaced to a cusp-to-cusp deviation from normal); extreme positive (more than one molar in buccal cross-bite or the deviation is worse than cusp-to-cusp deviation); slight negative (lingual cross-bite of one tooth) or extreme negative (severe lingual cross-bite or more than one molar involved).

4. *Buccal segment relation (BSR):* First molar anterior-posterior relation scored as normal (first maxillary molar mesiobuccal cusp overlaps the first mandibular molar buccal groove); slight positive (distoclusion or Angle Class II; maxillary mesiobuccal cusp is displaced anteriorly to overlap with the mandibular mesiobuccal cusp); extreme positive (maxillary molar more anterior than cusp-to-cusp deviation or more than one molar tooth is in cusp-to-cusp deviation); slight negative (mesioclusion of one molar to cusp-to-cusp extent, that is Angle Class III); or extreme negative (severe deviation of one molar or noticeable deviation of several).
5. *Tooth displacement score:* The number of teeth noticeably displaced or rotated from ideal arcial arrangement viewed from the occlusal aspect, plus two times the number of teeth displaced more than 2 mm or rotated more than 45°. These variables are all consistent with illustrations in Kelley and Harvey (1977) and Baum *et al.* (1973). Additionally, the treatment priority index (TPI) is estimated (following Kelley and Harvey, 1977) as a continuously distributed measure of overall occlusal variation spanning the values 0 (perfect, ideal) to 10 (theoretically indexed as severe malocclusion with treatment rated mandatory according to the United States orthodontic concensus). Our computation of the TPI is only intended to carry internal meaning as a morphological variable, however.

Maxillary arch length was next recorded with point calipers accurate to 0.05 mm as the distance from the point between the mesial-incisal edge of right and left central incisors to the wax-bite fossa depicting the mesiolingual cusp apex of the first molar. Maxillary arch breadth was taken between mesiolingual cusp apexes of left and right first molars.

As the interviews for social and epidemiological data were conducted in Hindi and recorded separately from the Western observers scoring occlusal variables, the latter were collected with no knowledge of the exact SEG or other provenience.

Statistical methods to compare these groups for these data are as follows. Ratio-interval variables, such as geographic or morphological measurements, are compared between the three SEGs by *f* tests (variance ratios) and *t* tests (of mean difference) using 95% confidence intervals. Ordinal or nominal variables are contrasted by X^2, whereas all variables are analyzed by three-group two-way analysis of variance (Croxton, 1953), employing 97.5% confidence intervals to protect against Type I error. Interaction among variables is assessed by pairwise product-moment correlation, substituting the phi coefficient for discontinuous variables (Nunnally, 1967; Thomas, 1976), which is essentially equivalent but has a different probability distribution.

3. Results

First, it was determined that sex was not significantly associated with any occlusal variables except maxillary size measures. Therefore, males and females were treated together in the SEG samples. At any rate, the sex proportion did not vary significantly from random among the three groups. The only other significant association of sex was with the age of the subjects—males were older.

Table I shows statistical results for discontinuously scored variables. Overjet, particularly of the mandibular incisors, is fairly frequent. Occlusal variation beyond normal limits does not differ significantly among the three SEG. However, the high SEG differs from the others in the *type* (though not undesirable extent) of overjet, having significantly more anterior maxillary incisors. Treating

Table I
Frequencies of Discontinuous Variables

Variable	Frequency (%)			F	χ^2
	Positive	Normal	Negative		
Overjet					
High SEG	13	63	24	5.56[a]	3.8
Mid SEG	8	48	44		
Low SEG	3	66	31		
Overbite					
High SEG	12	88	0	5.06[a]	5.0
Mid SEG	3	96	1		
Low SEG	0	100	0		
Cross-bite					
High SEG	18	82	0	2.52	14.0[a]
Mid SEG	18	82	0		
Low SEG	6	94	0		
BSR					
High SEG	9	60	31	0.70	18.9[a]
Mid SEG	9	66	25		
Low SEG	3	93	4		
	Extreme	Observable	None		
Gingivitis					
High SEG	1	23	76	10.08[a]	18.3[a]
Mid SEG	0	37	63		
Low SEG	4	54	42		

[a]χ^2 (df = 2) and/or variance ratio (df = 2, 262) rejects null hypothesis of no difference among the groups.

the Indian youths as a single sample, some 45.7% differ from the occlusal ideal. This compares with 33.7% of American youths in the same age range (Kelley and Harvey, 1977). This comparison is highly distorted, however, by the orthodontically influenced definition of *ideal incisor relation*. In fact, in aboriginal societies an edge-to-edge bite between incisors is the norm, which is perhaps related to the functional use of these teeth (Hinton, 1981). This results in less than the 2–4 mm maxillary overjet orthodontists like to see. When a maxillary overjet of from 0 to 4 mm is accepted instead, only 12.5% of Indian youths are "maloccluded" compared with 29.7% for Americans.

The overbite–openbite trait shows gradation from the high (most variation) to the low (least variation) SEGs. The high SEG differs the most—in showing larger vertical overbite of the maxillary incisors. Again, this is not necessarily considered undesirable by orthodontic consensus (Kelley and Harvey, 1977), although preliterate human groups show little overbite. The low SEG is significantly better occluded in this regard. About 15.5% of American youths have undesirable over-bite–open-bite amounts, which is much more than the Indians (4.9%).

The cross-bite type does not differ among the SEGs; all show only buccal mandibular deviations. The frequency of these is significantly lower in the low SEG. The proportion of American youths with cross-bite is 17.1%, which is comparable to high- and middle-SEG Indians, but much more than the low-SEG Indians.

The BSR also shows a significant dichotomy between the low SEG and the high and middle SEGs. Mesioclusion occurs more frequently than distoclusion in all world populations except Western Europeans and American whites. The figure of 46.5% of American youths with BSR discrepancies is most comparable to the high-SEG Indians.

Periodontal disease is significantly more frequent in the lower SEG youths as compared with either middle or high SEGs.

Among continuously distributed variables (Table II), the tooth displacement score exhibits a very strong and significant trend toward higher values in the higher two SEGs than in the lowest SEG. Because this variable has the highest correlation with the overall treatment priority measure as well as a direct visual influence on lay-person assessments of malocclusion, this result is compelling. American youths average 5.1 for the tooth displacement score, somewhat higher than all the Indian samples.

The TPI is designed to gauge total variation from occlusal norms. The low SEG is quite significantly lower than the middle and high SEGs, whereas the highest SEG is significantly lower than the middle SEG. The mean TPI of 5.0 for American youths is generally comparable to the figures for high- and middle-SEG Indians, but this index can only be compared within very broad limits among different observers. It must also be noted that the TPI is incremented

Table II
Descriptive Statistics of Continuous Variables

	High SEG		Mid SEG		Low SEG		
Variable	mean	(s.d.)	mean	(s.d.)	mean	(s.d.)	F
Tooth displacement	3.7	(2.0)	4.3	(2.1)	2.8	(1.8)	10.85[a]
TPI	4.6	(2.8)	5.7	(3.2)	3.4	(2.4)	9.37[a]
Arch length	37.5	(3.0)	37.6	(2.7)	37.8	(1.9)	0.20
Arch breadth	40.8	(2.8)	41.8	(2.8)	42.0	(2.7)	4.31[a]
Age	14.2	(0.9)	13.6	(1.3)	13.2	(1.0)	14.05[a]
Migration distance	457.0	(870)	225.0	(385)	177.0	(524)	4.88[a]
PBD (km)	483.0	(906)	466.0	(1349)	280.0	(686)	0.83
Carious teeth	0.35	(1.06)	0.17	(0.62)	0.09	(0.28)	2.61

[a]Partition of variance rejects null hypothesis of no difference among the groups.

somewhat when an individual has a maxillary overjet between 0 and 2 mm in spite of the fact that this condition is actually morphologically normal in nonindustrialized populations. Thus, the TPI has been increased disproportionately, especially in the low and middle SEGs; despite this, the low SEG is much less variable occlusally.

Maxillary arch length and breadth were taken to describe palate shape and to examine the phenomenon of palatal narrowing or the maxillary collapse syndrome noted in other rural and immigrant studies (Goose, 1972; Lavelle, 1973). The only significant finding is with respect to arch breadth, which is smaller in the high SEG when compared to either middle or low SEGs. The low SEG is significantly less variable in arch length than is the middle SEG. However, these measures are influenced by sex of the subjects; males are larger. We therefore compared palatal shape by regression analysis. First, we determined that males and females within samples were quite homogeneous with respect to correlation and slope between arch length and breadth. The resulting least squares regressions predicting breadth from length for the combined sex samples are as follows:

High SEG ($r = +0.624$): $B = 18.9 + 0.584(L)$
Middle SEG ($r = +0.547$): $B = 19.8 + 0.583(L)$
Low SEG ($r = +0.631$): $B = 8.8 + 0.876(L)$

The correlation coefficients signifying morphological integration of arch size are not significantly different. The low SEG, however, differs significantly in having a steeper slope. In other words, arch breadth maintains a relatively larger proportion compared to arch length in lower SEG subjects.

Among the epidemiological variables, the following results are noted. Age shows a highly significant rising trend going up the SEGs, perhaps because of earlier school dropout age among poorer children. Subject migration distance (from birthplace to Chandigarh) is significantly greater in the highest SEG, reflecting the occupational mobility of this group; also, the high and middle SEGs are much more variable in migration distance than is the low SEG. This is not to say the low-SEG subjects are not immigrants; they are, but they come from relatively near areas. Parental birthplace distance is lower in the low SEG but not significantly so. This distance is significantly more variable in the middle SEG than in the high or the low SEGs and is more variable in the high than the low SEG. The distribution of caries does not differ more than can be ascribed to chance variation in the three SEGs, and all have low caries prevalence.

4. Discussion

Significant differences in pattern and variability of occlusion are found according to SEG. In particular, the lowest SEG, which is predominantly rural in origin, differs from the higher, mainly urban SEGs in having less variable and more ideal occlusal relations in all regards except overjet, and in having broader maxillary arches. Because this finding of better rural occlusal health is now approaching a generality, we must consider some of the possible etiological explanations.

4.1. Age

There is an artificial relation between age and occlusal variation; the best occluded low SEG was younger. There is, however, no significant correlation of age with any occlusal variable (even the arch size measurements) *within* any of the three SEG samples. Arch breadth alone shows a significant *negative* correlation with age in the total sample, but this is an artifact of sample heterogeneity.

4.2. Gene Frequencies

Orthodontic researchers generally believe in a predominantly genetic basis for malocclusions (Smith and Bailit, 1977). Following this line, we would expect to detect significant gene frequency differences among the SEGs, implying that they are separate breeding populations. In fact, such evidence is lacking. Despite socioeconomic variation, the people in this region largely belong to one caste group—the Jats. Furthermore, the caste situation has been particularly fluid historically in the Punjab with much exogamy. Accordingly, various serologic and dermatoglyphic investigations (Bhalla, 1966; Seth, 1968; Seth, Bansal, and Seth, 1971; Singh, Sareen, and Goedde, 1974a, 1974b; Sunderland, Sawhney, Cartwright, and Jolly, 1976; Gill, 1981) show no variation among known genetic markers in these groups. In fact, from a long-term view, the caste situation in India is genetically fluid. It has been found repeatedly (Bowles, 1977) that differences among castes within a region are less than differences between equivalent castes in different regions. This "looseness" of caste endogamy over time is especially evident in northwestern India, as compared with the Ganges Basin (Bowles, 1977). At any rate, our Punjabi sample is taken from a single interbreeding population. As may easily be true in other studies of rural-urban differences in occlusion, the differences we found cannot reasonably be ascribed to simple genetic difference.

4.3. Inbreeding

Inbreeding theoretically increases the probability of deleterious gene homozygosity, and it has been linked with an endless series of diseases. In the present study, parental birthplace distance (PBD) serves as a correlate of inbreeding coefficients, and this variable does not significantly differ between the SEG, despite sharp differences in occlusion. Furthermore, the most inbred subgroup—the low SEG—has the least occlusal variation (cf. results of Corruccini and Whitley, 1981). Correlational analysis shows no positive relation, either between or within SEGs of PBD with occlusal variables or the TPI.

4.4. Racial Crossing

No concept has been more overused or abused by orthodontists than that of outbreeding causing mismatches between occluding parts (Horowitz and Osborne, 1971), for example a large maxilla from one parent with a small mandible from the other. This idea is rejected by geneticists because it is illogical in view of the principles of polygenic linkage and developmental canalization with stress-induced symmetry (Chung *et al.*, 1971; Lombardi and Bailit, 1972; Corruccini and Whitley, 1981). We have recorded subject migration distance as one measure of the probability of social mobility and significant heterozygosity, although PBD might also be looked upon as indicative of outbreeding. Neither of these epidemiological variables correlates with any occlusal variables, either within the aggregate sample or in the three separate samples; in fact, their only significant correlation was a positive one among themselves. Furthermore, the high SEG would have the highest probability of outcrossing but is significantly lower in TPI than the middle SEG that is overwhelmingly of Punjab origin and has shown no recent trend toward reduced endogamy.

4.5. Caries

Caries activity (causing arch space loss, irregular contacts, or irregular eruption succession) has long been supposed to influence occlusal variation, even though statistical epidemiological evidence is largely lacking. In the present study, the number of carious teeth failed to correlate with any occlusal variable or measurement, either over the entire sample or within SEG. Furthermore, the overall caries rate is very low in permanent teeth (confirmed by V. Kaul, 1980; S. Kaul, personal communication) and shows no trend by SEG or age. On the other hand, Sushma (1972) demonstrated much greater *deciduous* caries rates in rural children as opposed to urban, and he assigned this to the Punjabi habit of giving children many sweets, especially in the rural areas. Sushma found almost no decayed or missing permanent teeth in youths aged 12–16, but he found a 30% rate in deciduous teeth between ages 9 and 11. Sushma also detected more Class II malocclusion in the high SEG. Saxena (1972) likewise documented slightly greater malocclusion in higher SEGs in Chandigarh; yet the lower SEG had more caries. Thus, we feel we can reject caries as a causal factor in our observed occlusal differences, although it probably is a contributing factor (the caries–TPI correlation approaches significance, explaining 4% shared variance).

4.6. Premature Deciduous Tooth Loss

As with caries, this factor has been suggested, but positive epidemiological tests of association with malocclusion in populations are absent. One of our motives in choosing Chandigarh schools for sampling occlusal variation was that this group has already been thoroughly surveyed for permanent tooth eruption (Kaul, 1975; Kaul *et al.*, 1975). The high-SEG children have earlier gingival emergence, and this also seems characteristic of urban children as opposed to rural children in other societies (cf. Kaul *et al.*, 1975). Thus, early deciduous shedding, premature permanent eruption, and an anomalous time gap between these events (all of which are related; see Miller *et al.*, 1965; Singh, 1980), is likely a correlate of increased occlusal variation. Furthermore, earlier deciduous shedding is related to the secular trend (in Western societies) of increasingly early puberty (Miller *et al.*, 1965; S. P. Singh, 1980), and this secular phenomenon is demonstrably correlated with nutritional factors (Garn, 1966). Thus, the fact that the Chandigarh high SEG is better nourished probably relates to accelerated dental eruption. More study of the tooth replacement occlusion relation on a longitudinal basis is badly needed. Another factor possibly influencing premature deciduous tooth loss is caries; as we have seen, deciduous caries are more prevalent in the lower SEG; thus, the observed permanent eruption pattern occurs in spite of, not because of caries activity. This also appears to be the case among the Pima Indians in the Southwest of the United States (Corruccini *et al.*, 1983).

4.7. Periodontal Disease

Davies (1983) and others suggest that "facial degeneration" through periodontal destruction as well as caries and functional influences underlies rising malocclusion rates. In fact, Davies states that mouth breathing is caused by rather than results in narrowing of the middle third of the face. We know of little previous evidence of a positive correlation between periodontal disease and malocclusion in human populations (Poulton and Aronson, 1961; Bilmoria, 1963; Morris, 1966; Paunio, 1973; Katz, 1977). Rather, most researchers refer to a contrary causal process, with more tooth displacements creating a greater chance for the development of periodontal infections. In our data, periodontal disease was greater in the sample with the *least* occlusal variation—our low SEG. However, these are probably unrelated variables; no significant correlations result between gingivitis and any occlusal trait within any of the three SEGs.

4.8. Nutrition

Garn (1961) lists hormonal or endocrine disturbances (leading to erratic, accelerated, or nonintegrated growth) as possible malocclusion factors; these in turn might be related to excessive food additives, protein, sodium, or sugar intake in children. It is logical to expect such effects in our highest SEG, but that group could not have any relation to the highest TPI occurring in the middle SEG. One problem in our data is the inseparability of the SEG (nutritional) and rural origin (dietary consistency) factors, which are virtually absolutely correlated. Future research with human ethnic groups or experimental animals should be directed toward testing the effects of very early nutritional (especially sugar) variation.

4.9. Mouth Breathing

Related to allergy, which is itself another "disease of civilization," just like malocclusion, habitual oral breathing can cause palatal distortion (Harvold *et al.*, 1973) and abnormal chewing and swallowing action. Goose *et al.* (1957) also suggest urban pollution and respiratory infection as possible correlates. This complex of factors is likely involved in the Indian rural-urban occlusal epidemiological transition, but we instituted no control in the experimental design to measure its effect. Furthermore, two possible reasons for higher urban allergy prevalence are hyperactive and antigenic reactions that result from food additives or excess sugar intake in young children. This resembles the nutritional mechanism cited previously. Thus, the allergy and nutrition factors may be interrelated.

4.10. Habits

Thumb sucking and bottle feeding in infants may affect occlusion of the deciduous dentition, but probably not in the full permanent dentition we observed in Indian youths. Posture, sleeping attitudes, and abnormal muscle, tongue thrust, or swallowing habits, have all been suggested at one time or another, but are unlikely as well as difficult to control for in any experimental or epidemiological study.

4.11. Interproximal Attrition

Begg's (1954) theory for modern man's frequent malocclusion rested on the assumption that human teeth are genetically programmed to be slightly larger than the total space available to them in the jaws. In aboriginal societies, the rapid rate of interproximal attrition reduces tooth size to the extent that proper alignment can be maintained. In modern urban man, lack of attrition causes teeth to remain too large and crowding ensues. This theory probably deserves its very obscure level of recognition for two reasons. (1) It does not explain ontogeny of cross-bite, overbite, BSR, or spacing anomalies, all of which are frequent; it only applies to crowding displacement. (2) The adult pattern of malocclusion is firmly established by the age of 12, with the eruption of most of the permanent dentition, not only in this Indian population but in other groups used to document the sudden epidemiological transition in occlusion: rural Americans, American blacks, Melanesians, Pima Amerindians, Inuit, Chinese, Australian aboriginals (Corruccini, personal observation). At this age, even in coarse-diet, high-attrition populations, little if any interproximal attrition has occurred. Even among Inuit and Australian aboriginals, significant arch shortening begins at about age 20; well before this age, the rising incidence of malocclusion becomes evident in those groups eating a modern diet who live near urban settlements. In Chandigarh rurals also, visual inspection reveals little occlusal surface attrition before the age of 30, and significant interproximal space loss would occur even later. The low-SEG youths exhibited no shortening of the dental arch (Table II) as would occur with mesial tooth drift. We therefore consider the Begg model to be without merit; however, other dietary factors influencing earlier occlusal development have significant predictive value for occlusal variation.

4.12. Dietary Consistency and Its Relation to Functional Chewing Stress

Lombardi and Bailit (1972) have traced the history of this old anthropological idea about dietary consistency. It originated from observations of many aboriginal societies who developed high incidences of malocclusion within the first generation on a reservation, or in otherwise restricted residences with products being supplied from industrial areas thus replacing the raw, coarse natural foodstuffs (see Corruccini and Whitley, 1981, for review). Food toughness therefore should be highly predictive of the occlusal patterns in Indian youths. In the city, processed wheat *chapatis* and *dahl* tend to be the staples, whereas in the country corase millet and locally grown vegetables are staples. More importantly, raw sugar cane is widely chewed for enjoyment in rural areas. The few city dwellers who were acquainted with this habit had suffered from bleeding gums and could not chew and strip the material. Probably, the difference in habitual masticatory demand goes back far into childhood, perhaps to weaning. In the city, high-SEG children have access to professional dental care, whereas in the country this is wholly lacking; it is being substituted for by casual chewing on hard Acacia boughs that not only clean the teeth but are considered medicinal. Lack of functional stimulation explains the nonrandom aspects of occlusal changes that we have observed in world populations: Small jaws erupting normal-sized teeth resulted in crowding and maxillary narrowing (Watt and Williams, 1951) thus causing buccal cross-bite to be much more prevalent than lingual cross-bite. Furthermore, the chewing stress model leads one to expect early adolescent establishment of malocclusion patterns that are maintained into adulthood.

5. Conclusions

The Punjabis in and around Chandigarh are in the midst of a population-wide geographic and demographic transition, and as such, they offer unique opportunities and controls for studying aspects of the epidemiologic transition (Omran, 1971). The more recently rural component shows significantly better dental occlusion. This tendency has also been noted in several Western European-derived populations; additionally, it probably characterizes other Indian groups (Bilmoria, 1963; Sidhu and Shourie, 1970; Sidhu *et al.*, 1970; Reddy and Vijayakumar, 1978; Reddy, 1983). Genetically related causes of the difference (admixture, inbreeding) can be rejected, as can caries and other aspects of general oral health. We venture the opinion that this is also true of the other rural-urban studies, although none of them have attempted empirical analysis of correlative epidemiological factors. Orthodontic researchers need to look away from the prevalent genetic thinking to environmental causation (see also Harris and Smith, 1980; Corruccini and Potter, 1980; Potter, Corruccini, and Greene, 1981). Our present results suggest mouth breathing, premature deciduous tooth loss, nutritional heterostasis, and masticatory function as logical agents; furthermore, these factors are probably not separate but are interrelated by common influences from the diet and from hormonally guided and functionally stimulated orofacial growth.

We see future need for occlusal surveys in more distant and isolated Punjab communities, where even fewer urban influences will be encountered and where virtually all individuals will be West Punjab immigrants. Further comparative data in varying human populations would allow better understanding of environmental factors. This cross-cultural approach circumvents the problem of environmental homogeneity that negates epidemiological surveys of malocclusion in industrial societies.

ACKNOWLEDGMENTS

We thank S. P. K. Chopra, P. S. Gill, and N. S. Malhotra for assistance, the various schoolmasters for their permission to study subjects, and Drs. D. Johnson and F. Berkowitz for their help.

References

Barnard, P. D., 1956, Dental survey of state school children in New South Wales, *National Health and Medical Research Council Special Report Series* **8.**

Baum, L. J., *et al.*, 1973, A method for measuring occlusal traits, *Int. Dent. J.* **23:**530–537.

Begg, P. R., 1954, Stone Age man's dentition, *Am. J. Orthod.* **40:**298–312.

Bhalla, V., 1966, Blood group distribution pertaining to ABO, MNSs, and Rh-Hr systems in the Indian subcontinent, *Anthropologie* (Czechoslovakia) **4:**67–86.

Bilmoria, K. F., 1963, Malocclusion: Its role in the causation of periodontal disease, *J. All India Dent. Assoc.* **35:**293.

Bowles, G. T., 1977, *The People of Asia,* Weidenfeld and Nicolson, London.

Chung, C. S., Niswander, J. D., Runch, D. W., Bilben, S. E., and Kau, M. C. W., 1971, Genetic and epidemiologic studies of oral characteristics in Hawaii's schoolchildren. II. Malocclusion. *Am. J. Hum. Gen.* **23:**471–495.

Corruccini, R. S., and Potter, R. H. Y., 1980, Genetic analysis of occlusal variation in twins, *Am. J. Orthod.* **78:**140–154.

Corruccini, R. S., and Whitley, L. D., 1981, Occlusal variation in a rural Kentucky community, *Am. J. Orthod.* **79:**250–262.

Corruccini, R. S., Potter, R. H. Y., and Dahlberg, A. A., 1983, Occlusal variation across time in Pima Indians, manuscripts in preparation.

Croxton, F., 1953, *Statistics for Biomedical Science,* Dover, New York.

Davies, D. M., 1972, *The Influence of Teeth, Diet, and Habits on the Human Face,* W. Heinemann Medical Books, Ltd., London.

Garn, S. M., 1961, Research and malocclusion, *Am. J. Orthod.* **47:**661–673.

Garn, S. M., 1966, Nutrition in physical anthropology, *Am. J. Phys. Anthropol.* **24:**289–292.

Gill, P. S., 1981, A Study of Genetic Markers and Dermal Ridge Configuration in the Lowland Rajputs of Punjab, M.S. thesis, Punjab University, Chandigarh.

Goose, D. H., 1972, Maxillary dental arch width in Chinese living in Liverpool, *Arch. Oral Biol.* **17:**231–233.

Goose, D. H., Thomson, D. G., and Winter, F. C., 1957, Malocclusion in school children of the West Midlands, *Brit. Dent. J.* **102:**174–178.

Harris, E. F., and Smith, R. J., 1980, A study of occlusion and arch widths in families, *Am. J. Orthod.* **78:**155–163.

Harvold, E., Vargervik, K., and Chierici, G., 1973, Primate experiments on oral sensation and dental malocclusions, *Am. J. Orthod.* **63:**494–508.

Hinton, R. J., 1981, Form and patterning of anterior tooth wear among aboriginal human groups, *Am. J. Phys. Anthropol.* **54:**555–564.

Horowitz, S., and Osborne, R., 1971, The genetic aspects of cranio-facial growth, in: *Cranio-Facial Growth in Man* (R. E. Moyers and W. M. Krogman, eds.), Pergamon, Oxford, pp. 183–192.
Katz, R. V., 1977, Relationships of occlusal states with dental caries and periodontal disease, *J. Dent. Res.* **56:**A43.
Kaul, S. S., 1975, Estimation of age from the emergence of permanent teeth, *Ind. Ped.* **13:**233–235.
Kaul, S. S., Saini, S., and Saxena, B., 1975, Emergence of permanent teeth in schoolchildren in Chandigarh, India, *Arch. Oral Biol.* **20:**587–593.
Kaul, V., 1980, Ph.D. thesis, Panjab University, Chandigarh.
Kelley, J. S., and Harvey, C. R., 1977, An assessment of the occlusion of youths 12–17 years, *U.S.P.H.S. Vital and Health Statistics,* Series 11, no. 162, Washington, D.C.
Lavelle, C. L. R., 1973, Variation in the secular changes in the teeth and dental arches, *Angle Orthod.* **43:**412–421.
Lombardi, A. V., and Bailit, H. L., 1972, Malocclusion in the Kwaio, a Melanesian group on Malaita, Solomon Islands, *Am. J. of Phys. Anthropol.* **36:**283–294.
Miller, J., Hobson, P., and Gaskell, T. J., 1965, A serial study of the chronology of exfoliation of deciduous teeth and eruption of permanent teeth, *Arch. Oral Biol.* **10:**805–818.
Morris, M. L., 1966, Orthodontic-periodontic relationships, in: *The Nature of Orthodontic Diagnosis* (S. L. Horowitz and E. H. Hixon, eds.), C. V. Mosby, St. Louis, pp. 192–216.
Nunnally, J., 1967, *Psychometric Theory,* McGraw-Hill, New York.
Omran, A. R., 1971, The epidemiologic transition, *Milb. Mem. Fund Quart.* **49:**509–538.
Paunio, K., 1973, The role or malocclusion and crowding in the development of periodontal disease, *Int. Dent. J.* **23:**470–475.
Potter, R. H. Y., Corruccini, R. S., and Greene, L. J., 1981, Variance of occlusion traits in twins, *J. Craniof. Gen. Dev. Biol.* **1:**217–227.
Poulton, D. R., and Aaronson, S. A., 1961, The relationship between occlusion and periodontal status, *Am. J. Othod.* **47:**690–699.
Reddy, V. Rami, 1983, Dental occlusion among the people of Gulbarga, Karnataka, *Anthrop. Contemp.*
Reddy, V. Rami, and Vijayakumar, M., 1978, Caries and some dental features among the Vysyas of southeastern Andhra Pradesh, *Acta Anthropogen.* **2:**63–72.
Saxena, B., 1972, Eruption of permanent teeth, state of dental health and body size of school-going girls in Chandigarh, M.S. thesis, Panjab University, Chandigarh.
Seth, S., 1968, A study of the A_1A_2BO blood groups system and ABO(H) secretion in six endogamous groups of Punjab. *Am. J. Phys. Anthropol.* **29:**387–396.
Seth, S., Bansal, I. J. S., and Seth, P. K., 1971, Studies on haptoglobin and transferrin types in Khatris and Aroras of Punjab, India, *Humangenetik* **14:**44–49.
Sidhu, S. S., and Shourie, K. L., 1970, Morphology of Class II Division 1 malocclusion—a cephalometric study, *J. Ind. Orthod. Soc.* **2:**1–6.
Sidhu, S. S., Shourie, K. L., and Shaikh, H. S., 1970, The facial skeleton and dental patterns in India—a cephalometric study, *J. Ind. Orthod. Soc.* **2:**7–13.
Singh, S., Sareen, K. N., and Goedde, H. W., 1974a, Investigation of some biochemical genetic markers in four endogamous groups from Punjab (N.W. India). I. Protein and enzyme polymorphisms in serum, *Humangenetik* **21:**341–346.
Singh, S., Sareen, K. N., and Goedde, H. W., 1974b, Investigation of some biochemical genetic markers in four endogamous groups in Punjab (N.W. India). II. Red cell enzyme polymorphisms, *Humangenetik* **22:**133–138.
Singh, S. P., 1980, Eruption of permanent teeth in Gaddi Rajput males of Dhaula Dhar Range of the Himalayas, *Zeit. Morph. Anthropol.* **70:**295–301.
Smith, R. J., and Bailit, H. L., 1977, Problems and methods in research on the genetics of dental occlusion. *Angle Orthod.,* **47:**65–77.

Sunderland, E., Sawhney, K. S., Cartwright, R. A., and Jolly, J. G., 1976, Studies of haptoglobin and transferrin types in four castes of the Punjab, Northern India, *Hum. Hered.* **26**:16–24.

Sushma, S., 1972, Order and Eruption Times of Permanent Teeth, State of Dental Health, Height and Weight of School-Going Boys in Chandigarh, M.S. thesis, Panjab University, Chandigarh.

Thomas, D. H., 1976, *Figuring Anthropology,* Holt, Rinehart & Winston, New York.

Watt, P. G., and Williams, H. M., 1951, The effects of the physical consistency of food on the growth and development of the mandible and maxilla of the rat, *Am. J. Orthod.* **37**:895–928.

World Health Organization, 1971, *Oral Health Surveys—Basic Methods,* Geneva.

CHAPTER 10

Current Status of Dermatoglyphic Studies in South Asia

P. DASH SHARMA

1. Introduction

The ridged skin of palmar and plantar surfaces (often termed *friction skin*) is a specialized characteristic of all primates. This specialized character is also observed in an incompletely developed form in some mammals like the common squirrel, hedgehog, kinkajou (of South America) and some marsupials. The prosimians, unlike human beings, apes, and the majority of monkeys, exhibit large areas in which ridge formation is incomplete. Continuously ridged skin is a characteristic feature of the palmar and plantar surfaces of monkeys, apes, and *Homo sapiens*.

The individual variations in epidermal ridge configurational arrangements are greatest in apes and humans. The word *dermatoglyphics* (*derma*-skin, *glyphe*-carve) was proposed in 1926 by Cummins and Midlo (1926). The term embraces all the features of the epidermal ridges (except flexion creases and other secondary folds) of the palmar and plantar surfaces of the hands and feet of humans as well as other primates. The epidermal ridges become evident by the 12th to 13th week of gestation; they are well developed by the 4th fetal month, and the process is completed sometime between the 4th to 6th month (Patten, 1953).

The configurations of the epidermal ridges on fingers, palms, and soles of humans have attracted the attention of many physical anthropologists and geneticists for the study of ethnic variation and inheritance of the trait. Of late, the

P. DASH SHARMA • Reader in Physical Anthropology, University of Ranchi, Ranchi 834 001, India.

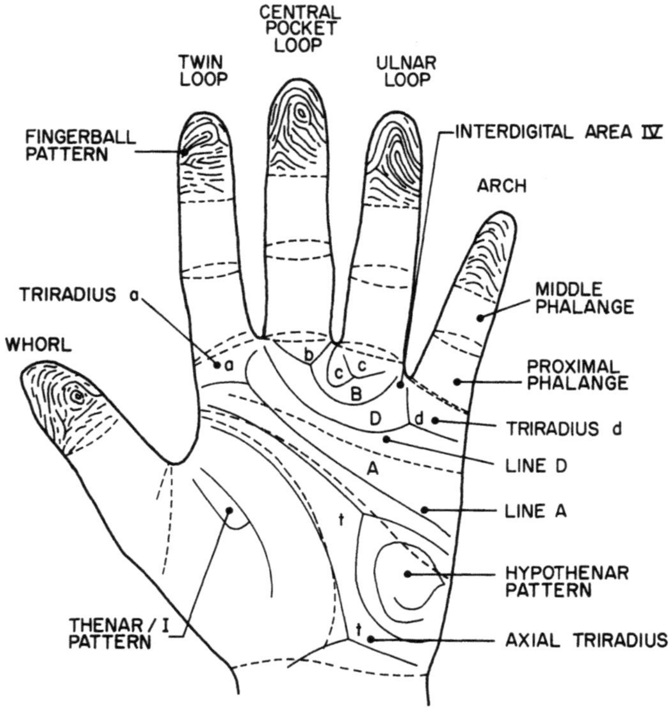

Figure 1. Dermatoglyphic features of finger and palmar surfaces.

significance of the dermatoglyphic studies in chromosomal and developmental defects has drawn the attention of many cytogeneticists, human biologists, and medical personnel. We presume that the reader has a basic understanding of dermatoglyphics, and we will proceed with a discussion of the dermatoglyphic studies in South Asia, with particular reference to India. For easy reference, however, a few illustrations (see Figures 1 and 2) show the dermatoglyphic features discussed in the text.

2. The Formative Stage

Starting with Risley's classic attempt to classify the people of India in 1915 and with the subsequent publication of Guha's report in 1935, many scholars have devoted their energies to the problem of the "origin, migration, and classification of the Indian population." The primary research tool available to these scholars was anthropometry. A large number of similar studies followed Guha's classification. I. P. Singh in his presidential address to the anthropology and

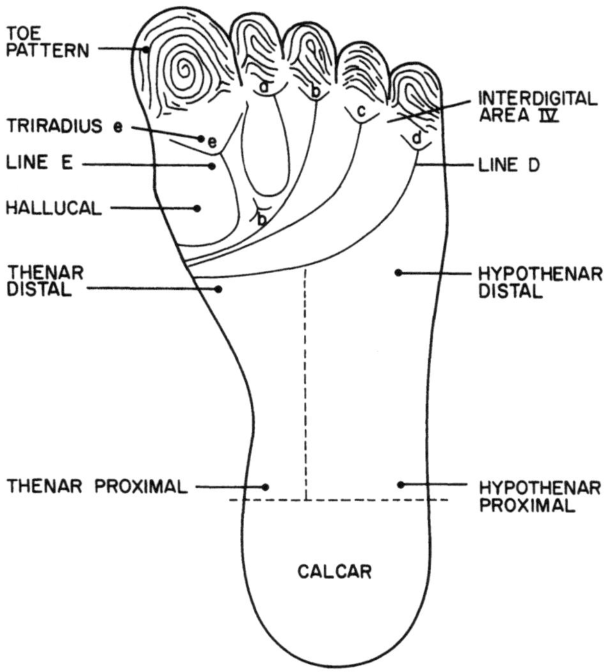

Figure 2. Dermatoglyphic features of sole.

archaeology section of the 56th Indian Science Congress in Bombay in 1969 stated:

> Most of these studies end up with either examining Guha's classification for various unstudied populations or describing the same population with added morphological and/or genetical markers. Addition of blood groups and dermatoglyphic factors gained popularity in these series of ethnic discrimination studies. The works of Biswas (1936) and Sarkar (1936) deserve special mention here for their attempt at popularizing dermatoglyphics and multiple genetic studies respectively." (Singh, 1969, p. 3.)

P. C. Biswas did pioneering work in the field of dermatoglyphic research in India. In the mid-1930s in Germany, he worked under Fischer in Berlin. Soon after completing his thesis he had to leave Germany because of the impending World War. His thesis, entitled "Uber Hand und Fingerleisten von Indern," appeared in *Ztschr. f. Morphul. u. Anthropol.* in 1936. Biswas's work was referred to by Cummins and Midlo (1943) in their chapter on racial variation. This was the only reference to a South Asian scholar mentioned in the bibliography. The 50 samples on which Biswas's thesis was based represented a heterogenous group of Indians living in Germany at that time. If we compare Biswas's thesis with the titles of papers presented at the International Symposium of Dermatoglyphics in Delhi in 1966, we realize the striking differences in the units of analyses employed in these ethnic variation studies. The shift was from a heterogenous population group to a more homogenous one based on a definite mating unit. Indian researchers were beginning to realize the importance of the mating unit in population studies, which resulted in sampling specific groups like the Lahulis, Kashmiri Muslims, and Pasis.

I. P. Singh was the first student to receive a Ph.D. under Biswas at Delhi (1959), and he was also the first student to write a thesis on dermatoglyphics under the guidance of an Indian thesis adviser. The subject of the thesis was not ethnic variation, but, as stated in the title, it was on inheritance of fingerball patterns. Thus, Biswas introduced new areas of research to his students, a trend he continued until his retirement from active service in 1968.

Another important landmark for dermatoglyphics research in India was Biswas's participation in the Second International Congress of Human Genetics in Rome in 1961 along with his student A. Sharma. They took the initiative in founding the International Conferences on Dermatoglyphics, and convened its first meeting in Rome in 1961 (organizer D. C. Rife). During the fourth meeting held in Paris in 1971, the name was changed to the International Dermatoglyphics Association. In Rome, Prof. Biswas presented a paper entitled "Ethno-Geographic Variation in Dermatoglyphics." In this paper, he (Biswas, 1961) reported on 43 Indian population samples and compared them with other world population samples for which data were available. During the two decades between 1961 and 1981, over 500 reports on ethnic variation in dermatoglyphics have been published for Indian populations alone (Dash Sharma, ms.). We are often confronted with questions regarding the utility of these numerous reports on Indian samples. This question is answered in the concluding part of this chapter.

3. International Symposium on Dermatoglyphics (1966)

P. C. Biswas opened the first session of the International Symposium on Dermatoglyphics (February, 1966) with the following remarks.

> The growing development and utility of dermatoglyphics in various fields and disciplines urged us on the need of organizing an International Symposium on Dermatoglyphics in India. . . . Dermatoglyphics in earlier days were known as a police science, as this was mainly used for criminal identification. In the beginning of the twentieth century, its importance in other disciplines was realized, particularly in Anthropology, Human Biology, and Medical Genetics. Anthropologists have been using it as one of the physical criteria for ethnic differentiation and classification as it has given a valuable clue for the study of racial stratification in racially composite populations . . . (Biswas and Sharma, 1968, p. 4).

The articles contained in the proceedings volume (Biswas and Sharma, 1968) revealed that the emphasis of these studies on dermatoglyphics was largely confined to the frequency distribution of dermatoglyphic traits in different Indian populations. Of the 34 scientific papers presented in the symposium, 7 were on research methodology and contested paternity, 6 were on inheritance and disease, 1 was on forensic science and the value of dermatoglyphics, and 20 papers were on the dermatoglyphics of Indian populations. Thus, about 59% of the papers were on ethnic variation studies. This trend toward ethnic studies in dermatoglyphics abated in later years—a fact revealed in the papers presented at the 10th International Congress of Anthropological and Ethnological Sciences (New Delhi, 1978) and at the International Symposium on Dermatoglyphics (Patiala, 1980). Before we discuss these two international meetings, it is necessary to discuss the papers presented in the 1966 International Symposium on Dermatoglyphics.

In the section *Research Methodology and Contested Paternity* (no paper was presented on "contested paternity"), a few of the papers were noteworthy. One paper by P. C. Biswas and D. K. Bhattacharya, entitled "Deviation Quotient of Digital Triradii, a New Variable in Palmar Dermatoglyphics," was left without much discussion, and we have not come across any other paper addressing the suggestions put forth by the authors. Apparently, this deviation was not taken seriously by other researchers of ethnic variation. Another paper, by P. K. Chattopadhyay and entitled "Quantitative Estimation of the Position of Axial Triradius and its Radio-Ulnar Deviation," generated much heated discussion during the session. Unlike the Biswas and Bhattacharya paper, this paper was heavily criticized by the senior scholars present in the audience, even though both these papers were based on similar methodologies—one suggested "deviation quotient" and the other "deviation index."

We now realize that simple or even complex methods, if based on arbitrary measures, do not lead to a meaningful conclusion in the study of ethnic variation. The methodology of dermatoglyphics is based mostly on conventions that are being followed almost universally and are rapidly developing into standardized rules. All over the world, almost, researchers in dermatoglyphics have been following Cummins and Midlo (1943) and the earlier works of these authors for about half a century. In India, Abhimanyu Sharma did extensive work on the methodological aspects of palmar dermatoglyphics, mostly based on a single sample of 400 Burmese (Kachin) males.

Sharma devised the *t* index (Sharma, 1962) (see Figure 3) and established in his paper (Sharma, 1968, p. 60) that "angle *atd* is an altogether different metric concept relative to *t*-index and one must not be considered to be synonymous with the other". Sharma based his *t* index on the proximo-distal positioning of axial triradius, that is, "longitudinal locationing of *t*- positions," whereas the angle *atd* is connected more with "the relative positioning of digital triradii *a* and

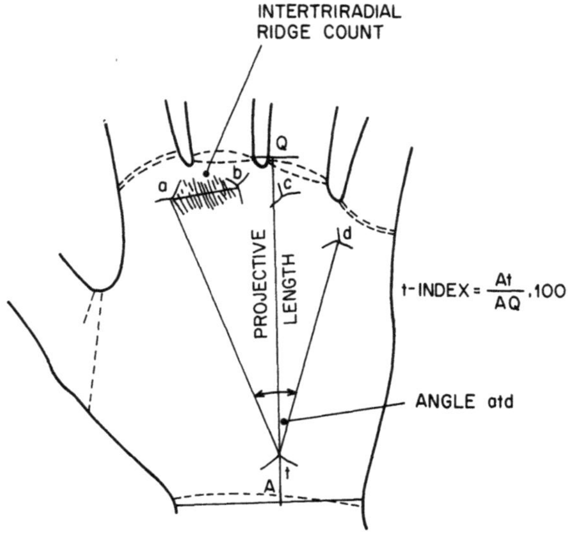

Figure 3. Intertriradial ridge count *a-b* and diagrammatic representation of *t* index and angle *atd* in palm.

d and the axial triradius (*t*, *t'*, or *t''*)." According to Sharma (1968), the latter is the "transversal measure of maximal angle *atd*." He also proposed a few other indexes and angles (breadth–height index, modified positional index, flexion angle) in later publications (Sharma and Taneja, 1968).

Sharma was indeed innovative in devising indexes based on new methodologies in palmar dermatoglyphics (Sharma, 1966; Sharma and Taneja, 1968). However, these methods were followed only by Sharma's students at Delhi and were not adopted by students of dermatoglyphics at other important centers of physical anthropology in India (Calcutta, Chandigarh, Pune, and Waltair). Sharma compared his work on the *atd* angle (Sharma, 1968) with the methods and results of Penrose (1954) and Mavalwala (1963). Penrose used the angle as a criterion to identify mongolism, not simply as a tool for ethnic discrimination. Sharma's impact on the field of palmar dermatoglyphics can be assessed by reviewing the abstracts of papers presented in the anthropology and archaeology sections of the Indian Science Congress (Bangalore, 1971). Of the 20 abstracts on dermatoglyphics, 10 were by Sharma and his students. These papers discussed the modified positional index, correlation matrices, and association between various longitudinal and quantitative transverse trends in palms and soles. The untimely death of Sharma in September, 1978, left a void in the development of dermatoglyphic research methodology in India. Bhanu has recently discussed the methodological aspects of dermatoglyphics in various conferences and seminars (Bhanu, 1973, 1978, 1980).

Only six papers were presented in the section on inheritance and disease, and the papers discussing statistical treatment and analysis were of limited scope. The analytical part was limited to "occurrence and non-occurrence of various pattern types in parents and their offspring," particularly in studies on fingerball and toe patterns. Bali (1968) presented an interesting paper that discussed the relationship between finger and toe patterns in the same individual. The toes showed a definite tendency to exhibit types of patterns often present on fingers of the same individual. An increase in whorls on fingerballs was associated with an increase in their frequency on the toes. Bali (1968) further noted that when whorls are absent on fingers, arches appear twice as frequently as whorls on the toes of the same individual. The other papers were on such topics as inheritance of loop patterns on toes (25 families); inheritance of the palmar hypothenar area (98 families); inheritance of palmar main lines (53 families); inheritance of right and left combinations of fingerball patterns (25 families). Though all these reports were based on a small number of families and simple analytical methods

Table I
Finger Pattern-type Indexes among Some Indian Populations[a]

Populations	Sex	Number	Pattern intensity index	Dankmeijer's index	Furuhata's index
Mongoloid					
Lahuli	Male	100	14.30	5.00	112.0
Ladakhi	Male	55	15.42	3.25	132.76
	Female	45	15.53	1.56	131.06
Bhutane	Male	69	15.29	1.40	115.32
Raji	Male	62	14.50	3.13	89.50
Abor	Male	147	15.08	4.46	120.23
Bhotia	Male	36	14.85	4.30	108.00
Riang	Male	68	14.23	5.28	84.44
Australoid					
Kadar	Male	—	15.88	0.99	148.11
	Female	—	14.72	1.07	92.18
Urali	Male	—	15.39	0.02	115.07
	Female	—	14.31	2.86	81.57
Paniyan	Male	—	15.20	8.98	138.42
Pahira	Male	—	15.23	6.49	138.42
	Female	—	14.18	3.32	78.42
Adiyan	Male	—	14.72	9.62	122.23
Koya Dora	Male	71	14.21	6.31	97.04
	Female	39	14.81	1.02	103.33

[a]From Biswas and Sharma 1968, pp. 196, 212.

were used, they stimulated much discussion among the participants in the symposium.

As mentioned previously, 59% of the papers presented in the symposium were on ethnic variation studies. The papers were grouped under the topics of fingers, palms, and soles, and both qualitative and quantitative dermatoglyphic traits were reported. In Table I, the values of the fingerball indexes (Pattern intensity index, Dankmeijer's index, and Furuhata's index) have been given on some Indian populations that were reported on in the symposium. The values of the indexes on some northern and northeastern Indian populations having mongoloid features were reported by Bhasin (1968), whereas Rao (1968) reported on the values observed in some populations of southern India having australoid features. It is evident from Table I that there is much overlap in fingerball indexes of the mongoloid and australoid populations of India. In the other quantitative trait, the *a-b* ridge count (see Table II), no distinct ethnic differentiation was observed in the values among the Indian populations reported on (Dash Sharma, 1968). Bhattacharya (1968) stated that "I have used absolutely no statistical tools whatsoever to avoid a forced ethnic conclusion as *a-b* ridge count has yet to enter into the horizon of established taxonomic character taken for ethnic evaluation and discrimination purposes." This statement reflects the general impression on the *a-b* ridge count prevalent in the mid-1960s. The trend setters in palmar intertriradial ridge count studies in India are P. K. Dutta (1961) and P. K. Seth (1963), both of whom have worked on palmar *a-b* ridge

Table II
Mean a-b Ridge Count in Some Indian Populations[a]

Populations	Sex	Number	Mean ± S.E.	Investigators
Indian (Andhra Pradesh)	Male	80	76.92 ± 0.91	Datta, 1961
Indian (Punjab)	Male	62	76.42 ± 1.60	Seth, 1963
	Female	38	80.68 ± 1.49	
	Total	100	78.04 ± 1.14	
Anglo-Indian	Male	48	80.16	Bhattacharya, 1966
Bengali				
Bagdi	Male	33	81.80 ± 2.21	Chattopadhyay and Dash Sharma, 1966
Duley	Male	9	76.66 ± 2.83	
Rarhi Brahmins	Male	104	77.22 ± 1.05	
Ladakhi	Male	54	80.95 ± 1.22	Dash Sharma, 1966

[a]From Dash Sharma, 1968, p. 269.

counts. In the International Symposium on Dermatoglyphics in Patiala in 1980, the intertriradial ridge counts in palms were discussed in 12% of the papers presented in the symposium by Indian scholars. The increasing interest in palmar ridge count studies among Indian scholars suggests the importance of this dermatoglyphic trait, an absolute quantitative value that has greater genetical significance than an index value. An important outcome of the symposium was that scholars understood the meaning and significance of the *Mendelian population* concept in the Indian context. This is crucial in India where there is a caste system, within which are subcaste and sub-subcaste groupings. This 4-day symposium at Delhi was indeed the central pillar supporting the superstructure of Indian dermatoglyphics that developed in later years.

4. Calcutta—The Other Center

Since the inception of the Anthropological Survey of India in 1947, Calcutta has proven to be a major center of physical anthropological studies under the leadership of such scholars as B. S. Guha and S. S. Sarkar. In the anthropological survey and in the Department of Anthropology of Calcutta University, the primary emphasis in dermatoglyphic studies has been on ethnic variation. M. R. Chakravartti (in some papers his surname is spelled differently) and D. P. Mukherjee did extensive investigation among northeastern Indian populations in the early 1960s (Chakraborty and Mukherjee, 1961; Mukherjee and Chakravartti, 1964). The Chakravartti–Mukherjee bond was severed in 1964 and 1965 when Mukherjee went to London to work with S. B. Holt at Galton Laboratory and Chakravartti went to Heidelberg to work under Prof. Vogel. Though Mukherjee continued his interest in the dermatoglyphics of Indian populations (Mukherjee, 1965), he broadened his research focus to include genetical investigations in dermatoglyphics under the guidance of S. B. Holt, an authority on the genetics of dermal ridges (Holt, 1968). Mukherjee published an excellent contribution entitled "Inheritance of Total Number of Triradii on Fingers, Palms, and Soles" in 1966 while at the Galton Laboratory (University College of Science, London). The following year he presented his thesis at the University of London, which was entitled "Quantitative Genetics of Dermal Ridges with Special Reference to an Indian Population" (Mukherjee, 1967). These two papers are the most important landmarks in dermatoglyphics research in India since Biswas's first publication in 1936 when dermatoglyphics was in its formative stages. Thus, since the mid-1960s, Indian scholars have begun to investigate the inheritance of dermatoglyphic traits seriously (Tiwari, 1965; Mitra *et al.*, 1966; Dash Sharma, 1971; Bansal and Bhattacharya, 1972, etc.).

The first report on inheritance of middle phalangeal and basal phalangeal configurations among families (70 Punjabi families with 236 children) and twin

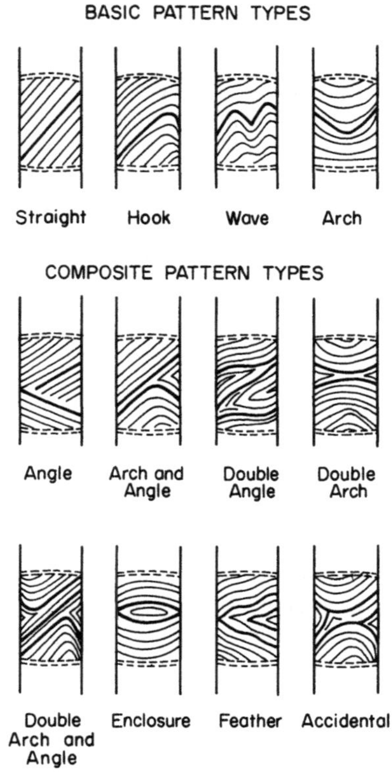

Figure 4. Diagrammatic representation of middle and proximal (basal) phalangeal pattern types.

pairs (14 MZ and 26 DZ pairs) was by S. K. Basu (Basu, 1968). He found that both middle and basal phalangeal patterns (see Figure 4) showed high concordance values (92.86% and 96.71%, respectively) in MZ twins, whereas DZ twins showed much lower concordance values (33.17% and 39.23%, respectively). Using the formula suggested by Rife (1959), the heritability estimate (*H*) was calculated by Basu who found that the estimate for the middle phalanges (89.3%) was slightly lower than that for basal phalanges (92.9%). No other reports on heritability estimates for the basal and middle phalanges are available for Indian populations. Because little work has been done on the dermatoglyphics of this trait in India, the nature of variation in these phalangeal regions is not fully understood. Dash Sharma (1973) also worked on the dermatoglyphics of the basal and the middle phalanges among the Oraons of Ranchi and found that the hook pattern (see figure 4) is 3 times more frequent on the basal phalanges than on the middle phalanges, whereas the angle type shows 10 times the increased occurrence on the middle phalanges than on the basal phalanges. We have yet to determine if this is a general trend in the dermatoglyphics of this region.

5. Dermatoglyphics and Chromosomal Studies

Following the retirement of Biswas from Delhi University in 1968, dermatoglyphic research in India has advanced significantly with the publication of two articles. "Finger Dermatoglyphics of Mentally Retarded Children in North India" by Bandyopadhyay (1969) and "Dermatoglyphics in Childhood Cirrhosis" by Chandra (1969). These contributions appeared simultaneously in the same volume of the same journal. From the 1970s onward, students in the field of dermatoglyphics took increasing interest in the study of associations between dermatoglyphic traits, specific diseases, and chromosomal aberrations. In July, 1970, the Anthropological Survey of India (Calcutta) organized a 3-day seminar on physical anthropology and allied disciplines, and there were five papers presented in the session on dermatoglyphics. Four papers were on ethnic variation and one was entitled "Dermatoglyphics Associated with Congenital Malformations and Chromosomal Anomalies" (by Dash Sharma, 1970). This paper was an exhaustive review of the literature on dermatoglyphics and congenital diseases. The review covered a span of over three decades, beginning with the first publication of Cummins in 1939, "Dermatoglyphic Stigmata in Mongoloid Imbeciles." Prior to the 1970s very few Indian scholars worked in the field of dermatoglyphics and diseases. Notable among them are Mruthyunjaya (1968) who worked in California; Chandra (1969) and Bandyopadhyay (1969) who worked at New Delhi; and Mavalwala and associates (1969) who worked on chromosomal anomalies in California at Santa Barbara. Mruthyunjaya and Chandra are both pediatricians, whereas Bandyopadhyay and Mavalwala are anthropologists. Some physical anthropologists at Delhi University have been developing a focus on cytogenetics following training received in West Germany in the early 1970s. We hope that in the near future their contributions to the field of dermatoglyphics will shed new light on the relationship between chromosomal anomalies and dermatoglyphics. Recently, many doctors in the medical colleges of Delhi, Bangalore, Hyderabad, Pune, and Calcutta are investigating the dermatoglyphic features of their patients independently or in collaboration with physical anthropologists. Thus, physical anthropologists are no longer considered "untouchables" in the eyes of medical researchers and pediatricians in the medical colleges of India. Table III shows the association of dermatoglyphic features with some diseases. The table is based on the reports (except that of Bandyopadhyay, 1969, and Chandra, 1969) presented in two recent meetings held at Patiala and Ranchi in 1980. It is encouraging to note that in one single year so many reportings were made on dermatoglyphics and diseases by Indian

Table III
Association of Dermatoglyphic Features with Some Diseases

Diseases	Sample Size and locality	Dermatoglyphic features (fingers and palms only)	Investigators
Mental disorder	104 patients (children–72 males and 32 females), Delhi	Increased composite whorls in all the digits, on digits II and IV there is rise in the frequency of arches with corresponding decrease in whorl frequency	Bandyopadhyay, 1969
Childhood cirrhosis	43 patients (children—31 males and 12 females), New Delhi	High value of TRC in fingers and mean total *a–b* ridge count. High incidence of pattern in III interdigital area, significantly larger *atd* angle	Chandra, 1969
Diabetes mellitus	76 patients (58 males and 18 females), Hyderabad	In right hand of males: Increase in the frequency of whorls and decrease in the frequency of ulnar loops, higher value of pattern intensity index, increased value of TFRC and ridge counts on II, III, and IV fingers, higher value of palmar *c–d* and *a–d* ridge counts	Ahuja *et al.*, 1980[a]
Tuberculosis	47 patients (females), Patiala	Abstract does not state specific observations	Bhatnagar, 1980[a]
Asthma	62 patients, Patiala	Higher incidence of monomorphic hands for whorls	Bhatnagar *et al.*, 1980[a]
Retinitis pigmentosa	89 patients (60 males and 29 females), New Delhi	Higher incidence of whorls in I, II, and IV fingers. Lower frequency of patterns in hypothenar, II, and III interdigital areas	Deshmukh *et al.*, 1980[a]
Schizophrenia	112 patients (61 males and 51 females), Calcutta	Significant differences in *a–b*, *b–c*, and *c–d* ridge counts, *atd* angle, simian crease types, and incidence of pearl line	Karmakar and Malhotra, 1980[a]
Congenital heart disease	80 patients, Pune	Among Cyanotic category: increased frequency of whorls and arches on digits, higher frequency of proximal and absent types of C-line terminations,	Kulkarni *et al.*, 1980[a]

Table III (*Continued*)

Diseases	Sample Size and locality	Dermatoglyphic features (fingers and palms only)	Investigators
		more radial loops on hypothenar area. Among Acyanotic category: higher frequency of loops on digits. Higher frequency of ulnar and proximal types of C-line terminations, Decrease of radial loops in hypothenar area	
Stein-Leventhal syndrome	33 patients, Kolhapur	Abstract does not state specifically the distinctive features of the patient group	Nagaonkar, 1980[a]
Down's syndrome	Sample size not stated, Bangalore	Greater frequency of ulnar loops, large *atd* angle, increased frequency of simian crease	Narayanan, 1980[a]
Manic depressive psychosis	Sample size not stated, Bangalore	Patient group showed significant differences in frequencies of ulnar loops, whorls, and arches	Narayanan and Mallikarjunaiah, 1980[a]
Childhood cirrhosis	51 patients (children), Patiala	Preponderance of ulnar loops, low frequency of arches, low values of total ridge count and pattern intensity index, high value of angle *atd*, lower value of a–b and c–d ridge counts	Kumar *et al.*, 1980[a]
Mental retardation	Sample size not stated, Delhi	Abstract does not state specific observations	Roy *et al.*, 1980[a]
Psoriasis	63 patients (46 males and 17 females), Waltair	Higher frequency of whorls particularly on V finger, much less frequency of ulnar loops	Satyanarayana, 1980[a]
Tuberculosis	50 patients (females), Patiala	Abstract does not state specific observations	Singal *et al.*, 1980[a]
Partially deaf	41 patients (male), Hyderabad	Increased frequency of ulnar loops in digits, higher incidence of patterns in thenar/I interdigital area, high value of t–d ridge count	Sujetha *et al.*, 1980[b]

(*continued*)

Table III (*Continued*)

Diseases	Sample Size and locality	Dermatoglyphic features (fingers and palms only)	Investigators
Retinitis pigmentosa	200 patients, New Delhi	Abstract does not state specific observations	Grewal *et al.*, 1980[b]
Congenital heart disease	160 patients, Hyderabad	Significant increase in the frequency of arches and corresponding decrease in the frequency of radial loops in fingers, significant increase in the mean values of *a–b*, *b–c*, *c–d*, and *a–d* ridge counts, high value of *atd* angle	Sundari and Ahuja, 1980[b]

[a]International Symposium on Dermatoglyphics (Abstracts), Patiala, February, 1980.
[b]*Seventh Annual Conference of Indian Society of Human Genetics (Abstracts)*, Ranchi, December, 1980.

researchers. It is hoped that in the near future Indian scholars will make commendable contributions on this aspect of dermatoglyphics.

6. Some New Trends

Bali and Chaube (1971) continued the analysis of palmar flexion creases (see Figure 5) that was initially investigated by Büchi (1954) and Sarkar (1961). Thus, after a decade, analysis of this trait was conducted seriously by Bali and his students who discussed the formulation of palmar creases on the basis of population, family, and twin studies (Bali and Chaube, 1971). In the International Symposium on Dermatoglyphics in Patiala in 1980, there were seven papers on palmar creases by Bali and his students. The range of their studies includes formulation, classification, ethnic variation, and inheritance studies of palmar creases.

After the first publication by Plato (1970), "Polymorphism of the C line of palmar dermatoglyphics," we find a number of papers on C line reported by Indian investigators (Bansal and Bhattacharya, 1972; Bhanu and Malhotra, 1972). In the 10th International Congress of Anthropological and Ethnological Sciences (New Delhi, 1978) and in the International Symposium on Dermatoglyphics (Patiala, 1980), there were six papers presented on C-line polymorphism. This suggests the importance attributed by Indian researchers to the C line in palmar dermatoglyphics. An interesting paper on triradius *c* and main line

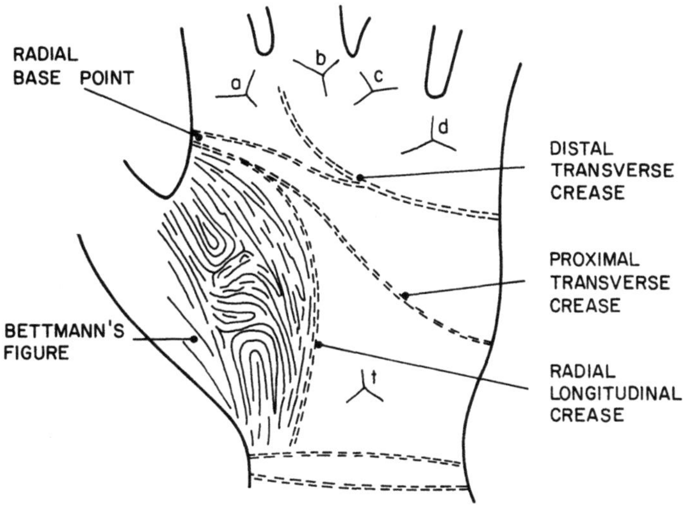

Figure 5. Diagram showing Bettmann's figure in thenar/I interdigital area of palm and palmar creases.

C by Mahapatra (1971) reported the absence of triradius *c* up to 2 to 3 generations in three families and assessed the inheritance as dominant. Patel (1971) reported on Bettmann's figure (see Figure 5) on the palms of both the parents and the children in a Tibetan family.

Two interesting investigations deserve special mention because they effectively redirected dermatoglyphic research in India. The first study, by Basu and Namboodiri (1971), explored the functional relationship between total ridge count (TRC) and the pattern intensity index (PII) by using the least square regression line (linear and quadratic). They showed that the relationship between these variables might be different in different ethnic groups. Later, other scholars (Malhotra *et al.*, 1978, 1980) worked on this problem and presented their findings at two international meetings. Their papers were of an exploratory nature, however, and the relationship between TRC and PII needs further investigation. The second study, by Holt and Dash Sharma (1977), was the first to report the absence of triradius *d* in two Nicobarese sisters living on Nancowry Island. That such a rare phenomenon occurs in two sisters suggests that the absence of triradius *d* is genetically determined, possibly by a rare recessive gene. This initial report and one appearing subsequently (Dash Sharma, 1979) on the absence of triradius *d* has evoked interest among students of dermatoglyphics. This is evident from the presentation of papers on the absence of triradius *d* at symposia and seminars in India.

Due to limited space, it is not possible to discuss individual papers critically; rather, subsequent discussion will be limited to the nature of papers presented at conferences and seminars held in India during the 1975 to 1980 period that will help us in understanding the trend in research on dermatoglyphics in India.

7. Present Status of Dermatoglyphic Studies

The Indian Society of Human Genetics convened for its second annual conference in Calcutta during November, 1975. Of the seven papers presented on dermatoglyphics, three dealt with ethnic variation studies, one with inbreeding effects, one with the relationship between digital ridge counts, and two with dermatoglyphic association with diseases. The general trend emerging from these papers was encouraging, in that the reports focused on specific problems rather than on stereotypic descriptive accounts of ethnic variation in dermatoglyphics. The most significant paper was that on inbreeding effects and dermatoglyphics. The authors (Sabarni and Mukherjee, 1975) suggested that a significant excess of whorls occurs in inbred populations along with a high frequency of arches and radial loops on individual fingers of each hand. They concluded that this significant excess is possible only if there is a recessive or additive inheritance of the trait. These results support the earlier observations on the genetics of finger pattern types. Although ample opportunity for investigating dermatoglyphic characteristics of inbred populations exist in India, very few reports are available at this time. Two other papers that deserve mention investigated the dermatoglyphics of congenital heart disease (Annapurna *et al.*, 1975) and carcinoma of the cervix (Reddy *et al.*, 1975). In both papers, significant differences were reported between the samples and control groups for certain dermatoglyphic parameters like increased frequency of whorls on digits, higher frequency of patterns in interdigital areas III and IV, and lower values of the *d-t* ridge count as well as *atd* angle for carcinoma of the cervix. For all categories of congenital heart disease there was considerable decrease in the *d-t* ridge count.

Out of the 140 scientific papers presented at the fourth annual conference of the Indian Society of Human Genetics in Madras in 1977, only about 7% were on dermatoglyphics. These studies deviated strikingly from the general trend. All but three papers dealt with dermatoglyphic features of deaf mutes, mentally retarded individuals, and patients with congenital heart disease or cataracts; furthermore, all samples were compared with the control groups. This was indeed a welcome change in dermatoglyphic research trends in India. It should be noted that the average sample size for the seven papers is about 100 individuals. This is indeed a small sample for association studies of a multifactorial trait like dermatoglyphics. This is a reflection of the financial and other limitations of physical anthropologists in India. They are not directly affiliated with medical colleges or hospitals, which puts them at a certain disadvantage for long-term projects on specific diseases. We hope that in the near future there will be much more cooperation between medical colleges/hospitals and physical anthropologists in India for long-term projects on dermatoglyphics and diseases.

In the three abstract volumes of the 10th International Congress of Anthropological and Ethnological Sciences (10th ICAES, New Delhi, 1978) the total number of papers on dermatoglyphics contributed by Indian scholars was 38 out of 319 papers (about 12%) abstracted in physical anthropology. These papers can be grouped into the following categories: population studies on dermatoglyphics, 21 (55%); dermatoglyphics and diseases, 7 (19%); association among dermatoglyphic traits, 5 (31%); methodology/formulation, and so forth, 3 (8%); and genetical investigations in dermatoglyphics, 2 (5%).

Thus, it is evident that Indian researchers in the field of dermatoglyphics primarily contributed to the understanding of population variation with much less emphasis on relations with diseases, association among traits, and other aspects of dermatoglyphics. One significant revelation of this world anthropological congress was that there was no representation from Sri Lanka, Bangladesh, or Pakistan for any aspect of physical anthropology. This is probably due to the fact that in these countries, there are few anthropology departments and thus few physical anthropologists. Kennedy (1980) mentioned one biological anthropologist in Quaid-I-Azam University in Islamabad, but so far no research presentation from Pakistan has been given at any recent international gathering of physical anthropologists. The most widely acclaimed paper in the session on dermatoglyphics in the 10th ICAES (New Delhi, 1978) was entitled "Decoding Dermatoglyphics" by A. G. de Wilde. De Wilde, who worked in the Netherlands, presented a new concept of ridge pattern formation on basal and middle phalanges and on the palm that was based on embryological development. Other innovative papers were also presented in the session on dermatoglyphics, such as "Dermatoglyphics of Palmar Prints with Absent *c* Triradius"; "Correlation between Ridge Counts on Different Fingers and the Relationship between TFRC, ATFRC and FPII: Indian Data"; and "Genetic Interrelationship between Ridge Counts on Fingers." In addition to those dealing with dermatoglyphics and disease, these showed a distinct deviation from traditional dermatoglyphic research in India.

The International Symposium on Dermatoglyphics in Patiala in 1980 that was organized one and one-half decades after Prof. Biswas's 1966 symposium further revealed the trend in Indian dermatoglyphic research. There were 73 papers presented at Patiala; 63 were contributed by Indian scholars and 10 by foreign scholars. The 63 abstracted papers contributed by Indian scholars, can be grouped as follows: population studies in dermatoglyphics, 28 (44%); dermatoglyphics and diseases, 18 (29%); association among dermatoglyphic traits, 8 (12%); methodology/formulation, and so forth, 3 (5%); and genetical investigations in dermatoglyphics, 6 (10%).

When this distribution is compared to that for the 10th ICAES at New Delhi, it becomes evident that the researchers gave more attention to other aspects of the dermatoglyphic studies than to general population studies. That studies by Indian scholars are branching out from traditional dermatoglyphic research is commendable and promises to lead toward a greater understanding of the biomedical, psychological, and behavioral aspects of dermatoglyphics.

From 1966 to 1980, within a span of one and one-half decades, the status of dermatoglyphics research in India passed through the adolescent stage. We are eagerly looking forward to its further development when our knowledge of dermatoglyphics will be utilized for screening patients for specific diseases before taking up the highly expensive medical and clinical investigations. In order to achieve this stage we must have the basic understanding of the nature of variation of different dermatoglyphic parameters and the associations among the different dermatoglyphic patterns and configurational areas of fingers, palms, and soles of different ethnic groups. Much of the applied aspects of dermatoglyphics depends on the understanding of the variations, associations, and the genetics of dermatoglyphics.

Now is the time when we should pause, ponder, and plan out our next program collectively, if this tiny group engaged in the study of dermatoglyphics is to contribute in a meaningful way to the benefit of South Asian populations.

ACKNOWLEDGMENTS

The author is deeply indebted to Dr. Kailash C. Malhotra of the Indian Statistical Institute in Calcutta for his very helpful suggestions during the preparation of this chapter.

References

Annapurna, V., Ahuja, Y. R., Reddi, Y. R., Reddi, G. D., Rao, V. S., and Rao, N., 1975, Dermatoglyphics in congenital heart disease, *2d Annu. Conf. Indian Soc. Hum. Genet.* (Abstract No. 16), Indian Statistical Institute, Calcutta.

Bali, R. S., 1968, Some genetic observations on dermatoglyphic traits, in: *Proc. Vol. of Int. Symp. on Dermatoglyphics* (P. C. Biswas and A. Sharma, eds.), Department of Anthropology, University of Delhi, Delhi, pp. 85–104.

Bali, R. S., and Chaube, R., 1971, On the formulation of palmar creases, *Z. Morph. Anthropol.* **63:**121–130.

Bandyopadhyay, M., 1969, Finger dermatoglyphics of mentally retarded children in North India, *Hum. Hered.* **19:**410–414.

Bansal, I. S., and Bhattacharya, D. K., 1972, Inheritance of C-line in palmar dermatoglyphics, *Z. Morph. Anthropol.* **63:**385–390.

Basu, S. K., 1968, Inheritance of middle phalangeal and basal phalangeal configurations by twin and family studies, *Z. Morph. Anthrop.* **60:**85–99.

Basu, A., and Namboodiri, K. K., 1971, The relationship between total ridge count and pattern intensity index of digital dermatoglyphics, *Am. J. Phys. Anthropol.* **34:**165–174.

Bhanu, B. V., 1973, Course of the Pattern Radiants: Classification, Paper presented at the Ninth Int. Congr. Anthropol. Ethnol. Sci., Chicago.

Bhanu, B. V., 1978, Whorls: ulnar, radial and median, *10th Int. Congr. Anthropol. Ethnol. Sci., New Delhi,* Abstracts **2:**2–3.

Bhanu, B. V., 1980, Transverse axis and longitudinal mid-axis of the palm: A method to construct them on prints, *International Symposium on Dermatoglyphics,* Punjabi University, Patiala, Abstracts:5–6.

Bhanu, B. V., and Malhotra, K. C., 1972, Palmar C-line polymorphism among Gadvas of Goa and Ezhavas of Kerala, *Man in India* **52:**261–267.

Bhasin, M. K., 1968, A study of finger dermatoglyphics of Bhutanese, in: *Proc. Vol. of Int. Symp. on Dermatoglyphics,* (P. C. Biswas and A. Sharma, eds.), Department of Anthropology, University of Delhi, Delhi, pp. 193–209.

Bhattacharya, D. K., 1968, A note on the *a-b* ridge count of the Anglo-Indians of India, in: *Proc. Vol. of Int. Symp. on Dermatoglyphics* (P. C. Biswas and A. Sharma, eds.) Department of Anthropology, University of Delhi, Delhi, pp. 251–253.

Biswas, P. C., 1936, Uber Hand-und Fingerleisten von Indern, *Ztscher. f. Morph. u. Anthropol.* **35:**519–550.

Biswas, P. C., 1961, Ethno-geographic variations in dermatoglyphics, *Proc. Second Int. Congr. Hum. Genet.* Rome, pp. 1430–1449.

Biswas, P. C., and Sharma, A. (eds.), 1968, *Proceedings Vol. of Int. Symp. on Dermatoglyphics (Delhi, 1966),* Department of Anthropology, University of Delhi, Delhi.

Büchi, E. C., 1954, The simian crease in India, *Bull. Dept. Anthropol.* **3:**39.

Chakraborty, M. R., and Mukherjee, D. P., 1961, Dermatoglyphic study of tribes and castes of the state of Assam, *Science and Culture* **27:**584–585.

Chandra, R. K., 1969, Dermatoglyphics in Indian childhood cirrhosis, *Hum. Her.* **19:**540–545.

Cummins, H., 1939, Dermatoglyphic stigmata in mongoloid imbeciles, *Anat. Rec.* **73:**407–415.

Cummins, H., and Midlo, C., 1926, Palmar and plantar epidermal ridge configurations (dermatoglyphics) in European-Americans, *Am. J. Phys. Anthropol.* **9:**471–502.

Cummins, H., and Midlo, C., 1943, *Fingerprints, Palms and Soles: An Introduction to Dermatoglyphics,* Blakiston Co., Philadelphia. (Reprinted, 1961, Dover, New York.)

Dash Sharma, P., 1968, The *a-b* ridge count of the Ladakhis, in: *Proc. Int. Symp. Dermatoglyphics* (P. C. Biswas and A. Sharma, eds.), Department of Anthropology, University of Delhi, Delhi, pp. 267–270.

Dash Sharma, P., 1970, Dermatoglyphics associated with congenital malformations and chromosomal aberrations, in: *Bio-anthropological Research in India* (Hirendra K. Rakshit, ed.), Anthropological Survey of India, Calcutta, pp. 178–184.

Dash Sharma, P., 1971, Quantitative genetics of *a-b* ridge count in human palms, *J. Anthrop. Soc. Nippon.* **79:**375–376.

Dash Sharma, P., 1979, Further observations on absence of palmar triradius *d* in normal people, *Am. J. Phys. Anthropol.* **50:**213.

Dash Sharma, P., and Sahu, B., 1973, Finger, palmar, middle and basal phalangeal dermatoglyphic study of the Oraons of Ranchi, India, *J. Anthropol. Soc. Nippon.* **81**(4):260–267.

Dutta, P. K., 1961, A study on the quantitative value of palmar digital triradii: The *a-b* ridge count in the people of Andhra Pradesh, *Sagar Univ. J. (Sci.),* 1961.

Guha, B. G., 1935, The racial affinities of the peoples of India, *Census of India,* 1931, Volume I, Part III, Delhi.

Guha, B. S., 1935, The racial affinities of the peoples of India, *Census of India,* Vol. I, Part III, Delhi.

Holt, S. B., 1968, *The Genetics of Dermal Ridges,* Charles C Thomas, Springfield, Ill.

Holt, S. B., and Dash Sharma, P., 1977, Absence of triradius *d* on the palms of normal people, *Ann. Hum. Genet., Lond.* **41**:195–197.

Kennedy, K. A. R., 1980, Integration of Western and Indian patterns of biological anthropology: An historical study, *South Asian Anthropol.* **1**(1):1–9.

Mahapatra, Usha, D., 1971, Inheritance of absence of triradius *c, Man in India* **51**:54–59.

Malhotra, K. C., Chakraborty, R., Bhanu, B. V., and Kazi, R. B., 1978, The correlation between ridge-counts on different fingers, and the relationship between TFRC, ATFRC and FPII: Indian data, *10th Int. Congr. Anthropol. Ethnol. Sci., New Delhi,* Abstracts **2**:25.

Malhotra, K. C., Chakraborty, R., and Bhanu, B. V., 1980, Quantitative analysis of digital dermatoglyphics of 20 Dhanger castes of Maharashtra, *Int. Symp. on Dermatoglyphics, Patiala,* Abstracts, p. 16.

Mavalwala, J., 1963, The utility of the angle *atd* in dermatoglyphics, *Am. J. Phys. Anthrop.* **21**:77–80.

Mavalwala, J., Parker, C. E., and Melnyk, J., 1969, Dermatoglyphics of the XYY syndrome, *Am. J. Phys. Anthrop.* **30**:209–214.

Mitra, A. K., Chattopadhyay, P. K., Dash Sharma, P., and Bardhan, A., 1966, Inheritance of *a-b* ridge count in human palms, *Humangenetik,* **2**:25–27.

Mruthyunjaya, G. T., 1968, Essay on Dermatoglyphic Patterns of Mid-line Defects, Paper read at Irvine, California College of Medicine, California.

Mukherjee, D. P., 1965, Anthropological observations on toe print patterns among the hill tribes of north-east India, *Z. Morph. Anthrop.* **56**:217.

Mukherjee, D. P., 1966, Inheritance of total number of triradii on fingers, palms and soles, *Ann. Hum. Genet.* **29**:349–353.

Mukherjee, D. P., 1967, Quantitative Genetics of Dermal Ridges with Special Reference to an Indian Population, Ph.D. thesis, University of London.

Mukherjee, D. P., and Chakravartti, M. R., 1964, A dermatoglyphic approach to the Mundari ethnic problem, *Z. Morph. Anthrop.* **55**:32–45.

Patel, S., 1971, Inheritance of Bettmann's figure among Tibetan refugees, *Man in India* **51**:67–70.

Patten, B. M., 1953, *Human Embryology,* Blakiston, New York.

Penrose, L. S., 1954, The distal triradius *t* on the hands of parents and sibs of Mongol imbeciles, *Ann. Hum. Genet.* **19**:10.

Plato, C. C., 1970, Polymorphism of the C line of palmar dermatoglyphics with a new classification of the C line terminations, *Am. J. Phys. Anthropol.* **33**:413–420.

Rao, M. B., 1968, Finger dermatoglyphics study of the Koya Doras of Andhra Pradesh, in: *Proc. Int. Symp. on Dermatoglyphics* (P. C. Biswas and A. Sharma, eds.), Department of Anthropology, University of Delhi, Delhi, pp. 205–214.

Reddy, S. S., Ahuja, Y. R., and Reddy, O. S., 1975, Dermatoglyphics in carcinoma of the cervix, *2d Annu. Conf. Indian Soc. of Hum. Genet.,* Abstract **17,** Indian Statistical Institute, Calcutta.

Rife, D. C., 1959, *Heredity and Human Nature,* Vantage Press, New York.

Risley, H. H., 1915, *The People of India,* Thacker, Spink, Calcutta.

Sabarni, P., and Mukherjee, D. P., 1975, Inbreeding effects of finger print patterns, *2d Annu. Conf. Indian Soc. Hum. Genet.,* Abstract **107,** Indian Statistical Institute, Calcutta.

Sarkar, S. S., 1935–1936, The racial affinities of the inhabitants of Rajmahal Hills, *Trans. Bose Res. Inst.* **11.**

Sarkar, S. S., 1961, The simian crease, *Z. Morph. Anthrop.* **51**:212–219.

Seth, P. K., 1963, The *a-b* ridge count in palmar dermatoglyphics of the Indians of Punjab, *Man* **242**:189–190.

Sharma, A., 1962, A Study of Palmar Dermatoglyphics of Burmans: Certain Fresh Methodological Approaches as Based on Burman Data, Ph.D. thesis, University of Delhi.

Sharma, A., 1966, Axial triradii formulation and certain fresh indices giving metric expression of variable positioning of axial triradii and digital triradii *c* and *b*, in: *Proc. Summer School of Anthropology* (Dalhousie, 1964), Department of Anthropology, University of Delhi, Delhi, pp. 81–92.
Sharma, A., 1968, A methodological study of cotangent groupings of angle *atd*, in: *Proc. Int. Symp. Dermatoglyphics* (P. C. Biswas and A. Sharma, eds.), Department of Anthropology, University of Delhi, Delhi, pp. 57–68.
Sharma, A., and Taneja, K., 1968, A methodological study of 'flexion angle' in quantitative palmar dermatoglyphics, *The Eastern Anthropologist* **21**:257–266.
Singh, I. P., 1959, Inheritance of fingerball patterns in human populations, Ph.D. thesis, University of Delhi.
Singh, I. P., 1969, Physical anthropology in India: Retrospect and prospects, Presidential Address to the Section of Anthropology and Archaeology of the 56th Indian Science Congress, Bombay.
Tiwari, S. C., 1965, Genetical analysis of *a-b* ridge counts, *The Anthropologist* **12**:125–128.

CHAPTER 11

Inbreeding in India: Concepts and Consequences

P. S. SUNDAR RAO

1. Introduction

India is one of the very few countries in the world today where consanguineous marriages are still practiced extensively. This custom varies, of course, among the multitude of subgroups within its population, and it can be traced back to ancient cultures and traditions. Social and economic changes, migrations, and newer religions have all had some influence in shaping the present levels of consanguinity. Some of the earlier reasons for preferring such marriages may no longer be valid, but nevertheless they remain popular in various sections of the country.

The impact of long-term and varied practices of inbreeding vis-à-vis short-term effects on human biology have not been fully investigated, and they require urgent attention. Since inbreeding produces an increase of homozygosity, recessive genes are expressed much more, and, when deleterious, the fitness of an individual may be affected. Another consequence is greater genetic variability within a population. On the other hand, in the presence of selective forces, the frequency of a specific bad gene might decline and the population would be rid of those genes. The Indian setting provides valuable opportunities to obtain empirical data that are necessary to test these various theoretical models of population genetics.

In this chapter, the concepts of inbreeding and the methodology of its measurement, both in terms of the level and in the expression of the homozygosity, are presented. This is followed by describing the extent of inbreeding in India and the consequences of such inbreeding on the basis of available data.

P. S. SUNDAR RAO • Department of Biostatistics, Christian Medical College, Vellore 632 002, India.

2. Definitions

2.1. Consanguinity

Marriages between "blood" relatives are termed *consanguineous*. The term *blood relative* refers to a person related through a common ancestor. Related individuals may have more than one common ancestor.

2.2. Inbreeding

The offspring of consanguineous matings are said to be *inbred*. The extent of inbreeding depends on the amount of common ancestry shared by the parents of the inbred child. In other words, it depends on the proportion of genes that the parents have in common. When parents have one or more common ancestors, they are more likely to possess the same genes, and thus the inbred individual is often homozygous at various loci.

2.3. Autozygosity

An individual whose two homologous genes at any given locus are identical by descent from common ancestors of his or her parents is said to be *autozygous*. When such homozygosity arises out of independent ancestry, then he or she is said to be *allozygous*.

3. Measurement of Inbreeding

3.1. Frequency of Incidence of Inbreeding

The extent of consanguinity in a population can be expressed as a ratio of such marriages to the total of the number of marriages contracted during any given time period. The different types of consanguineous marriages can also be stated as a proportion of total marriages or of total consanguineous marriages during the specified time period.

3.2. Types of Consanguineous Marriages

Blood relatives can be grouped into categories or degrees based on their closeness to an individual. The extent of consanguinity can thus be expressed in terms of those categories. For an individual, his or her relationship to parents and full sibs is called *first degree;* to his or her sib's offspring, *second degree;* to first cousins as *third degree* and so on, the number increasing with each step-generation removed from an individual. Children of sibs are called first cousins and with each generation removed beyond this, the relatives are termed one and one-half cousins or first cousins once removed, second cousins, two and one-half cousins, and so forth, increasing by one half each time another generation is involved. In each of these various degrees, distinction is made in terms of the kind of alliance resorted to.

For example, the pairs of first-degree relatives could be listed as follows: father–daughter, mother–son, and brother–sister pairs. Among second-degree relatives, there would be four pairs as follows: brother–sister's daughter; brother–brother's daughter; sister–brother's son; and sister–sister's son. Among third-degree (first cousin) relatives there are four types of marriages for men: mother's brother's daughter (MBD); father's sister's daughter (FSD); mother's sister's daughter (MSD); and father's brother's daughter (FBD). The first two pairs are called *cross-cousins*—matrilateral (MBD) and patrilateral (FSD), whereas the latter two are called *parallel cousins.* This distinction at times has no apparent biological implications, but it will have great social significance.

3.3. Inbreeding Coefficient

Although the frequency data are interesting and useful, the need for a coefficient that could quantify the degree of inbreeding was felt as early as 1913 (Pearl, 1914). Several investigators have attempted to define such an inbreeding coefficient that falls under one of two approaches: correlation analysis or probability rules.

Wright (1921, 1923) defined the inbreeding coefficient, F, as the correlation between uniting gametes. Such a correlation could also exist if there is assortative mating from any cause (Wahlund, 1928; Wright, 1931; Yasuda, 1968; Reid, 1973). Malecot (1948) defined the inbreeding coefficient based on the probability that the homologous genes of uniting gametes are identical by descent (Haldane and Moshinsky, 1939; Cotterman, 1940). Thus, f is the probability of autozygosity.

In the estimation of inbreeding coefficients based on parental consanguinity these two approaches can be used interchangeably. The inbreeding coefficient of an individual is the same as the coefficient of consanguinity of his or her parents, coefficient of parents (Malecot, 1948) or coefficient of co-ancestry (Kempthorne, 1957; Falconer, 1960).

A different measure of relatedness, introduced much earlier and still widely used, is Wright's (1922) coefficient of relationship, r_{IJ}, defined as

$$r_{IJ} = \frac{2f_{IJ}}{\sqrt{(1 + f_I)\ \ (1 + F_J)}}$$

For two individuals that are not inbred, the coefficient of relationship is exactly twice the coefficient of consanguinity.

3.4. Computation of Inbreeding Coefficient

Consider the following diagram (Figure 1) depicting an offspring I of a first-cousin marriage. One of the common ancestors is E (great grandfather of I).

The inbreeding coefficient of I, f_I is the same as the coefficient of consanguinity of the parents (f_{AB}) and denotes the probability that I is autozygous, or the probability that A and B contribute the same gene to I, if gametes are denoted by lowercase letters, then we need to determine $P(a = b)$, which will be the product of probabilities $P(c = a)$, $P(e = c)$, $P(e' = d)$, $P(d = b)$ and $P(e = e')$, each of which is ½, if E is *not* inbred.

If E is inbred, then we need to add the probability that the two alleles are identical by descent to ½. Thus if f_E is the inbreeding coefficient of E, then $P(e = e') = ½ + ½F_E = ½(1 + f_E)$. So, because of common ancestor E,

$$f_I = f_{AB} = P(a = b) = (½)^5(1 - f_E)$$

Likewise, if we consider the great grandmother, G (wife of E), then the contribution to $f_{I'}$ will be another $(½)^5(1 + f_G)$, where f_G is the inbreeding coefficient of G. Thus,

$$f_I = (½)^5(2 + f_E + f_G)$$

If $f_E = f_G = 0$, that is, if the common ancestors are *not* themselves inbred, then

$$f_I = (½)^5\ (2) = (½)^4 = \frac{1}{16}$$

Thus, the inbreeding coefficient of a first-cousin marriage is 1/16. In general, each path of relationship to a common ancestor is

$$(½)^n(1 + f_c)$$

where n is the number of individuals in the path from one parent to the ancestor and back through the other parent, and f_c is the inbreeding coefficient of a common ancestor. If there are several common ancestors, then the various contributions are summed and the inbreeding coefficient is given by

$$f_I = \Sigma[(½)^n\ (1 + f_c)]$$

where f_c is the inbreeding coefficient of a common ancestor.

Although not specifically stated, the preceding formula is applicable only for genes on autosomes. A gene on the X chromosome that is in a gamete produced by a male must be the same as was in the egg from which this male came. Therefore, the probability of identity by descent in these two gametes is 1, rather than ½ as it would be for a female or an autosomal locus. The effect is thus as if the males were not counted at all. Also, a path involving two successive males makes no contribution to the probability of identity of X-chromosomal

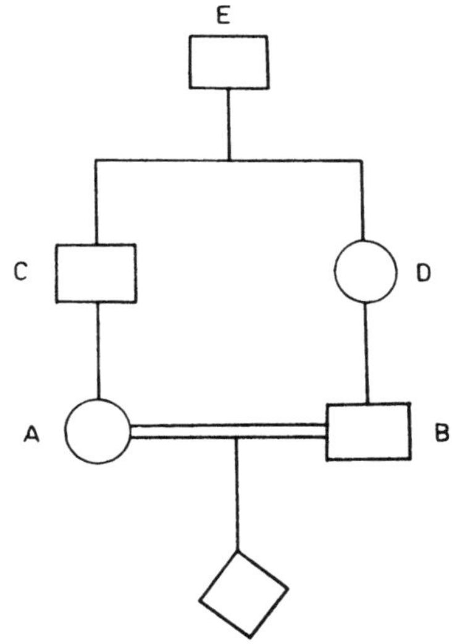

Figure 1. Pedigree of a first-cousin marriage.

loci. Thus the rule for obtaining the inbreeding coefficient for a sex-linked locus in females is to count only females in a path and to omit completely the path with two successive males.

Thus, among the first-cousin marriages, the f_I for X-linked gene will be for MBD: 1/8; for FSD: 0, for MSD: 3/16 and for FBD: 0.

An overall measure of inbreeding in a population may be obtained as a weighted mean of the various values of f_i (including $f = 0$) where f_i is the inbreeding coefficient in the ith subgroup who constitute proportion c_i in the population. This is characterized as α (or F), where

$$\alpha \text{ or } F = \Sigma\, c_i f_{i'} \text{ with } \Sigma\, c_i = 1$$

4. The Extent of Inbreeding in India

4.1. General Observations

India is a very large country with an impressive historical background that is characterized by political upheavals and the intermingling of a variety of castes, tribes, and religions. It is no wonder that only broad generalizations are possible, and a certain amount of intracaste and interreligious variations are to be expected, even among peoples living in specified geographic areas.

The regulation of consanguineous marriages is one of the three important regulations governing marriages among Hindus in India; the other two are the controls on endogamous and exogamous marriages. The Hindu community is structured into several hierarchical groups (varnas, castes, and subcastes), each with its own rights, duties, and privileges. Regardless of the origin of the Hindu caste system (Karve, 1961), each individual belongs by birth to one of four hierarchial groups known as *varnas,* with Brahmins at the top, followed by Kshatriyas, Vaishyas, and lastly by Shudras. Each varna is subdivided into castes (or jāti) that are endogamous. The various caste names are derived from the principal professions or crafts practiced by their members. Thus, in former times the Brahmins conducted prayers and religious rituals and were involved in teaching; the Kshatriyas were rulers and warriors. The potters, blacksmiths, carpenters, washermen, and the like each had their own caste names. The castes at the top had power and privileges that were denied to the lower castes who were tenants, servants, landless laborers, and clients of the higher castes. In recent years, the lower castes have shown an increasing desire to free themselves from the control of the locally dominant castes, and they have been assisted by political forces operating at higher levels. However, the social status of an individual is still dependent on his or her caste.

Each caste is further split into subcastes (*gotra*) that are exogamous. The gotra is transmitted through the male line; hence the exogamous regulation prevents marriages between children of two brothers but not those between children of two sisters or a brother and a sister. In its strictest form, the regulation on consanguinity prohibits marriages between two persons related through a common male up to the seventh generation on the father's side and to the fifth generation on the mother's side. Although such restrictions on consanguinity were scrupulously followed in the northern part of India, the population failed to do so in the south, apparently due to the earlier Dravidian culture prevalent there that preferred consanguineous marriages (Sastri, 1976). Thus, even Brahmins in southern India indulged in some consanguineous marriages. As members of the top hierarchy, the Brahmins greatly influenced the marriage patterns in their geographical areas, not only among other castes but among members of other later religions.

The origin of the taboos against consanguinity can be found in several religious and mystical ideas, but the taboos can also be shown to be related to a desire for preserving the function of families, or to enlarge the single nuclear family into a wider group for mutual aid, collective economic security, internal peace, and sharing of cultural innovations (White, 1948; Murdock, 1949; Selligman, 1950).

No one theory seems to be sufficient to explain the origin of the consanguinity regulations or incest taboos (Lévi-Strauss, 1956; Schechner, 1971). What is striking, however, is that the very same reasons stated for the taboos are also used by the proponents encouraging consanguineous marriages. In the study of mating customs of the Andhra Pradesh people, Dronomraju (1964) cites five reasons stated by the respondents for preferring consanguineous marriages: (1) to keep the cultivable land in larger subdivisions; (2) parental influence; (3) mutual knowledge of families; (4) economic benefit, pooling resources, and sharing the expenditure; and (5) the extreme youth of the brides. Centerwall and Centerwall (1966) conclude that consanguineous marriage is practiced in order to minimize the amount of dowry to be given and to arrange the best possible marriage of a girl with the same social status as the man. Centerwall *et al.* (1969) also state that the practice of marriage between younger brother and elder sister's daughter (uncle–niece marriage) is a traditional method by which property that went to an elder sister by the ancient matrilineal custom actually got passed on to her brother. Reid (1973) is of the opinion that the major motivation for consanguineous marriage is to promote better interpersonal relationships between a new wife and her mother-in-law with whom she is likely to live.

In India, as in many other Eastern cultures, the family is a very important social entity, and marriage is an important part of the family system that cannot be left to the will of the young. A large proportion of the marriages in India are still arranged by the parents, for whom the perpetuation and prosperity of the family takes precedence over the individual preferences of the bride and the groom. Even in urban areas, there is still a significant proportion of marriages arranged with these considerations in mind, and, wherever it is possible, consanguineous marriages are preferred. This situation is somewhat similar to that documented in the Japanese studies reported by Schull and Neel (1965).

The present status of inbreeding in India is thus fashioned through historical events, traditional culture, and socioeconomic considerations. In certain instances, isolation and restrictions within specific geographic localities, as in the case of several tribals and scheduled castes, have led to inbreeding.

Whereas most countries have shown a decline in consanguineous marriages with increase in literacy and the knowledge of the genetic consequences of inbreeding, industrialization, greater mobility, and breakdown of traditions, such changes are not seen except in certain parts of India.

4.2. Geographic Variations

During the 1961 decennial census of India, an attempt was made to assess the incidence of inbreeding in rural areas through a survey of 587 villages spread all over the country. The number of villages included in each state varied from 2 to 48, and the survey may not be entirely representative because it was based on 330 of all these villages (Government of India, 1974). The survey confirmed that inbreeding was quite popular in southern India in most religious groups; Hindus showed the highest inbreeding coefficients (Figure 2). It was practically nonexis-

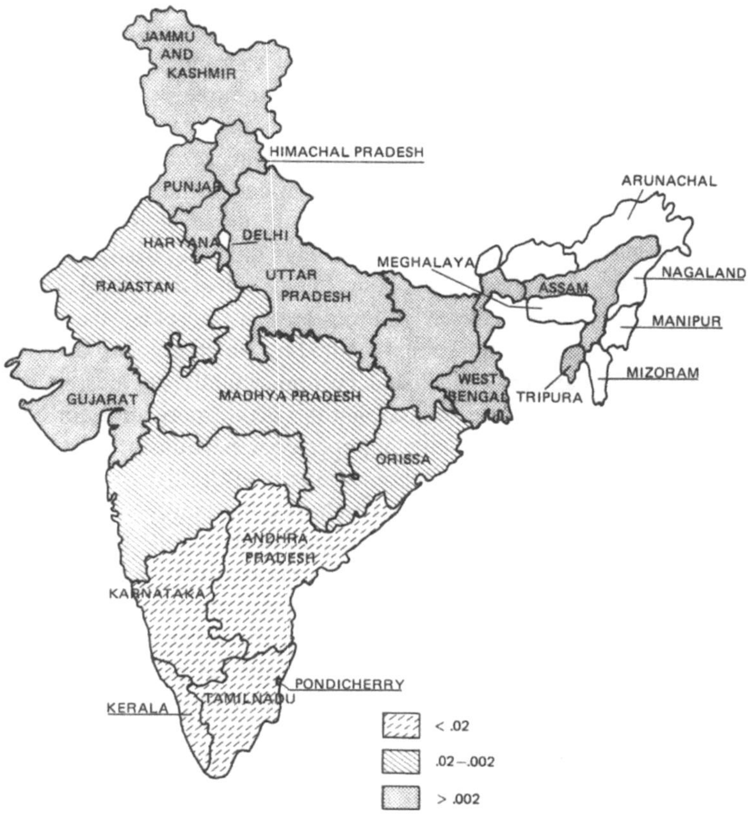

Figure 2. Extent of inbreeding in India.

tent among the rural Hindus in the north, whereas other religious groups showed some practice of inbreeding. Tribals had, in general, maximal inbreeding coefficients (Roychoudhury, 1976).

Although the north-south differential in inbreeding levels is quite striking within any northern or southern state, wide variations are reported. Among the 12 districts of Tamilnadu state in South India, South Arcot had the highest level (0.038) of inbreeding coefficients and Kanyakumari (0.013) had the lowest. The other districts had values varying between 0.018 and 0.034 (Roychoudhury, 1980).

In a consanguinity survey of 6745 marriages during 1957–1958 in 39 villages spread over 14 districts of Andhra Pradesh (Sanghvi, 1966), there was a gradual decline in the inbreeding levels away from the coast. The average coefficients of inbreeding were 0.032 for autosomal genes and 0.051 for sex-linked genes. This excess for the sex-linked genes is due entirely to matrilateral cross-cousin marriages. There was a high proportion of uncle–niece marriages in the coastal areas, which have the highest coefficients of inbreeding. Such geographical variations were confirmed by other studies (Veeraraju, 1973).

4.3. Social Variation

Within any geographical boundaries, there are variations in inbreeding due to religious affiliations, social status, and educational levels. Among the southern states, Kerala shows the lowest rates, between 0.002 and 0.011; Christians showed the lowest and Muslims the highest. This progressive state has high literacy rates and a higher percentage of orthodox Christian population than any other state. Based on the census survey of Tamilnadu, significant variation in inbreeding coefficients are observed among the communities within each category. In upper castes, the inbreeding coefficient was high (0.035–0.043) in Lingayat and Reddy/Reddiar, low (0.011–0.015) in Brahmin and Asari, and intermediate (0.023) in Mudaliar. Among four communities of scheduled castes, Adi-Dravida showed the highest value (0.030) of inbreeding coefficients. It was followed by Chakkiliyan, Pallan, and Parayan. The inbreeding coefficient varied from 0.012 to 0.033 among five communities of backward castes. Among the scheduled tribes, it was high (0.041) in Pulayan, low (0.011) in Karalan, and intermediate (0.026–0.028) in three other communities. Small sample size might be responsible for the high value of inbreeding coefficients in the Pulayan tribe (Roychoudhury, 1980).

In a sample of 6597 marriages from 12 endogamous groups based in Bombay, Maharashtra state, among the Marathi-speaking Hindus, the Brahmans and Prabhus, the inbreeding coefficients varied from 0.001 to 0.003, whereas it varied from 0.005 to 0.007 among Marathas, Agris, and Mahars. The coefficients varied from 0.006 to 0.013 among the Muslims and the Parsis, and only 0.001 among Roman Catholics. Whereas only matrilateral cross-cousin mating was most popular among the Hindus, all of the four possible first-cousin marriages were common among the non-Hindus. There was evidence of decline in inbreeding among the Parsis, but this was not the case in any other group.

In an analysis of data according to occupations, there were comparatively low levels of inbreeding among Brahmins (0.019) and traders (0.022), whereas shepherds (0.038) and fishermen (0.047) showed the highest. The large group of farmers (0.033), artisans (0.033), and Harijans (0.029) were intermediate and reflected the average values for the region. Muslims (0.025) and Christians (0.029) had comparatively lower values, and like the Hindus in this region, they practiced uncle–niece and cross-cousin marriages, but did not permit the two types of parallel-cousin marriages, as in the Maharashtra study.

The tribal populations generally have higher inbreeding levels regardless of their geographic location, as compared to any other religious or social subgroups in the population. The tribals in Andhra Pradesh (0.023–0.041), Madhya Prasesh (0.037), and Maharashtra (0.017–0.025) demonstrate this fact. Nevertheless, there are variations among the different tribes, and some even show very low rates, for example, in the northeastern parts of India, where this situation was perhaps due to the higher literacy rates prevalent there (Roychoudhury, 1976a).

Among the Muslims also, there are variations between the Sayyad Shias of Lucknow (0.020) and the Sunnis of Delhi (0.010) (Basu, 1975). Even within the Sunni sect, those people living in villages nearer Calcutta have a lower degree of inbreeding than those in interior villages (Barua, 1976). Similarly in Maharashtra, the inbreeding levels among the three Muslim groups—Memons, Bhoras, and Khojas—varied between 0.006 to 0.013 (Sanghvi, 1966).

The Parsis, who are descendants of the Zoroastrians, migrated from Iran and settled on the western coast of India some 1300 years ago. Another group of Zoroastrians, numbering about 5000, migrated to India from central Iran during the last 100–150 years. They are commonly known as Iranis and are mostly found in Bombay, Pune, and Dahanu. In a study of 3141 fertile Parsi couples and 195 fertile Irani couples married during the period from 1939 to 1972, Undevia and Balakrishnan (1978) reported a consanguinity of 7.8% and 6%, respectively. Though reduction was seen after the earliest period, there is no significant difference in the rate of consanguineous marriages or in the rates for the different types of consanguineous marriages. All of the four types of first-cousin marriages are prevalent in both communities. Moreover, the rates for parallel cousin (51.6% and 52.4%) and cross-cousin (48.4% and 47.6%) marriages are also the same in both communities. However, there seems to be a greater preference for union between the children of two sisters among the Parsis and for union between a man and his maternal uncle's daughter among the Iranis.

4.4. Vellore Studies

Much of the data on the extent of inbreeding in different parts have been collected from patients in hospitals or as part of morbidity surveys. Only a few studies have taken adequate precautions to ascertain true consanguinity of marriage. Information based on verbal statements or marriage relationships are prone to error, unless they are verified by drawing pedigrees. Consanguineous marriages are often confounded with affinal ones, and, similarly, full blood relations with stepkin. Sometimes the fact of consanguinity may not be revealed. Much caution is therefore necessary before one attempts to generalize incidence even in any one part of the country. Further, sample sizes are inadequate in some instances or are confined only to specific subgroups of a population in that area.

During 1969–1975, a population-based prospective study was established in North Arcot district of Tamilnadu state, the demographic characteristics of which are fairly typical of those prevailing in other parts of the state. The principal local language is Tamil. About 91% of the population is Hindu, 6% is Muslim, and 2% is Christian. Other religious groups (mostly Jains and Buddists) make up the remaining percentages. One-third of the town of Vellore, the headquarters of the district, was selected through stratified random sample procedure to provide the urban sample of 40,000 persons. A typical village development block, 18 mi. (30 km) from Vellore, was chosen to provide the rural sample of 50,000 persons.

All the married women in the selected areas were contacted by the research team to collect relevant data on consanguinity and other pertinent socioeconomic and demographic data. For each marriage, a family pedigree was drawn extending upward two earlier generations on the side of each spouse in order to determine the existence and type of consanguinity involved. This procedure was followed uniformly for all marriages. Five percent of all married women were later reinterviewed by supervisory personnel to check the validity of the pedigrees.

The results revealed that nearly 47% of rural women and 29% of urban women were consanguineously married. The common types of such marriages are shown in Table I.

In over 80% of the consanguineous marriages, the spouses were first cousins or more closely related. Among the uncle–niece matings, 98% or more were between a man and his sister's daughter. Among first-cousin marriages, marriages between children of different-sexed sibs (cross first cousins) were significantly more frequent than those between children of like-sexed sibs (parallel first cousins) as is shown in Figure 3.

Figure 2 also reveals that parallel first-cousin marriages were seen relatively

Table I
Frequency of Consanguineous Marriages in Rural and Urban Areas of Tamil Nadu

	Percentage of all marriages	
Type of consanguinity	Rural	Urban
	(11,628)	(8,998)
Nonconsanguineous	53.1	70.9
Consanguineous	46.9	29.1
Uncle niece and aunt nephew	15.8	6.6
First cousins	24.8	17.5
First cousins once removed	3.4	3.0
Second cousins	2.3	1.6
Beyond second cousins	0.6	0.5

Type of first-cousin marriage	Inbreeding coefficients: f Autosomal	Inbreeding coefficients: f Sex-linked	Area	Percentage of all marriages in each religion: Hindu	Muslim	Christian	All
FSD	$\frac{1}{16}$	0	Rural	35.1	31.1	41.7	35.3
			Urban	32.1	22.7	36.7	30.2
MBD	$\frac{1}{16}$	$\frac{1}{8}$	Rural	63.0	48.9	58.3	62.5
			Urban	66.2	31.3	63.3	59.3
FBD	$\frac{1}{16}$	0	Rural	1.0	11.1	0.0	1.1
			Urban	0.6	22.1	0.0	4.8
MSD	$\frac{1}{16}$	$\frac{3}{16}$	Rural	1.0	8.9	0.0	1.1
			Urban	1.2	24.0	0.0	5.7

Figure 3. Preference to the four types of first-cousin marriages in rural and urban areas by religion.

more frequently among Muslims than among Hindus or Christians. In fact, among urban Muslims, all four types of first-cousin marriages seem preferred. The average inbreeding coefficients, F, in the rural and urban areas were 0.0371 and 0.0204, respectively. These are significantly higher than those prevalent in most parts of the world, and they confirm what was revealed through earlier surveys done in this part of India.

The coefficients of inbreeding in the rural areas were around 0.038 among the illiterates, and they declined to about 0.03 when the spouses were educated beyond the secondary-school level (see Table II). In the urban areas, the coefficients of inbreeding were lower at both extremes of education status. However,

Table II
Inbreeding Coefficients in Rural and Urban Areas by Educational Attainment of Husband and Wife

	Rural				Urban			
	No. observed		F		No. observed		F	
Level of education	Wife	Husband	Wife	Husband	Wife	Husband	Wife	Husband
Illiterate	9802	7369	0.038	0.038	4966	2897	0.020	.018
Primary school	917	1959	0.033	0.036	1427	1141	0.027	.025
Middle school	637	1394	0.035	0.037	1516	1904	0.020	.024
Secondary school and over	272	907	0.028	0.032	1089	2782	0.016	.018

Table III
Inbreeding Coefficients by Religious Affiliation

Religious affiliation	No. observed		Inbreeding coefficients			
			Rural		Urban	
	Rural	Urban	Autosomal	Sex-linked	Autosomal	Sex-linked
All	11,628	8998	0.037	0.041	0.021	0.023
Hindu	11,288	6765	0.037	0.042	0.023	0.027
Muslim	212	1960	0.020	0.025	0.011	0.015
Christian	126	264	0.022	0.026	0.012	0.014

the inbreeding levels of couples who had only a primary school education were higher than those of couples with more education.

Differentials by occupational categories were more pronounced in the rural than in the urban areas and showed patterns similar to those seen in Table II. In certain occupational groups, such as agricultural laborers, semiskilled workers in cottage industries, and service workers, there were significantly higher coefficients of inbreeding as compared to those in the white-collar groups in both the rural and urban areas ($P < 0.05$).

The highest coefficients of inbreeding were seen for Hindus (rural: 0.037; urban: 0.023) which were nearly 1.5 times those seen among Muslims or Christians (rural: 0.02; urban: 0.01) (Table III).

Among the Hindus, the inbreeding coefficients varied by caste from 0.05 to less than 0.02. In general, the coefficients in the urban areas were significantly lower than those in the rural areas for each of these castes ($P < 0.05$). The "backward" communities show the highest coefficients of inbreeding (Table IV).

Table IV
Inbreeding among Hindu Castes

Hindu caste group	No. observed		Inbreeding coefficients			
			Rural		Urban	
	Rural	Urban	Autosomal	Sex-linked	Autosomal	Sex-linked
Forward	1849	4210	0.032	0.035	0.022	0.025
Backward	6536	3262	0.040	0.045	0.026	0.030
Scheduled	2957	634	0.037	0.040	0.016	0.019

The lowest F values are seen in the "forward" communities in the rural areas, but in the scheduled communities in the urban areas. The inbreeding coefficients in the rural and urban areas reveal no significant decline over the past five decades: They were 0.0297 and 0.0189, respectively, for those married in 1919 or earlier, as compared to 0.0304 and 0.0173 for those married in 1960 or later. Data based on similar studies in other parts of India are lacking.

5. Consequences

5.1. Theoretical Considerations

5.1.1. Short-term effects. An immediate consequence of inbreeding will be an increase in homozygosity and a decrease in heterozygosity. Recessive genes, whose effects were subsumed by their dominant partners, will thus be expressed. If such genes are deleterious, inbreeding will lead to a decrease in the fitness of the individual. If there are heterotic effects in which the heterozygote is fitter than either of the homozygotes, then inbreeding will lead to decreased fitness. Because similar genes tend to be concentrated in the same individuals, genetic variability within a population will increase, as will the phenotypic variation. This is shown in the following example.

Suppose the frequency p of a recessive gene causing some disorder was approximately 1/200. Then, with random mating, the frequency of individuals homozygous for this gene will be 1/40,000. On the other hand, if the parents were first cousins (f = 1/16), then the probability of an *affected* child will be $p^2\,(1 - f) + pf$, or $\left(\frac{1}{40{,}000} \times \frac{15}{16}\right) + \left(\frac{1}{200} \times \frac{1}{16}\right) = \frac{215}{640{,}000}$. Thus, the probability or risk will be approximately 13 times more than when the parents are not related.

The rarer the recessive genes, the greater will be the probability that the affected individuals are inbred. On the other hand, if the recessive gene is common, consanguinity plays a minor role in the frequency of the disease concerned.

When dealing with quantitative traits, the phenotypic consequences depend on the extent of dominance and epistasis. The mean values are not affected if there is no dominance regardless of epistasis. If there is dominance but no epistasis, the effect of inbreeding on the mean will be linear to f, and on the variance, a quadratic. If there is both dominance and epistasis, the inbreeding effect on the mean will be quadratic or higher orders in f, depending on the number of loci involved.

The effect of any inbreeding that is of a type that divides the population into isolated groups will be to decrease the variance within groups, to increase the variance between groups, and to increase the total variance. When there are recessive alleles of low frequency, variance within a subpopulation increases during the early stages of the inbreeding process until it is offset by the increasing homogeneity in gene content from individual to individual within the subpopulation. Reliable data on the results of inbreeding that are uncomplicated by the effects of selection are rare.

5.1.2. Long-term effects. If a random mating population that has reached an equilibrium for a certain lethal homozygote "*aa*" resorts to inbreeding, the frequency of "*aa*" will show a sudden increase. If this inbreeding is continued over a period of generations with a constant intensity (F), the incidence of the trait (aa) and the frequency (q) of this lethal gene (a) will continue to diminish. If the gene in the original population was maintained by mutation (rate, u), a new equilibrium will eventually be reached. If the gene was maintained by selective advantage of the heterozygote, it will ultimately be lost (Sanghvi, 1966) as is shown later.

Combining two separate formulas normally used for mutational and segregational loci, the frequency for each genotype of the first-generation offspring of a population that had just resorted to inbreeding will be:

Genotype	Frequency	Relative fitness
AA	$p^2 + Fpq$	1
Aa	$2pq(1 - F)$	$1 + kt$
aa	$q^2 + Fpq$	$1 - t$

where $kt \geqq -1$ and $0 \leqq 1$.

The variables k and t, respectively, replace variable h and s used in the mutational formula and are related to the variables t_1 and t_2 in segregational formulas by the following relations:

$$k = \frac{t_1}{t_2 - t_1}; \qquad t = \frac{t_2 - t_1}{1 - t_1}$$

If q_o was the initial frequency of the lethal gene ($t = 1$) and inbreeding (f) continued for "n" generations, the gene frequency q_n in the nth generation will be given by the following two equations.

Under the mutation hypothesis:

$$q_n = xq_o - x(1 - x)\frac{q_o^2}{F} + (1 - x)\frac{u}{F} \tag{1}$$

where

$$x = (1 - F)^n$$

Under the selection hypothesis:

$$q_n = yq_o - y(1 - y)\frac{q_o^2}{F_1} \tag{2}$$

where

$$y = (1 - F_1)^n \qquad \text{and} \qquad F_1 = F - k + Fk$$

The terms of third and higher order of q are neglected, under the assumption of small values of q.

With the help of these equations, the fate of a gene under inbreeding over a period of generations was estimated under specified rates of mutation and selection. For example, if a gene is comparatively common ($q = 0.01$) and is maintained by an advantage of the heterozygote, then, at an inbreeding level of $F = 0.05$, the incidence declines from a value of 591 affected per million to six per million in 100 generations and only one per million in 150 generations. If this gene is, however, maintained by mutation, its frequency will be stabilized at its new equilibrium value, giving 100 affected per million. Thus, the results under the selection and mutation hypotheses are very different. Similar but somewhat less striking results are obtained for $q = 0.005$. For very rare genes ($q = 0.001$), there is a decline in gene frequency, but the differential effects of mutation and selection are not so marked as to be of practical significance.

On the other hand, if $F = 0.03$ and gene frequency $q = 0.005$, the incidence of the trait would have stabilized at a level of one in 40,000 under the mutation hypothesis and would have become less than one in a million under the selection hypothesis after 200 generations of inbreeding. If the initial gene frequency was high ($q = 0.01$), the results are more striking.

Thus, long-term practices of inbreeding could reduce the frequency of deleterious alleles in a population. Interpretation of the effects of inbreeding should therefore take into account the historical background and duration of inbreeding.

5.1.3. Concepts of genetic loads and their measurement. Another approach to the study of relationship between inbreeding and certain of the presumed effects lies in the estimation of *genetic load*. Genetic load is defined as the relative decrease in the average fitness of a population if all individuals in that population had the genotype that has the maximum fitness (Crow, 1958).

Genes that are deleterious when homozygous can belong to either of the following major classes:

1. Genes that are not (or are only moderately) deleterious when heterozygous. The fitness of the genotypes *AA* and *Aa* are hence almost the same, and it is the genotype *aa* that is at a disadvantage. Under such

conditions, the gene frequency of "a" will be kept very low by the balance between mutation and selection.

2. Genes for which the heterozygote is the fittest genotype and is therefore more fit than either homozygote. Such genes become polymorphic so that either allele can attain a relatively high frequency. They are often called *overdominant*.

For both types of genes, homozygotes will occur with increased frequency in the progeny of consanguineous matings, and thus the average fitness of the population will decrease with inbreeding. The concept of *load* was first introduced by Muller (1950) and was applied to genes maintained in equilibrium by mutation–selection balance. The loss of zygotes due to such loci is called the *mutational* load. The genetic load due to overdominant loci is known as the *segregational* load.

In general, if w_{max} is the maximum fitness and $\bar{w}$ the average fitness, the load is defined by the quantity $[w_{max} - \bar{w}]/w_{max}$. When the optimum genotype is assigned a fitness of 1 ($w_{max} = 1$), then the genetic load is simply equal to $(1 - \bar{w})$.

The estimation of the genetic load due to the combined effects of several loci is based on the assumption that the corresponding decrease of fitness is entirely accounted for by some fraction of, perhaps all of, the prereproductive mortality. The following is further assumed by Morton *et al.* (1956):

1. Since the various genetic causes of death act independently, the probability of surviving the deleterious effects of two loci is equal to the product of the probabilities of surviving the effects of each.
2. Genetic causes of death act independently from environmental causes. These two assumptions are critical to the subsequent development of the load theory.

The probability of death due to deleterious alleles present at a given ith locus is the genetic load at the locus L_1. Thus, the probability of survival will be given by

$$p_i = 1 - L_i$$

Because of the first assumption, the probability of survival, considering all possible loci, will be

$$P = p_1 p_2 p_3 \,.\,.\,.\,.\,.\, p_n = \pi\, p_i\, (1 - L_i)$$

where π indicates the product over all loci.

Because of the second assumption, if the probability of surviving all of the environmental causes of death is P_a, then the overall probability or survival is given by

$$P_s = P_a P$$

Taking logarithms of both sides,

$$\log P_s = \log P_a + \log P = \log P_a + \Sigma \log(1 - L_i)$$

where the summation is extended over all loci.

Morton, Crow, and Muller (1956) advocate a method of analyzing the genetic load that distinguishes the relative importance of the two classes of genes—deleterious recessives and overdominants—in determining the genetic load.

In general, the overall probability of survival can be stated as

$$-\log P_s = X + \Sigma a_i + F \Sigma b_i = A + BF$$

Thus, a simple linear relationship is expected between the logarithm of the probability of survival P and the inbreeding coefficient F.

These considerations of the genetic load lead to the expectation that B/A will be high for genes maintained by mutation–selection balance and low for those maintained through heterozygote advantage. Thus, in principle, an estimate of the B/A ratio based on the relationship between P_s and F should tell us whether the load is mainly mutational or mainly segregational. For multiple allelic loci, it has also been estimated that the B/A ratio for overdominant loci can be as high as the number of alleles.

This concept and measurement of genetic load has been discussed at length because of the great importance and implications they have for the interpretation of inbreeding effects. Objections have been raised about the underlying assumptions made by Li (1963), Sanghvi (1963), Crow (1963), and Sutter and Goux (1964) on the independence of gene action and on the basis for using different standards of comparison for the mutational and segregational models. Instead of using the B/A ratio, Sanghvi (1963) suggests the ratio $(1 - B)/(1 - A)$ for distinguishing between the mutation and segregational models.

5.2. General Findings from Indian Studies

Much of the Indian data on the effects of inbreeding are based on hospital admissions or from retrospective studies. Hospital data should have accurate medical diagnoses and perhaps a reasonably correct assessment of consanguinity, but due to the selective nature of the hospital clientele, the difficulty lies in generalizing the findings beyond the hospital and in choosing controls for valid comparisons and hence to measure the true effect of inbreeding, if any. Retrospective studies have an inherent recall bias and also have the problem of getting the proper controls for comparisons.

A survey of 3433 outpatients in a pediatric clinic in Tamilnadu showed that, of the children from consanguineous parents, 9.1% had congenital anomalies as compared to 5.3% from nonconsanguineous parents (Centerwall and Centerwall, 1966). Another survey taken during the same time on 1037 newborn children in that hospital revealed that the risk of consanguineous parents having a child with a major anomaly was 4.1% compared to 1.1% for a nonconsanguineous parent. In a study of 23,000 consecutive births in 1972–1974 in a hospital in Madras, it was found that consanguineous parents had a significantly higher rate of malformed offspring (Kesavan *et al.*, 1978). In a study done in Bangalore, Karnataka state (Narayan and Rama Rao, 1978), on 2400 cases of mental retardation, the consanguinity rate was 30%. However, the consanguinity rate was also found to be 30% on cases other than mental retardation. And in a sample survey on the general population, the authors found the frequency of consanguinity varied from 30 to 60%. Sinclair (1972) found only 7% parental consanguinity among 470 cases of mental retardation; of the 32 whose parents were consanguineously married, 7 were from South India and 25 from the North. In a review of records of nearly 24,000 singleton births from one hospital in Bombay, no significant differences could be detected between offspring born of consanguineous and nonconsanguineous parents (Sanghvi, 1974). This is in contrast to another hospital study in Bombay itself, where inbred offspring showed a significantly higher rate of major anomalies compared to the noninbred (Chakraborty and Chakravarti, 1975).

In a study of newborn children in Hyderabad (Andhra Pradesh), Murty and Jamil (1972) found significantly higher rates for mortality and congenital anomalies in offspring of consanguineous unions as compared to that found in the nonconsanguineous unions. In-depth studies on a few endogamous caste groups in Andhra Pradesh have shown that inbreeding was associated with higher childhood and fetal losses and, at the same time, with higher fertility (Reid, 1973; Mukherjee, 1974; Lakshmanudu and Mukherjee, 1975; Rao and Mukherjee, 1975; Rami Reddy and Padmanabha Naidu, 1978). In another hospital-based study in Kerala state, the 83 patients who had married first cousins and 8 to their second cousins and 185 to unrelated persons had significantly higher fetal and infant mortality rates as compared to the losses in 185 patients who had married unrelated persons (Kumar *et al.*, 1967). In a follow-up study on a cohort of 183 families in Vellore, Tamilnadu, John, and Jayabal (1971) found that the rates of abortion, perinatal death, deaths up to 1 year, and deaths up to 10 years among the progeny of consanguineous matings did not differ significantly from the losses of offspring of the nonconsanguineous matings.

In a study of inpatients admitted to one hospital in Andhra Pradesh, the mean coefficient of inbreeding among the parents of 38 patients with pulmonary tuberculosis was 0.033, which was significantly higher than that in the rest of the patients. The value for abortions was 0.03 and for congenital malformations, 0.031; these were also higher but failed to achieve statistical significance (Dronamraju and Meera Khan, 1963). In the same hospital, out of 81 gynecological patients, 22% of women who had married consanguineously were sterile as compared to 16.6% who were not; this difference also was not statistically significant. Lakshmanudu (1980) carried out a study to determine the effects of inbreeding on physical measurements of 1200 adult males from two endogamous populations in Chittoor district of Andhra Pradesh state, the Gampasati Kammas and the Telagas, and on 355 Nulia fishermen from neighboring Orissa State. He found appreciable inbreeding depressions on stature, trunk height, lower limb length, and chest girth. The amount of change was, however, not proportional to the intensity of inbreeding. The author emphasizes the roles of selection factors, epistasis, and perhaps the historical background of the population investigated to explain the variable nature of inbreeding effects Mukherjee and Lakshmanudu (in press).

In a study on the effects of consanguinity among Muslims, Basu (1978) reported significantly higher fertility rates with inbreeding in Sayyad Shias and Shiekh Sunnis but not among Dawoodi Bohras. Basu comments on whether such variations could be due to the different inbreeding histories among the Muslims. All these groups showed significantly higher child mortality and morbidity with inbreeding.

It is seen that the findings are not consistent and at times they are quite contradictory. Part of these inconsistencies could perhaps be due to the great differences in the populations surveyed, definitions adopted, methodologies used, and types of controls used. Further, rigorous statistical treatment is lacking in most studies. Unless adequately designed and unless community-based population samples are prospectively and intensively followed up by qualified investigators, the crucial issues on inbreeding effects will remain unresolved. The findings from one such study done at Vellore are briefly summarized in the next section.

5.3. Vellore Studies on Effects of Inbreeding

The setting for the Vellore studies was described in section 4.4. All data were personally collected by qualified women investigators and included a general profile of each household on social, economic, and demographic aspects, and for each married women, a pedigree of her marriage and a detailed account of her past reproductive performance. Married women in the age range of 15–44 years who were living with their husbands were visited once every 5 weeks to obtain details of outcome on every pregnancy that occurred during 1969–1973. Birth measurements and detection of externally manifested congenital malformations were done within 48 hours after birth (Rao and Inbaraj, 1977a). For purposes of statistical analysis, parental consanguinity was classified into four types: (1) spouses related closer than first cousins, mostly uncle–niece unions (UN); (2)

Table V
Pregnancies Observed in Prospective and Retrospective Studies According to Parental Consanguinity in Rural and Urban Areas

	Rural		Urban	
Parental consanguinity	Prospective	Retrospective	Prospective	Retrospective
Nonconsanguineous	4449	20,606	4251	2116
Consanguineous	3889	19,438	1654	9001
Uncle and niece	1308	6,109	371	2001
First cousin	1991	10,722	989	5488
Beyond first cousin	590	2,607	294	1512
Total	8338	40,044	5905	30117

spouses who were first cousins (FC); (3) spouses whose relationships were beyond that of first cousins (BFC); and (4) spouses who were unrelated or nonconsanguineous (NC).

A series of 14,243 pregnancies were registered and followed up during the prospective study. The retrospective study on past reproductive histories yielded data on over 70,000 pregnancies. The numbers in various parental consanguinity groups are given in Table V. Inbreeding effects on fertility based on prospective study are shown in Table VI.

The mean levels of fertility were slightly but significantly elevated among the consanguineous marriages in the rural groups but not in the urban groups. Among women married at least 20 years, the means of live-born in noncon-

Table VI
Infant Mortality Rates per 1000 Live-born by Parental Consanguinity

	Mortality rates per 1000					
	Neonatal		Postneonatal		Infant	
Consanguinity	Rural	Urban	Rural	Urban	Rural	Urban
Nonconsanguineous	46.8	33.7	47.7	58.8	93.6	93.3
Consanguineous	54.6	46.4	54.1	60.3	106.7	106.9
Uncle and niece	56.1	44.4	48.2	90.9	102.4	133.9
First cousin	53.5	55.7	61.3	46.0	112.6	102.4
Beyond first cousin	55.3	17.9	44.3	70.2	95.1	88.5

sanguineous and consanguineous marriages in the rural areas were 5.43 and 5.63, and in the urban areas, 5.64 and 5.47. These are small differences in opposite directions that nonetheless attained statistical significance in view of the large sample sizes. The frequency of primary sterility among women married for at least 20 years was less in the consanguineous marriages (rural: 3.1%; urban: 3.6%) as compared to that of the nonconsanguineous marriages (rural: 3.7%; urban: 4.8%). However, these differences were not statistically significant. The frequencies of secondary sterility did not differ significantly in either the rural or the urban areas. No significant trends in sterility were seen by degree of consanguinity. Thus, either marginal or no significant effects of inbreeding are observed on the fertility of women. Inbreeding effects on fetal losses based on prospective studies are displayed in Figure 4.

The total fetal loss rates were 21.9% in the rural areas and 21.2% in the urban, with over 80% occurring prior to 20 weeks of gestation. The differences between the consanguineous and nonconsanguineous marriages in early, intermediate, and late fetal losses were generally not statistically significant. Only the total fetal loss rate in the rural areas for the consanguineous marriages was significantly higher than that for the nonconsanguineous marriages ($p < 0.05$); the margin of differences was only 1.8%. Further analyses made by birth order and maternal age for each of the specific rates as well as for the total did not reveal any significant differences due to consanguinity. The same results were true for perinatal mortality, combining late fetal deaths and first-week neonatal losses. The neonatal, postneonatal, and infant mortality rates by types of marriages of the parents are given in Table VII.

In general, although the differences were minor, the rates were significantly higher among the consanguineous marriages as compared to the noncon-

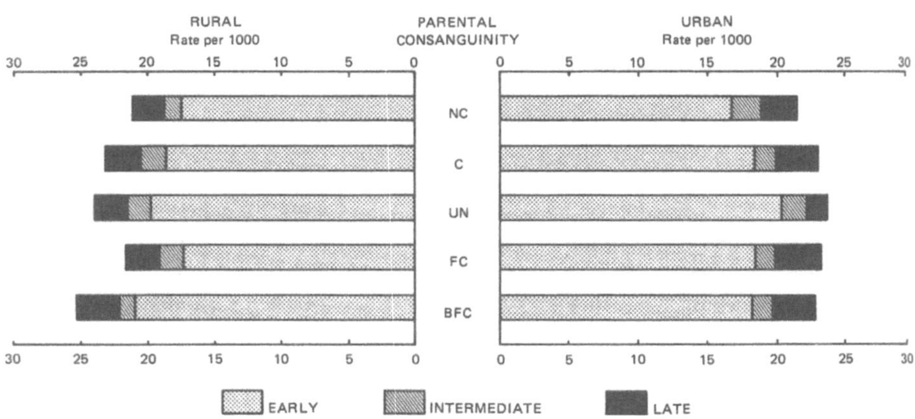

Figure 4. Early, intermediate, and late fetal death rates by parental consanguinity.

sanguineous marriages. Perhaps this was due to the large sample sizes observed. There were no consistent monotonic changes by degree of relationship in either area.

These findings on fetal and infant mortality based on a prospective survey may be compared with those from the past reproductive histories. The data are displayed in relation to birth cohort of women in Figures 5 and 6.

Here again, the differences between consanguineous and nonconsanguineous marriages in terms of total fetal loss, perinatal, neonatal, postneonatal, and infant mortality rates showed only marginal differences that attained statistical significance only because of the large sample sizes involved. No consistent relationships were observed between the degree of consanguinity and these reproductive losses. These actual differences were more marked in the older-age groups of women and declined to rather insignificant proportions as the age groups became younger. The overall infant mortality rates and their components during neonatal and postneonatal periods were significantly higher among offspring of consanguineous marriages as compared to those of nonconsanguineous marriages in retrospective study; and in the prospective survey, much narrower differentials are seen. The incidence of congenital malformations and sex ratios at birth in relation to consanguinity are given in Table VIII.

A little over 51% (51.2) of the rural births and 51.1% of the urban births were male. The differences in the sex ratios among the consanguineous and

Table VII
Inbreeding Effects on Fertility (Prospective Survey)

	Pregnancies		Live births		Living	
Parental consanguinity	Mean	SEM	Mean	SEM	Mean	SEM
			Rural			
Nonconsanguineous	3.3	0.04	3.2	0.03	2.5	0.03
Consanguineous	3.6	0.04	3.4	0.04	2.6	0.03
Uncle and niece	3.3	0.06	3.2	0.06	2.4	0.05
First cousin	3.7	0.05	3.6	0.05	2.7	0.04
Beyond first cousin	3.6	0.11	3.4	0.10	2.6	0.08
			Urban			
Nonconsanguineous	3.3	0.04	3.1	0.03	2.4	0.03
Consanguineous	3.4	0.06	3.2	0.05	2.4	0.04
Uncle and niece	3.4	0.12	3.2	0.11	2.3	0.09
First cousin	3.5	0.07	3.3	0.07	2.4	0.05
Beyond first cousin	3.3	0.13	3.1	0.13	2.4	0.10

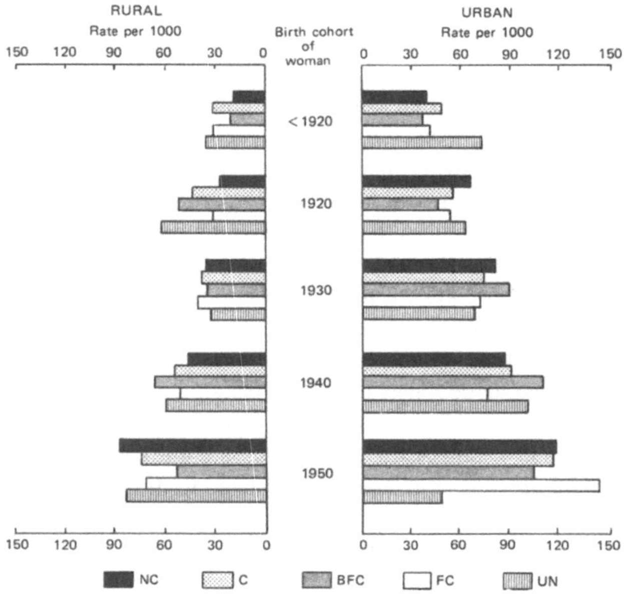

Figure 5. Fetal-loss rates by type of consanguinity and birth cohort of women—rural and urban.

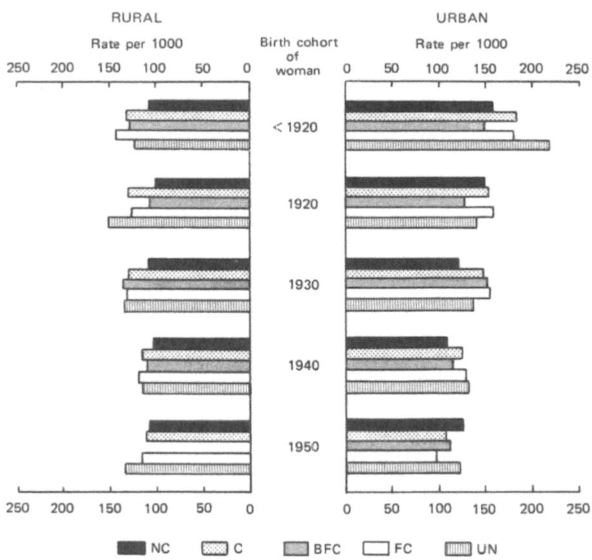

Figure 6. Infant mortality rates by type of consanguinity and birth cohort of woman—rural and urban.

Table VIII
Sex Ratio and Incidence of Congenital Malformations by Parental Consanguinity

Parental consanguinity	Sex ratio (Number of males per 100 live-born)		Congenital malformations	
	Rural	Urban	Rural	Urban
Nonconsanguinity	51.2	51.5	7.7	9.7
Consanguinity	51.1	50.2	5.9	12.2
Uncle and niece	52.5	47.9	6.2	11.1
First cousin	50.8	50.4	7.3	10.9
Beyond first cousin	48.6	52.5	0.0	17.9

Table IX
Type of Congenital Malformation by Parental Consanguinity

Congenital malformation	Rural		Urban	
	NC	C	NC	C
Polydactyly	11	5	5	—
Club foot	5	3	6	5
Cleft lip, with or without palate	3	3	1	2
Imperforate anus with or without other anomaly	2	1	5	—
Anomalies of musculoskeletal system	1	1	3	1
Hydrocephalus	1	1	1	1
Anomalies of ear, eye, or face	—	1	2	1
Anomalies of genitals	2	—	1	—
Absence of fingers or toes	—	—	1	2
Anomalies of the tongue	—	1	1	—
Anomalies of skin	—	—	2	—
Ancencephalus	—	—	—	1
Cleft palate	—	1	—	—
Down's syndrome	—	—	—	1
Congenital blindness	—	—	—	1
Indeterminate sex	—	—	1	—
Other specific anomalies	1	—	2	—
Total	26	17	31	15

Table X
Effect of Inbreeding on Birth Measurements in Rural Areas: Mean ± Sem

Parental consanguinity	Birth weight (g)	Crown heel length (cm)	Crown rump length (cm)	Head circumference (cm)	Chest circumference (cm)
Nonconsanguineous	2772 ± 12.4	47.5 ± 0.09	31.1 ± 0.07	33.7 ± 0.05	32.5 ± 0.06
Consanguineous	2740 ± 13.4	47.3 ± 0.09	31.1 ± 0.08	33.5 ± 0.05	32.3 ± 0.06
Uncle and niece	2730 ± 9.1	47.3 ± 0.16	30.9 ± 0.13	33.5 ± 0.09	32.3 ± 0.09
First cousin	2737 ± 18.7	47.2 ± 0.13	30.9 ± 0.11	33.5 ± 0.08	32.2 ± 0.09
Beyond first cousin	2775 ± 33.7	47.7 ± 0.24	31.5 ± 0.20	33.4 ± 0.14	32.3 ± 0.16
Total	2757 ± 9.1	47.4 ± 0.06	31.1 ± 0.05	33.6 ± 0.04	32.4 ± 0.04

nonconsanguineous marriages were not statistically significant. No significant differences existed in the incidence of congenital anomalies among offspring between the consanguineous and nonconsanguineous marriages in the rural or in the urban areas. Nor were any significant trends seen by degree of consanguinity, by birth order, or by the different age groups. The types of congenital malformations seen are displayed in Table IX.

With the small sample sizes, it is difficult to compute type-specific rates and expect statistical significance. A perusal of Table IX shows, however, that the types of malformation seen in the consanguineous marriages are similar to, and occur no more often than, those seen in the nonconsanguineous group.

The birth measurements in relation to parental consanguinity are given for rural areas in Table X and for the urban areas in Table XI. No significant

Table XI
Effect of Inbreeding on Birth Measurements in Urban Areas: Mean ± SEM

Parental consanguinity	Birth weight (g)	Crown heel length (cm)	Crown rump length (cm)	Head circumference (cm)	Chest circumference (cm)
Nonconsanguineous	2867 ± 13.0	48.2 ± 0.09	31.7 ± 0.07	33.9 ± 0.05	32.6 ± 0.06
Consanguineous	2883 ± 20.6	48.4 ± 0.12	31.6 ± 0.10	33.9 ± 0.07	32.5 ± 0.08
Uncle and niece	2877 ± 37.7	47.9 ± 0.27	31.6 ± 0.06	33.9 ± 0.14	32.7 ± 0.18
First cousin	2885 ± 28.2	48.4 ± 0.16	31.5 ± 0.13	33.9 ± 0.09	32.5 ± 0.11
Beyond first cousin	2883 ± 47.0	49.0 ± 0.26	31.9 ± 0.22	34.0 ± 0.14	32.4 ± 0.18
Total	2872 ± 11.0	48.3 ± 0.07	31.7 ± 0.06	33.9 ± 0.04	32.6 ± 0.05

Table XII
Regression Analyses of Inbreeding Effects on Reproductive Performance
Estimates of α and β

	Rural		Urban	
Reproductive performance	A	B	A	B
Primary sterility	0.037	0.052	0.049	0.155
All fetal loss	0.240	0.200	0.234	0.204
Late fetal loss	0.020	0.002	0.024	0.023
Perinatal loss	0.063	0.030	0.056	0.259
Neonatal loss	0.048	0.084	0.034	0.200
Infant loss	0.106	0.395	0.098	0.046
Sex ratio at birth	0.688	0.495	0.662	0.474
Congenital malformations	0.069	0.0171	0.0102	0.0158

differences are observed by types of marriages in both areas in any of the birth measurements.

Assuming an exponential model of inbreeding effects on the several aspects of human reproduction, regression analyses were carried out using the model

$$P_i = 1 - \exp[-(\alpha + \beta F_i)]$$

where P_i is the estimated proportion of subjects with, for example, congenital malformation, neonatal mortality, and so forth, in the subgroup based on type of parental consanguinity, and F_i is the coefficient of inbreeding for that subgroup. The maximum likelihood estimates of α and β were obtained through weighted regression techniques using iterative procedures. The estimated values *A* and *B* are shown in Table XII for the rural and urban areas, using data from prospective studies. None of the regression coefficients attain statistical significance. Similar results were seen in retrospective survey data.

In summary, the differences between the consanguineous and nonconsanguineous marriages with respect to fertility, sterility, fetal, perinatal, and infant losses were quite small and attained statistical significance mainly due to the large sample sizes involved. Also, differences in sex ratios, incidence of congenital malformations, and birth measurements were not statistically significant.

Taking into account the background of the population studied, the methodology adopted, and the lack of significant patterns by type of parental consanguinity, the most reasonable conclusion is that the continuing practices of consanguinity over several generations have narrowed the differentials of human reproduction and of its wastage among various types of marriages based on parental consanguinity.

6. Conclusions

The picture of inbreeding in India is kaleidoscopic. A number of studies have been done throughout the country, but with varying sample sizes, definitions, and methodologies for ascertaining consanguinity and its effects. These studies were analyzed using different statistical techniques. How much of the diversity of conclusions reached are due to these factors and whether the differences observed are real cannot be easily answered; yet one could venture to make the following general observations.

1. The custom of consanguineous marriages is still very popular in South India and is relatively rare in the North; however, there exists significant variations between different regions and within each region.
2. Both the practice of consanguinity and the types of matings preferred conforms more to the culture in the south than to religious beliefs.
3. The patterns and varieties of consanguineous marriages have shown little change over the past few decades in the various religious and social groups.
4. The effects of inbreeding in India depend on the history of such practices over past generations; where there is a long history, the effects tend to be marginal.
5. More studies must be undertaken with a uniform methodology on a prospective basis throughout the country. This seems urgently needed, not only to complement or corroborate the conclusions arrived at in small ad hoc surveys done in the past but to determine current gene frequencies and the spatial, social, and temporal trends in gene frequencies according to the levels of inbreeding practiced.

References

Barua, S., 1976, Selection intensity among the consanguineous and nonsanguineous groups of a Muslim population of 24-Parganas, West Bengal, *Third Annu. Conf. Indian Anthropol. Soc., August 14–15.*

Basu, S. K., 1975, Effect of consanguinity among north Indian Muslims, *J. Pop. Res.* **2:**57–68.

Basu, S. K., 1978, Effects of consanguinity among Muslim Groups of North India, *Med. Genet. in India* **2:**173–187.

Bhalla, V., and Bhatia, K., 1974, Analysis of migration effect on mating system of a north Indian inbred Hindu community—the Bhatias of Garhi-Dhaneta, *Proc. First Conf. Ind. Soc. Hum. Genet.* **1:**147–156.

Centerwall, W. R., and Centerwall, S. A., 1966, Consanguinity and congenital anomalies in South India: A pilot study, *Indian J. Med. Res.* **54:**1160–1167.

Centerwall, W. R., Savarinathan, G., Mohan, L. R., Booshanam, V., and Zachariah, M., 1969, Inbreeding patterns in rural south India, *Soc. Biol.* **16:**81–91.

Chakravartti, M. R., 1968, Consanguinity in India. *Z. Morph. Anthropol.* **60:**170–183.

Chakraborty, R., and Chakravarti, A., 1975, On Consanguineous marriages and the genetic load, *Proc. of Second Conf. Ind. Soc. Hum. Genet.*, Calcutta.
Cotterman, C. W., 1940, A Calculus for Statistico-Genetics. Unpublished thesis, Ohio State University, Columbus, Ohio.
Crow, J. F., 1958, Some possibilities for measuring selection intensities in man, *Hum. Biol.* **30:**1–13.
Crow, J. F., 1963, The concept of genetic load: A reply. *Am. J. Hum. Genet.* **15:**310–315.
Dronamraju, K. R., and Meera Khan, P., 1963, The frequency and effects of consanguineous marriages in Andhra Pradesh, *J. Genet.* **58:**387–401.
Dronamraju, K. R., 1964, Mating systems of the Andhra Pradesh people, *Cold Spring Harbor Symposia on Quantitative Biology* **29:**81–84.
Falconer, D. S., 1960, *Introduction to Quantitative Genetics,* The Ronald Press Co., New York.
Goswami, H. K., 1970, Frequency of consanguineous marriages in Madhya Pradesh, *Acta Genet. Med. Gemellol.* **19:**486–490.
Government of India, 1974, Marriage with Consanguineous and Affinal Relations (mimeographed), Census of India, 1961, Office of the Registrar General, New Delhi.
Government of India, 1975, Polygamous Marriage in India—A Survey, Census of India, 1971, Office of the Registrar General, New Delhi.
Haldane, J. B. S., and Moshinsky, P., 1939, Inbreeding in Mendelian populations with special reference to human cousin marriage. *Ann. Eugen.* **9:**321–340.
John, R. J., and Jayabal, P., 1971, Foetal and child loss in relation to consanguinity in southern India, *Indian J. Med. Res.* **59:**1050–1053.
Karve, I., 1961, *Hindu Society: An Interpretation,* Deshmukh and Co., Pune.
Kempthorne, O., 1957, *An Introduction to Genetic Statistics,* Wiley, New York.
Kesavan, P., Uma Nataraja, Murugesan, K., and Ramakrishnan, M. S., 1978, Congenital malformations and consanguinity, *Medical Genetics in India* **1:**65–69.
Kumar, S., Pai, R. A., and Swaminathan, M. S., 1967, Consanguineous marriages and the genetic load due to lethal genes in Kerala, *Ann. Hum. Genet.* **31:**141–145.
Lakshmanudu, M., 1980, Inbreeding Effects on Physical Measurements in Some Indian Populations, Ph.D. thesis, University of Calcutta.
Lakshmanudu, M., and Mukherjee, D. P., 1975, Pregnancy spacing in inbreeding, *Second Annu. Conf. Indian Soc. Hum. Genet.* Calcutta.
Lévi-Strauss, C., 1956, The family, in: H. L. Shapiro (ed.), *Man, Culture and Society,* Oxford University Press, New York.
Li, C. C., 1963, The way the load ratio works, *Am. J. Hum. Genet.* **15:**316–321.
Malecot, G., 1948, *Les mathematiques de l'heredite,* Masson et Cie, Paris.
Morton, N. E., Crow, J. F., and Muller, H. J., 1956, An estimate of the mutational damage in man from data on consanguineous marriages, *Proc. Natl. Acad. Sci. (USA)* **42:**855–863.
Mukherjee, D. P., 1974, Final report of ICMR project on genetic studies in relation to fertility, New Delhi, ICMR.
Mukherjee, D. P., and Lakshmanudu, M. (in press). Inbreeding depression on stature, in: D. P. Mukherjee (ed.), *Human Variation in India,* Anthropological Survey of India, Calcutta.
Muller, M. J., 1950, Our load of mutations, *Am. J. Hum. Genet.* **2:**111–176.
Murdock, G. P., 1949, *Social Structure,* Macmillan, New York.
Murty, J. S., and Jamil, T., 1972, Inbreeding load in the new born of Hyderabad, *Acta Genet. Med. Gemellol.* **21:**327–331.
Narayanan, H. S., and Rama Rao, B. S. S., 1978, Parental consanguinity and mental retardation, *Med. Genet. India* **2:**141–144.
Pearl, R., 1914, On the results of inbreeding a Mendelian population: A correction and extension of previous conclusions, *Am. Natural.* **48:**57–62.

Rami Reddy, V., and Padmanabha Naidu, G., 1978, Effect of consanguinity on fertility and mortality in the Gampasati Kammas of Andhra Pradesh, *Med. Genet. India.* **2:**151–156.

Rao, A. P., and Mukherjee, D. P., 1975, Consanguinity and inbreeding effects on fertility, mortality and morbidity in a small population of Tirupati, *Proc. Second Conf. Ind. Soc. Hum. Genet.*, Calcutta.

Rao, P. S. S., and Inbaraj, S. G., 1977a, Inbreeding effects on human reproduction in Tamil Nadu of South India. *Ann. Hum. Genet.* **41:**87–98.

Rao, P. S. S., and Inbaraj, S. G., 1977b, Inbreeding in Tamil Nadu, South India, *Soc. Biol.* **24:**281–288.

Rao, P. S. S. S., and Inbaraj, S. G., 1979, Trends in human reproductive wastage in relation to long-term practice of inbreeding, *Ann. Hum. Genet.* **42:**401–413.

Reid, R. M., 1973, Social structure and inbreeding in a south Indian caste, in: N. E. Morton (ed.), *Genetic Structure of Populations,* University of Hawaii, Honolulu, pp. 92–99.

Roychoudhury, A. K., 1976a, Incidence of inbreeding in different states of India, *Demography of India* **1, 2:**108–119.

Roychoudhury, A. K., 1976b, Inbreeding in Indian population. *Trans. Bose Res. Inst.* **39:**65–76.

Roychoudhury, A. K., 1980, Consanguineous marriages in Tamil Nadu, *J. Indian Anthropol. Soc.* **15:**167–174.

Sanghvi, L. D., 1963, The concept of genetic load: A critique, *Am. J. Hum. Genet.* **15:**298–309.

Sanghvi, L. D., 1966, Inbreeding in India, *Eug. Quart.* **13:**291–301.

Sanghvi, L. D., 1974, The genetic consequences of inbreeding and outbreeding, in: *The Role of Natural Selection in Human Evolution,* Burg Wartenstein Symposium **63.**

Sanghvi, L. D., Verde, D. S., and Master, H. R., 1956, Frequency of consanguineous marriages in twelve endogamous groups in Bombay, *Acta Genet. Stat. Med.* **6:**41–49.

Sastri, K. A. N., 1976, *A History of South India,* 4th ed. Oxford University Press, Madras.

Schechner, R., 1971, Incest and culture—A reflection on Claude Lévi-Strauss, *Psychoanal. Rev.* **58:**497–510.

Schull, W. J., and Neel, J. V., 1965, *The Effects of Inbreeding on Japanese Children,* Harper & Row, New York.

Selligman, B. Z., 1950, The problem of incest and exogamy: A restatement, *Am. Anthropol.* **52:**309–316.

Sinclair, S., 1972, Familial mental retardation and consanguinity, *Indian J. Med. Res.* **60:** 1718–1723.

Sutter, J., and Goux, M., 1964, Lethal equivalents and demographic measures of mortality, Cold Spring Harbor Symp. *Quant. Biol.* **29:**41–50.

Undevia, J. V., and Balakrishnan, V., 1978, Temporal changes in consanguinity among the Parsi and Irani communities of Bombay, *Med. Genet. India.* **2:**145–150.

Veerraju, P., 1973, Inbreeding in Coastal Andhra Pradesh, in: *Proc. Int. Sym. of Hum. Genet. at Waltair, India (1971).*

Wahlund, S., 1928, Zuzammensetzung von Populationen and Korrelationserscheinungen vom Standpunkt der Vererbungelehre aus betrachtet, *Hereditas* **11:**65–106.

White, L. A., 1948, The definition and prohibition of incest, *Am. Anthropol.* **50:**416–434.

Wright, S., 1921, Systems of mating, *Genetics* **6:**111–143.

Wright, S., 1922, Coefficients of inbreeding and relationship, *Am. Natural.* **56:**330–8.

Wright, S., 1923, Mendelian analysis of the pure breeds of livestock. I. The measurement of inbreeding and relationship, *J. Hered.* **14:**339–348.

Wright, S., 1931, Evolution in Mendelian populations, *Genetics* **16:**97–159.

Yasuda, N., 1968, Estimation of inbreeding coefficient from phenotype frequencies by a method of maximum likelihood scoring, *Biometrics* **24:**915–936.

CHAPTER 12

Taxonomic Distance and Human Populations of South Asia

RUSSELL M. REID

1. Introduction

With the emergence of what has been called *genetic anthropology* or *anthropological genetics* since the early 1950s, the traditional interest of physical anthropologists in human population affinities has persisted. The older paradigm of racial classification has, however, been largely replaced by other models. These include the use of branching tree models called *dendrograms* that graphically represent the general degree of genetic or anthropometric similarity or dissimilarity between populations. Such measures of taxonomic distance mathematically reduce multivariate data on population differences to single measures of the relative degree of difference between pairs of populations.

Methods of taxonomic distance and related graphic representations of such distances have been applied to questions of human affinities at many levels ranging from the local to the global. At the global level, issues of "racial affinities" have been addressed. In such studies, a few populations from each major region of the world have been selected for comparison. At an intermediate or regional level questions about the population history of the region or about its ties to the populations of adjacent regions are addressed. Studies at this intermediate level sometimes link the analysis of biological distance with linguistic, archaeological, or historical data on group affinities or with patterns of geographic proximity. A third or local level to which taxonomic distance analysis has been applied involves the examination of degrees of biological similarity between

RUSSELL M. REID • Department of Anthropology, University of Louisville, Louisville, Kentucky 40292.

endogamous groups living in a very restricted area or between subdivisions of a single population. In such studies the examination of taxonomic distance may be part of a more general study of the *genetic structure* of a population. The label *genetic structure* is applied to any or all of the phenomena that structure mating and reproduction and thus are determinants of such forces of genetic evolution as genetic drift, gene flow, and inbreeding. The global, regional, and local levels of study are arbitrary divisions of a continuous range of possibilities.

This chapter reviews the general features of measures of taxonomic distance in contrast to traditional racial taxonomies, examines the use of these models in the literature on India and adjacent areas of South Asia, and outlines problems on which further work is needed. Given the regional nature of this volume, it is also important to note that Indian geneticists and statisticans have not only played a central role in the empirical research on the region, but they have also been major contributors to the theoretical and analytical tools of taxonomic distance analysis.

2. Taxonomic Distance

2.1. Measures of Distance

The groundwork for the development of our contemporary approaches to the study of human population affinities was begun long before physical anthropologists began to question the utility of the traditional techniques of racial taxonomy. Beginning in the mid 1920s, P. C. Mahalanobis (1925, 1936) and K. Pearson (1926) developed measures of taxonomic distance between populations that used data on mean values of measurable anatomic traits. When applied to data on human populations, such taxonomic measures are frequently referred to as measures of *anthropometric distance*. The development of such analytical tools was continued by R. A. Fisher (1936) and C. R. Rao (1952) in the decades that followed. These techniques involve the use of differences between mean values of a list of anthropometric variables for pairs of populations in order to quantify the relative degree of similarities or differences between such pairs. A small distance between two populations would result if their means are similar for most of the list of anthropometric variables, or a large value results if the two populations display more significant differences in their means for a majority of the empirical variables.

In the early 1950s, L. D. Sanghvi (1952, 1953) proposed analogous multivariate measures of population similarity or dissimilarity to be applied to nonmetric, Mendelian traits rather than measurable anatomical features. Sanghvi's and other subsequent approaches using genetic data are based either on gene frequency differences between pairs of populations or on probabilities of gene identity (a function of gene frequencies). Such measures of taxonomic distance are frequently referred to as *genetic distance* measures. As in the case of anthropometric distances, genetic distance measures reduce to a single value the degree to which a pair of populations are biologically similar to or different from each other.

Any analytical approach that reduces a longer list of empirical variables to a smaller number of derived measures, as in the case of taxonomic distances, will, to some degree, oversimplify and introduce bias into our view of diversity. Much of the literature that debates the relative merits of the various measures of taxonomic distance is devoted to the issue of what sorts of biases and how much oversimplification are acceptable. Such an evaluation is not the purpose of this chapter; however, several comparative studies published over the past decade are recommended to the interested reader (Gower, 1972; Sanghvi and Balarishnan, 1972; Latter, 1973; Balakrishnan, 1974; Goodman, 1974; and Lalouel, 1980). Two measures, one using anthropometric data and another using gene frequencies are provided as illustrative examples of the general approach of taxonomic distance analysis. They were selected for use here because of their simplicity. Pearson's coefficient of racial likeness (1926), simplified by the use of standardized units of measure,

$$\mathrm{CRL}_{jk} = \frac{1}{\nu} \sum_{i=1}^{\nu} (\bar{x}_{ij} - \bar{x}_{ik})^2$$

may be thought of as the average of the square of the differences between mean values of ν different variables for two populations, j and k. If, by contrast, we were to compare gene frequencies in two populations, then an analogous and equally simple approach would be to define the distance between two populations as the

$$d_{jk}^2 = \frac{1}{\nu} \sum_{i=1}^{\nu} (p_{ij} - p_{ik})^2$$

average of the square of the differences between the two populations in the frequencies of ν different genes. Although these two measures of taxonomic distance may not be the most satisfactory that are available, they serve as useful illustrations because of their simplicity. Table I illustrates a hypothetical set of gene frequency data for three populations of the sort that might be used to calculate genetic distances. The gene frequencies in this table were selected so that a quick inspection would reveal that while populations P1 and P2 are relatively similar to each other, P3 is quite different. This pattern of population similarity and difference is continued in the table and figure that follow.

2.2. Distance Matrices

Because taxonomic distances are not measured in absolute units, but rather will vary depending on one's choice of distance measures and on the particular

Table I
A Hypothetical Set of Gene Frequencies on Three Populations

	Populations		
Genes	P1	P2	P3
G1	0.239	0.317	0.624
G2	0.542	0.702	0.297
G3	0.910	0.789	0.583
—	—	—	—
—	—	—	—
Go	0.717	0.802	0.467

set of variables to which they are applied, the distance between any two populations is not meaningful except in relation to comparable measures on other pairs of populations. When comparable genetic or anthropometric data are available for three or more populations, then taxonomic distances can be calculated between all possible pairs of such populations and summarized in a "distance matrix" that looks much like the mileage table on a road map. Table II indicates the general form of a distance matrix. As in the gene frequencies in the previous table we see a relatively small distance separating populations P1 and P2 and larger distances between each of them and P3.

2.3. Graphic Representation of Taxonomic Distance

Oversimplification results not only from the reduction of multivariate data to single measures of similarity but also from the graphic representation of a set of such measures. If the distance between two populations was never greater than the sum of their respective distances to a third population, then the distances between three populations could be represented by the three sides of a triangle. To do the same with four populations would require a three dimensional space,

Table II
Matrix of Genetic Distances between Three Populations

Populations	P1	P2	P3
P1	—	0.132	0.401
P2	—	—	0.439
P3	—	—	—

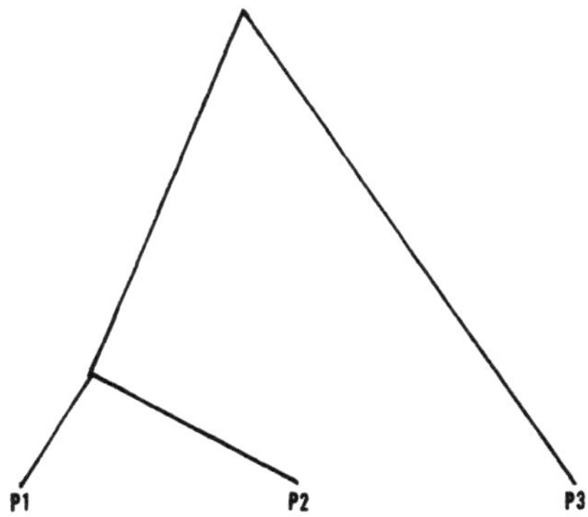

Figure 1. Dendrogram representing the genetic distances between three populations.

and in general an $n-1$ dimensional space is required to represent the taxonomic distances between n populations. An alternative manner of graphic representation of taxonomic distances involves the construction of dendrograms—branching tree diagrams. The distances presented in the previous table are represented by such a dendrogram in Figure 1. Again, we see the representation of the relatively smaller difference between populations P1 and P2 as compared to the differences between either of them and P3. Even with dendrograms we run into limitations on the representation of distances between more than a few populations in a two-dimensional space. It is for precisely this reason that graphic representations of a set of taxonomic distances results in oversimplification. Principal components analysis and other related methods of multivariate analysis provide alternative approaches to the quantification of similarity and its graphic representation. For a very useful recent summary of methods of distance analysis and multidimensional scaling the reader is directed to the work of J. M. Lalouel (1980).

2.4. Taxonomic Distance and Racial Classification

In traditional racial taxonomies, each taxon in the hierarchy of progressively more general or inclusive categories is described in stereotypic terms, an approach that is referred to as *typological.* As a result of those stereotypical descriptions, such taxonomies are, at best, classifications of individuals rather than of populations. Even as classifications of individuals, they are not necessarily very successful. In Hooton's and Dupertuis's (1955) analysis of 10,000 Irishmen it was found that very few could be described by the stereotypical descriptions of the presumed races of Europe. Even hyphenated categories combining pairs of such presumed races could include only about half of the individuals in the sample. Variation within populations resulting from independently assorting traits simply does not sort individuals into racial types. Although a classification of populations rather than individuals is desired, the variation within populations precludes the use of stereotypical descriptions.

In traditional racial taxonomies it is necessary to make arbitrary choices about which biological traits will be used to contrast more general divisions of the species and which will be reserved to contrast the included subdivisions. The resulting patterns of group affinities depend on the arbitrary choices that are made. For example, in traditional racial classifications such traits as skin color and hair form were usually used to distinguish the major human races, and features such as the Cephalic index (head shape) were used to separate minor subdivisions. The resulting patterns of racial affinities would have been quite different if the cephalic index had been used to distinguish major divisions and skin color and hair form had been reserved for separating the minor subdivisions of the human species. I suspect that these arbitrary choices were guided by the desire to contrast populations of European origin to those of the rest of the world. As such, they did little more than provide a scientific veneer of Latin labels to what was otherwise a folk classification.

While the graphic representation of taxonomic distances by the use of dendrograms is superficially similar to the product of racial classification, the underlying methods are quite different. The methods of taxonomic distance dealt with in this chapter use either phenotypic means or gene frequencies from populations that ideally have been defined by their mating behaviors. This consequently shifts us to population taxonomy rather than individual taxonomy and acknowledges individual diversity within populations. Further, there is no assignment—arbitrary or otherwise—of empirical variables to different levels in the classification. Because of the very different methods employed in racial classification and taxonomic distance analysis, the visual similarity and shared interest in biological affinities of human groups are about all they have in common.

3. Taxonomic Distance Studies in South Asia

Much of the literature that applies taxonomic distance analysis to empirical data on human variation does so to demonstrate the analytical technique rather than to learn something about the populations from which the data were drawn. Although this is somewhat frustrating, it reflects both the fact that the analytical techniques are still being refined and the difficulty involved in obtaining comparable data on an appropriate range of populations so that interesting questions may be addressed. Some important insights may be obtained nonetheless. L. D. Sanghvi (1952, 1953) was one of the first to develop measures of genetic distance and to apply them to human data. Drawing on data from western India

(1953), he showed that anthropometric and genetic data produced the same patterns of population affinities when applied to a regionally restricted set of populations. However, when later investigations at a more global level were subsequently conducted, it was found that the population affinities resulting from anthropometric distance studies were often quite different from those resulting from genetic distance studies. Specifically, when allele frequencies from five blood group systems (ABO, Rh, MNS, Di, and Fy) were subjected to genetic distance analysis, the major division of the species contrasted a Western cluster composed of Europe and Africa with an Eastern cluster including Asia, the Pacific area, and pre-Columbian American (Edwards and Cavalli-Sforza, 1964; Cavalli-Sforza and Edwards, 1965). By contrast, the analysis of anthropometric data resulted in a clustering of nontropical populations of Europe, East Asia, and pre-Columbian America that were contrasted with tropical populations of Africa and the Pacific area (Cavalli-Sforza and Edwards, 1965; Howells, 1973). The apparent conflict between population affinities as revealed by anthropometric versus those revealed by blood group data was resolved by a more elaborate analysis of anthropometric data in which the raw data were corrected for their correlations with climatic conditions. When the anthropometric variation that correlated with climatic variables was removed, the residual variation produced taxonomic distances and resultant dendrograms in which the major contrast was, as with the blood groups, the West versus the East (Guglielmino-Matessi *et al.*, 1979). Unfortunately, that important study included no populations of India or of continental Asia. It remains to be seen if the East versus West contrast is as clear when geographically intermediate populations are considered.

Data-oriented studies focused on populations of a single region have somewhat different objectives. These studies often reflect an interest in the culture history of the region, and the potential exists for the integration of genetic distance analysis into broader studies making use of data on linguistic and cultural diversity, written and traditional histories, and archaeological materials. Roychoudhury (1974) has applied Nei's (1973) method of measuring genetic distance to previously published data (Blake *et al.*, 1970, 1971) on populations around Delhi and Bombay, India. In both locations he found that only about 1% of the genetic diversity, measured as heterozygosity, represented differences between populations of the same region. The remaining heterozygosity resulted from genetic diversity within populations. Consequently, the genetic distances between populations of a single region are minute to the point that it is difficult to measure them reliably. In the case of the data from Bombay the problem may be that the units of study were defined linguistically (Marathas and Gujaratis), and thus they may represent the pooling of genetically diverse endogamous caste groups. This was not, however, the case for the data Roychoudhury used for Delhi, and his results have been replicated by others. Mukherjee and his associates (1979) applied Nei's distance measure to genetic data on nine endogamous groups in Maharashtra, the state in India where Bombay is located. These groups included four Hindu castes (Deshasta Rigvedi, Chitpavan Brahmin, Maratha, Chandrasenya Kayastha Prabhu, and Nava Budha), three tribal groups (Bhil, Pawara, and Katkari) as well as a sample of Parsis. The tribal groups are presumed to have inhabited the area for the longest period of time and the Parsis to have arrived most recently. Although it was found again that the between-population component of genetic diversity was very small relative to the within-population variation, and that the standard errors of the genetic distance estimates were large compared to the values of those distances, the method did differentiate the tribal from the nontribal groups. Among the tribals, the Katkari, who are removed both linguistically and geographically from the other two tribes, were found to be the most genetically divergent group. Das *et al.* (1978) have also applied such techniques to a sample of five endogamous castes in Delhi. Using data on the ABO, MN, Rh, P, and Hp loci, they found significant gene frequency differences between castes only for the MN, Rh, and P blood group systems. Further, it was found that intercaste variation accounted for only about 3% of the total heterozygosity. Again, the standard errors of the estimated genetic distances between castes were large, relative to the small values of those distances. These standard errors in fact ranged from 35 to 84% of their associated distance estimates. What clusters do emerge from this genetic distance analysis do not reflect patterns of caste ranks.

The application of genetic distance analysis to the Dhangar caste cluster of Maharashtra (Malhotra *et al.*, 1978) represents an extreme in the application of the approach to minimally differentiated groups. The Dhangar are a cluster of 23 endogamous groups scattered throughout Maharashtra, most of whom have traditionally herded sheep or woven woolen blankets. In most cases, these are highly localized castes; however, a few are scattered over several districts. In this instance the between-caste component of total genetic diversity was only 1%. With so little genetic differentiation of castes, one must be cautious in interpreting the clusters that emerge from the analysis. However, it is significant that the castes that appear to be the most genetically divergent also seem to have migrated into the area from surrounding states.

At the other extreme is a study by Kirk (1976) that computes genetic distances between six widely separated populations from India and Sri Lanka. The purpose of Kirk's study was to identify the origins of the Sinhalese—the major ethnic group of Sri Lanka (Ceylon)—and to evaluate interpretations of the legend of Prince Vijaya, the legendary founder of the Sinhalese. The genetic samples used are identified either by their regional language or state (Sinhalese, Tamils, Keralites, Bengalis, Punjabis, and Gujaratis) and probably represent the pooling of data from several endogamous groups. The Sinhalese speak an Indo-European language that is closely related to the languages of northern India (including the Bengalis, Punjabis, and Gujaratis), whereas their kinship and marriage systems as well as other aspects of their culture more closely resemble those of their Dravidian-speaking neighbors in southern India (including the Tamils and Keralites). The distinction between Indo-European-speaking versus Dravidian-speaking populations was not reflected in the genetic distances in Kirk's study. Although the Sinhalese were found to most closely resemble genetically the Bengalis with whom they also have close linguistic ties, that pair was found to have its next closest genetic ties to the two Dravidian-speaking groups rather than to the remaining Indo-European-speaking groups. This serves as a reminder that the patterns of linguistic, cultural, and genetic affinities need not parallel each other. (See Shaffer, this volume—Ed.)

Even with populations that are geographically separated, as in Kirk's study, there remains the problem of standard errors that are large as compared to their associated distance estimates. Kirk's best results came from the use of Cavalli-Sforza's (1969) distance measure in which case all but one of the population comparisons produced an estimated distance at least twice as large as its standard error. Using Latter's (1972) and Nei's (1972) methods, only about one third of the comparisons produced estimated distances that were at least twice as large as their standard errors.

The techniques of genetic distance analysis applied at the regional level have yet to be conducted to greatest advantage. Malhotra (1974) has, for example, drawn attention to the contrast between the classical model of caste history and that proposed by Karve (1958, 1961) as a problem amenable to analysis using genetic distances. By the classical model, the hierarchy of subdivisions within Hinduism into universal *varnas,* regional castes, and local subcastes is viewed as having resulted entirely from a process of caste and population fission. Thus, it is expected that hierarchical proximity between endogamous groups is of more importance to genetic distance than is geographic proximity. By Karve's model, subcastes of separate regional origins but comparable ritual or social functions and status might fuse to form a common caste or *varna* even though they might have closer genetic affinities to hierarchically separate subcastes of their own locality. This model suggests a greater role of geographic proximity between endogamous groups as a determanent of their relative genetic similarities. At least two studies (Gulati, 1971; Malhotra, 1974) do indeed support the Karve model of caste history. Their findings emphasize the need for the units of study in genetic surveys to be local endogamous units rather than more general caste or linguistic groups that could include genetically diverse populations.

Thus, the major efforts over the past several decades have been directed toward the development of measures of genetic distance. Additional work of a more empirical nature has been conducted. However, in the case of South Asia this has primarily involved comparisons between populations with close geographic proximity and/or recent historical ties. As we have seen, these populations were genetically quite similar to each other, so that the estimated genetic distances between them were often not much larger than the standard errors of those distance estimates. This was even seen to be the case in the study by Kirk (1976) that was based on more geographically separated populations. Any interpretation of patterns of population clustering as illustrated in dendrograms must, therefore, be tempered by an appreciation of this limitation.

4. The Future for Taxonomic Distance Studies

The emergence of studies that apply genetic distance measures has been hindered by the limited availability of appropriate data. Comparisons are limited to populations that have been surveyed for the same set of genes and should be limited further to samples including persons from a single endogamous group. Data from blood banks or hospitals are often heterogeneous in terms of the geographic and caste origins of the individuals tested. Even survey populations identified by language or by such general caste labels as *Brahmins* are likely to include a variety of potentially genetically differentiated endogamous groups. This pooling of endogamous groups will bring each sample nearer the gene frequency averages for the region and thus minimize the estimated genetic distances between such samples. As more genetic surveys are conducted on the populations of South Asia, it is important that the units surveyed be defined by patterns of endogamy, that the largest possible number of genes be studied, and that the sample sizes be adequate to provide reliable estimates of gene frequencies. This will maximize their utility for genetic distance analysis.

As more high-quality data become available, it is also important that more emphasis must be placed on the use of genetic distance to answer questions about the history of the populations of South Asia. The previous works of Malhotra (1974) and of Kirk (1976) are important contributions of this sort; however, there remain many questions to which genetic distance analysis could be applied. For example, is the pattern of genetic distinctiveness of tribal versus nontribal populations seen in Maharashtra (Mukherjee *et al.*, 1979) general to South Asia? Do the Austro–Asiatic-speaking groups of eastern India have closer genetic ties to their Indo-European and Dravidian-speaking neighbors in India or to the Austro–Asiatic-speaking groups of southeastern Asia? Is there, as Kirk's (1976) work would suggest, no genetic separation of Dravidian from Indo-European-speaking groups of South Asia? What are the external affinities of the populations of South Asia?

Although it would require much more genetic data than is now available, a useful approach to the study of South Asia and adjacent regions would be the approach applied by Menozzi and his associates (Menozzi *et al.*, 1978) to data on Europe and the Middle East. Their approach overcomes one of the weaknesses of genetic distances and dendrograms—the inability to represent clinal gradations across a geographic space conveniently. Rather than compute genetic distances between pairs of populations and graph the resulting dendrograms, Menozzi and colleagues used the multivariate statistical technique of principal components analysis. Where comparable data is available on a series of correlated variables from a number of different populations, the technique of principle components analysis can reduce these empirical variables to a shorter list of hypothetical or synthetic variables, each of which is statistically independent of the others. These synthetic variables, or principal components, are ranked in their decreasing order of contribution to the variance of the empirical variables. The intent is to reduce a rather long list of variables to a few principal components that collectively account for most of the variance of the empirical variables. The study by Menozzi and his associates (1978) was based on the analysis of data on 38 alleles from blood groups and other systems, including 21 alleles from the HLA-A and HLA-B loci. Geographic variation in the frequencies of these genes was subjected to principal components analysis. The authors then superimposed gradations in the intensity of each of the first three principal components onto a map of Europe and the Middle East. The first principal component, which accounted for 27% of the variance in all data and 31.8% of the variance in the HLA data, displayed a pattern of intensities that grade from the Middle East at one extreme to northwestern Europe at the other. The authors point out that this pattern of gradation parallels the presumed radiation of agricultural peoples from the Middle East into Europe after the rise of domestication. The second principal component also produced an east-west gradient, but it is much more irregular than the first. The third component, however, shows a pattern of gradations radiating outward from the Ukraine region. Although the authors attribute this third principal component to "the invasion of 'barbarians' of central and eastern Europe," it is worth noting that the center of radiation corresponds to the area tentatively identified as the center of origin of the Indo-European languages by Friedrich (1970). His conclusions were based on an historical linguistic analysis of the Indo-European vocabularies referring to trees. Others (Thieme, 1964) studying a wider range of vocabularies have placed that homeland further to the west but still not dramatically different from the center of radiation of the third principal component of the genetic analysis. The linguistic analysis provided by Thieme (1964) supports the view that the proto-Indo-European speakers had a herding rather than an agricultural economy. Herding is a custom that is now viewed as having developed subsequent to and out of settled agricultural cultures. Perhaps the patterns displayed in the principal components analysis of genetic variation in Europe reflect a major contribution resulting from the radiation of agricultural peoples out of the Middle East, followed by a later spread of pastoralists from the area north of the Black Sea speaking early forms of Indo-European languages.

With the accumulation of additional genetic data on the region from the

Middle East to southeastern Asia, it will be possible to extend the approach taken by Menozzi and his associates (1978) to that region. This could provide major new insights into the population history of South Asia and its relations with the surrounding regions.

References

Balakrishnan, V., 1974, Comparisons of some commonly used genetic distance measures, in: *Human Population Genetics in India: Proc. First Conf. Indian Soc. Hum. Genet.*, Volume 1 (L. D. Sanghvi, V. Balakrishnan, H. M. Bhatia, P. K. Sukumaran, and J.V. Undevia, eds.), Orient Longman, New Delhi, pp. 173–186.

Blake, N. M., Kirk, R. L., and Baxi, A. J., 1970, The distribution of some enzyme group systems among Marathis and Gujaratis in Bombay, *Hum. Hered.* **20**:409–416.

Blake, N. M., Kirk, R. L., McDermid, E. M., Omoto, K., and Ahuja, Y. R., 1971, The distribution of serum protein and enzyme group systems among north Indians, *Hum. Hered.* **21**:440–457.

Cavalli-Sforza, L. L., 1969, Human diversity, *Proc. 12th Intern. Congr. Genet.*, Volume 3, pp. 405–416.

Cavalli-Sforza, L. L., and Edwards, A. W. F., 1965, Analysis of human evolution, *Genetics Today, Proc. 11th Intern. Congr. Genet.*, Volume 3, pp. 923–933.

Das, S. K., Mukherjee, B. N., Malhotra, K. C., and Majumder, P. P., 1978, Serological and biochemical investigations among five endogamous groups of Delhi, India, *Ann. Hum. Biol.* **5**:25–31.

Edwards, A. W. F., and Cavalli-Sforza, L. L., 1964, Reconstruction of evolutionary trees, in: *Phenetic and Phylogenetic Classification* (W. E. Heywood and J. McNeil, eds.), The Systematics Association, London.

Fisher, R. A., 1936, CRL and the future of craniometry, *J. R. Anthropol. Inst.* **66**:57–63.

Friedrich, P., 1970, *Proto-Indo-European Trees*, University of Chicago Press, Chicago.

Goodman, M. M., 1974, Genetic distance: Measuring dissimilarity among populations, *Yearbook of Physical Anthropology 1973* **17**:1–38.

Gower, J. C., 1972, Measures of taxonomic distance and their analysis, in: *The Assessment of Population Affinities in Man*, (J. S. Weiner and J. Huizinga, eds.), Oxford University Press, London, pp. 1–24.

Guglielmino-Matessi, C. R., Gluckman, P., and Cavalli-Sforza, L. L., 1979, Climate and the evolution of skull metrics in man, *Am. J. Phys. Anthropol.* **50**:549–564.

Gulati, R. K., 1971, Inter-group Differences in an Artisan Caste of Maharashtra, Field Research Projects, Coral Gables, Florida.

Hooton, E. A., and Dupertuis, C. W., 1955, The physical anthropology of Ireland, *Pap. Peabody Mus. Archaeol. Ethnol., Harvard University* **30**:1–2.

Howells, W. W., 1973, Measures of population distance, in: *Methods and Theories of Anthropological Genetics* (M. H. Crawford and P. L. Workman, eds.), University of New Mexico Press, Albuquerque, pp. 159–176.

Karve, I., 1958, What is caste?: (I) Caste as extended kin, (II) Caste and occupation, (III) Caste as a status group, *Economic Weekly* **10**:125–138, 401–407, 881–888.

Karve, I., 1961, *Hindu Society: An interpretation*, Deshmukh and Co., Pune.

Kirk, R. L., 1976, The legend of Prince Vijay: A study of Sinhalese origins, *Am. J. Phys. Anthropol.* **45**:91–99.

Lalouel, J. M., 1980, Distance analysis and multidimensional scaling, in: *Current Developments in*

Anthropological Genetics, Volume 1 (J. H. Mielke and M. H. Crawford, eds.), Plenum Press, New York, pp. 209–250.
Latter, B. D. H., 1972, The island model of population differentiation: A general solution, *Genetics* **73**:147–157.
Latter, B. D. H., 1973, Measures of genetic distance between individuals and populations, in: *Genetic Structure of Populations*, Population Genetics Monographs, Volume 3 (N. E. Morton, ed.), University of Hawaii Press, Honolulu, pp. 27–37.
Mahalanabis, P. C., 1925, Analysis of race mixture in Bengal, *J. Asiat. Soc. Beng.* **26**:541–588.
Mahalanabis, P. C., 1936, On the generalized distance in statistics, *Proc. Natl. Inst. Sci. India* **12**:49–55.
Malhotra, K. C., 1974, Some models for the study of human population genetics in India: A review, in *Human Population Genetics in India: Proc. 1st Conf. Indian Soc. Hum. Genet.*, Volume 1 (L. D. Sanghvi, V. Balakrishnan, H. M. Bhatia, P. K. Sukumaran, and J. V. Undevia, eds.), Orient Longman, New Delhi, pp. 157–172.
Malhorta, K. C., Chakraborty, R., and Chakravarti, A., 1978, Gene differentiation among the Dhangar caste-cluster of Maharashtra, India, *Hum. Hered.* **28**:26–36.
Menozzi, P., Piazza, A., and Cavalli-Sforza, L., 1978, Synthetic maps of human gene frequencies in Europeans, *Science* **201**:786–792.
Mukherjee, B. N., Majumder, P. P., Malhotra, K. C., Das, S. K., Kate, S. K., and Chakraborty, R., 1979, Genetic distance analysis among nine endogamous population groups of Maharashtra, India, *J. Hum. Evol.* **8**:567–570.
Nei, M., 1972, Genetic distance between populations, *Amer. Nat.* **106**:283–292.
Nei, M., 1973, The theory and estimation of genetic distance, in: *Genetic Structure of Populations*, Population Genetics Monographs, Volume 3 (N. E. Morton, ed.), University of Hawaii Press, Honolulu, pp. 45–54.
Pearson, K., 1926, On the coefficient of racial likeness, *Biometrika* **18**:105–117.
Rao, C. R., 1952, *Advanced Statistical Methods in Biometrical Research*, Wiley, New York.
Roychoudhury, A. K., 1974, Gene differentiation among caste and linguistic populations of India, *Hum. Hered.* **24**:317–322.
Sanghvi, L. D., 1952, Biological Studies on Some Endogamous Groups in Bombay, India, Ph.D. thesis, Columbia University, New York.
Sanghvi, L. D., 1953, Comparison of genetical and morphological methods for a study of biological differences, *Am. J. Phys. Anthropol.* **11**:385–404.
Sanghvi, L. D., and Balakrishnan, V., 1972, Comparison of different measures of genetic distance between human populations, in: *The Assessment of Population Affinities in Man* (J. S. Weiner and J. Huizinga, eds.), Oxford University Press, London, pp. 25–36.
Thieme, P., 1964, The comparative method for reconstruction in linguistics, in: *Language in Culture and Society* (D. Hymes, ed.), Harper & Row, New York.

CHAPTER 13

Genetic Relationships between Indian Populations and Their Neighbors

A. K. ROYCHOUDHURY

1. Introduction

The Indian population may be divided into two main divisions, tribal and nontribal. About 450 tribes and subtribes, constituting about 7% of the total population are distributed in five regions, namely, the Northeast, the sub-Himalayan region of the North and Northwest, eastern and central, western, and southern India (Roy Burman, 1972). Morphologically, the tribals are different from the nontribal populations in stature and in cephalic, nasal, and facial indexes. The tribes in central and southern India are of short stature, have curly hair, dark pigmentation, are dolichocephalic, and have broad depressed noses when compared to the nontribal populations (Malhotra, 1978). Anthropometric measurements of five tribes in western India show that they have much in common racially and, as a group, differ from neighboring nontribal populations more than from each other (Shah, 1962). Differences in fingerprint patterns between tribal and nontribal populations are found in one state of southern India. Nontribal samples with high frequencies of loops and relatively low frequencies of whorls are markedly different from most of the other tribal samples (Basu, 1980).

The genetic differentiation between tribal and nontribal populations in India is also conspicuous. The tribal populations in middle and southern India are, in general, characterized by the presence of the sickle-cell trait (Saha and Banerjee,

A. K. ROYCHOUDHURY • Biometry and Population Genetics Unit, Bose Institute, Calcutta 700 009, India. The study was partly supported by grants from the National Institutes of Health to Professor M. Nei.

1973), and this characteristic differentiates them from neighboring nontribal populations. Tf-D_{Chi}, a variant of transferrin, is found with higher frequencies among the Koya Dora tribe in southern India (Rao *et al.*, 1979) and the Oraon tribe in eastern India (Kirk *et al.*, 1962) than among nontribal neighboring populations. Saha *et al.* (1976) and Ghosh *et al.* (1977) studied genetic relationships of tribal and nontribal populations in southern India using a number of serological and biochemical markers. Four tribes, namely, the Irula, Kurumba, Kadar, and Malayarayan, are genetically closer to each other than they are to the neighboring nontribal populations. Mukherjee *et al.* (1979) found by genetic analysis that three tribes in Maharashtra, the Bhil, Pawara, and Katkari groups belong to one cluster, whereas six nontribal neighboring populations belong to another cluster. It has been shown recently that the genetic differentiation between tribal and nontribal populations is larger than the differentiation among tribal or nontribal populations in western, eastern, and southern India (Roychoudhury, 1982).

2. Genetic Relationships between Tribal Populations in India and Their Neighbors

Though opinions differ, the tribes are said to be either autochthons or the first migrants to India. Guha (1937) referred to the tribes in central and southern India as protoaustraloids, because they show a physical resemblance to the Australian aboriginals with respect to sunken nasal root, head shape, skin color, and structure of hair. Apparently, there is no evidence to prove that the Australian aboriginals came to India or that the Indian tribes of South India migrated to Australia in prehistoric times. Although there is no such evidence, it is worthwhile to examine whether there exists any genetic affinity between the tribal populations in South India and those in Sri Lanka, Malaya, Australia, and New Guinea.

Three tribal populations living in the Nilgiri Hills of South India, namely, the Toda, Irula, and Kurumba were selected to be studied with respect to their genetic relationships with the neighboring tribal populations living outside India—namely, the Veddah in Sri Lanka, the Senoi in Malaya, Australian aboriginals, and groups in New Guinea. All the tribes were selected in such a way that the number of common genetic loci available for comparison was maximum. The Veddah are a small hunting group in Sri Lanka. The Senoi are one of the three main groups of Malay aborigines in the Malay Peninsula. The other two groups are the Negritos and the Aboriginal Malay. Genetically, the Senoi are closer to the aboriginal Malay than to the Negritos (Lie-Injo, 1976). The Australian aboriginals and the New Guinean groups are represented by the people living in the northern territory of Australia and in western New Guinea, respectively.

Surveying the literature, gene frequency data of 10 common loci—

A_1A_2BO, MNS, Rh, P, Fy, Lu, Hp, Tf, Hbβ, and Gm—for seven populations were collected. The data for the Toda, Irula, and Kurumba were taken from Saha *et al.* (1976); those for the Veddah from Wickremasinghe *et al.* (1963) and Kirk *et al.* (1962); and those for the Senoi from Polunin and Sneath (1956) and Lie-Injo (1976). Because no other sources of data were found, many of these data were collected from old literature. The gene frequencies of the Duffy blood group and hemoglobin were not available for the Senoi; they were taken from the aboriginal Malay (Polunin and Sneath, 1956). Most of the data for the Australian aboriginals were taken from the Malag tribe on Elcho Island (Simmons and Cooke, 1969). In the case of the New Guineans, average gene frequency data of the southern coastal plain, central highlands, and lake plain in western New Guinea were used (Gajdusek *et al.*, 1978). The gene frequency data for gamma globulin (gm) for all the tribes were taken from Vos *et al.* (1963), Steinberg and Lie-Injo (1972), and Steinberg *et al.* (1972). Except for Lutheran (Lu), all the loci are polymorphic for at least one population.

Nei's formula for standard genetic distance was applied to study the genetic relationships among the populations (Nei, 1972), and the standard error of the distance was computed following the method given by Nei and Roychoudhury (1974). Finally, the unweighted pair group method was used to construct the dendrogram from the matrix of genetic distances (Sneath and Sokal, 1973).

The average heterozygosity per locus and the genetic distances among seven tribal populations are shown in Table I. The average heterozygosity varies from 35 to 38% among the four tribal populations of the Indian subcontinent and 24 to 28% among the three tribal populations in southeastern Asia and Oceania. Low heterozygosity in the latter populations is caused by random genetic drift; because these populations are relatively small and isolated. The genetic distances among the Toda, Irula, Kurumba, and Veddah are small, but their distances from the Senoi in Malaya, Australian aboriginals, and the New Guineans are large. The distance between the Senoi in Malaya and the Veddah in Sri Lanka is small in comparison with that between the Senoi and the Australian aboriginals, but this is not clear from the dendrogram (Figure 1). This anomaly of relationship can be explained by the fact that the average distance of the Senoi from the Australian aboriginals and New Guineans is smaller than that from the other tribes under study. Complete dichotomy of seven tribal populations can be seen in the dendrogram. Three tribes in South India and the Veddah in Sri Lanka cluster together, as do the tribal populations in southeastern Asia and Oceania.

It is to be noted that the ratio of interpopulational genic variation (genetic distance) to the intrapopulational genic variation (mean of the average heterozygosities for the two populations concerned) is generally small (Nei and Roychoudhury, 1982). In the present investigation, this ratio is 0.39 between the Irula and Australian aboriginals and 0.07 between the Irula and Kurumba, thus indicating that the gene differentiation between the South Indian tribes and the Australian aboriginals is larger than that between the two South Indian tribes.

Table I
Average Heterozygosities and Genetic Distances (D × 10²) among 3 South Indian Tribes, 1 Sri Lankan Tribe, 1 Malay Tribe, and 2 Oceanic Tribes Based on 10 Genetic Loci[a]

	(1)	(2)	(3)	(4)	(5)	(6)	(7)
(1) Toda	34.77 ±7.93						
(2) Irula	2.19 ±0.97	37.66 ±8.47					
(3) Kurumba	4.30 ±1.77	2.57 ±1.35	37.49 ±7.75				
(4) Veddah	2.68 ±1.14	2.07 ±0.97	2.33 ±1.09	35.82 ±6.80			
(5) Senoi	15.21 ±13.07	14.45 ±11.61	15.16 ±11.92	12.95 ±11.96	28.41 ±6.95		
(6) Australian aboriginal	15.91 ±8.09	12.52 ±4.74	13.72 ±6.24	8.57 ±4.16	14.99 ±8.04	25.97 ±5.78	
(7) New Guinean	22.77 ±12.26	25.14 ±12.44	24.18 ±12.10	18.34 ±10.63	11.60 ±6.05	8.52 ±5.46	24.43 ±4.99

[a]The figures on the diagonal are the average heterozygosity per locus in percentages.

The South Indian tribes and the Australian aboriginals differ in the incidences of some genes. A critical examination of the gene frequencies of different systems of blood groups and proteins in two groups of tribal populations reveals that except for $CDE(R_z)$ of the Rh system, there is not much similarity in their distribution. The A_2 and *cde(r)* are present in most of the tribes of South India and in the Veddah of Sri Lanka, but they are completely absent in the Senoi of Malaya and Oceanic people (Wickremasinghe *et al.*, 1963; Simmons and Cooke, 1969; Saha *et al.*, 1976; Gajdusek *et al.*, 1978). The *S* antigen occurs with high

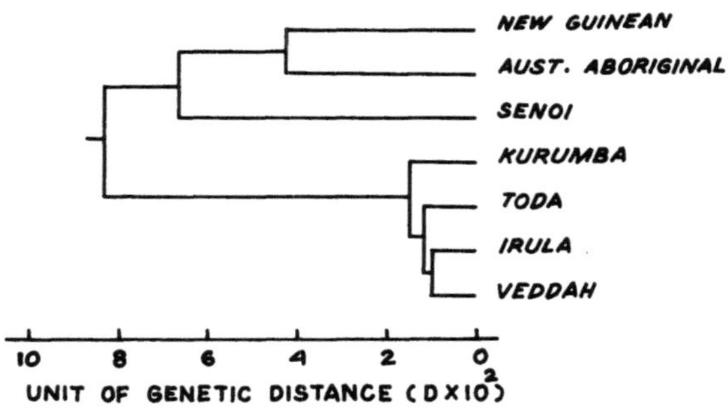

Figure 1. Dendrogram of three South Indian tribes, the Veddah of Sri Lanka, the Senoi of Malay, Australian aboriginals, and New Guineans.

frequency in the tribes of South India and Sri Lanka, but it is rarely present in Australian aboriginals or New Guineans. High frequency of *M* in southern Indian tribes is in contrast to the low frequency found in Australian aboriginals and New Guineans (Kirk *et al.*, 1962). Sanghvi (1976) compared allelic variability between 10 tribes of western India and 10 populations of Australian aboriginals and found that the variation in allele frequencies between India and Australia is the highest for *B* and *M* and the lowest for *A* and $cDe(R_0)$. The Tf^{D_1} allele of transferrin is present in Australian aboriginals and New Guineans (Omoto, 1974; Gajdusek *et al.*, 1978), but it has not been detected in any tribal population of South India (Saha *et al.*, 1976). By contrast, the Veddah of Sri Lanka have a small incidence of $Tf^{D_{Chi}}$. Abnormal hemoglobin is not found in the Australian aboriginals or New Guineans but *HbS* and *HbE* occur with appreciable frequencies in the South Indian tribes and the Veddah, respectively. The Veddah seem to have received the $Tf^{D_{Chi}}$ and *HbE* genes from the people of southeastern Asia or northeastern India in the past (Mourant *et al.*, 1976; Kirk, 1976a). With respect to gamma globulin, the tribal populations in South India and Sri Lanka have Gm^1, $Gm^{1,2}$ and Gm^5 haplotypes, whereas the Senoi in Malaya, the Australian aboriginals, and New Guineans have Gm^1, $Gm^{1,2}$ and $Gm^{1,5}$ haplotypes (Vos *et al.*, 1963; Steinberg and Lie-Injo, 1972; Steinberg *et al.*, 1972). Lastly, the variant genes Gc^{Ab} of group specific component and CA_1^9 and CA_2^4 of carbonic anhydrase I and II are present in the Australian aboriginals but are absent in the Indian populations (Cleave, 1974; Ghosh, 1977; Blake, 1978). It therefore appears that there are no common and specific markers by which the tribes of South India and the Veddah of Sri Lanka can be linked with the Australian aboriginals (Kirk, 1976b). On examining the distribution of gene frequencies of ABO, MNS, and Rh, a similar conclusion had been made previously by Simmons (1976).

Despite morphological similarity, the tribes in South India and the aboriginals in Australia are genetically diverse. In their survey on genetic relationships of human populations, Nei and Roychoudhury (1982) found that the Asian Negritos and African Pygmies are genetically different but morphologically alike. Coon (1965) postulated that the morphological similarities between the two groups of people might have developed independently in similar environmental conditions rather than because of common descent.

3. Genetic Relationships between Nontribal Populations in India and Their Neighbors

Attempts have already been made to study the genetic relationships of Indian nontribal populations with their neighbors. It has been demonstrated that the Sinhalese in Sri Lanka are closer to the Tamils and Keralites of South India and to the upper castes of Bengal than they are to the populations of Gujarat and Punjab (Kirk, 1976a). Migrant populations like the Parsis and Iranis in western India have been shown to be genetically affiliated with the Parsian and Turkoman-speaking peoples in Iran, respectively (Kirk *et al.*, 1977). Except for these, no other studies seem to have been made to determine the degree of genetic affinity of Indian nontribal populations with their neighbors. This section has been devoted to this aspect of study in a more comprehensive way than has been done in the past.

Four nontribal populations of India, namely, northern Indians, Marathis, southern Indians, and Bengalis living in northern, western, southern, and eastern India, respectively, and six neighboring populations, namely, the Iranians and Afghans in the northwest, the Sinhalese in the south, the Bhutanese in the north and the Malay and the Chinese in southeastern Asia were selected. The gene frequency data of 10 common loci (ABO, MN, Rh, Hp, Tf, ACP, AK, 6PGD, PGM-1, and G6PD) for 10 populations were obtained from the literature. All the loci are polymorphic for at least one population. The data for nontribal Indian populations were collected from Blake *et al.* (1970, 1971), Ananthakrishnan and Kirk (1969), Das *et al.* (1970), Mukherjee and Das (1970), and Mourant *et al.* (1976). The Iranians were represented by the people living in the northern part of Iran (Kirk *et al.*, 1977) and the Afghans by the people belonging to the Pushtun and Dari linguistic groups of Kabul (Papiha *et al.*, 1977). The data for the Bhutanese, Sinhalese, and Malay were taken from their respective countries (Kirk *et al.*, 1962; Kirk, 1968a,b; Roberts *et al.*, 1972; Blake *et al.*, 1973; Mourant *et al.*, 1969, 1976). Due to the nonavailability of the data for the Chinese in mainland China, they were collected from Chinese residing in Calcutta and Singapore (Chaudhuri *et al.*, 1967; Blake *et al.*, 1973).

The average heterozygosity per locus and genetic distances among four nontribal populations of India and their six neighboring populations are shown in Table II. The average heterozygosities of the Iranians and Afghans are slightly higher than those of the Indian populations, whereas those of the remaining four neighboring populations fall within the range of the Indian populations. The genetic distances among five populations of the Indian subcontinent from the Iranians and Afghans are generally small when compared to their distances from the Bhutanese, Malay, and Chinese. This indicates that the people of the Indian subcontinent have had gene exchange more with the former populations than with the latter populations. In other words, the people of the Indian subcontinent show a smaller amount of gene differentiation from their neighbors in the Northwest than from those in the North and in southeastern Asia.

For a long period of time, the people from South India migrated and settled in the northern part of Sri Lanka. It is, therefore, logical that southern Indians are found to have a close affinity with the Sinhalese. Also, there is historical evidence that the people in northeastern India had contact with the Sinhalese. Two

Table II
Average Heterozygosities and Genetic Distances ($D \times 10^2$) among 4 Indian Populations and Their 6 Neighboring Populations Based on 10 Genetic Loci[a]

	(1)	(2)	(3)	(4)	(5)	(6)	(7)	(8)	(9)	(10)
(1) Iranian	32.03 ± 6.97									
(2) Afghan	0.33 ± 0.13	32.10 ± 7.21								
(3) North Indian	0.31 ± 0.17	0.35 ± 0.18	30.86 ± 7.18							
(4) Marathi	0.42 ± 0.19	0.56 ± 0.34	0.21 ± 0.09	28.93 ± 7.01						
(5) South Indian	0.60 ± 0.23	0.57 ± 0.33	0.32 ± 0.09	0.21 ± 0.19	25.49 ± 7.02					
(6) Bengali	0.49 ± 0.25	0.75 ± 0.50	0.26 ± 0.25	0.43 ± 0.40	0.47 ± 0.32	29.94 ± 6.86				
(7) Sinhalese	0.27 ± 0.16	0.40 ± 0.23	0.15 ± 0.11	0.18 ± 0.11	0.08 ± 0.06	0.20 ± 0.18	28.99 ± 6.39			
(8) Malay	0.84 ± 0.54	1.13 ± 1.07	0.89 ± 0.68	1.35 ± 0.92	0.94 ± 0.76	0.49 ± 0.19	0.67 ± 0.46	27.63 ± 6.44		
(9) Chinese	0.90 ± 0.37	1.11 ± 0.74	1.14 ± 0.57	1.50 ± 0.80	1.10 ± 0.69	0.73 ± 0.29	0.68 ± 0.39	0.36 ± 0.19	28.53 ± 6.27	
(10) Bhutanese	1.91 ± 0.75	1.80 ± 0.88	2.09 ± 0.91	1.97 ± 1.01	1.44 ± 0.90	1.44 ± 0.68	1.56 ± 0.78	1.13 ± 0.50	1.11 ± 0.50	27.29 ± 6.59

[a]The figures on the diagonal are the average heterozygosity per locus in percentages.

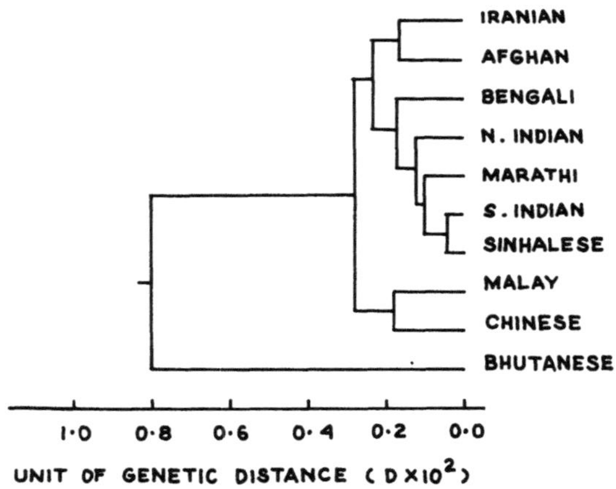

Figure 2. Dendrogram of four Indian populations and their six neighboring populations.

common traits, namely, hemoglobin E and hairy pinnae found in both the populations, may provide evidence for their contact in the past (Kirk, 1976a).

The overall pattern of genetic relationships among 10 populations is shown in the dendrogram (Figure 2). In the first instance, the Bhutanese are separated from the remaining 9 populations that form two clusters. The Malay and Chinese belong to the first cluster, and the remaining 7 populations to the second cluster. The Bhutanese seem to have been more isolated than the Malay and Chinese who had some degree of admixture with the Indians in the past (Teng and Tan, 1979). The 5 populations of the Indian subcontinent, namely, northern Indians, Marathis, southern Indians, Bengalis, and Sinhalese and two other populations, namely, Iranians and Afghans, group separately in the second cluster.

Questions may be asked about the inclusion of the loci HbS and G6PD that are subject to natural selection. Similarly, justification may be sought for the inclusion of the P blood group, because of its poor repeatability in determination (Osborne, 1958; Mourant *et al.*, 1976). Excluding all the loci from tribal and nontribal data, genetic distance analysis was redone. Although the magnitude of the genetic distances had been changed, the topologies of both the dendrograms remained unaffected (not shown).

Acknowledgment

Part of the study was done during the author's tenure at the Center for Demographic and Population Genetics, University of Texas Health Science Center in Houston, Texas.

References

Ananthakrishnan, R., and Kirk, R. L., 1969, The distribution of some serum protein and enzyme group systems in two endogamous groups in South India, *Indian J. Med. Res.* **57:**1011–1017.

Basu, A., 1980, Dermatoglyphic Variation in Six Endogamous Castes of Mysore, Ph.D. Thesis, Calcutta University, Calcutta.

Blake, N. M., 1978, Genetic variants of carbonic anhydrase in the Asian-Pacific area, *Ann. Hum. Biol.* **5:**557–568.

Blake, N. M., Kirk, R. L., and Baxi, A. J., 1970, The distribution of some enzyme group systems among Marathis and Gujaratis in Bombay, *Hum. Hered.* **20:**409–416.

Blake, N. M., Kirk, R. L., McDermid, E. M., Omoto, K., and Ahuja, Y. R., 1971, The distribution of serum protein and enzyme group systems among north Indians, *Hum. Hered.* **21:**440–457.

Blake, N. M., McDermid, E. M., Kirk, R. L., Ong, Y. W., and Simons, M. J., 1973, The distribution of red cell enzyme groups among Chinese and Malays in Singapore, *Singapore Med. J.* **14:**2–8.

Chaudhuri, S., Mukherjee, B., Ghosh, J., and Roychoudhury, A. K., 1967, Blood groups of the Chinese in Calcutta, *Nature* **213:**1245.

Cleave, H., 1974, The variants of the group-specific component, in: *Genetic Polymorphisms and Diseases in Man* (B. Ramot, ed.), Academic Press, New York.

Coon, C. S., 1965, *The Living Races of Man,* Knopf, New York.

Das, S. R., Mukherjee, B. N., Das, S. K., Blake, N. M., and Kirk, R. L., 1970, The distribution of some enzyme group systems among Bengalis, *Indian J. Med. Res.* **58:**866–875.

Gajdusek, D. C., Leyshon, W. C., Kirk, R. L., Blake, N. M., Keats, B., and McDermid, E. M., 1978, Genetic differentiation among populations in western New Guinea, *Am. J. Phys. Anthropol.* **48:**47–64.

Ghosh, A. K., 1977, The distribution of genetic variants of glyoxalase 1, esterase D and carbonic anhydrase I and II in Indian populations, *Indian J. Phys. Anthropol. and Hum. Genet.* **3:**73–83.

Ghosh, A. K., Kirk, R. L., Joshi, S. R., and Bhatia, H. M., 1977, A population genetic study of the Kota in the Nilgiri Hills, South India, *Hum. Hered.* **27:**225–241.

Guha, B. S., 1937, An outline of the racial ethnology of India, in: *An Outline of the Field Sciences of India,* Indian Science Congress Association, Calcutta, pp. 125–139.

Kirk, R. L., 1968a, Haptoglobin groups in man, *Monogr. Hum. Gen.* **4,** Karger, Basel.

Kirk, R. L., 1968b, The world distribution of transferrin variants and some unsolved problems, *Acta Genet. Med. Gemellol.* **17:**613–640.

Kirk, R. L., 1976a, The legend of Prince Vijaya—A study of Sinhalese origins, *Am. J. Phys. Anthropol.* **45:**91–100.

Kirk, R. L., 1976b, Serum protein and enzyme markers as indicators of population affinities in Australia and the western Pacific, in: *The Origin of the Australians* (R. L. Kirk and A. G. Thorne, eds.), Australian Institute of Aboriginal Studies, Canberra, pp. 329–346.

Kirk, R. L., Lai, L. Y. C., Vos, G. H., Wickremasinghe, R. L., and Perera, D. J. B., 1962, The blood and serum groups of selected populations in South India and Ceylon, *Am. J. Phys. Anthropol.* **20:**485–497.

Kirk, R. L., Keats, B., Blake, N. M., McDermid, E. M., Ala, F., Karimi, M., Nickbin, B., Shabazi, H., and Kmet, J., 1977, Genes and people in the Caspian littoral: A population genetic study in northern Iran. *Am. J. Phys. Anthropol.* **46:**377–390.

Lie-Injo, L. E., 1976, Genetic relationships of several aboriginal groups in southeast Asia, in: *The Origin of the Australians* (R. L. Kirk and A. G. Thorne, eds.), Australian Institute of Aboriginal Studies, Canberra, pp. 277–306.

Malhotra, K. C., 1978, Morphological composition of the people of India, *J. Hum. Evol.* **7:**45–53.

Mourant, A. E., Godber, M. J., Kopec, A. C., Lehmann, H., Steele, P. R., and Tills, D., 1969, The hereditary blood factors of some populations in Bhutan, *Anthropologist* (special volume), pp. 29–43.

Mourant, A. E., Kopec, A. C., and Domaniewska-Sobczak, K., 1976, *The Distribution of the Human Blood Groups and Other Polymorphisms,* Oxford University Press, London.

Mukherjee, B. N., and Das, S. K., 1970, The haptoglobin and transferrin types in West Bengal and a case of haptoglobin "Johnson," *Hum. Hered.* **20:**209–214.

Mukherjee, B. N., Majumder, P. P., Malhotra, K. C., Das, S. K., Kate, S. L., and Chakraborty, R., 1979, Genetic distance analysis among nine endogamous population groups of Maharashtra, India, *J. Hum. Evol.* **8:**567–570.

Nei, M., 1972, Genetic distance between populations, *Am. Nat.* **106:**283–292.

Nei, M., and Roychoudhury, A. K., 1974, Sampling variances of heterozygosity and genetic distance, *Genetics* **76:**379–390.

Nei, M., and Roychoudhury, A. K., 1982, Genetic relationship and evolution of human races, in: *Evolutionary Biology* **14:**1–59.

Omoto, K., 1974, Polymorphic traits in peoples of eastern Asia and the Pacific, in: *Genetic Polymorphisms and Diseases in Man* (B. Ramot, ed.), Academic Press, New York, pp. 69–89.

Osborne, R. H., 1958, Serology in physical anthropology: Technical problems as revealed by repeated blood determinations in twins, *Am. J. Phys. Anthropol.* **16:**187–196.

Papiha, S. S., Roberts, D. F., and Rahimi, A. G., 1977, Genetic polymorphisms in Afghanistan, *Ann. Hum. Biol.* **4:**233–241.

Polunin, I., and Sneath, P. H. A., 1956, Studies of blood groups in south-east Asia, *J. R. Anthropol. Inst. Gr. Br. Ir.* **83:**215–251.

Rao, P. R., Goud, J. D., and Rama Swamy, B., 1979, The occurrence of D_{Chi} and new D and B transferrin variants among caste groups of Andhra Pradesh (South India), *Hum. Genet.* **48:**235–239.

Roberts, D. F., Papiha, S. S., and Abeyaratne, K. P., 1972, Red cell enzyme polymorphisms in Ceylon Sinhalese, *Am. J. Hum. Genet.* **24:**181–188.

Roy Burman, B. K., 1972, Tribal demography: A preliminary appraisal, in: *Tribal Situation in India* (K. Suresh Singh, ed.), Indian Institute of Advanced Study, Simla, pp. 39–50.

Roychoudhury, A. K., 1982, Genetic Relationships of Indian Populations, paper presented to the Golden Jubilee Celebration of Indian Statistical Institute, Calcutta.

Saha, N., and Banerjee, B., 1973, Haemoglobinopathies in the Indian subcontinent, *Acta Genet. Med. Gemellol.* **22:**117–138.

Saha, N., Kirk, R. L., Shanbhag, S., Joshi, S. R., and Bhatia, H. M., 1976, Population genetic studies in Kerala and the Nilgiris (Southwest India), *Hum. Hered.* **26:**175–197.

Shah, P. G., 1962, Racial surveys in Gujarat, in: *Indian Anthropology* (T. N. Madan and G. Sarana, eds.), Asia Publishing House, Bombay, pp. 150–162.

Sanghvi, L. D., 1976, Comparative genetic studies between some groups of Australian aboriginals and certain tribal peoples of India, in: *The Origin of the Australians* (R. L. Kirk and A. G. Thorne, eds.), Australian Institute of Aboriginal Studies, Canberra, pp. 401–410.

Simmons, R. T., 1976, The biological origin of Australian aboriginals, in: *The Origin of the Australians* (R. L. Kirk and A. G. Thorne, eds.), Australian Institute of Aboriginal Studies, Canberra, pp. 307–328.

Simmons, R. T., and Cooke, D. R., 1969, Population genetic studies in Australian aborigines of the Northern Territory—Blood group genetic studies in the Malag of Elcho Island, *Arch. Phys. Anthropol. in Oceania* **4:**252–259.

Sneath, P. H. A., and Sokal, P. R., 1973, *Numerical Taxonomy,* W. H. Freeman, San Francisco.

Steinberg, A. G., and Lie-Injo, L. E., 1972, Immunoglobulin G allotypes in Malayan aborigines, *Hum. Hered.* **22:**254–258.

Steinberg, A. G., Gajdusek, D. C., and Alpers, M., 1972, Genetic studies in relation to Kuru. V. Distribution of human gamma globulin allotypes in New Guinea populations, *Am. J. Hum. Genet.* **24**(Suppl.):95–110.

Teng, Y. S., and Tan, S. G., 1979, Genetic evidence of gene flow from Indians to Malays, *Japanese J. Hum. Genet.* **24**:1–8.

Vos, G. H., Kirk, R. L., and Steinberg, A. G., 1963, The distribution of the gamma globulin types Gm(a), Gm(b), Gm(x) and Gm-like in South and Southeast Asia and Australia, *Am. J. Hum. Genet.* **15**:44–52.

Wickremasinghe, R. L., Ikin, E. W., Mourant, A. E., and Lehmann, H., 1963, The blood groups and haemoglobins of the Veddahs of Ceylon, *J. R. Anthropol. Inst. Gr. Br. Ir.* **93**:117–125.

CHAPTER 14

Population Structure among the Dhangar Caste-Cluster of Maharashtra, India

KAILASH C. MALHOTRA

1. Introduction

1.1. Relevance of Population Structure

The interpretation of the temporal and spatial variation of gene frequencies in populations is one of the main aims of population genetics. Aside from the systematic evolutionary processes (mutation, selection, and admixture), non-systematic factors such as size, density, and distribution of a population, the nature of mate selection within a population, and differential fertility and viability also influence the genetic composition of a population. These non-systematic factors are generally referred to as *population structure,* that is, the way in which two haploid individuals produce a diploid individual. It is now well known that very different patterns exist in human populations by which this process is achieved. The pattern of choice of mates provides a fair amount of insight into the generational and spatial dynamics of a gene in a population (see among others, Cavalli-Sforza, 1958, 1962; Boyce *et al.*, 1967; Malhotra and Majumder, 1974; Majumder, 1977; Wolanski, 1977; Majumder and Malhotra, 1979). Aspects of nature and history in the Indian subcontinent have provided circumstances of control and variation that, in many ways, approximate laboratory conditions (Karve, 1965). In fact, the nature and extent of diversity observed

KAILASH C. MALHOTRA • Indian Statistical Institute, Calcutta 700 035, India. The study was sponsored by the University Grants Commission, New Delhi.

in Indian populations is unparalleled in the world and should more aptly be described as a *living laboratory* for conducting a wide array of experiments in human population structure.

1.2. Population Structure in India

The people of India are estimated to consist of over 40,000 Mendelian populations (Gadgil and Malhotra, 1982). An estimated 37,000 endogamous groups are structured in a system commonly referred to as *Hindu caste system*. Individually, each population in the system is called a *jati* or a caste (Karve and Malhotra, 1968). There are some 3000 Mendelian populations that, strictly speaking, are outside the caste system. These populations include tribal autochthonous groups and religious communities. The main features of the Indian population structure are summarized in Figure 1.

As noted, Hindu society is composed of over 30,000 discernible endogamous castes; 2378 castes were actually counted in the Indian census of 1901 (Hutton, 1963, p. 149). Hutton's estimate is low, because in the census returns many different castes belonging to a caste-cluster were shown as a single caste. Each caste theoretically belongs to one of the five *varnas:* Brahmin, Kshatriya, Vaishya, Sudra, and Pancham. In a majority of the cases the varna affiliation of a caste is quite clear.

The five varnas are arranged in a hierarchical order, the Brahmin varnas are at the top of the hierarchy and are followed by the Kshatriya, Vaishya, Sudra, and Pancham varnas. The social stratification of the society is not only hierarchical, but the hierarchy is rationalized by ritual and religious criteria. The system has been strengthened by an elaborate philosophy. Traditionally, the members of each caste followed a particular profession, practiced endogamy, and had elaborate rules for selecting mates.

Some of the more notable consequences of the Hindu caste system, in terms of evolutionary implications, have been (1) the entire population has been divided into a number of endogamous groups and the system does not permit large-scale intercaste marriages, whereby the gene pool of each caste has evolved over at least the last 3000 years; (2) the population sizes of the castes show enormous variation; there are several castes that number below 1000 persons, whereas many others number over 100,000 people; (3) several castes are located in rather small territories, often only in a single village, whereas many others are found in several districts; (4) apart from the ecological considerations, the caste system promotes an uneven geographical distribution among many castes because of occupational differences (Malhotra, 1980b); and (5) the system encouraged retention of diversity in many sociocultural practices including those related to the choice of mates among different castes.

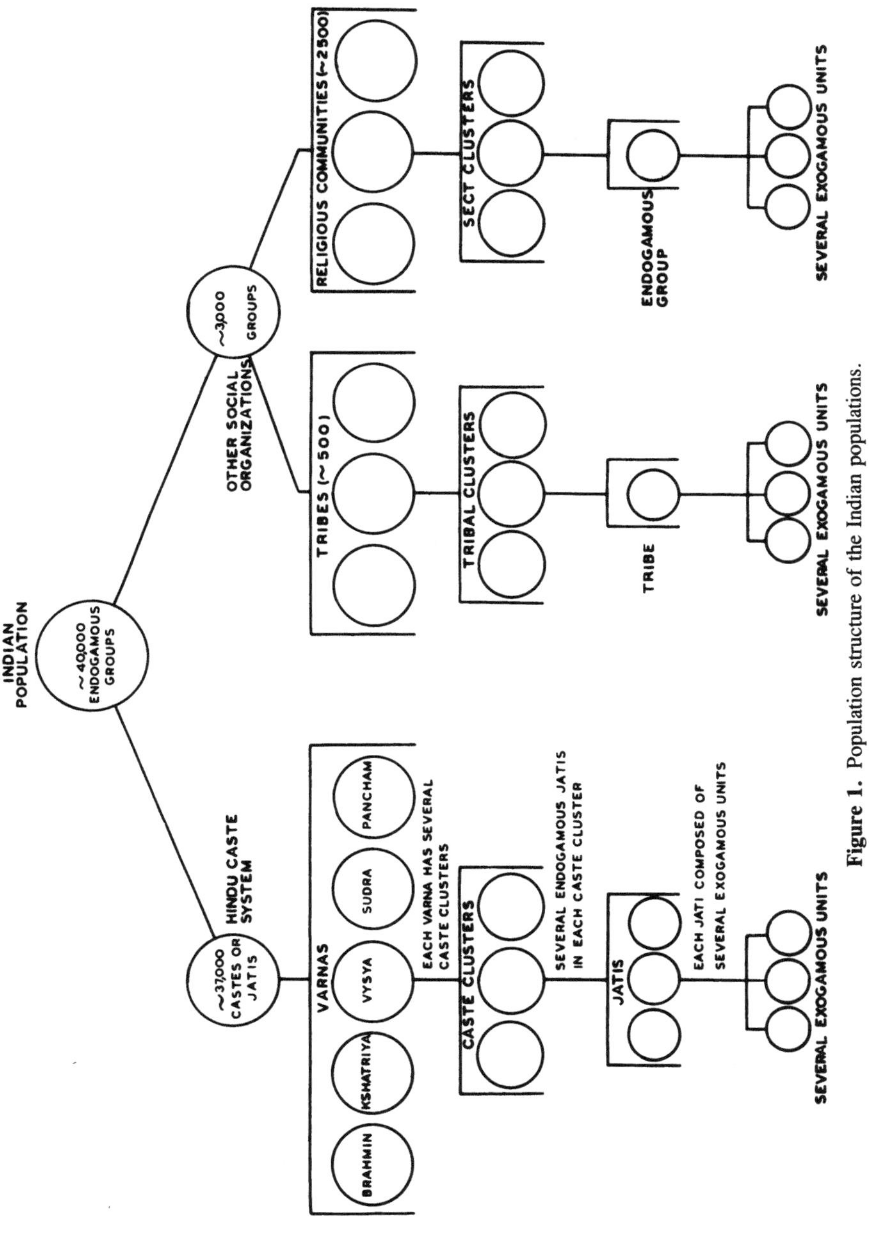

Figure 1. Population structure of the Indian populations.

1.3. Population Structure in Western India

Western India, in particular the state of Maharashtra, presents a unique geographical position that is not shared by many other Indian states. It is a territorial gateway between the two very diverse kinship systems—the Dravidian (southern) and Indo-Aryan (northern). Whereas in the former system consanguineous marriages are preferred and are often prescriptive, in the latter there is a strong taboo against them (Karve, 1953). It is, therefore, to be expected that population groups in this region will exhibit wide diversity in many cultural practices, including the question of who marries whom. To the autochthonous tribal populations, castes, and communities with a long history in this region have recently been added a number of immigrant populations from western Asia. As a result, the population structure of this region is fairly complex and of great interest to the anthropologist and geneticist.

2. Objectives

The purpose of this chapter is to assess the nature and extent of social and spatial variation with respect to three components of population structure, namely, (1) inbreeding, (2) village endogamy, and (3) matrimonial distances among the Dhangar caste-cluster of Maharashtra. The data are analyzed with a view to finding differences in these three components within and between the Dhangar castes and to examine the nature of the relationship between coefficient of inbreeding (α), mean matrimonial distances (MMD), and rates of village endogamy. The chapter further examines the differences in these three components in terms of sociocultural norms regulating choice of mates, geographical distribution of the population, migration history, and the influence of Indo-Aryan and Dravidian cultural practices. Lastly, the implications of these findings for gene differentiation among the Dhangar castes are discussed briefly.

3. The Dhangar Castes

It is estimated that the Dhangar caste-cluster numbers over 3 million souls. These castes-clusters are found in all of the 26 districts of Maharashtra and one composed of 23 endogamous castes (Figure 2). They are in different stages of sedentary life: The Khatik, Shegar, and Zende are sedentary, parts of the Hatkar and Thellari are true nomads, and the rest are seminomads. Some of them are highly localized whereas others, like the Hatkar and Khutekar in particular, are found widely distributed in several districts. They show considerable variation in population size. The Gadhari-Nikhar, Thellari, Ladshe, Hande, Kannade, Kur-

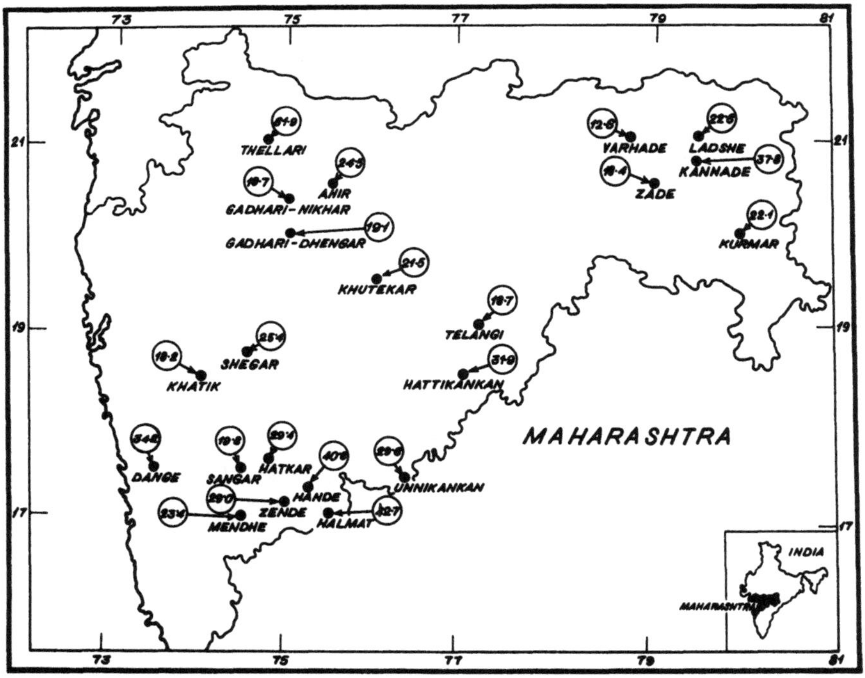

Figure 2. Geographical distribution of 22 Dhangar castes of Maharashtra, India. Figures in circles give the incidence of total consanguineous marriages for each caste.

mar, Telangi, and so forth, number a few thousand, whereas a few, such as the Hatkar, Ahir, Khutekar, and Dange, number over 100,000. Although the popular connotation of the word *Dhangar* is shepherd, the Dhangar caste-cluster includes castes with varied traditional occupations; sheep rearing (Hatkar, Ahir, Thellari), sheep rearing and woolen-blanket weaving (Khutekar, Kannade), woolen blanket weaving only (Sangar), buffalo rearing (Dange), agriculturists (Zende), and meat selling (Khatik). The Dhangar castes differ markedly with respect to language (at least four different languages are spoken by these people—Marathi, Kannada, Telugu, and Hindi), food habits, and other cultural traits.

Some of the castes have been living in their present habitats for the last several centuries, whereas a few, such as the Thellari and Kurmar, are recent immigrants. The estimated rate of admixture between these castes is of the order of 1 in 10,000 marriages. Ethnographic data show that at least some of the castes have arisen due to fission, for example, the Thellari and Hatkar. Archaeological evidence in the form of sheep bones suggests that the present-day Dhangars migrated into this western state of India from the northwestern-part of the country *ca.* 5000–10,000 years B.P., and that possibly more than one wave of migration was involved. For further details on the ethnography, biological variables, and population structure, I refer readers to, among others, Chakraborty *et al.* (1977), Majumdar and Malhotra (1979), Malhotra (1978, 1979a, 1979b, 1979c, 1980a, b), Malhotra and Gadgil (1981), Malhotra *et al.*, 1977a,b), and Mukherjee *et al.* (1976, 1977).

4. Methods and Materials

The materials presented in this chapter were generated using a multistage sampling design developed by T. V. Hanurao and R. Chakraborty of the Indian Statistical Institute in Calcutta. In brief, the sampling design was as follows: For each of the 26 districts, a random sample of *talukas* (geographical administrative units) was chosen. Within each taluka, all villages where Dhangar castes were available (based on the directory we prepared in the first phase of the project), were stratified into one of two categories, large or small, depending on population sizes; the sizes of the villages, in most part, were obtained from 1961 census reports. The final sample subjects were chosen from a stratified random sample of villages drawn from the selected talukas. The number of samples to be selected from the chosen villages was decided upon by making a proportional allocation of the total sample size to villages. Thus altogether, data on the three variables (mentioned previously) were collected from 103 *talukas* (Tehsil) in 24 districts in Maharashtra state. The number of couples interviewed for each of the variables and for each caste are indicated in relevant tables in the text.

For ascertaining consanguinity status, the following procedure was followed: There were six investigators. Four of them were trained anthropologists and the other two were trained for the purpose of this project. No major difficulty was encountered in ascertaining consanguinity. Vernacular expressions like *mame behini lagn* (matrilateral cross-cousin marriage), *ate behini lagn* (patrilateral cross-cousin marriage) and *mama bhachi lagn* (materal uncle–niece marriage) were extremely helpful in establishing accurately the type of consanguineous mating, and expression like *sakhi* (first cousin), *chult* (second cousin), and *lamcha nata* (distantly related) clearly differentiated the degree of relatedness. As a check, genealogies were also taken.

The responses were entered as (1) unrelated (where no consanguinity could be established); (2) distantly related (all related marriages other than first cousins); (3) first cross-cousin matrilateral and patrilateral marriages; and (4) maternal uncle–niece marriages. In order to retain strict comparability with earlier studies, in the present analysis category 2 was grouped with category 1.

Data related to the distances between the villages of the spouses were collected personally by the interview method. The distances between those two places as reported by the respondents were later cross-checked. Sometimes, when errors were detected upon cross-checking they were corrected to the actual distances. It is important to note that the distances reported here are along the *travel route* between the spouses' villages and are *not* direct map distances.

The population estimates for these castes are based on figures provided mostly by the leaders of these castes. In cases where the population sizes are less than 20,000, the estimates are highly reliable (over 95%). Most of these castes have their own associations or societies, and they could provide reliable figures. But in the case of castes numbering over 100,000, the estimates may not always be very reliable. In each case of these various estimates provided, we have accepted the lowest figure because the leaders generally tried to inflate the figures for political reasons.

5. Results

5.1. Inbreeding

5.1.1. Caste-cluster variation. There are three types of consanguineous matings that occur at nontrivial frequencies. Both types of cross-cousin (matrilateral and patrilateral) and maternal uncle–niece unions are encountered in varying degrees among the Dhangar caste-cluster (Table I), but both types of parallel-cousin marriages are absent.

Matrilateral cross-cousin marriages are the most preferred and are found in all the castes. The frequency varies from 10.6% to 59.67% with a series average of 21.5%. The next preferred type is patrilateral cross-cousin marriage. It is absent among three castes (the two Gadhari castes and the Telangi), but among other castes it varies from 0.21% to 17.78% with a series average of 3.35%. It is certain that the Gadhari, who migrated from the north, have a taboo against this type of marriage, but the Telangi attach no such stigma to it. The variation in maternal uncle–niece marriages is striking. Such marriages are absent in 11 castes, and among the remainder, the frequency ranges from 0.60% to 14.29% with a series average of 1.53%. The castes in whom it is absent are located in the northern districts of Maharashtra.

Over a quarter (26.39%) of all marriages are consanguineous. The intercaste variaion with respect to total consanguineous marriages is large; it ranges from 18.18% to 61.88%. Broadly speaking, consanguineous marriages are more frequent among the castes of southern Maharashtra (see Figure 2). Intercaste comparisons suggest much heterogeneity; out of 231 caste-pair comparisons, 96 pairs show differences significant at the 5% level and 69 of these at the 1% level.

The mean coefficient of inbreeding (α) for autosomal genes varies from 0.008 to 0.039 with a series average of 0.017. The Dhangar castes living in the

Table I
Inbreeding among the Dhangar Castes of Maharashtra

		Consanguineous marriages (%)				
Dhangar castes	*N*	Matrilateral	Patrilateral	Uncle–niece	Total	α
Ahir	473	24.31	0.21	0.00	24.52	0.015
Dange	383	26.89	6.27	1.04	34.20	0.022
Gadhari-Dhangar	131	19.08	0.00	0.00	19.08	0.012
Gadhari-Nikhar	64	18.75	0.00	0.00	18.75	0.012
Halmat	21	14.29	14.29	14.29	42.86	0.036
Hande	76	31.58	2.63	6.58	40.79	0.030
Hatkar	978	23.01	17.78	2.25	29.35	0.020
Hattikankan	47	19.15	6.38	6.38	31.91	0.024
Kannade	111	35.13	2.70	0.00	37.84	0.024
Khatik	253	15.87	2.37	0.00	18.18	0.011
Khutekar	827	18.86	2.06	0.60	21.52	0.014
Kurmar	163	20.86	1.23	0.00	22.08	0.014
Ladshe	133	18.80	3.76	0.00	22.56	0.014
Mendhe	333	15.31	3.30	4.80	23.42	0.018
Sangar	232	12.93	6.03	0.86	19.83	0.013
Shegar	165	21.82	3.03	0.61	25.45	0.016
Telangi	75	18.67	0.00	0.00	18.67	0.012
Thellari	181	59.67	2.21	0.00	61.88	0.039
Unnikankan	81	14.81	9.88	4.94	29.63	0.022
Varhade	151	10.61	1.99	0.00	12.58	0.008
Zende	252	15.08	7.54	6.35	28.97	0.022
Zade	152	13.82	4.60	0.00	18.42	0.011
Total	5282	21.51	3.35	1.53	26.39	0.017

southern districts of Maharashtra have high values (generally above 0.020), and so do—strangely—the Thellari (0.039) from northwestern Maharashtra. The mean inbreeding estimates obtained here are based on first cross-cousin and uncle–niece marriages only, and are, therefore, minimal estimates. The actual estimates based on pedigrees will be higher, because 1533 (29.40%) marriages, considered in this preliminary analysis as unrelated, were between distantly related individuals. This, however, does not invalidate the interpretation of the castes and geographical differences observed here.

5.1.2. Geographical variation. Data on the spatial distribution of consanguinity in 2827 marriages among Dhangar castes are shown in Table II and Figures 3–6. Although it would have been of interest to analyze the data at village levels separately for each caste and to bring out details of geographical

Table II
Inbreeding in Districts of Maharashtra: Pooled Dhangar Data

District	N	Consanguineous marriages (%)				α
		Matrilateral	Patrilateral	Uncle–niece	Total	
Ahmadanagar	145	28.28	2.76	0.00	31.03	0.021
Akola	70	10.00	1.43	0.00	11.43	0.021
Amravati	90	11.11	2.22	0.00	13.33	0.008
Aurangabad	94	14.89	0.00	0.00	14.89	0.009
Bhandara	55	23.64	7.27	0.00	30.91	0.019
Bhir	74	12.16	1.35	0.00	13.51	0.008
Buldhana	15	46.67	0.00	0.00	46.67	0.029
Chanda	70	20.00	2.86	0.00	22.86	0.014
Dhulia	137	44.52	0.00	0.00	44.53	0.028
Jalgaon	44	25.00	0.00	0.00	25.00	0.016
Kolaba	48	31.25	4.17	0.00	35.42	0.022
Kolhapur	262	16.03	9.16	4.20	29.39	0.021
Nagpur	171	16.96	5.85	0.00	22.81	0.014
Nanded	54	12.96	5.55	5.55	24.07	0.018
Nasik	133	21.80	0.00	0.00	21.80	0.013
Osmanabad	69	8.69	1.45	5.80	15.94	0.013
Parbhani	70	20.00	2.86	0.00	22.86	0.014
Poona	331	20.85	3.02	0.30	24.17	0.015
Ratnagiri	30	20.00	0.00	0.00	20.00	0.012
Sangli	157	10.19	9.55	7.64	27.39	0.022
Satara	337	12.17	5.64	0.89	18.69	0.012
Sholapur	239	15.06	5.44	2.09	22.59	0.015
Wardha	65	9.23	3.08	0.00	12.31	0.008
Yeotmal	67	14.92	1.49	0.00	16.42	0.010
Total	2827	18.15	4.10	1.38	23.63	0.016

variation, if any, within single castes, this was impractical because of the small sample size. Therefore only data pooled into districts have been considered. In this analysis, the matrilateral type of marriage, as was expected, is present in all 24 districts and ranges in frequency from 8.69% to 46.67%. An increasing trend from south to north is obvious. In the northwestern districts (Dhulia, Jalgaon, Buldhana, Nasik, and Aurangabad) adjacent to Gujarat and Madhya Pradesh, only this type is present (Figure 3). The patrilateral type is absent in the five northwestern districts and in Ratnagiri, a coastal district, and its incidence elsewhere ranges up to 9.55%. By contrast to the matrilateral type, its incidence decreases from south to north, though there are notable frequencies in Nagpur and Bhandara districts in the northeast (Figure 4). The uncle–niece type is

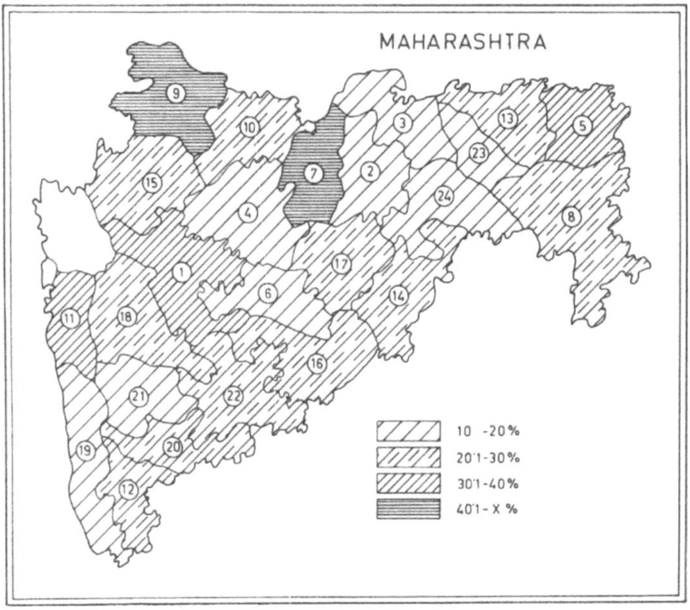

Figure 3. Incidence of matrilateral cross-cousin marriages in different districts of Maharashtra.

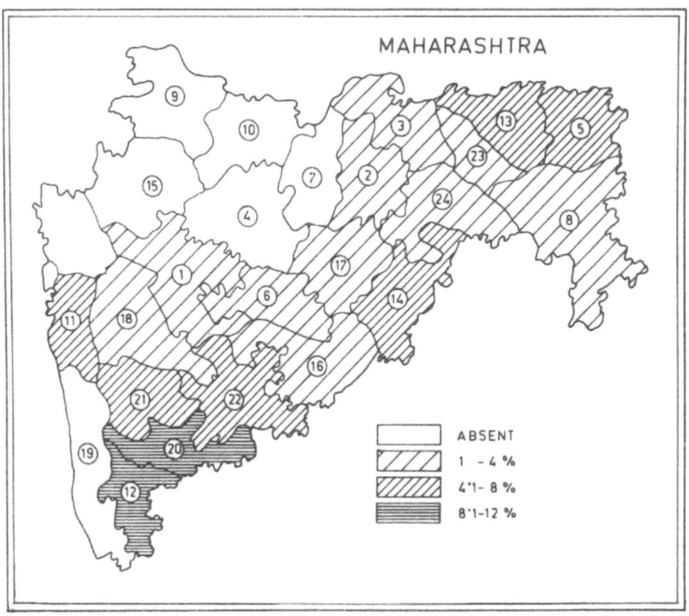

Figure 4. Incidence of patrilateral cross-cousin marriages in different districts of Maharashtra.

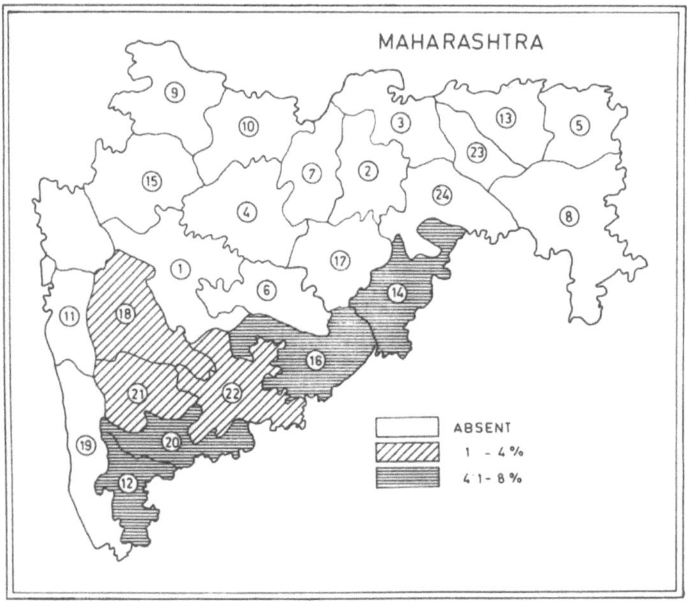

Figure 5. Incidence of uncle–niece marriages in different districts of Maharashtra.

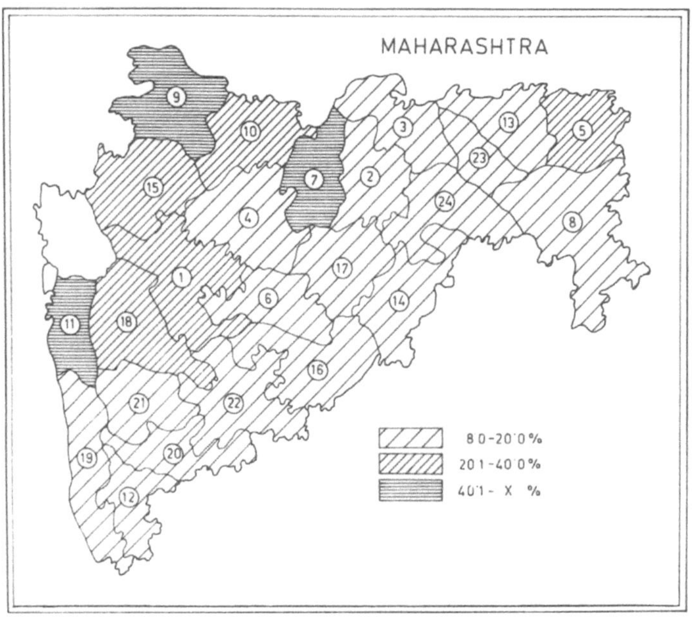

Figure 6. Incidence of total consanguineous marriages in different districts of Maharashtra.

present in only seven districts, and all of them, except Pune, are adjacent to Karnataka and Andhra Pradesh. In these districts the incidence ranged up to 7.64%, and also decreased from south to north (Figure 5).

District differences in incidence of total consanguineous marriages, like those between castes, are quite pronounced, ranging from 11.43% to 46.67%. Out of 276 district–pair comparisons, 73 pairs showed differences significant at 5% and 44 of these at 1%. Unlike the individual marriage types, the distribution of total related marriages shows no clear-cut spatial pattern, though, broadly speaking, the northwestern and northeastern districts have higher incidences than do southern districts (Figure 6). Several of the central districts have low levels. This does not fully agree with the caste distribution, perhaps because of the fact that 10 separate castes were sampled in each district.

The mean coefficient of inbreeding (α) for autosomal genes in the districts varies from 0.008 to 0.029, with a series average of 0.016. These estimates by district vary slightly from those obtained by caste; this may be because the samples for the two series were different and all the villages were not the same in both series. The values, in general, tend to be lower in the north-central districts, except in Buldhana (Figure 7).

5.1.3. Geographical variation within castes. A few of the Dhangar castes have a wide geographical distribution. It would be of interest to examine

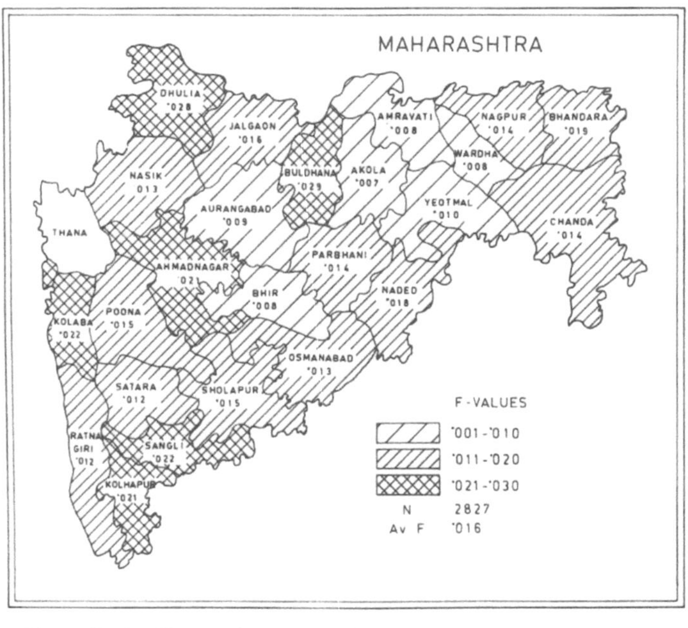

Figure 7. Coefficient of inbreeding in different districts of Maharashtra.

whether the results, mentioned previously, would be observed within a single endogamous, widely distributed caste. For the present analysis, four castes—Hatkar, Khutekar, Ahir, and Dange—that were sampled in at least four districts were selected. A total of 987 Hatkars, 827 Khutekars, 473 Ahirs, and 383 Danges were sampled from 14, 15, 8, and 6 districts, respectively. The names of the districts, their geographical locations, and the number of persons investigated for each caste separately are given in Tables III to VI and in Figures 8, 9, 10, and 11.

The incidence of different types of related marriages, total consanguineous marriages, and the coefficient of inbreeding (α) for each district—separately for each of the four castes—are given in Tables III–VI and Figures 8–11. These tables reveal pronounced differences in the rate of consanguineous marriages between the districts for each caste. Among the Hatkars, the consanguineous marriages range from 20.97% to 42.06% (average 28.67%); the Khutekars have a range from 6.84% to 38.16% (average 21.52%); the Ahirs reveal a range from 12.94% to 50.88% (average 24.52%), and the Danges show a range of 11.92% to 45.57% (average 34.20%).

Several of the differences among the districts are statistically significant. From these results it is clear that significant interdistrict differences exist within all the four castes; the level of interdistrict variation, however, varies among

Table III
Percentage Frequency of Consanguineous Marriages and Coefficient of Inbreeding (α) among the Hatkar Dhangars Sampled in 14 Maharashtrian Districts

District	*N*	Matrilateral	Patrilateral	Uncle–niece	Total	α
Ahmadnagar	107	38.32	3.74	0.00	42.06	0.026
Aurangabad	9	22.22	0.00	0.00	22.22	0.014
Bhir	38	21.05	2.63	0.00	23.68	0.015
Dhulia	57	29.82	0.00	0.00	29.82	0.019
Jalgaon	16	37.50	0.00	0.00	37.50	0.023
Nanded	18	6.25	0.00	18.75	25.00	0.024
Nasik	104	26.92	0.00	0.00	26.92	0.017
Osmanabad	54	12.96	7.41	7.41	27.78	0.022
Parbhani	24	25.00	4.17	0.00	29.17	0.018
Poona	135	30.37	3.70	0.00	34.07	0.021
Sangli	9	0.00	22.22	11.11	33.33	0.028
Satara	124	13.71	7.26	0.00	20.97	0.013
Sholapur	220	14.09	5.91	6.36	26.36	0.020
Yeotmal	72	22.22	1.39	0.00	23.61	0.015
Total	987	23.39	4.05	2.23	28.67	0.019

Table IV
Percentage Frequency of Consanguineous Marriages and Coefficient of Inbreeding (α) among the Khutekar Dhangars Sampled in 15 Maharashtrian Districts

Districts	N	Matrilateral	Patrilateral	Uncle–niece	Total	α
Ahmadnagar	169	29.58	0.09	0.00	30.18	0.019
Akola	1	—	—	—	—	—
Amraoti	117	5.13	1.71	0.00	6.84	0.004
Aurangabad	17	23.53	0.00	0.00	23.53	0.015
Bhir	76	38.16	0.00	0.00	38.16	0.024
Jalgaon	14	21.43	0.00	0.00	21.43	0.013
Nanded	69	20.20	4.35	0.00	24.64	0.015
Nasik	34	20.59	0.00	0.00	20.59	0.013
Osmanabad	68	5.88	4.41	2.94	13.23	0.010
Parbhani	31	9.68	3.22	0.00	12.90	0.008
Poona	64	10.94	4.69	0.00	15.62	0.010
Satara	65	12.31	3.08	0.00	15.38	0.010
Sholapur	55	14.54	3.64	5.45	23.64	0.018
Wardha	4	—	—	—	—	—
Yeotmal	43	23.25	0.00	0.00	23.25	0.014
Total	827	18.86	2.06	0.60	21.52	0.014

these castes. In Table VII mean consanguineous marriages per district and their standard deviations are given for each caste. The Danges appear to be most variable; the Ahirs the least variable.

5.1.4. Geographical variation in uncle–niece marriages. Among three

Table V
Percentage frequency of Consanguineous Marriages and Coefficient of Inbreeding (α) among the Ahir Dhangars Sampled in 8 Maharashtrian Districts

Districts	N	Matrilateral	Patrilateral	Uncle–niece	Total	α
Ahmadnagar	57	50.88	0.00	0.00	50.88	0.032
Akola	85	11.76	1.18	0.00	12.94	0.008
Amraoti	67	13.43	0.00	0.00	13.43	0.008
Aurangabad	22	36.36	0.00	0.00	36.36	0.023
Buldhana	71	21.13	0.00	0.00	21.13	0.013
Dhulia	33	18.18	0.00	0.00	18.18	0.011
Jalgaon	56	19.64	0.00	0.00	19.64	0.012
Nasik	82	32.93	0.00	0.00	32.93	0.021
Total	473	24.31	0.21	0.00	24.52	0.015

Table VI
Percentage Frequency of Consanguineous Marriages and Coefficient of Inbreeding (α) among the Dange Dhangars Sampled in 6 Districts of Maharashtra

Districts	*N*	Matrilateral	Patrilateral	Uncle–niece	Total	α
Aurangabad	1	—	—	—	—	—
Kolaba	79	40.51	3.80	1.26	45.57	0.029
Kolhapur	194	22.68	8.25	0.51	3.44	0.020
Poona	2	—	—	—	—	—
Ratnagiri	43	20.93	2.32	0.00	23.26	0.014
Satara	64	8.81	2.07	1.04	11.92	0.023
Total	383	26.89	6.27	1.04	34.20	0.022

castes—the Hatkar, Khutekar, and Dange—although uncle–niece marriages do occur, their incidence is rather low, 2.23%, 0.60%, and 1.04%, respectively. The Ahirs who live in northwestern Maharashtra completely lack such marriages; in fact, in this caste there is a strong taboo against such marriages. An examination of seven districts in which such marriages have been encountered in the three castes shows that, except Kolaba, all other districts (Nanded, Osmanabad, San-

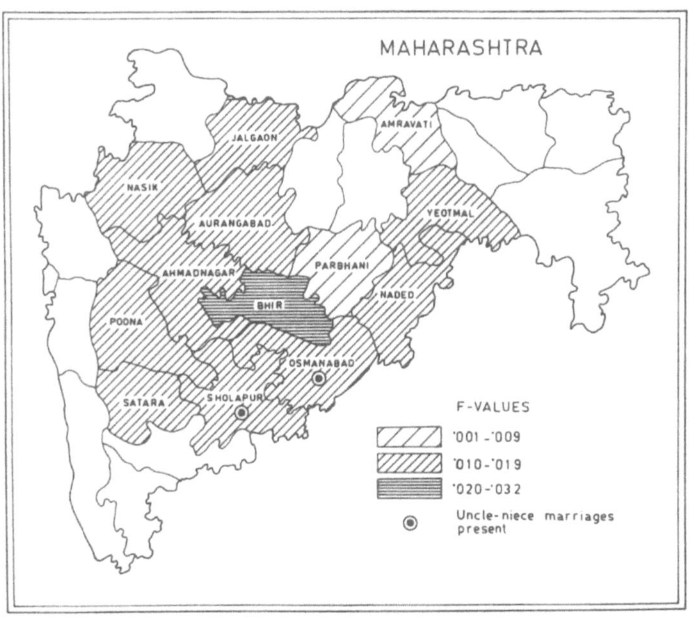

Figure 8. Spatial variation in the coefficient of inbreeding among the Hatkars.

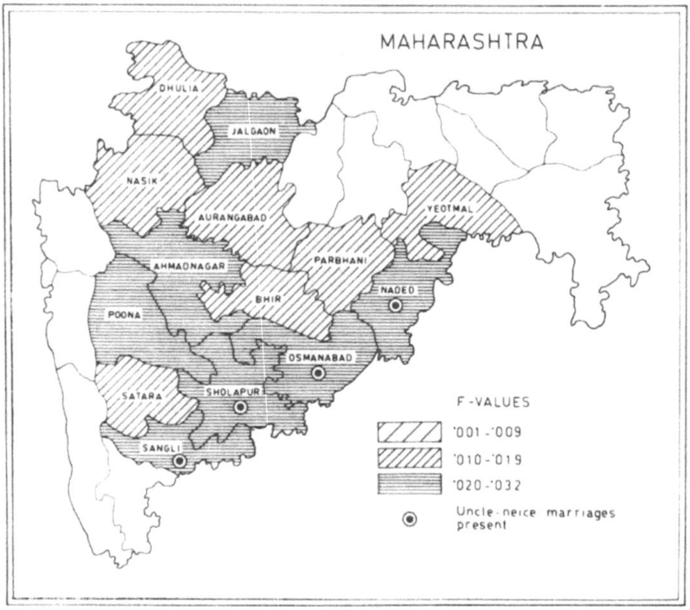

Figure 9. Spatial variation in the coefficient of inbreeding among the Khutekars.

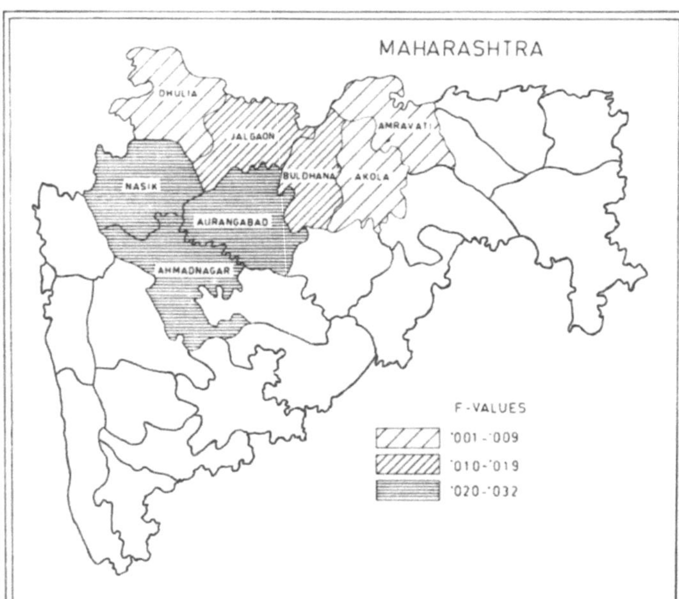

Figure 10. Spatial variation in the coefficient of inbreeding among the Ahirs.

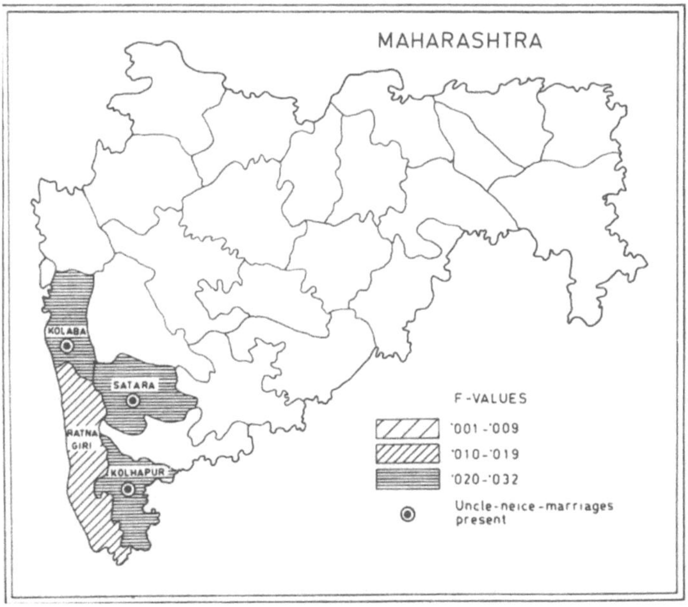

Figure 11. Spatial variation in the coefficient of inbreeding among the Dange.

gli, Sholapur, Kolhapur, and Satara) share a border with the two Dravidian-speaking states, Andhra Pradesh and Karnataka (for details, see Figures 8, 9, and 11). In these two states uncle–niece marriages are not only preferred, but they are prescriptive (Karve, 1953). In Andhra Pradesh, 9.65% of 6374 Hindu marriages were of this type (Sanghvi, 1966). Another noteworthy aspect about these

Table VII
Mean Consanguineous Marriages at District Level among the Four Dhangar Castes

Dhangar castes	Total consanguineous marriages	Number of districts	Mean ± S.E.	S.D.
Hatkar	283	14	20.21 ± 1.20	18.06
Khutekar[a]	175	13	13.46 ± 1.02	13.16
Ahir	116	8	14.50 ± 1.35	8.75
Dange[b]	130	4	32.50 ± 2.85	21.76

[a]Because of small sample sizes, the districts Akola and Wardha are not included in these computations.
[b]The districts of Aurangabad and Poona are excluded from these computations.

Table VIII
Analysis of Variance (Three Castes—Hatkar, Khutekar, Ahir; Four Districts—Ahmadnagar, Aurangabad, Jalgaon, and Nasik)

	df	SS	MS	F
Between districts	3	2618.25	872.75	9.38
Between populations	2	32.67	16.33	0.18
Residual	6	558.00	93.00	—
Total	11	3208.92		

marriages is that although Hatkar and Khutekar do practice them, they are confined only to the residents of southern districts.

5.1.5. Analysis of consanguinity rates between castes and between districts. As noted previously, geographical proximity had a profound effect on the prevalence of the types of consanguineous marriages. In order to examine whether this also holds true with respect to the total rate of related marriages, the data were further analyzed as follows: In four districts, Ahmednagar, Aurangabad, Jalgaon, and Nasik, all the three castes, namely, Hatkar, Khutekar, and Ahir, were sampled. Analysis of variance showed that although the differences between the districts were significant (*f* ratio, 9.38; *df* 3 and 6; these were significant at the 5% level), the differences between the castes were nonsignificant (Table VIII). These results clearly establish the fact that geographical proximity does play an important role in shaping mating patterns.

5.1.6. Geographical variation in coefficient of inbreeding. To evaluate whether the coefficient of inbreeding (α) decreases as one moves from southern to northern districts in Maharashtra, the α values have been plotted for each district and for each caste separately in Figures 8–11. Generally speaking, all four castes show higher values of α in southern districts and the values decrease in northern districts. The result that even in a single endogamous caste the α decreases in northern districts supports the earlier conclusions reached on pooled district-wide distribution of α among 22 Dhangar castes.

5.2. Mean Matrimonial Distances (MMD)

5.2.1. Distribution. The distribution of matrimonial distances for the 21 Dhangar castes are all apparently extremely skewed positively. Values of β_1, β_2, W_1 and W_2 are in Table IX, from which it is very clear that all the distributions are positively skewed, and most of them (except 4) are leptokurtic too.

Although the distributions of *MMD* are all similar—in the sense that they are positively skewed and leptokurtic—there are some striking differences. For

Table IX
Mean Matrimonial Distances, Variances and Measures of Skewness and Kurtosis of the Distributions of Matrimonial Distances of 21 Dhangar Castes

		Matrimonial distance (miles)					
Population group	Sample size[a]	Mean	Variance	Skewness	Kurtosis	W_1	W_2[b]
Ahir	253 (11.19)	14.36	166.54	3.44	7.70	12.19	15.58
Dange	160 (7.08)	7.17	426.70	85.76	101.75	48.72	261.52
Gadhari-Dhengar	72 (3.19)	22.94	893.94	0.99	2.73	3.59	−0.34[b]
Hande	59 (2.61)	16.74	539.04	5.07	7.88	7.43	8.36
Hatkar	231 (10.22)	10.53	191.55	5.80	10.57	15.14	23.98
Hattikankan	50 (2.21)	10.34	72.94	1.99	4.78	4.32	2.97
Kannade	55 (2.43)	16.35	344.30	12.07	18.54	11.10	25.47
Khatik	111 (4.91)	50.29	3429.03	0.85	2.66	4.07	−0.64[b]
Khutekar	358 (15.84)	16.77	1196.57	108.68	132.54	81.20	505.99
Kurmar	89 (3.94)	11.57	303.55	10.81	16.74	13.09	27.81
Ladshe	89 (3.94)	18.29	952.77	6.62	10.83	10.25	15.90
Mendhe	98 (4.34)	6.91	48.84	1.84	4.39	5.65	3.05
Sangar	62 (2.74)	18.27	797.20	9.86	16.36	10.59	23.07
Shegar	61 (2.70)	13.72	189.41	1.80	4.83	4.49	3.27
Telangi	59 (2.61)	9.66	131.75	10.70	3.44	10.79	0.91[b]
Thellari	103 (4.56)	6.42	76.75	8.66	6.11	12.55	6.82
Unnikankan	55 (2.43)	10.02	111.40	66.35	4.87	26.03	3.22
Varhade	50 (2.21)	23.42	537.76	2.83	4.82	5.15	3.03
Zende	126 (5.58)	8.51	100.68	2.40	5.20	7.27	5.32
Zade	52 (2.30)	22.31	688.83	3.89	7.09	6.15	6.68
Gadhari-Nikhar	67 (2.96)	18.10	237.29	1.14	3.74	3.73	1.47[b]

[a]Figures in parentheses are percentage sample sizes out of a total of 2260.
[b]These figures are insignificant at 5% level. All remaining values are significant at 5% level. All the W_1 values are significant at 5% level.

the purpose of elucidating some of these differences, I have selected five castes: one from northwestern Maharashtra (Ahir), one from northeastern (Varhade), one from the southwestern coast (Dange), one from the central area (Khatik), and one caste (Khutekar) that is spread over 17 districts of the state. The distributions of *MMD* for these five castes are given in Figure 12. Whereas, among the Danges, 70% of marriages take place at a distance of $\leq$ 5 mi, the corresponding figures for Ahirs and Varhades are 22.92% and 12.0%, respectively. The distribution of *MMD* for Khatik is bimodal (highly noteworthy), one mode lying near 0 and the other at a distance of about 90 mi. The distribution for Khutekars, although leptokurtic, tapers off more gradually than the distributions of the other groups. The distribution of matrimonial distances for the pooled series is also positively skewed and leptokurtic (Figure 12).

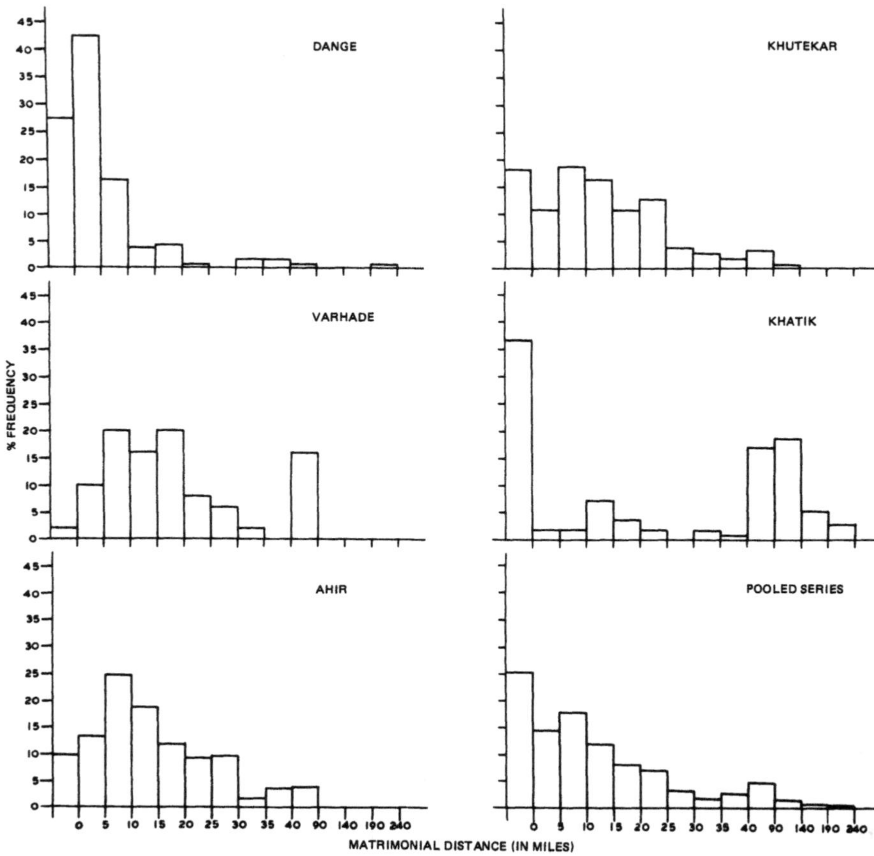

Figure 12. Distribution of matrimonial distances for five Dhangar castes and Dhangar pooled data.

Considerable variation is observed in the *MMD* (Table IX). It varies from 6.42 mi (Thellaris) to 50.29 mi (Khatiks). It appears that the *MMD* increase as one moves from south to north. A pairwise comparison of *MMD* indicates that most of the castes are different from each other (120 out of 210 pair comparisons turned out be significant at the 5% level). Only one small cluster of similar mean values is discernible, which consists of Varhade, Ladshe, Kannade, and Zade.

5.2.2. Variation between districts. This analysis has been attempted on the four widely distributed castes, namely, the Hatkar, Khutekar, Ahir, and Dange. A total of 471 Hatkars, 309 Khutekars, 273 Ahirs, and 146 Danges were sampled from eight, seven, five, and three districts in Maharashtra, respectively. Names of the districts along with the number of persons investigated for each caste are given separately in Tables X–XIII and Figures 13–16. Considerable

Table X
Incidence of Intravillage Marriages and Mean Matrimonial Distances among Eight Subsamples of Hatkar Dhangars[a]

Districts in Maharashtra	Sample size	Marriages within the village: Number	Marriages within the village: Percentage	Mean marriage distance: Mean ± S.E.	Mean marriage distance: S.D.
Ahmadnagar	30	8	26.67	11.37 ± 1.82	9.98
Dhulia	36	4	11.11	10.89 ± 1.35	8.10
Nasik	74	21	28.38	16.00 ± 2.02	17.40
Osmanabad	38	7	18.42	12.76 ± 2.14	13.22
Poona	53	10	18.87	11.41 ± 1.54	11.21
Satara	69	21	30.43	8.28 ± 1.02	8.49
Sholapur	139	63	45.32	8.56 ± 1.24	14.64
Yeotmal	32[1]	5	15.62	24.72 ± 3.53	19.99
Total	471	139	29.51		

[a]There was one marriage at the distance of 400 mi that has been excluded.

variation is observed in *MMD* in different districts inhabited by a single caste. Among the Hatkars the *MMD* varies from 8.28 mi in Satara district to 24.72 mi in Yeotmal district; the Khutekars show a range of 7.89 mi in Nanded district to 16.89 mi in Nasik district. Ahirs and Dange show relatively less variation; the range is 10.97 mi to 16.50 mi, and 4.50 mi to 6.58 mi, respectively.

Table XI
Incidence of Intravillage Marriage and Mean Matrimonial Distances (*MMD*) among Seven Subsamples of Khutekar Dhangars

Districts in Maharashtra	Sample size	Intravillage marriage: Number	Intravillage marriage: Percentage	Mean marriage distance: Mean ± S.E.	Mean marriage distance: S.D.
Ahmadnagar	104	26	25.00	14.92 ± 1.35	13.81
Amraoti	66	3	4.54	15.17 ± 1.38	11.25
Aurangabad	18	3	16.67	12.67 ± 1.88	7.97
Bhir	34	9	26.47	12.03 ± 1.88	10.98
Nanded	36	12	33.33	7.89 ± 1.15	6.89
Nasik	19	3	15.79	16.89 ± 3.86	16.83
Osmanabad	32	4	12.50	11.84 ± 2.08	11.75
Total	309	60	19.42		

Table XII
Incidence of Intravillage Marriages and Mean Matrimonial Distances *MMD* in Five Subsamples of Ahir Dhangars

Districts in Maharashtra	Sample size	Intravillage marriage		Mean marriage distance	
		Number	Percentage	Mean ± S.E.	S.D.
Ahmadnagar	51	3	5.88	13.23 ± 1.53	10.93
Akola	44	0	0.00	16.50 ± 1.65	10.97
Buldhana	61	6	9.84	10.97 ± 1.16	9.09
Jalgaon	42	8	19.05	15.45 ± 2.59	16.77
Nasik	39	7	17.95	13.18 ± 1.97	12.32
Total	237	24	10.13		

A pairwise comparison of the *MMD* between districts, as expected, revealed significant differences within the Hatkars and Khutekars. Ahirs who were sampled in five districts revealed significant difference only for one pair of districts, that is, Akola and Buldhana. The Dange sampled in three districts show homogeneous distribution for *MMD*. It is clear from Tables X–XIII and Figures 13–16 that the *MMD* increases as one moves from southern districts to northern ones.

5.3. Intravillage Marriages

5.3.1. Intercaste variation. The frequency of intravillage marriages shows considerable variation among the castes and varies from 2% (Varhade) to

Table XIII
Incidence of Intravillage Marriages and Mean Matrimonial Distances (*MMD*) among Three Subsamples of Dange Dhangars

Districts in Maharashtra	Sample size	Intravillage marriage		Mean marriage distance	
		Number	Percentage	Men ± S.E.	S.D.
Colaba	36	8	22.22	4.50 ± 0.80	4.80
Kolhapur	79	25	31.64	4.90 ± 0.82	7.33
Satara	31	11	35.48	6.58 ± 2.64	14.72
Total	146	44	20.14		

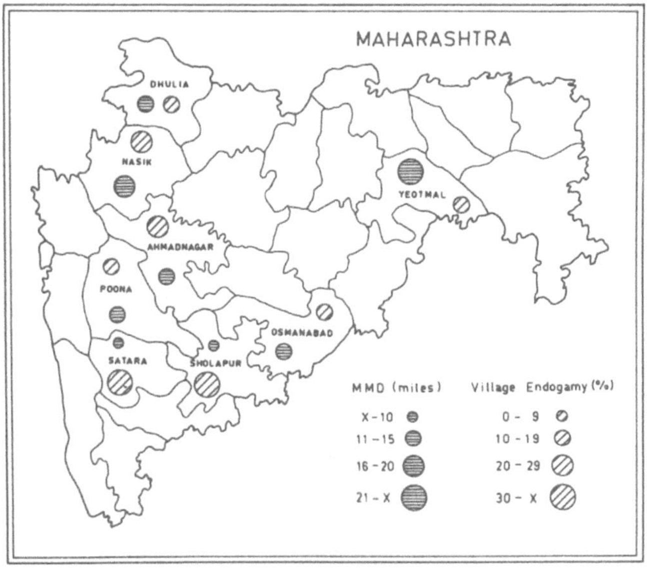

Figure 13. Spatial variation in *MMD* (mean matrimonial distance) and village endogamy within the Hatkar Dhangars.

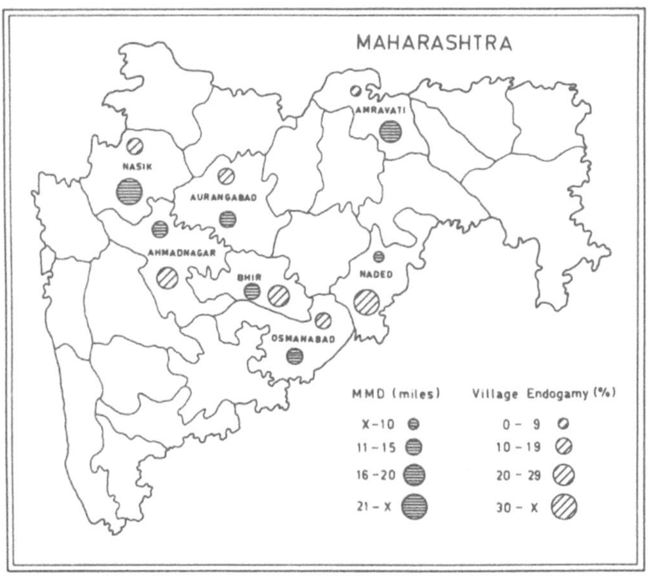

Figure 14. Spatial variation in *MMD* and village endogamy within the Khutekar Dhangars.

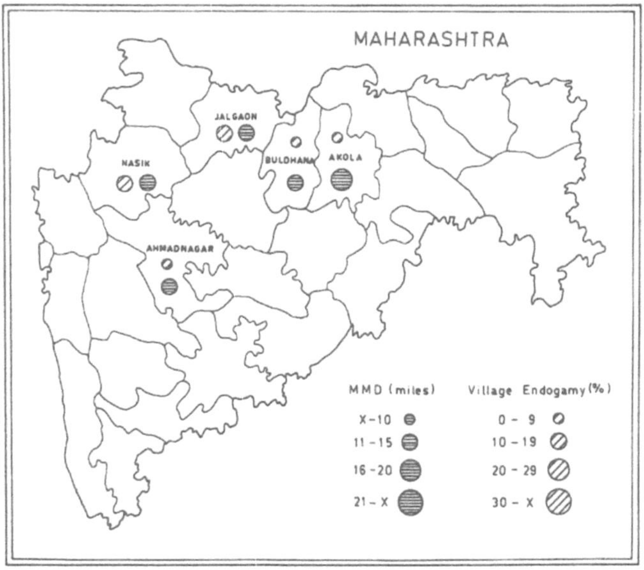

Figure 15. Spatial variation in *MMD* and village endogamy within the Ahir Dhangars.

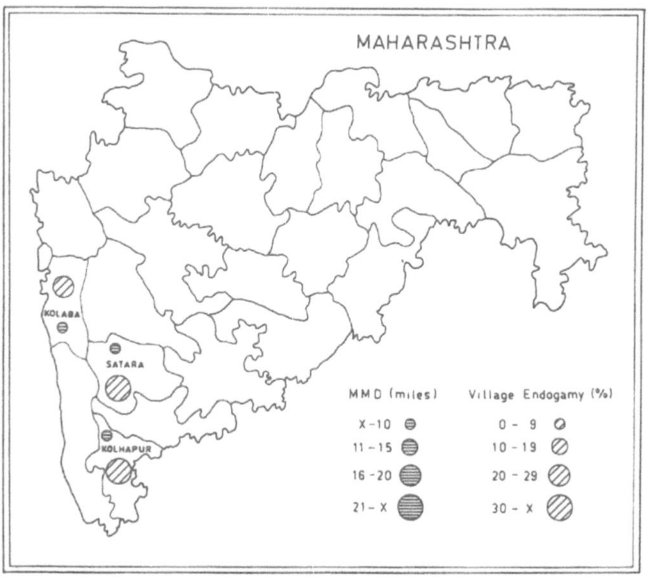

Figure 16. Spatial variation in *MMD* and village endogamy among the Dange.

47.22% (Gadhari Nikhar); the series average is 25.44% (Table VIII). Generally speaking, it appears that as one moves northward, the frequency of village endogamy decreases.

5.3.2. Variation between districts. As in the case of *MMD*, here also, four castes, Hatkar, Khutekar, Ahir, and Dange, have been studied for variation between districts with respect to intravillage marriages. The frequency of intravillage marriages, for each district and for each caste separately, are given in Tables X–XIII and Figures 13–16. All four castes reveal varying degrees of variation between the districts. Among the Hatkars, intravillage marriages range from 11.11% in Dhulia district to 45.32% in Sholapur district (average 29.51%); the Khutekars reveal a range of 4.54% in the Amraoti district to 33.33% in the Nanded district (average 19.42%); Ahirs show a range of 0% in Akola district to 17.95% in Hasik district (average 10.13%), and the Danges, a range of 22.22% in Kolaba district to 35.48% in Satara district (average 30.14%).

It is noteworthy that the two castes, Hatkar and Khutekar, who have a much wider geographical distribution, also reveal a larger variation in the incidence of intravillage marriages. It is also obvious that the frequency of village endogamy is higher in the southern districts and decreases as one moves northward.

5.4. Relationship between α, *MMD* and Village Endogamy

5.4.1. Relationship between α and *MMD*. Data on α and *MMD* are available on 20 samples at caste level and 23 samples at district level (Figure 17). The distribution, generally speaking, shows a negative relationship between

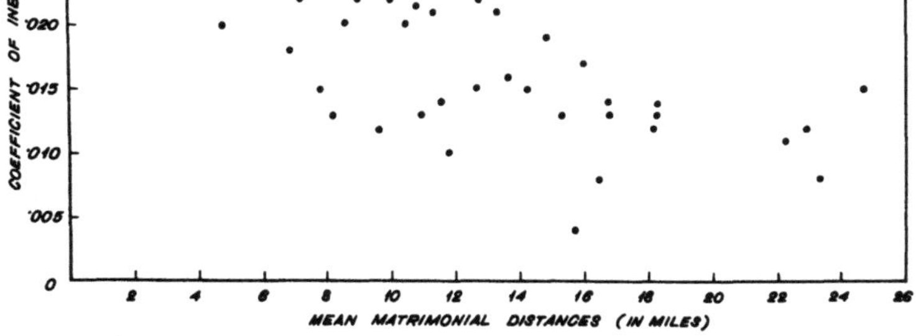

Figure 17. Joint distribution of matrimonial distances and coefficient of inbreeding in 43 samples.

these two variables. The value of coefficient of correlation (r), -0.684, is significant ($t = 6.0$; $df = 41$). The relationship appears to be linear.

5.4.2. Relationship between α and village endogamy. A joint distribution of the frequency of village endogamy and α among the 43 samples reveals that these two variables do not conform to any definite pattern. It is therefore obvious that rates of village endogamy do not influence the α in any regular fashion, or, at least, it is not discernible in the present population samples.

5.4.3. Relationship between village endogamy and *MMD*. Because the level of village endogamy and *MMD*, as observed earlier, show considerable variation, it was found desirable to examine the relationship between these two variables. For this analysis, data on both these variables were available also for 43 population samples. An examination of the joint distribution between these two variables suggests that although in some samples the *MMD* decreases with an increase in village endogamy, for the majority of the samples it is not true. Thus, we may conclude that like α, village endogamy does not influence *MMD* in any definite predictable direction.

6. Discussion

From the analysis presented in the preceding section the following main points emerge.

1. The frequency of consanguineous marriages in the Dhangar caste-cluster are fairly high, and pronounced intercaste variations exist.
2. All three types of matings show definite spatial patterns—matrilateral unions increase northward, whereas patrilateral and uncle–niece unions decrease northward. Castes inhabiting the southern districts of Maharashtra, in general have a higher mean coefficient of inbreeding for autosomal genes.
3. Considerable amount of variation in the rate of consanguineous matings between the districts in a single widely distributed caste has been shown.
4. It has been observed that geographical proximity had profound effect on the prevalence of the types and magnitudes of consanguineous marriages and, consequently, upon the coefficient of inbreeding.
5. The general form of the distribution of matrimonial distances is one that is extremely skewed positively and leptokurtic (with the exception of Khatiks where it is bimodal).
6. Considerable variation is observed in the mean matrimonial distances (range 6.4 mi to 50.29 mi).

7. The mean matrimonial distances are smaller in castes in the southern districts of Maharashtra when compared to the castes of northern districts.
8. Pronounced variation exists in matrimonial distances in different districts inhabited by a single caste.
9. Even within a single widely spread caste, the matrimonial distances tend to be shorter in southern districts as compared to the northern districts.
10. The frequency of intravillage marriages shows considerable variation among the castes (range 2% to 47.22%).
11. The frequency of village endogamy decreases as one moves northward; this feature is also seen within a single widely distributed caste.
12. The two variables, matrimonial distance and coefficient of inbreeding, show a negative relationship between them ($r = -0.684$).
13. The relationship between coefficient of inbreeding and rate of intravillage marriages and between intravillage marriages and matrimonial distances is weak and no pattern is discernible.

The preceding results can be best understood and interpreted by keeping in view the unique geographical position of the state of Maharashtra. In the north, it borders with Madhya Pradesh and Gujarat where predominantly Indo-Aryan languages are spoken. In the south, it shares a border with two Dravidian-speaking states, Karnataka and Andhra Pradesh. The kinship system and consequently the marriage patterns in the Indo-Aryan and Dravidian-speaking states are quite different. Broadly speaking, the Hindu castes in the former system have a strong taboo against village endogamy and consanguineous marriages, whereas in the latter system, there is no taboo against village endogamy, and certain types of consanguineous marriages are not only preferred but are also prescriptive. Thus, it was expected that the caste Hindus, depending upon where they resided in Maharashtra (north, central, south, or east), would reveal in varying intensities elements of both Dravidian and Indo-Aryan marriage customs. It was also further expected that the influence of Dravidian norms would be maximum in the populations of the southern districts of Maharashtra, whereas the maximum impact of Indo-Aryan customs would be seen in the populations of northern districts. More precisely, in terms of the three components of social structure considered here, our expectations were as follows: (1) the Dhangar caste-cluster, because of its wide geographical spread in Maharashtra, would show a large amount of variation in the three variables considered; (2) castes or parts thereof found in northern districts would depict a low frequency of intravillage marriages, low rates of consanguinity, and larger matrimonial distances; and (3) castes of southern districts would be characterized by a high frequency of intravillage marriage, high rates of consanguinity and consequently high α, and shorter matrimonial distances. It was further assumed that decreased rates of village endogamy and reduced rates of inbreeding would lead people to marry at greater distances, resulting in higher values of matrimonial distances.

Let us now examine whether these expectations are fulfilled in the present data. The results show that much variation occurs among the Dhangar castes with respect to the three components of social structure mentioned previously and that castes residing in southern Maharashtra and castes known to have migrated to northern districts from southern Maharashtra (like the Thellari) and from Mysore State (like the Kurmar and probably Kannade) have a higher incidence of consanguineous marriages, high rates of intravillage marriages, and shorter matrimonial distances. It is noteworthy that a similar situation is noticed even within a single caste distributed over a wide territory. With a few exceptions, the present results satisfy most of our expectations, and, therefore, the observed geographical pattern clearly demonstrates the influence of both Indo-Aryan and Dravidian marriage customs.

Let us now examine the results obtained with respect to the relationship between village endogamy, matrimonial distance, and coefficient of inbreeding. It is reasonable to assume that, generally speaking, in rural India close kin would be found within close geographical proximity. And, if the consanguineous marriages are preferred and/or prescriptive, this will have two effects: First, the incidence of consanguineous marriages would be higher, and second, the matrimonial distances would tend to be shorter. Thus, a linear negative relationship is expected between matrimonial distances and α. The obtained value of $r(-0.684)$, its significance level, and the joint distribution of these two variables indicate that the relationship is mostly linear. Similar negative relationship has also been found among Brazilian populations (Salzano and Freire-Maia, 1970) and in certain other populations of Maharashtra (Mukherjee *et al.*, 1980). Morton (1964) found a leptokurtic regression between these two variables.

Contrary to our expectations, however, the relationship between village endogamy and α and village endogamy and matrimonial distances in the present population samples reveal no definite pattern. Thus, it is seen that differential rates of village endogamy do not substantially affect α and matrimonial distances.

The observed relationship might be due to the fact that the populations included in the present study actually differ widely with respect to marriage customs. Our expectations about the castes where consanguinity is prescriptive were that a large number of such marriages would be between close relatives, whereas among castes who barely tolerate such marriages only a few marriages would be consanguineous.

It is, therefore, suggested that future work among the Dravidian-speaking states will probably reveal predictable relationships between these parameters of population structure.

The variations observed in the three components of social structure among the Dhangar caste-clusters would have differential effects on the temporal and local gene differentiation.

The analysis of the biological data collected on the Dhangar castes in the light of the present results is in progress, and the findings will be reported in a subsequent publication. However, on the basis of the present results, it can be stressed, though only qualitatively, that the extent and nature of local gene differentiation within and between the Dhangar castes will be quite variable. In general, the castes having shorter matrimonial distances will have smaller effective population sizes compared to castes having larger matrimonial distances (this will be true only if the population densities in all the castes are alike), and the variability in effective population sizes, coupled with variable coefficients of inbreeding, will lead to differential effects on the local gene differentiation among and within the Dhangar castes.

ACKNOWLEDGMENTS

I am grateful to Mrs. S. Kirtane, Mrs. K. Patkar, and Mrs. A. Kelkar of Decan College, Pune, who helped in the analysis of the data. Thanks are also due to Mrs. Awati, Miss V. Shirole, Mrs. U. S. Shastree, Mr. S. B. Khomne, and Dr. B. V. Bhanu who helped in collection of the data.

References

Boyce, A. J., Kuchemann, C. F., and Harrison, G. A., 1967, Neighbourhood knowledge and the distribution of marriage distances, *Ann. of Hum. Genet.* **30**:335–338.

Cavalli-Sforza, L. L., 1958, Some data on the genetic structure of human populations, *Proc. of the 10th Int. Congr. Genet.*, Toronto, Toronto University Press, Volume I, pp. 389–407.

Cavalli-Sforza, L. L., 1962, The distribution of marriage distances: Models and applications to genetics, in: *Les Deplacements Humains* (T. Sutter, ed.), Monaco Science Humains, Entret, pp. 139–158.

Chakraborty, R., Chakravarti, A., and Malhotra, K. C., 1977, Variation in allele frequencies among caste groups of the Dhangars of Maharashtra, India: An analysis with Wright's F_{st} statistics, *Ann. of Hum. Biol.* **4**:275–280.

Gadgil, M., and Malhotra, K. C., 1982, Adaptive Significance of the Indian Caste System: An Ecological Perspective (submitted for publication).

Hutton, J. H., 1963, *Caste in India,* Bombay, Oxford University Press.

Karve, I., 1953, *Kinship Organization in India,* Pune, Deccan College.

Karve, I., 1965, Research needed, *Curr. Anthropol.* **6**:332–333.

Karve, I., and Malhotra, K. C., 1968, Biological comparison of eight endogamous groups of the same rank, *Curr. Anthropol.* **9**:109–124.

Majumder, P. P., 1977, Matrimonial migration: A review, with special reference to India, *J. Biosoc. Sci.* **9**:381–401.

Majumder, P. P., and Malhotra, K. C., 1979, Matrimonial distance, inbreeding coefficient and population size: Dhangar data, *Ann. Hum. Biol.* **6**:17–27.

Malhotra, K. C., 1978, Natural selection and colour blindness: Fresh data on Indian castes, *Genet. Res.* **31**:203–207.

Malhotra, K. C., 1979a, Inbreeding among Dhanger castes of Maharashtra, India, *J. Biosoc. Res.* **11**:397–409.

Malhotra, K. C., 1979b, Inbreeding among four Dhangar castes of Maharashtra, India: Differences among districts, *Collegium Antropologicum* **3**:19–28.

Malhotra, K. C., 1979c, Qualitative finger dermatoglyphic variation among 21 endogamous Dhangar castes of Maharashtra, in: *Dermatoglyphics—50 years later* (W. Wertelecki and C. C. Plato, eds.) Birth defects, *Original Article Series* **15**:335–345.

Malhotra, K. C., 1980a, Matrimonial distances among the four Dhangar (shepherd) castes of Maharashtra, India: differences among districts, *South Asian Anthropol.* **1**:25–34.

Malhotra, K. C., 1980b, Gene dispersion in man: The Indian case, *Curr. Anthropol.* **21**:135–136.

Malhotra, K. C., and Majumder, P. P., 1974, A prospectus for studying the effects of marriage distance on genetic distance, *The Anthropologist,* **19**:33–40.

Malhotra, K. C., Chakraborty, R., and Chakravarti, A., 1977, Gene differentiation among the Dhangar caste-cluster of Maharashtra, India, *Hum. Hered.* **28**:26–36.

Malhotra, K. C., Das, S. K., Mukherjee, B. N., Bhanu, B. V., Undevia, J. V., Yee, S., and Majumder, P. P., 1977, Distribution of blood groups among 21 Dhangar castes of Maharashtra, *Indian J. Phys. Anthropol. Hum. Genet.* **3**:141–159.

Malhotra, K. C., and Gadgil, M., 1981, The ecological basis of the geographical distribution of the Dhangars: A pastoral caste-cluster of Maharashtra, *South Asian Anthropol.* **2**:49–60.

Mukherjee, B. N., Das, S. K., and Malhotra, K. C., 1976, Serum protein and enzyme polymorphism in the Dhangars of Maharashtra, *Indian J. Med. Res.* **64**:1240–1244.

Mukherjee, B. N., Das, S. K., Malhotra, K. C., and Das, S. R., 1977, Haptoglobin and acid phosphatase gene distribution in Dhangars of Maharashtra, India, *J. Genet.* **63**:39–44.

Mukherjee, B. N., Malhotra, K. C., Pakrasi, K., and Kate, S. L., 1980, Inbreeding, village endogamy and marriage distances: Spatial, temporal and social variation, *Homo* **31**:21–38.

Morton, N. E., 1964, Genetic studies of north eastern Brazil. *Cold Spring Harbor Symp. Quantit. Biol.* **29**:69–79.

Salzano, F. M., and Freire-Maia, N., 1970, *Problems in Human Biology: A study of Brazilian populations,* Detroit, Wayne State University Press.

Sanghvi, L. D., 1966, Inbreeding in India, *Eugenics Quarterly* **13**:291–301.

Wolanski, N., 1977, Selective migration: Mating distance and outcrossing, *Collegium Antropologicum* **1**:41–44.

CHAPTER 15

The Impact of Irrigation on the Demographic Structure of the Peshawar Basin of Northwest Pakistan

CHARLES A. WEITZ

1. Introduction

The neo-Malthusian perspective common in ecology suggests that populations possess the potential to increase geometrically until they reach some environmental limit. This limit constrains population growth beyond what is referred to as the *carrying capacity*. In human populations, it has been common to associate carrying capacity with food resources (Zubrow, 1976; Hassan, 1979), and to view increases in population as consequences of technological changes that increase food production (Watson and Watson, 1969). This perspective competes with the nearly opposite notion that population increases are the cause of agricultural intensification (Boserup, 1965; Cohen, 1977) as well as with the idea that the relationship between population sizes and resources is structured by social, political, and economic conditions (Zubrow, 1975; Hassan, 1979; Orlove, 1980).

The use of historical demographic data, particularly if they span some clear alteration in food supplies, would help clarify the relationship between resources and population growth. Such data exist during the latter part of the 19th century in western India where the British colonial government began the construction of

---

CHARLES A. WEITZ • Department of Anthropology, Temple University, Philadelphia, Pennsylvania 19122. This chapter is based on research supported by grants from the American Institute of Pakistan Studies, the American Philosophical Society, and Temple University.

irrigation canals on a truly massive scale. Because these irrigation networks abruptly increased food production, an excellent opportunity exists to test both the Malthusian and population pressure models.

2. The Peshawar Basin

2.1. Conditions Prior to Irrigation

Part of this construction occurred in the Peshawar region of what is presently northwestern Pakistan. Peshawar is a natural basin surrounded by mountains, except for a gap in the southeastern area that is closed by the Indus River (see Figure 1). When the British assumed control from the Sikhs in 1848–1849, the area was in considerable political and economic disarray. The Siekhs had, in reality, only governed the western part of the valley. The rest of the area was subject to periodic punitive raids, which were used by the Siekhs as a means of revenue collection (Bellew, 1864).

The first 20 to 30 years of British colonial rule did not necessarily improve the situation. A Western notion of land ownership was imposed with mixed results on a population where property was often held collectively. Class distinctions based on land ownership emerged as the British granted tracts of land to important individuals in return for their cooperation, or awarded the revenue

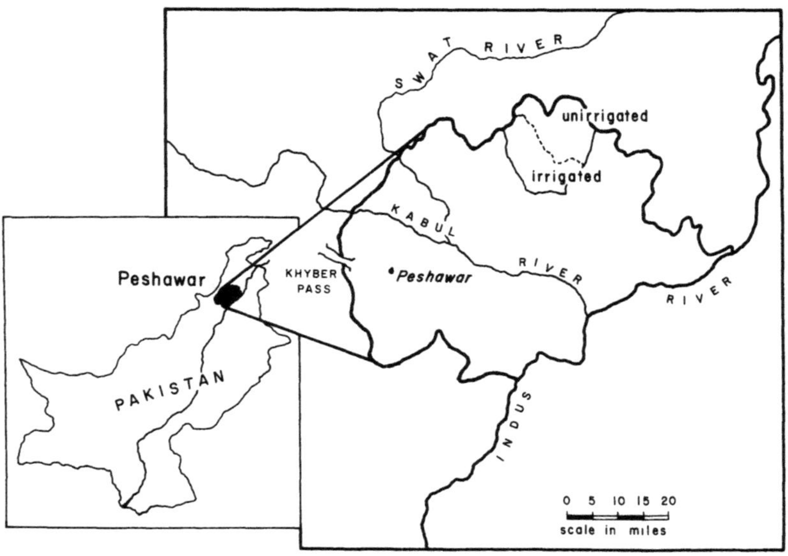

Figure 1. Map of the Peshawar region of northwestern Pakistan. Irrigated and unirrigated zones of field research area are also indicated.

produced by one or a number of villages to inhabitants who assisted them militarily, politically, or socially (Hastings, 1878; Dane, 1898).

When relative political stability was achieved, a systematic assessment of land types, land ownership, crop production, livestock, and human population was undertaken. This elaborate survey lasted 7 years (1869 to 1876), and it marks the beginning of reliable record keeping in the area (Hastings, 1878). The results substantiated earlier impressions that Peshawar was an area whose agricultural potential was virtually undeveloped. At that time, 137,471a, or 13.9% of the cultivable land (986,936 a), was canal irrigated. Most of this land was located near the confluence of the Swat and Kabul Rivers in the western part of the basin; but another 37,544 a (3.8% of all cultivable land) were also irrigated by wells, springs, or by diverting seasonal torrents near the hills. Rainfall-dependent agriculture was practiced on 655,164 a (66.4% of all cultivable land); and 15.5% of all cultivable land was simply unused (Hastings, 1878).

Rainfall-dependent agriculture in Peshawar was, and continues to be, an extremely risky business. There are significant annual, seasonal, and regional variations in the basin's climate. Mean monthly temperatures during the winter average about 55°F (daily highs are about 65°F and nighttime lows are about 35°F). During the summer, mean monthly temperatures vary between 87°F and 93°F (nighttime lows are about 80°F and daytime highs are between 100° and 110°F). Figure 2 shows the means and standard deviations of monthly rainfall (from 1881 and through 1970) in the eastern and western parts of the basin. Rainfall is heaviest in the eastern area along the Indus River (annual mean = 24.9 inches per year) and lowest in the western and southern areas (annual mean = 10.7 inches per year). Summer monsoon rainfall, the heaviest experienced by the basin, is carried on easterly air currents and is greatest along the Indus River. Winter rainfall, only half that of summer, is carried on westerly air currents and is heaviest in the western area. The capricious nature of both winter and summer air currents in the region has a tremendous effect on annual rainfall. During the years when the monsoon and winter rainfall are both heavy, the region receives between 37.5 inches (in the eastern area) and 22.5 inches (in the west). During poor rainfall years, the area receives between 15.2 inches (in the east) and 3.5 inches (in the west).

Most of the rainfall-dependent area was monocropped. A major sowing of wheat and barley took place during October or November. After these crops were harvested in April or May, about one third to one half of the land would be resown with maize or millet. Because of the unpredictable rainfall, a large percentage of both the winter and summer crops failed each year. During the last quarter of the 19th century, crop failures occurred on about 30% of all rainfall-dependent agricultural land every year (Dane, 1894, 1896a, 1896b). Figure 3 shows the frequency with which failures occurred in one unirrigated area in the northern part of the basin (about 114,000 culturable a) during the 29 winter

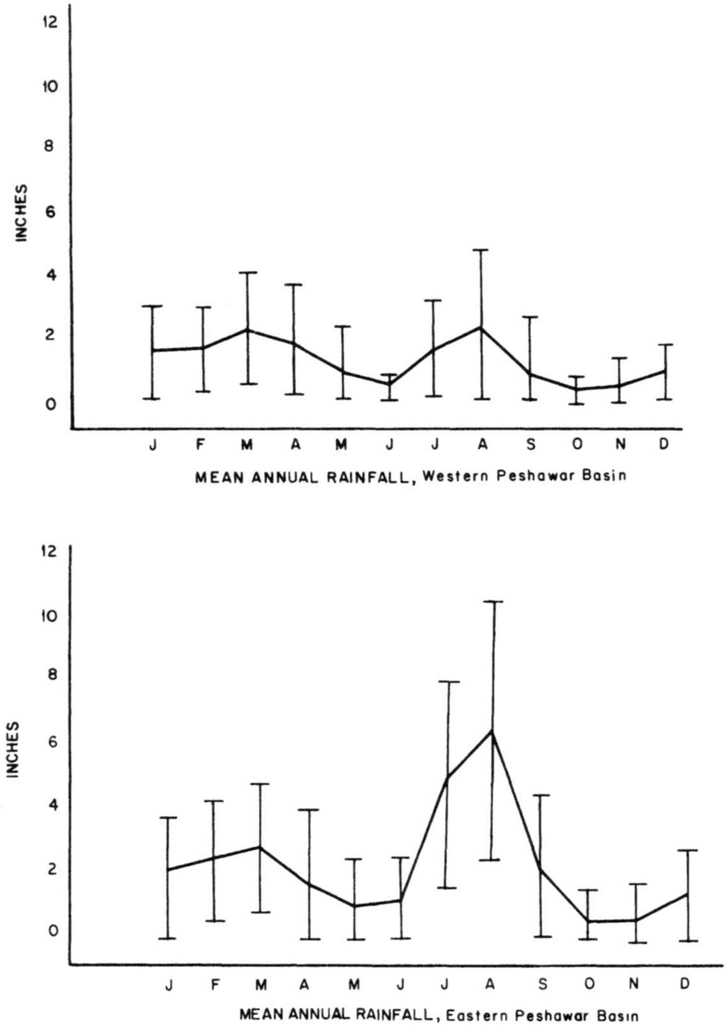

Figure 2. Mean annual rainfall in the eastern and western parts of the Peshawar Basin.

seasons between 1895–1896 and 1923–1924. During the same period, an average of 25% of the summer crops failed each year (Wylie, 1926b).

The impact of fluctuating food supplies on fertility and mortality during the last half of the 19th century is difficult to assess. The best statistics are available for the least affected areas (i.e., those in the more irrigated western portion of the valley). In the north, south, and east, registration of births and deaths only began in the late 1870s and early 1880s and did not become reliable until the 1890s.

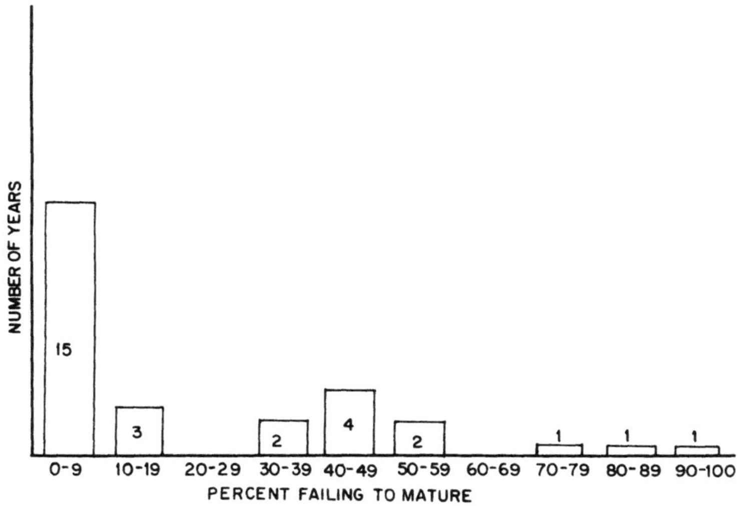

Figure 3. Crop failures in an unirrigated region of the Peshawar Basin.

Census data indicates that the population grew at an average annual rate of about 0.9% between 1868 and 1881. This, however, may overstate the growth rate because the 1881 census was carried out far more deliberately than the 1868 census. More likely, the population changed little, if at all, during this time.

In 1881, the rural population density of the basin was a comparatively low 200 persons/mi^2. In the generally unirrigated portions of Peshawar, it varied between 70 and 150 persons/mi^2. But even the more irrigated areas were not densely populated. For the most part, population density in these regions varied between 200 and 300 persons/mi^2. Only in the area between the confluence of the Swat and Kabul rivers did the density reach about 450 persons/mi^2 (Dane, 1894, 1896a, 1896b).

2.2. Conditions after Irrigation

In the 1880s, the British began the construction of massive irrigation networks. The Lower Swat Canal was opened for the 1887–1888 seasons, and irrigated the area east of the Swat River and north of the Kabul River. The Kabul River Canal was opened in 1903–1904, and irrigated the area south of the Kabul River. In 1914–1915, the Upper Swat Canal began irrigating the area north and west of that irrigated by the Lower Swat Canal.

Land utilization figures following the construction of these large irrigation networks are not always comparable with earlier data. Changes in boundaries and improved surveying techniques in the 50 to 55 years between the first systematic assessment of the basin's agriculture (1869–1876) and the third (1923–1929) added approximately 250,000 a to the district. The latter assessment reported the existence of 1,201,185 a of cultivable land (an increase of 21.7% over the 1869–1876 figure). Most of the "added" lands fell into the unused-but-cultivable category, which increased to about 30% of the cultivable area. Canal-irrigated land increased over three times to 423,908 a, or 35.5% of all cultivable land. The area on which rainfall-dependent agriculture was practiced declined to 369,027 a. The remainder was irrigated by wells, springs, or seasonal torrents (Wylie, 1926a, 1926b, 1927, 1928, 1929).

These three canals profoundly affected the economic life of the basin's population. They created vast new tracts of irrigated land, altered property values and, in some cases, caused the creation of new villages and the physical relocation of others. Cropping patterns also changed. Prior to irrigation, barley was a popular winter crop, primarily because of its hardiness. Wheat, which brought a higher cash return, was more sensitive to rainfall fluctuations and was consequently more prone to failure. Between 1869–1876 and 1926–1929, however, barley acreage declined from 246,000 to about 158,000. Wheat acreage increased to about as much as the barley acreage declined. Maize became the most important summer crop, increasing from about 64,000 a prior to irrigation to about 166,000 a in the late 1920s. The amount of land used to grow fodder, fruits, and vegetables also increased (Dane, 1894, 1896a, 1896b; Wylie, 1926a, 1926b, 1927, 1928, 1929).

The change in per acre yields resulting from irrigation varied, depending upon the crop and the type of soil. In general, however, the per acre yield of maize increased between two and three times and the yield of wheat doubled. Between 1869–1876 and 1923–1929, the basin's wheat production increased from 68,662 tn to 110,207 tn annually. During the same time, the average annual production of maize increased from 39,118 tn to 105,240 tn (Dane, 1894, 1896a, 1896b; Wylie, 1926a, 1926b, 1927, 1928, 1929). But these figures do not reflect the truly remarkable increases in newly irrigated areas. In the northern area where fieldwork was carried out between 1974 and 1976 (about 114,000 cultivable a), average annual wheat production increased from 3,579 tn during the 1890s (before irrigation) to 12,092 tn during the late 1920s (after irrigation). During the same time, maize production increased from 659 tn to 6164 tn annually (Wylie, 1926b).

2.3. Demographic Data

Table I shows that these enormous increases in productivity were accompanied by a decline in the rate of population growth. Calculations of the intrinsic rate of natural population growth (r) are based on census enumerations of the nonimmigrant population (i.e., people born in Peshawar and listed in Peshawar

Table I
Changes in the Intrinsic Rate of Natural Population Growth (*r*) between 1881 and 1931

Decade	Intrinsic rate of natural population growth
1881–1891	0.0168
1891–1901	0.0104
1901–1911	0.0094
1911–1921	0.0046
1921–1931	0.0068

or in adjacent districts). They omit individuals born in Peshawar and listed outside western India. However, the number of individuals that fall into that category is small and should not effect the final computations. The accuracy of the census enumerations upon which these calculations are based increases progressively, particularly between 1881 and 1901 when several technical improvements were implemented (Davis, 1951). Consequently, the (*r*) values calculated for the early decades (1881 to 1891 and 1891 to 1901) overestimate the rate of population growth. But the degree of underenumeration (probably 7–10% in 1881 and 2–5% in 1891) is only sufficient to produce a slightly slower rate of decline than that noted in Table I (Census of India, 1881, 1891, 1901, 1911, 1921, 1931). In 1931, the noncooperation movement interfered with the census in some areas of India, but not greatly in Peshawar (Census of India, 1931). Therefore, the rate of population growth between 1921 and 1931 was probably characterized by the relatively small increase noted in Table I.

Three approaches to understanding population dynamics during and after the period of rising agricultural productivity can be employed: (1) an analysis of crude birth and death rates; (2) an analysis of age-specific mortality; and (3) an analysis of cohort survivorship. All three are based on vital statistics recorded at the village or town level. Data presented here are those that were compiled for Peshawar as a whole by district health officers and then reported in one of several serials *(Government of the Punjab [1881–1900], Government of the North-West Frontier Province [1901–1921], Government of the North-West Frontier Province [1922–1955] and Government of the North-West Frontier Province [1911–present])* or in unpublished documents at district health offices.

Figure 4 shows adjusted crude birth and death rates for the basin's natural population between 1881 and 1965. Significant problems with birth and death registration occurred in Peshawar, as in most of British India. Not all the population was under registration, and female births were underreported, as were

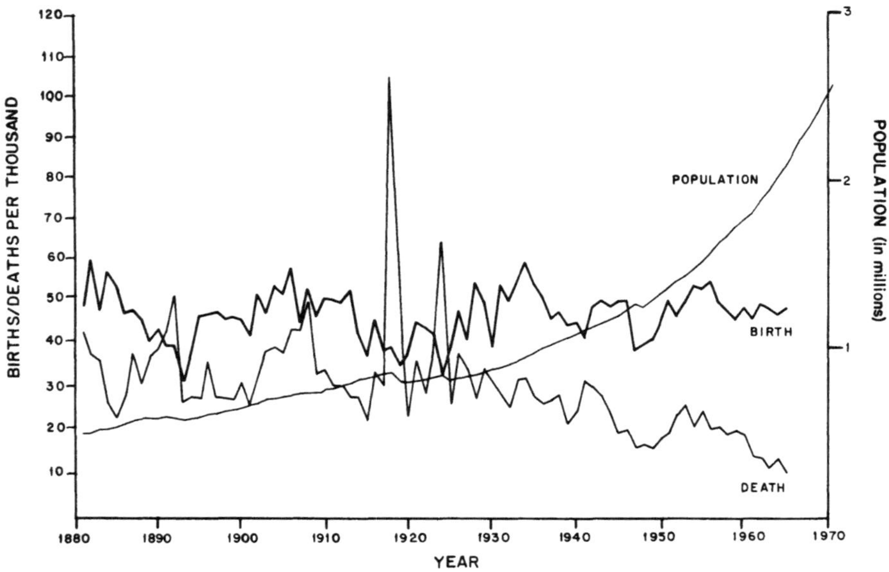

Figure 4. Adjusted birth and death rates for Peshawar's natural population and estimated population sizes between 1880 and 1970.

female infant and child deaths. Before 1901, the best reporting occurred among the stable rural population in the west, and along the irrigated belts just north and south of the Kabul River. Reports from the northern, southern, and eastern areas were less reliable. Assessments made after 1901 indicate that between 10 and 15% of all births and between 5 and 10% of all deaths were not reported. For these reasons, annual birth and death rates have been adjusted according to a method suggested by Demeny (1971) for statistically underdeveloped areas. This method generates average numbers of births and deaths based on comparisons of the more accurate decennial censuses. Because the degree of underreporting normally remained consistent from year to year, annual fluctuations in the registration of vital events reflect actual circumstances. Consequently, these data can be used to apportion the estimated decennial births and deaths computed by comparing censes.

Figure 5 shows unadjusted survivorship rates for males born between 1882 and 1961, arranged into 10-year cohorts. These data are based on annual reports of age and sex-specific mortality. Male survivorship is shown because the importance of sons in Peshawar's Pathan-dominated society increased the likelihood that male vital events would be reported. Because reporting female vital events was considered by many Pathans as an invasion of privacy, the accuracy of these data are poor (Census of India, 1891; Census of India, 1901). Although subject to reporting error, male survivorship data are likely to be internally consistent.

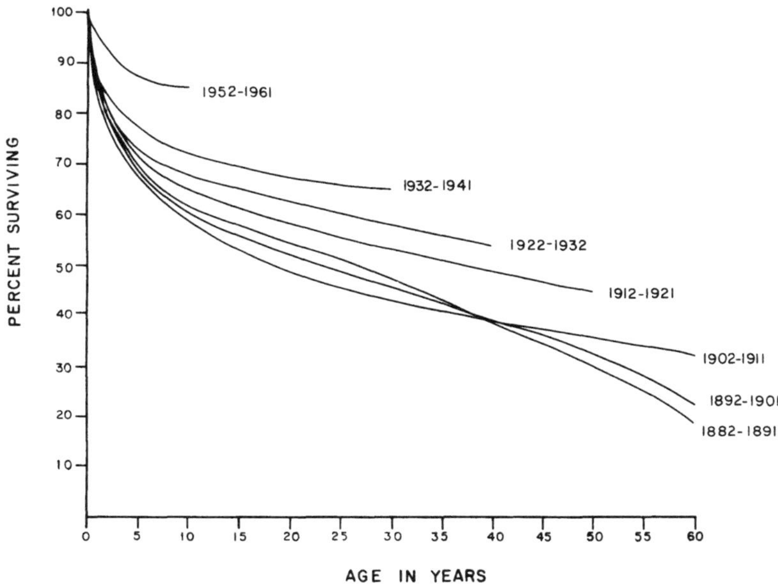

Figure 5. Unadjusted survivorship rates of seven cohorts of males born between 1882 and 1961.

The probability of reporting a death is much greater (as was discovered in a field analysis of one area's vital statistics) if the individual's birth was also recorded. This is particularly true for infant and child mortality. Consequently, these curves probably represent infant and child survivorship accurately. However, because deaths among older persons are more likely to be recorded regardless of whether their births were registered, the older parts of these curves are probably too low (i.e., survivorship was probably greater than indicated). Because longitudinal data only exist through the 1960s, the survivorship of males born after the 1902–1911 cohort is figured to a progressively younger age.

Figure 6 provides a closer examination of male infant mortality rates for most years between 1881 and 1965. In an analysis of records in the field, male infant mortality was found to be least affected by errors of age and reporting. It was extremely rare to find a male infant's death noted unless his birth was also recorded; and nearly all reported male infant deaths occurred among individuals whose birth had been recorded in the previous 12 months. Infant deaths are an important indication of changing morbidity patterns because infants are particularly susceptible to most of the diseases that affect the population. They also made up a large portion of the total deaths that occurred each year: about 13% of all deaths prior to irrigation; nearly 20% between 1891 and 1940; and about 12% in the 1950s and 1960s.

It seems clear that elevated mortality caused the declining rate of growth

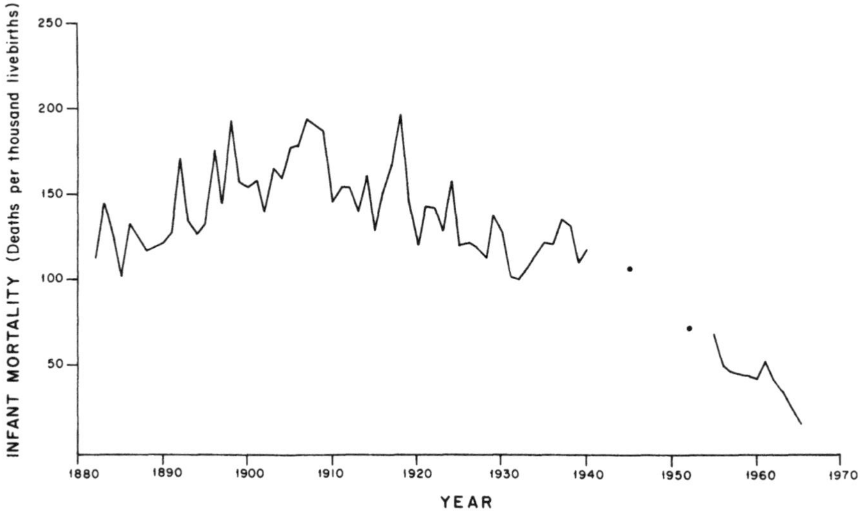

Figure 6. Unadjusted male infant mortality rates between 1881 and 1965.

mentioned earlier. Figure 4 shows that, between 1890 and 1930, the crude death rate was never below 25/1000 and, occasionally, it climbed to 50/1000 or more. Most of these mortality "spikes" resulted from diseases that were spread by contact or as a result of poor public health. The most common were cholera, plague, smallpox, and influenza. Except for smallpox, which was endemic, cholera, plague, and influenzas usually spread from urban to rural areas. This is reflected in the pattern of death registration during major epidemics—like the one caused by influenza during 1918. In the city of Peshawar, mortality from influenza began abruptly during the third week of October, apparently transmitted from an adjacent province. The registration of deaths indicate that a return to "normal" mortality occurred 3 to 4 weeks later, so that urban mortality peaked during October. The disease spread to rural areas about a week after it appeared in the city of Peshawar; therefore, influenza mortality increased the rural death rate only slightly during October. The epidemic was most severe in rural areas during November, but rural mortality also remained high in December, with some residual deaths reported in January, 1919.

Another cause of the high mortality between 1890 and 1930 was undoubtedly malaria. It was already common in the western part of the basin and along the Kabul River when the British annexed the area in 1848. Subsequently, the disease spread to almost all the remaining areas of the valley. As it did so, it was accompanied by substantial increases in mortality. Periodically, malaria would become epidemic, only to decline spontaneously or after the distribution of quinine.

Evidence from the villages in a single assessment circle in the northern part of the basin (see Figure 1 for location) indicates that mortality is inversely related to the degree of isolation. This area was chosen for analysis because it was bisected by the Upper Swat Canal in 1914–1915. Prior to irrigation, the inhabitants practiced rainfall-dependent, subsistence agriculture. Mortality at that time remained below, but close to, the crude birth rate, so that population size grew slowly. Subsequent to irrigation and increased commerce with market towns, mortality spikes frequently placed the death rate above the birth rate, and the population size remained almost constant between 1911 and 1931. Within the region, however, mortality was normally higher in the southernmost villages (those whose land became irrigated) than in the northernmost villages. These remained unirrigated in isolated locations adjacent to the northern hills.

Figure 5 shows that survivorship declined progressively from the 1882–1891 cohort through the 1902–1911 cohort. The decline in survivorship during the fourth decade among males born between 1882 and 1891 coincides with the enormous adult mortality caused by the 1918 influenza epidemic and those that followed in the 1920s. This same period is associated with low survivorship through the third decade among males born between 1892 and 1901, and low survivorship through the second decade among males born between 1902 and 1911.

The impact of early deaths on survivorship is indicated by the steady increases in infant mortality shown in Figure 6. During most of the 1880s, infant mortality remained between 100 and 125 deaths/1000 live births. In the subsequent 30 years (1891 to 1920), it was never below 125 deaths/1000 live births and was above 150 deaths/1000 live births 21 times.

Fertility fluctuates considerably during this period, showing no progressive increase or decrease. Of particular interest, however, are the declines in fertility that occur after periods of high mortality. The reason is not entirely clear. It may be related to the negative effect of disease on fecundity. In part, it also may be related to social factors surrounding adult male deaths. A significant negative correlation ($r = -0.7$) exists between adult male deaths in one year and the general fertility rate (number of live births to women aged 15–45) in the next. A case in point is the 1918 influenza epidemic. Over 25% of all deaths recorded in that year occurred among reproductively active males (aged 20 to 59), a particularly large number in view of the fact that over half the population was 19 years of age or younger. The next year saw a dramatic reduction in general fertility; and even the crude birth rate fell to under 40/1000. These two events may be related to the fact that adult male deaths produce an increase in the number of young widows who may not always remarry (or, if they do, may not remarry immediately) and thus will not bear children in the next year. In the field study area described previously, the decline in the general fertility rate is greater among women in irrigated villages than among women in unirrigated villages. This may be another reflection of the less severe effects of epidemics in more isolated zones.

Since the 1930s, death rates have gradually declined. Figure 4 probably does not show mortality during the 1940s accurately because World War II and Independence and Partition were enormously disruptive events. By the 1950s and 1960s, however, mortality had declined to between 10 and 20/1000—about the same as for Pakistan as a whole. These lower death rates resulted from a dramatic reduction in epidemic diseases. Plague ceased to exist. Malaria deaths declined due to the use of quinine and, later, antimalarial drugs. Improved urban water supplies cut cholera deaths in the cities and probably also reduced the disease's spread to rural areas. Only smallpox deaths remained unchanged, apparently because the vaccination program in rural areas was a victim of the "noncooperation movement" prior to Independence. After Independence, smallpox declined until it was eliminated in the 1970s.

Accompanying the lower mortality was an increase in survivorship. Figure 5 shows that survivorship to age 10 improved from 65% among males born between 1912 and 1921 to 85% among males born between 1952 and 1961. Although it is clear that declining infant mortality contributed to lower death rates and higher survivorship, Figure 6 probably overstates the rate of descent. Data from the 1950s and 1960s come disproportionately from urban areas where, compared to rural areas, health facilities are better and where mortality at all ages is lower.

Peshawar's declining death rate has been accompanied by persistently high fertility. The average birth rate of the natural population during the 1950s and 1960s, estimated by comparisons of the 1951, 1961, and 1972 census reports, was about 47/1000. This suggests that the mean annual increase in natural population size was on the order of 3.0 to 3.5%. When immigrants are added, the total population of the Peshawar Basin more than tripled in the 41 years between 1931 and 1972.

3. Discussion and Conclusions

A Malthusian relationship between production and population growth does not seem to have existed in Peshawar. During the time that agricultural production expanded most rapidly, increased mortality caused the rate of natural population growth to decline. The exponential increase in population growth that might be expected to follow a sudden increase in the carrying capacity (Schacht, 1980) did not materialize until two generations after the first irrigation project was completed. Even when it occurred, exponential population growth may not have been related to increased food availability. Food–grain production was already at modern levels between 1915 and 1930, a period of exceptionally high mortality. Between 1931 and 1971, when the basin's natural population more than tripled, there was only a 5% increase in the production of food grains, whereas the production of nonedible cash crops increased tenfold (Moeen-Ud-Din and Ikramullah, 1973; Wylie, 1926a, 1926b, 1927, 1928, 1929).

In the period prior to irrigation, Peshawar's population density was low, agricultural production was unstable, and the area was isolated by the Indus River. At the same time, India's northern region was densely populated. There, by the 1870s, population pressure had already led to agricultural intensification (irrigation, multiple cropping) and the exploitation of nearby marginal regions. Overcrowding and an unexpandable agricultural base, in combination with poverty, caused extremely high death rates from famines and infectious diseases (Klein, 1973, 1974). The official perception of a population at or near the carrying capacity led to the development of large irrigation and transportation schemes. Vast areas in the Punjab were opened to alleviate overcrowding in congested districts (Griffiths, 1952), and Peshawar was irrigated both to forestall the possibility of famine, and eventually, to produce surplus for export (Dane, 1898).

From this perspective, the Peshawar case would certainly seem to support the population pressure model. But, if the strain between food resources and population size was alleviated by increased productivity in Peshawar and the Punjab, it was not immediately detectable in the overcrowded areas of northern India. There, the population size increased only marginally during the latter part of the 19th century. And between 1901 and 1921, the size of the natural population actually declined (Klein, 1974). Furthermore, the population pressure model does not address itself to the demographic consequences of agricultural intensification in peripheral areas; and therefore offers no insight about why mortality should increase in the Peshawar region where there was no population pressure. The failure of the population pressure model to provide a completely satisfying explanation seems to stem from a combination of environmental and social factors that obscures any direct association between population and productivity.

In both northern India and Peshawar, environmental changes caused by irrigation promoted the spread of water-based disease vectors to areas where they previously had not existed. Among the most significant of these was the malaria-carrying anopheles mosquito. In Peshawar, a substantial portion of the progressive increases in mortality that occurred after the opening of the Lower Swat Canal in the late 1880s and the opening of the Kabul River Canal in 1903 was attributable to malaria. The most likely reason was the spread of the anopheles mosquitos to newly irrigated land. In each instance, public health officials tried to control the disease by distributing quinine; but in each instance the number of malaria cases increased and the residual mortality due to malaria remained high.

In modern Peshawar, the problem is ubiquitous in irrigated areas, although mortality is kept in check by antimalarial drugs.

Social factors are equally relevant. In northern India, the inequitable distribution of economic power led to the poverty of most rural peasants. Their access to land in the region they lived as well as to food and goods produced elsewhere was limited. This resulted in poor nutrition and increased their susceptibility to death by malaria and infectious diseases (Klein, 1974).

In Peshawar economic change caused by the increased production of food seems to link irrigation with high mortality. The abundance of wheat and maize grown on newly irrigated fields increased the opportunity for a large number of farmers to take part in the regional market economy. Before irrigation, most of these farmers engaged in subsistence agriculture on rainfall-dependent land. As evidence of this, the colonial government took note of the poor productivity in the north, south, and east and levied only nominal taxation in these areas in 1876 (Hastings, 1878). Following irrigation (and considerably increased revenue levies), farmers needed access to regional grain markets to sell their surplus crops. Access to the city of Mardan in the north-central region, the city of Peshawar in the west, and a number of smaller markets was made possible by roads constructed or improved when the canals were being built.

These marketplaces, particularly the cities, seem to have functioned as disease reservoirs. Hospital and dispensary records from the city of Peshawar indicate that sanitation prior to the 1930s was poor and public health was primitive. Diseases like tuberculosis, pneumonia, dysentary, and smallpox were common throughout the year, and epidemics of cholera and plague nearly always originated there. Periodic travel to and from these market towns, caused by the need to sell increasingly higher yields, could have broken down the protective isolation of Peshawar's rural population. Trade brought the rural population into closer and more continual contact with urban disease conditions, and these diseases were carried by farmers when they returned to their villages. The result was the spread of infectious diseases to a greater proportion of the basin's population.

Reasons for the steadily declining mortality that began during the 1930s are not entirely clear. Davis (1951) suggests that efficient transportation promoted the distribution of food to drought-stricken areas, thereby preventing or reducing famine mortality. Certainly there were also improvements in public health. Vaccinations succeeded in dramatically lowering smallpox mortality after independence, and the purification of water supplies reduced cholera. Other diseases, like plague, seem to have diminished spontaneously (Davis, 1951). In Peshawar during the 1930s and 1940s, the public health effort in urban areas was greater than in rural areas, but mortality declined in both regions. Perhaps the control of infectious diseases in the cities benefited the rural peasantry as well. It is also conceivable that selection favored the increase of less susceptible genotypes or that differences in immune response could have developed.

Population increases subsequent to 1930 resulted as much from the persistence of high fertility as from lowered mortality. The reasons behind such high birthrates seem basically economic (Elahi, 1975). Increased productivity in Peshawar's rural hinterlands during and after the construction of irrigation canals not only facilitated the spread of disease, but it also changed the way families used their land and deployed their working-age sons. In irrigated areas, there was a gradual shift from food cropping to cash cropping. By the 1920s, substantial increases in the area's two main cash crops, sugarcane and tobacco, were already underway. At the same time, there were increasing opportunities to engage in the emerging manufacturing and service sectors of the Indian economy. But, because of the high mortality, most males in Peshawar's patrilineal, extended-family system were needed at home to assist with agricultural tasks. When families could spare sons, they were encouraged to migrate, on a more or less permanent basis, to an urban area in Peshawar or elsewhere where they could get jobs as wage laborers. Afterward, they contributed to their families by returning a portion of their wages to the head of the household—usually the father. The increasing number of adult males that resulted from lower infant and child mortality rates during and after the 1930s has meant that a growing number of families could engage in this practice. Indeed, this view of male children as potential economic resources undoubtedly contributes to the continued preference for large families among poorly educated rural Pathans (Elahi, 1975).

That models relating resources and population growth do not consider social phenomena is not a new criticism. The Peshawar case merely provides an example of why such criticism is valid. It also serves to reiterate that social factors not only affect access to resources, but they may also influence susceptibility to disease. Because periods of high mortality may influence the course of social change, the impact of disease during episodes of agricultural intensification should clearly become part of any model relating population growth to changes in the resource base.

Acknowledgments

The author would like to express his appreciation to the North-West Frontier Province Archives, the India Office Library and the District Health Offices in Mardan and Peshawar for permission to review their historical records. A special debt of gratitude is due Professor Farzand A. Durrani and the faculty and staff of the Department of Archaeology at the University of Peshawar for their assistance in obtaining necessary permissions, as well as for their continuing support in the collection of field data.

References

Bellew, H. W., 1864, *A General Report on the Yusafzais,* The Government Press, Lahore.

Boserup, E., 1965, *The Conditions of Agricultural Growth,* Aldine, Chicago.

Census of India, 1881, *The Punjab,* Office of the Superintendent of Government Printing, Calcutta.

Census of India, 1891, Volume XIX, *The Punjab and its Feudatories,* Office of the Superintendent of Government Printing, Calcutta.

Census of India, 1901, Volume XVII, *The Punjab and its Feudatories,* Office of the Superintendent of Government Printing, Calcutta.

Census of India, 1911, Volume XIII, *North-West Frontier Province,* The Commercial Press, Peshawar.

Census of India, 1921, Volume XIV, *North-West Frontier Province,* North-West Frontier Province Government Press, Peshawar.

Census of India, 1931, Volume XV, *North-West Frontier Province,* Government Printing and Stationery, Peshawar.

Cohen, M. N., 1977, *The Food Crisis in Prehistory,* Yale University Press, New Haven.

Dane, L. W., 1894, Assessment report of the Charsadda Tahsil of the Peshawar District, *Proc. of the Government of the Punjab in the Revenue Department,* November, pp. 1–97.

Dane, L. W., 1896a, Assessment report of the Yusafzai Sub-Division in the Peshawar District, *Proc. of the Government of the Punjab in the Revenue Department,* January, pp. 1–104.

Dane, L. W., 1896b, Assessment report of the Peshawar and Nowshera Tahsils in the Peshawar District, *Proc. of the Government of the Punjab in the Revenue Department,* June, pp. 1–132.

Dane, L. W., 1898, *Final Report of the Settlement of Peshawar District,* Civil and Military Gazette Press, Lahore.

Davis, K., 1951, *The Population of India and Pakistan,* Princeton University Press, Princeton.

Demeny, P., 1971, Methods of Demographic Estimation for Statistically Underdeveloped Areas, Paper Number 10, East-West Center, Honolulu, Hawaii.

Elahi, K., 1975, Some aspects of socioeconomic change and fertility control among the emerging elite of the Pathans, in: *Population and Social Control* (M. Nag, ed.), Mouton Press, The Hague.

Government of the North-West Frontier Province, 1901–02—1920/21, *Report on Vaccination in the North-West Frontier Province,* The Commercial Press, Peshawar.

Government of the North-West Frontier Province, 1901–1921, *Report of the Sanitary Administration of the North-West Frontier Province,* The Commercial Press, Peshawar.

Government of the North-West Frontier Province, 1911–, *North-West Frontier Province Government Gazete,* Government Printing and Stationery, Peshawar.

Government of the North-West Frontier Province, 1922–1955, *Annual Public Health and Vaccination Reports of the North-West Frontier Province,* Government Stationery and Printing, Peshawar.

Government of the Punjab, 1881–1900, *Report of The Sanitary Administration of the Punjab,* The Government Press, Lahore.

Griffiths, P., 1952, *The British Impact on India,* MacDonald, London.

Hassan, F. A., 1979, Demography and archaeology, in: *Annual Review of Anthropology,* Volume 8 (B. J. Siegel, A. R. Beals, and S. A. Tyler (eds.), Annual Reviews, Inc., Palo Alto, Calif., pp. 137–160.

Hastings, E. G. G., 1878, *Report of the Regular Settlement of the Peshawar District of the Punjab,* The Central Jail Press, Lahore.

Klein, I., 1974, Population and Agriculture in northern India, 1872–1921, *Mod. Asian Stud.* **8**:191–216.

Klein, I., 1973, Death in India, 1871–1921, *J. Asian Stud.* **32**:639–659.

Moeen-Ud-Din, S., and Ikramullah, A., 1973, *Agricultural Statistics of the North-West Frontier Province,* 1945–70, Board of Economic Enquiry, North-West Frontier Province, Peshawar.

Orlove, B. S., 1980, Ecological Anthropology, in: *Annual Review of Anthropology,* Volume 8 (B. J. Siegel, A. R. Beals, and S. A. Tyler, eds.), Annual Reviews, Inc., Palo Alto, Calif., pp. 235–273.

Schacht, R. M., 1980, Two Models of Population Growth, *Am. Anthropol.* **82:**782–798.

Watson, R. A., and Watson, P. J., 1969, *Man and Nature: An Anthropological Essay in Human Ecology,* Harcourt, Brace and World, New York.

Wylie, E. V., 1926a, *Statements Relating to the Assessment Report of the Charsadda Tahsil of the Peshawar District,* Government of India, Central Publications Branch, Calcutta.

Wylie, E. V., 1926b, *Statements Relating to the Assessment Report of the Mardan Tahsil of the Peshawar District,* Government of India Central Publications Branch, Calcutta.

Wylie, E. V., 1927, *Statements Relating to the Assessment Report of the Swabi Tahsil of the Peshawar District,* Government of India Central Publications Branch, Calcutta.

Wylie, E. V., 1928, *Statements Relating to the Assessment Report of the Nowshera Tahsil of the Peshawar District,* Government of India Central Publication Branch, Calcutta.

Wylie, E. V., 1929, *Statements Relating to the Assessment Report of the Peshawar Tahsil of the Peshawar District,* Government of India Central Publication Branch, Calcutta.

Zubrow, E. B. W., 1975, *Prehistoric Carrying Capacity: A Model,* Cummings Publishing Co., Menlo Park, Calif.

Zubrow, E. B. W., 1976, Demographic Anthropology: An Introductory Analysis, in: *Demographic Anthropology* (E. B. W. Zubrow, ed.), University of New Mexican Press, Albuquerque, pp. 1–25.

CHAPTER 16

Anthropological Demography of Populations of the Eastern Himalayas

AMITABHA BASU, RANJAN GUPTA, AND BARUN MUKHOPADHYAY

1. Introduction

Between 20 and 30 million people live at altitudes above 2500 m and if all mountain dwellers are considered, the number would increase greatly, but still this number is a small proportion of the total population of the world. However, if mere numbers do not justify detailed study of these populations, the fact that high altitude people—and to a lesser extent all mountain dwellers—inhabit a narrowly specialized environment warrants that their responses to the stress components of this environment be studied comprehensively. The insights gained from such studies, apart from their intrinsic academic interest, may eventually help identify appropriate intervention points for maintenance of fertility at optimal levels, control of mortality and morbidity, and, in general, for promotion of the population health of these generally remote populations. The World Health Organization (WHO) (1971) has defined health in terms of "complete physical, mental and social well-being and not merely the absence of disease and infirmity." However, we shall be concerned in this chapter with the

---

AMITABHA BASU, RANJAN GUPTA, AND BARUN MUKHOPADHYAY • Human Adaptability Programme, Biological Sciences Division, Indian Statistical Institute, Calcutta 700 035, India. We wish to express our appreciation to the authorities of the Indian Statistical Institute for providing financial and logistical support for our research.

demographic variables of population growth, fertility, and mortality, that is, the ultimate indicators of well-being.

Studies on high altitude people have been carried out for over a century. Extensive studies were mainly conducted in the Andes (Cruz-Coke, 1967; Baker, 1969; Baker and Dutt, 1972; Hoff, 1974; Pawson, 1974; Frisancho, 1976; Schull and Rothhammer, 1977; Mirrakhimov, 1978; Weitz *et al.*, 1978; Bangham and Sacherer, 1980; Hu, 1981). These studies have indicated some generalities in the adaptive responses of human populations to the high altitude environment, for example, reduced fecundity/fertility, increased prenatal, neonatal, and infant mortality, reduced physical growth and adult body size, increased hematological values, and so forth, which have also been reported from animal experiments (Sundstroem and Michaels, 1942; Gordon *et al.*, 1943; Timiras, 1964; Weihe, 1964; Feigen and Johnson, 1964; Donayre, 1966; Hock, 1970; Lord and Murphy, 1973). However, having followed the set pattern of animal experiments and drawn inspiration from physiological investigations, the early studies on high altitude human biology generally neglected the whole range of interactions between sociocultural stresses and biological traits. These studies implicitly equated high altitude effects simply with effects of hypoxia via physiological functions so that studies on biocultural interactions in mountain and high altitude populations started rather late (Stycos, 1963; Rothhammer and Spielman, 1972; Haas, 1976; Mueller *et al.*, 1978; Weitz *et al.*, 1978; Weitz, 1980). The validity of the basic assumption regarding the high altitude environment's being a specialized niche thus remains open to verification. Finally, the Himalayas have remained a poorly studied mountain range from the viewpoint of human biology, in spite of the fact that the world's highest peak is located there, and one of the native populations of this region, the Sherpas, are internationally renowned for the efficiency of their working capacity at very high altitudes (Pugh, 1966; Weitz, 1973).

It is generally presumed that the basic demographic variables of fertility and mortality and the composite variable, population growth, are the ultimate indicators of a population's capacity for survival and, therefore, of its overall state of well-being, or its degree of adaptation to the environment. It is further assumed that although the mountain environment may have its own unique physical environmental and sociocultural characteristics when contrasted to other environmental extremes, for example, deserts, the tropics, polar areas, as has been pointed out by Brush (1976), Baker (1978), Pawson and Jest (1978), and others, environmental variations of smaller magnitudes do occur within each major niche to which human populations may also be sensitive.

In view of this, the purpose of this chapter is to (1) consider the fertility, mortality, and growth potentials of populations of the eastern Himalayas and their constituent political/administrative units vis-à-vis neighboring ones; and

(2) to inquire into the possible interrelations of physical environmental and sociocultural stresses with the basic demographic measures within political and administrative units, using both macro- and microlevel data.

2. The Eastern Himalayas

2.1. Definition and Physiographic Characteristics

According to the Gazetteer of India (1973) the western boundary of this region is the Singalila Mountain range and the Mechi River, both of which run along the eastern border of Nepal. The eastern boundary ends at the bend of the Brahmaputra River around Namcha Barwa in Tibet. Thus, the eastern Himalayas include Sikkim, Darjeeling, Bhutan Himalayas, and Assam Himalayas. For the purpose of this study, however, we have extended the western boundary to the eastern part of the Nepal Himalayas, which are conventionally a part of the central Himalayas, in view of the fact that the highest altitude permanent human settlements are found there (Figure 1).

2.1.1. Sikkim-Darjeeling Himalayas. This area is mainly drained by the Tista River and its tributary, the Rangit. Two transverse ranges running north to south, Singalila in the west and Dongkya in the east, with altitudes of 3679 and 7134 m, respectively, enclose the area. Here the great Himalayas run from west to east, from Kanchanjangha to Chomolhari. The Darjeeling Hills district is divided into two parts by the deep gorge of the Tista. To the east of the gorge are the Kalimpong Hills rising to a peak of 3200 m. Rivers flow in all directions from here, draining into the Tista River.

2.1.2. Bhutan Himalayas. The great Himalayan range runs along its northern border eastward from Chomolhari to Kula Kangri, the highest peak in Bhutan with an altitude of 7541 m. There are no large river basins in Bhutan. The northern half of Bhutan is fully glaciated.

2.1.3. Assam Himalaya. The great Himalayan range further east runs along the northern borders of Arunachal Pradesh, with the highest altitude being 7756 m. At many places the MacMohan Line—the international border—runs along the crest and ends in the massif of Namcha Barwa. It is called Assam Himalaya, although it is located in Arunachal Pradesh. A number of rivers flow across the MacMohan Line into Tibet.

2.1.4. Upper Khumbu (eastern part of the Nepal Himalayas). The Khumbu region lies immediately adjacent to the Tibetan border. In the triangle, enclosed by Dudh Kosi and Bhote Kosi, the Sherpa settlements are located (data on the Sherpa are presented in this chapter). The topographic features of this region are determined by the Dudh Kosi and Bhote Kosi river valleys. These two

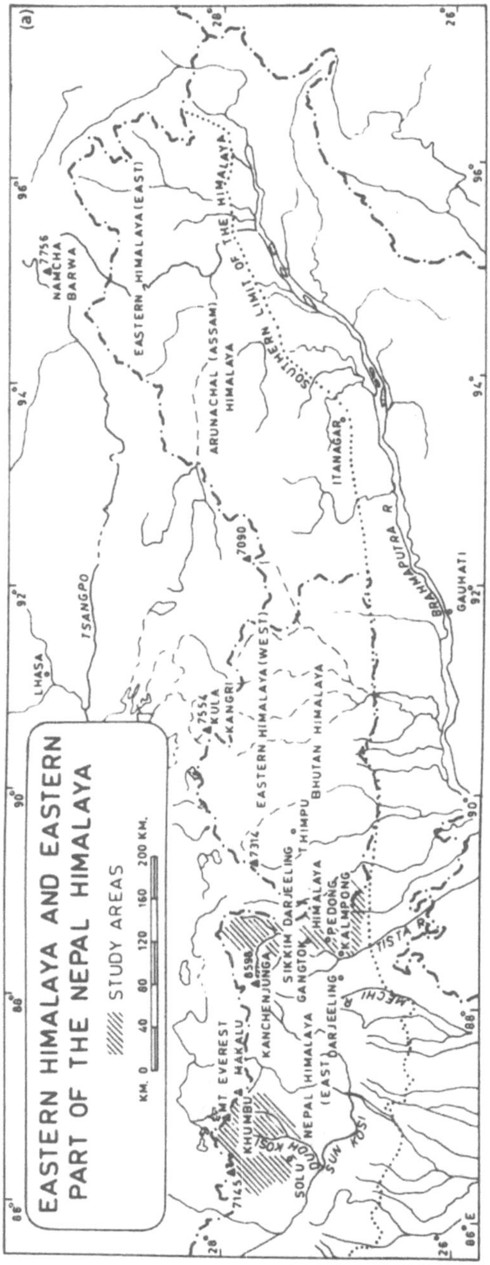

Figure 1. Map: (a) the eastern Himalayas, (b) the study areas, and (c) the study area in Kalimpong showing Sherpa and Lepcha villages.

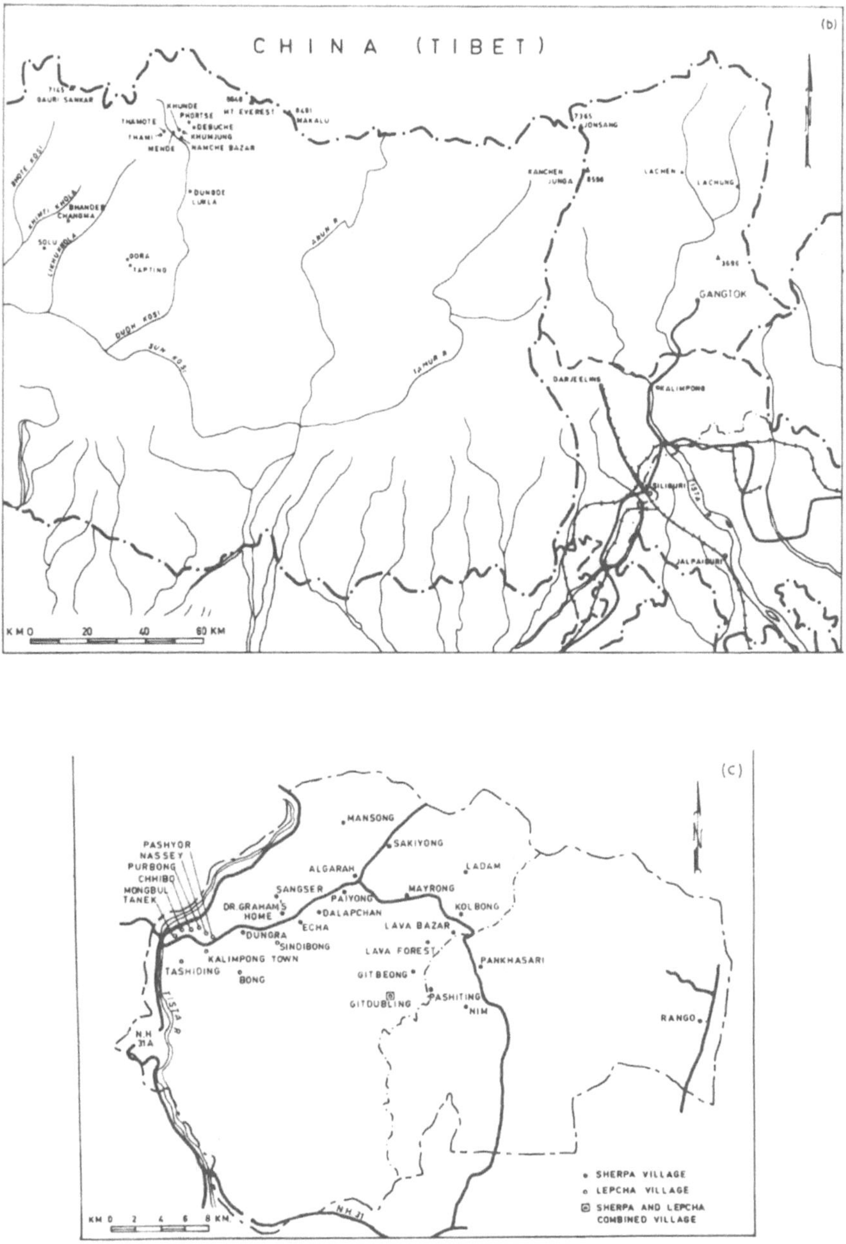

Figure 1. *(continued)*

Table I
Climatological Characteristics of the Western and Eastern Himalayas[a]

Region	Altitude (m)	Rainfall (mm)	Temperature (°C)	Total annual rainfall	Average monthly temperature (°C)	Humidity
Western Himalayas						
Leh	3522	5.1–12.7	+5.5–+21.1	84.0 mm	+10.0	Low
Simla	2130	1.2–52.7	+5.5–+20.0	198.2 cm	+13.3	Low
Eastern Himalayas						
Darjeeling	2130	0.5–80.7	+4.4–+16.6	307.7 cm	+14.4	High
Cherrapunji	1310	0.7–259	+11.7–+20.5	1142.0 cm	+17.0	High

[a]From Bose (1976).

rivers contribute to the formation of very steep valley sides and restrict access to the region. The highest Himalayan peak, Mount Everest, with an altitude of 8848 m, is located in this region. The eastern part of the Himalayas is a distinct physical unit; it is bounded by two north-south ranges, which are uncommon in the Himalayas.

2.2. Climatological Characteristics

Detailed data are not available, but Table I shows that the eastern Himalayas are characterized by relatively heavier rainfall and higher humidity than in the western Himalayas. Precipitation goes on increasing to about 2500 m. In summer, the monsoon from the southwest brings the major amount of rain. The eastern Himalayas have more rain and less snowfall, and they have the snowline at a higher level. Therefore the region has a richer and denser forest flora than the western Himalayas.

These generalities notwithstanding, wide variations exist within the eastern Himalayas and their constituent subregions with respect to physiographic and climatological characteristics. Data for the subregions from which microdemographic data are presented in this chapter can be seen in Table II.

3. Demographic Characteristics of the Eastern Himalayas and Neighboring Regions

Table III, which is based on macrolevel data, shows that population growth rates vary within the narrow range of 2–3% among the political/administrative units comprising the eastern Himalayas as well as the neighboring ones to the

Table II
Climatological Characteristics of the Study Areas

Area	Altitude (m)	Barometric pressure (mm/Hg)	Maximum temperature (°C)	Minimum temperature (°C)	Humidity (%)	Rainfall (mm)
Lachen	*ca.* 2600	550[e]	—	+7[f]	—	1270[f]
Kalimpong[a]	*ca.* 1200	655[e]	+15.5–+24.4[c]	+7.8–+19.3[c]	69–92[c]	4.9–635.0[c]
Upper Khumbu[b]	*ca.* 3500[d]	495[e]	+ 4.8–+16.2[d]	−11.5–+8.8[d]	68–88[d]	0.0–412.0[d]

[a]Because no meteorological data are available from the study areas, those from the town of Kalimpong are given.
[b]Because no meteorological data are available from all the study areas, those from Namche Bazar are given.
[c]Government of India, *Climatological Table of Observatories in India (1931–1960)*, Meteorological Department, Government of India Press, Nasik.
[d]His Majesty's Government of Nepal, *Climatological Records of Nepal (1971–1975)*, Volume 1, Department of Irrigation, Hydrology and Meteorology, His Majesty's Government of Nepal, Kathmandu.
[e]Estimated from Nomogram (Figure 2.3), Heath and Williams (1981).
[f]From Chopra (1979).

Table III
Macrodemographic Data, by Region/Country, on the Eastern Himalayan Populations

Region/country	Population 1961	Population 1971	Growth rate (*r*)	Population density/km²	Female literacy (%)	Source
Eastern Himalayas						
Arunachal Pradesh	337,000	468,000	0.0328	6[a]	3.71	Census, 1981
Nagaland	369,000	516,000	0.0335	31[a]	18.65	Census, 1981
Meghalaya	769,000	1,012,000	0.0275	45[a]	24.56	Census, 1981
Assam	10,837,000	14,625,000	0.0300	186[a]	18.63	Census, 1981
Bhutan	872,000	1,072,000	0.0206	46[b]	—	*World Population,* 1977
West Bengal (Darjeeling district)	624,640	781,777	0.0224	254[a]	23.23	Census, 1971
Sikkim	162,000	210,000	0.0260	30[a]	8.90	Census, 1981
Nepal (eastern region)	2,273,496	2,797,500	0.0207	81.2[a]	—	*Population of Nepal,* 1980
Tibet	1,500,000[c]	13,000,000	0.2160	—	—	Encyclopaedia Britannica, 1974

[a]1971 estimates.
[b]Per square mile.
[c]1951 estimates.

north, south, east, and west. Table III shows that neither the wide differences in physiographic and climatological characteristics nor in population density and sociocultural characteristics (e.g., GNP, per capita income/expenditure, female literacy, etc.) among these units and the constituent populations seem to make much impact at the macrolevel. The eastern Himalayan mountain dwellers seem to share their moderate (2–3%) growth rate with the Tibetans and the people of Nagaland, Meghalaya, and the Plains of Assam in the immediate neighborhood. The rate is not even strikingly different from the wider and much more diverse surrounding regions of India, Burma, mainland China, and Nepal as well as Asia as a whole (Table IV).

Such similarities, however, may be incidental and misleading, not only because large amounts of errors exist in census data from many "third world" countries, but also because finer variations among subareas/populations in relation to environmental stresses may be masked when data are pooled over wider areas/population aggregates. It was, therefore, considered desirable to compare and contrast subareas/populations within these political/administrative units that are characterized by differential physical environmental and/or sociocultural characteristics.

Table IV
Macrodemographic Data, by Country, on Neighboring Populations[a]

Country	Population 1961	Population 1971	Growth rate (r)
Burma	22,180,000	27,718,000	0.0223
Peoples' Republic of China	694,590,000	866,651,000	0.0221
India	454,946,000	566,180,000	0.0220
Nepal	9,417,000	11,566,000	0.0206
Bangladesh	54,992,000	71,556,000	0.0263

[a]From U.S. Bureau of the Census, *World Population* (1977).

4. Demographic Variations within Political/Administrative Units of the Eastern Himalayas

Demographic and environmental data are not available by subunits or populations for all the political/administrative units. However, the census data from Darjeeling district were broken down by the hill and plains subregions, and it appeared that the rate of population growth was much higher in the plains subregion than in the three hill subdivisions pooled together (Table V). The physiographic and climatological differences between the two subregions appear

Table V
Macrodemographic Data on the Plains and Hill Populations of the Darjeeling District[a]

Subregion	Population 1961	Population 1971	Growth rate (r)
Plains subdivision			
Siliguri	219,848	301,799	0.0317
Hill subdivisions			
Kalimpong	120,526	134,538	0.0110
Kurseong	8,074,300	100,233	0.0216
Darjeeling Sadar	203,523	245,207	0.0186
Pooled hill subdivisions	404,792	479,978	0.0170

[a]From Census (1971)

Table VI
Macrodemographic Data on the Bhutias and Lepchas[a]

	Population		
Social group	1961	1971	Growth rate (*r*)
Bhutia	23,595	33,912	0.0363
Lepcha	15,309	14,588	−0.0048

[a]From Das *et al.* (1978)

to provide a plausible explanation at first glance, but further breakdown of the data from the hill subdivisions shows considerable differences among themselves (Table V), suggesting that stresses other than, or in addition to, physical environmental ones need to be considered. The wide differences between the Bhutia and Lepcha tribal groups of the hill subregion in the rate of population growth (Table VI) may further substantiate the previously mentioned possibility. The lower developmental status of the Kalimpong subdivision when contrasted to Darjeeling Sadar, and Kurseong, as judged by sociocultural characteristics, for example, a higher percentage of agricultural laborers (landless peasants) in Kalimpong (11.10%) than in Darjeeling Sadar (6.70%) and Kurseong (7.36%) subdivisions (Census of India, West Bengal, 1971), may be related to its lower growth potentials (Table V).

Further corroboration of the intraregion variation in population growth rate is provided by analysis of population data on Scheduled tribes from Arunachal Pradesh. Excluding such populations for which the data seem to be grossly inaccurate (populations having annual growth rates higher than +5% or lower than −2% and female literacy above 10% were excluded), the population growth rate seems to be linearly related to female literacy (Figure 2).

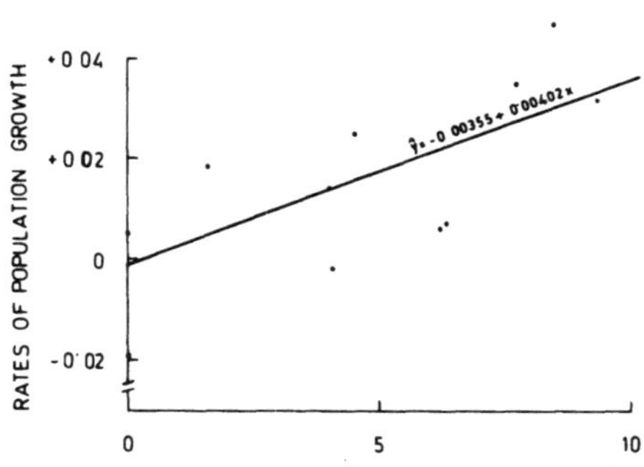

Figure 2. Population growth by female literacy.

Thus, the limited macrolevel data presented previously do show subregional and interpopulation variations in growth rates; these are presumably caused by region and community differentials in physical environmental, and sociocultural stresses. However, if such data are not amenable to any further, finer analyses, they nevertheless suggest that the apparent uniformity of the growth rates of populations of the eastern Himalayas and neighboring regions as well as those of the eastern Himalayan populations themselves may not be real and that intensive analyses of microlevel data from small, anthropological population units, which may conveniently be designated as *anthropological demography,* may yield useful results.

5. Anthropological Demography of Populations of the Eastern Himalayas

5.1. Anthropological Demography: Limitations and Advantages

Studies designated as *anthropological demography* are limited both in terms of their spatial coverage and the types of information collected; these studies are often conducted with very different and narrowly specialized objectives; their methodologies generally differ, and statistical methodologies are often far from rigorous, thereby rendering their utility suspect in the estimation of professional demographers. However, the intensive nature of the information collected and the scholar's personal, in-depth—even if subjective—knowledge of the people studied as well as of the totality of their environment may help one to comprehend the intricate interrelationships between the environmental stresses, on the one hand, and the demographic parameters, on the other.

A few illustrative examples are discussed later, mainly from our own studies on the *Sherpas* of Upper Khumbu, the northeastern Nepal and Kalimpong subdivisions, northern West Bengal, India, the *Lepchas,* also of the Kalimpong subdivision, northern West Bengal, India, and the *Bhutias* of northern Sikkim, India (Figure 1). The data are reviewed particularly from the physical environmental viewpoint (especially altitudinal) vis-à-vis sociocultural effects on the basic demographic variables of fertility and mortality.

5.2. Altitudinal Effects

In mountain-dwelling populations, the most obvious stress is what is called *altitude* in common scientific parlance, but what in reality is a set of stresses, that is, hypoxia, cold, terrain, high dosage of ultraviolet radiation, and iodine deficiency. Of all these stresses, hypoxia cannot yet be buffered by technological innovations and, therefore, is often treated as the most important altitudinal stress and is used almost synonymously by many. We shall speak of *altitude* as a

Table VII
Microdemographic Data on High and Low Altitude Sherpas[a]

Population	Altitude	Demographic measure: Completed family size (CFS)	Mean number of live births	Infant mortality rate	Source
High altitude					
Upper Khumbu	3500–4,050 m	4.77 (110)	3.11 (420)	15.78 (?)	Weitz *et al.*, 1978
Upper Khumbu	3500–4,050 m	4.53 (19)	4.06 (84)	7.21 (333)	Gupta, 1980
Low altitude					
Kalimpong	1000–1,500 m	7.44 (69)	5.00 (247)	6.58 (1186)	Gupta, 1980
Solu and Arun	ca. 1000–1,500 m	8.54 (26)	—	—	Bangham and Sacherer, 1980

[a]Figures in parentheses indicate number of women aged ≥ 45 years in case of CFS; number of women of all ages in case of mean number of live births and number of live births to mothers of all ages in case of IMR.

physiographic condition with which a multitude of stresses, including sociocultural ones, are associated. We shall not be able to isolate the effects of each of these stresses, but we shall try to evaluate the relative roles of, and interactions between, the two major sets of stresses, that is, physical environmental and sociocultural. The latter is presumably more variable than the former within a given ecological niche.

Several sets of fertility data are available from the high altitude region of Upper Khumbu as well as the lower altitude regions of Solu in eastern Nepal and Kalimpong (Table VII). Gupta (1980) in a comparative study between the high and low altitude Sherpas of Upper Khumbu and Kalimpong, respectively, has shown that fertility is considerably lower in the former than in the latter, judging by several fertility measures. Infant mortality is very similar between the two (Table VII and Figure 3). Completed family size in Weitz *et al.*'s (1978) sample of Upper Khumbu Sherpas is very similar to that in Gupta's (1980). Completed family size in Bangham and Sacherer's (1980) low altitude Sherpa sample from Solu is similar to that of Gupta's low altitude Kalimpong Sherpa sample, indicating the consistency of altitudinal difference in fertility reported by Gupta (1980). Gupta's report of low fertility in the high altitude Sherpas has been questioned by Goldstein *et al.* (1983) on the basis of possible underreporting, especially by old women due to recall lapse. Goldstein *et al.*'s (1983) own data from the population of Limi in western Nepal indicate that fertility is about as high as in Gupta's

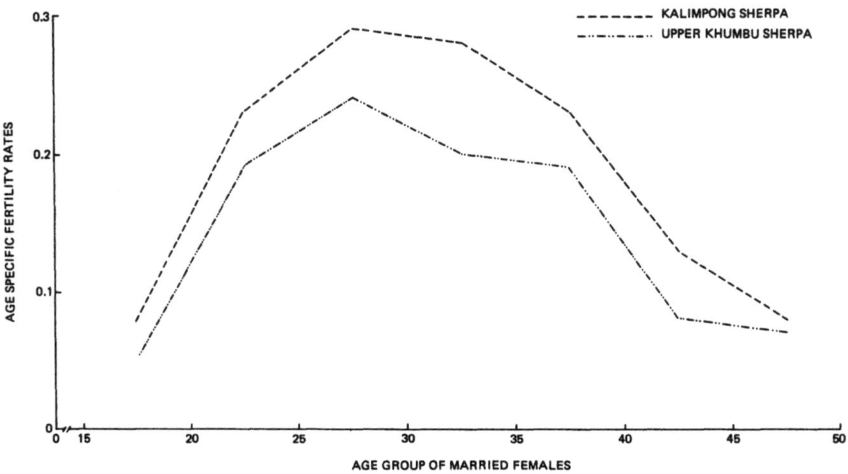

Figure 3. Age-specific fertility rates: High and low altitude Sherpas.

low altitude Sherpas. Gupta's (1980) data were collected by structured questionnaire schedules by the same investigator (R.G.) in both altitudinal subgroups, following all the standard methodological precautions used in anthropological field studies involving demographic and socioeconomic investigations. The possibilities of recall lapse and consequent underreporting cannot be incontrovertibly ruled out, but its magnitude is likely to be low and is unlikely to be very different among the several populations under consideration—including Goldstein *et al.*'s. The high fertility of Goldstein *et al.*'s (1983) Limi sample *per se* does not imply inaccuracy in Gupta's (1980) data that, corroborated as they are by Weitz *et al.*'s (1978) and Bangham and Sacherer's (1980) high and low altitude data, respectively, may still indicate a lower fertility at the high altitude. This pattern has also been suggested for Nepalese and Andean populations by Abelson (1982) who reviewed some extant data. Infant mortality, on the other hand, does not seem to differ between the high and low altitude Sherpas (Table VII). This is unlike the other populations studied (Baker and Dutt, 1972; Dutt, 1980).

5.3. Sociocultural Effects

Effects of sociocultural factors, for example, income/expenditure, education, and occupation, on fertility and mortality is wellknown (Whelpton and Kiser, 1950; Lorimer *et al.*, 1954; Nag, 1962; Mamdani, 1972; Stanhope and Hornabrook, 1974; Zodgekar, 1975; Chang *et al.*, 1979). That these factors operate in high altitude populations and perhaps override the effects of the narrowly specialized and relatively severe physical environmental stresses of hypoxia, cold, and terrain, has been shown by Baker to be true (1976) for an Andean population (the economic value of children might have promoted high fertility) and by Weitz *et al.* (1978) for a Himalayan population (modernization/acculturation might have led to low fertility). Data on infant mortality are not available for these populations, with the exception of Gupta's (1980); therefore, an analogous analysis of sociocultural effects cannot be done for them.

That sociocultural factors can also operate in the hill regions at a much lower altitude can be demonstrated using our own data from two subgroups of the low altitude Sherpas who inhabit similar altitudes of about 1500 m but which are distinguishable by their degree of urban contact (Basu and Mukhopadhyay, 1980). The data show (Table VIII) that both fertility and mortality are higher in the relatively remote subgroup working as laborers in the medicinal plantation of Rango than in the somewhat urbanized, pooled Sherpa subgroup. This confirms the sociocultural effects found in the high altitudes. Sociocultural effects are currently being investigated among the Lepchas who inhabit villages close to those of Sherpas in the Kalimpong subdivision. They are believed to be indigenous to these middle altitudes (Gorer, 1967; Das, 1978; Thakur and Lepcha, 1981). The data (Table VIII) show that both fertility and infant mortality are higher among the Buddhist than among Christian Lepchas. Presuming that the Christian Lepchas are economically better-off, more educated, and enjoy better living conditions due to missionary influence, this observation corroborates the finding of the effect of modernization on fertility among the Sherpas of both high (Weitz *et al.*, 1978) and low (Basu and Mukhopadhyay, 1980) altitudes.

The previously mentioned findings that the relationship between environmental stresses and demographic characteristics are not straightforward render suspect the common notion about the universality of the adverse effects of hypoxic stress on fertility. Indeed, the role of hypoxia (operating through phys-

Table VIII
Microdemographic Data on Sherpa and Lepcha Sociocultural Subgroups[a]

	Sherpa		Lepcha	
Demographic measure	More urbanized	Less urbanized	Buddhist	Christian
Completed family size	7.44	8.30	7.00	5.83
	(69)	(10)	(6)	(30)
Infant mortality rate	6.58	13.83	11.67	3.48
	(1186)	(253)	(240)	(517)

[a]Figures in parentheses indicate number of women aged ≥ 45 years in case of CFS and number of live births to mothers of all ages in case of IMR.

iologically determined processes of fecundity–inhibition) versus that of sociocultural stresses (operating through deliberate or incidental reduction of the exposure to the risk of pregnancy and/or its premature termination) is presently being debated (Bangham and Sacherer, 1981; Weitz, 1981). It seems more worthwhile to us, however, to evaluate the relative effects of the altitude-related physical environmental stress complex vis-à-vis the sociocultural one, of individual stresses within each complex, and of interactions between individual stresses as well as the stress complexes.

5.4. Effect of Interactions between Altitudinal and Sociocultural Stresses

Data from the Bhutias of two mountain villages, Lachung and Lachen, in northern Sikkim enable us to probe into the possible relationship between physical environmental and sociocultural stresses. Lachung is located at an altitude of about 2300 m and Lachen at about 2600 m. Both populations are generally believed to be of Tibetan origin; they speak a Tibetan dialect and follow the Tibetan sect of Buddhism (Chopra, 1979). Both villages are physically and culturally somewhat isolated. Transportation is limited to the southern area by infrequent bus service. Both populations are primarily agricultural. However, they differ remarkably with respect to their agricultural activity pattern: Whereas the people of Lachung travel to their agricultural fields at about 1200 m and stay there in temporary villages for sowing in April and May and for harvesting in August and September, the people of Lachen travel to about 4000 m and stay there to work their potato fields and to raise the crop during the same periods. Thus, although the people of Lachen are exposed regularly to the stressful physical environment of 4000 m twice a year, for a couple of months each time, those of Lachung enjoy the much milder physical environment at 1200 m for about the same period because of the differential locations of their agricultural fields.

Demographic data on the populations of Lachung and Lachen show that fertility is lower and infant mortality higher in the latter than in the former (Table IX). Figure 4 shows that age-specific fertility rates are higher in Lachen in the 15–19- and 20–24-year-old groups, but then decline as compared with Lachung, presumably due to the adverse effects of repeated exposures to high altitude stresses.

No definitive interpretations of the demographic differences between the two villages can be given with the data at our disposal, but plausible conjectures can be made. The ethnic origin and major sociocultural characteristics are similar between the Lachung and Lachen, and therefore, the demographic differences may be attributable to the only environmental differences existing between them,

Table IX
Microdemographic Data on the Populations of Lachung and Lachen[a]

Demographic measure	Population: Lachung	Lachen
Completed family size (CFS)	6.91 (22)[b]	3.80 (5)
Infant mortality rate (IMR)	7.63 (354)	22.34 (94)

[a]From Das *et al.* (1981).
[b]Figures in parentheses indicate number of women aged ≥ 45 years in case of CFS and number of live births to mothers of all ages in case of IMR.

namely, differential exposures to the high altitude environment, which in turn is determined by the differential transhumance pattern and differential frequency of polyandry (Lachung, 25.00%; Lachen, 42.11%). Considering that although polyandry is sometimes believed to reduce fertility at the population level, it is unlikely to do so at the individual level (Goldstein, 1976). This factor may be ruled out and the other alternative, that is, differential exposure to the altitudinal stresses, merits further consideration.

The high altitude environment is generally believed to adversely affect spermatogenesis and oogenesis, elevate the number of defective sperms, raise

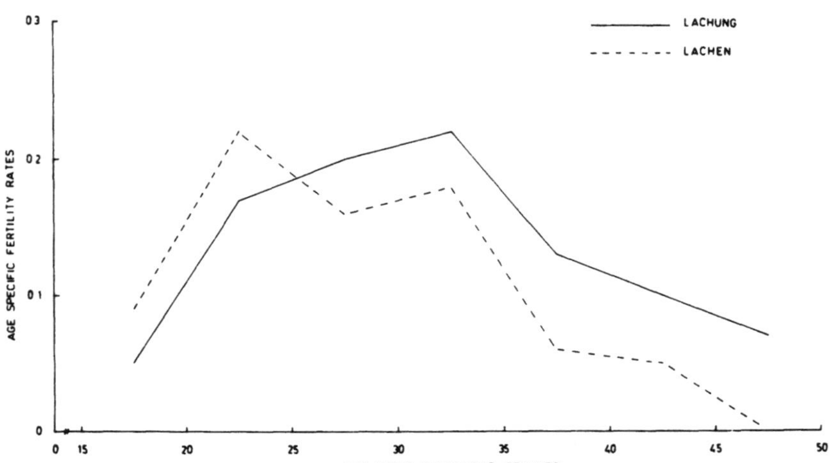

Figure 4. Age-specific fertility rates: Lachen and Lachung populations.

menarcheal age, hinder implantation, increase the chances of prenatal, neonatal, and perinatal mortality—in short, to inhibit fecundity and therefore fertility in animals and humans (Grahn and Kratchman, 1963; Mazess, 1965; Cruz-Coke *et al.*, 1966; Donayre, 1966; Donayre *et al.*, 1968; Frisancho and Baker, 1970; MacLennan *et al.*, 1972; Ward, 1975; Abelson 1976). These adverse effects are particularly noticeable intially when subjects from a lower altitude are taken to a high altitude habitat. Subsequently, however, the effects decline and stabilize at a somewhat lower level (Guerra-Garcia *et al.*, 1965; Hock, 1970). The adverse effects disappear, sometimes, when the subjects return to their native habitat, but the exact amount of time required for reversal to the original state is not well known. It is likely, however, that repeated exposures result in repeated adverse effects and do not permit acclimatization to occur. Therefore repeated exposures may be more harmful than prolonged exposure to high altitude stresses. It is also possible that once exposed to the high altitude environment, permanent damage is caused, and repeated exposures act as boosters. A plausible explanation of the fertility and mortality differences between the people of Lachung and Lachen may be as follows: The brief but repeated exposures to the high altitude environment at 4000 m where the potato fields are located adversely affects the reproductive system in the case of the Lachen people, reducing their fertility to the level of the high altitude Sherpas and increasing their mortality to even a higher level. In the case of the Lachung people, whose agricultural practices take them to a milder environment for similar periods, neither such damages nor the consequent fecundity/fertility reduction occur. The crucial point here is, if the sociocultural phenomenon of differential transhumance has caused differential exposure to the high altitude physical environmental stresses and thereby differentially affected fecundity/fertility between the people of Lachung and Lachen, then the controversy regarding physical environmental *versus* sociocultural stresses in the determination of human demographic characteristics becomes meaningless. It may, instead, render more meaningful the recognition of the complementarity of the two sets of variables, the study of their interactions in situations of the present kind and the identification and measurement of the relative individual effects as well as interaction effects on specific human traits/trait complexes in order that, eventually, the stress-effect relationship(s) can be formulated in somewhat general terms. Such studies may also help recognize the fact that hypoxia-induced fecundity inhibition due to the nature of the habitat, *deliberate* culturally induced reduction of exposure to the risk of pregnancy, and *incidental* culturally induced increased exposure to the high altitude stress in one but not another of a set of ethnically similar groups are all parts of a human population's total response—conscious or unconscious—to the totality of the stress complex associated with high altitudes. Such recognition may provide a broader understanding of the people–environment relationship than has so far been achieved, including a resolution of the crucial question regarding whether the mountain/high altitude environment should be treated at all as a specialized niche in the human situation.

6. Mountain/High Altitude Environment as a Specialized Niche

The basic question regarding the mountain/high altitude environment as a specialized niche in the human case cannot be definitively answered in this brief discourse, but it is, nevertheless, raised here if only to emphasize its vital importance. The following points, which are relevant in the context of this question, emerge tentatively from the preceding discussion.

1. The sociocultural factors that are widely known to affect demographic parameters at low altitudes (e.g., economic condition, occupation, urban contact, etc.) also operate in the mountain/high altitude environment.
2. In the human situation, altitudinal differences in demographic characteristics may not be attributable exclusively, or even mainly, to altitude-related physical environmental stresses; sociocultural stresses may be as effective in the mountain/high altitude environment as they are in low altitudes.
3. Interactions of physical environmental and sociocultural stresses and the demographic consequences thereof, as, for instance, in Lachen and Lachung, may form the crux of the problem at high altitudes as much as at the low altitudes.

It is to this last-mentioned aspect of the people–environment relationship that we plan to address ourselves to in future, applying a rigorous statistical methodology on detailed and extensive data that is collected by intensive, micro-level anthropological demographic techniques, with a view to evaluating and promoting population health and well-being of physiographically and/or socioculturally remote communities.

Acknowledgments

We are indebted to the people of our study areas, particularly to Dawa Tshering Sherpa, Pasang Tshering Sherpa, D. T. Tamsong, Tansing Lepcha, and Duk Tshering Lepcha of Kalimpong; and to Kami Doma, Konje Chunbi, and Ang Tshering Sherpa of Upper Khumbu for their help and cooperation to our studies. We are grateful to His Majesty's Government of Nepal, the Tribhuvan University, Kirtipur, the National Park and Wildlife Conservation Office, Kathmandu, and the Indian Embassy, Kathmandu, for providing permission and help to carry out fieldwork in Upper Khumbu. We wish to thank the subdivisional authorities, Kalimpong, Scheduled Castes and Tribes Welfare Department and the Directorate of Cinchona and Other Medicinal Plants, Government of West Bengal for organizational help in Kalimpong. We are indebted to Bhola Chatterjee and Professor B. P. Adhikari, ISI, for help and advice in organizing the work in Nepal; Ethnor, Ltd., Dolphin Laboratories, Ltd., East India Pharmaceutical Works, Ltd., Life Pharmaceuticals Pvt. Ltd., Ciba Pharmaceuticals Division, and Dey's Medical Stores for donating medicine to our projects. We also wish to thank Badal Dey for providing technical help, P. C. Kumar for preparing the diagrams, P. Adhikary for preparing the manuscript.

References

Abelson, A. E., 1976, Altitude and fertility, *Hum. Biol.* **48:**83–92.

Abelson, A. E., 1982, Altitude and Fertility: Biological and Cultural Effects, Paper presented to the Golden Jubilee Conference, Indian Statistical Institute, Calcutta.

Baker, P. T., 1969, Human adaptation to high altitude, *Science* **165:**1149–1156.

Baker, P. T. (ed.), 1978, *The Biology of High Altitude People,* Cambridge University Press, Cambridge.

Baker, P. T., and Dutt, J. S., 1972, Demographic variables as measures of biological adaptation: A case study of high altitude populations, in: *The structure of Human Populations* (G. A. Harrison and A. J. Boyce, eds.), Clarendon Press, Oxford, pp. 352–378.

Baker, T. S., 1976, Child care, child training and environment, in: *Man in the Andes: A Multidisciplinary Study of High Altitude Quechua* (P. T. Baker and M. A. Little, eds.), Dowden, Hutchinson and Ross, Pennsylvania, pp. 85–97.

Bangham, C. R. M., and Sacherer, J. M., 1980, Fertility of Nepalese Sherpas at moderate altitudes: Comparison with high altitude data, *Ann. Hum. Biol.* **7:**323–330.

Bangham, C. R. M., and Sacherer, J. M., 1981, Letter to the editor, *Ann. Hum. Biol.* **8:**385–386.

Basu, A., and Mukhopadhyay, B., 1980, Physical environmental and sociocultural correlates of demographic characteristics among the Sherpas, an indigenous high altitude population of the eastern Himalayas, *Arch. Biol. Andina* **10:**3–11.

Bose, S. C., 1976, *The Geography of the Himalaya,* National Book Trust, New Delhi.

Brush, S. B., 1976, Introduction: Cultural adaptations to mountain ecosystems symposium, *Hum. Ecol.* **4:**125–135.

Census of India, 1971, *District Census Handbook, Darjeeling District, West Bengal,* Series 22, Part X-A and B, Director of Census Operation, West Bengal.

Census of India, 1981, *Provisional Population Totals,* Ser. 1, India, Registrar General and Census Commissioner for India, Delhi.

Chang, G. C., Warren, R. D., and Pendleton, B. F., 1979, Testing and clarifying a macromodel of socioeconomic change and fertility, *Soc. Biol.* **26:**30–50.

Chopra, P. N., 1979, *Sikkim,* S. Chand and Co., New Delhi.

Cruz-Coke, R., 1967, Genetic Characteristics of High Altitude Populations in Chile, Paper presented at PAHO/WHO/IBP Meeting of Investigators on Population Biology of Altitude, November, 13–17, Washington, D. C.

Cruz-Coke, R., Cristoffanni, A. P., Aspillaga, A., and Biancani, F., 1966, Evolutionary forces in human populations in an environmental gradient in Arica, *Hum. Biol.* **38:**421–438.

Das, A. K., 1978, *The Lepchas of West Bengal,* Editions Indian, Calcutta.

Das, A. K., Chowdhuri, M. K., Basu, S. K., Saha, R. N., and Khan, N. C., 1978, *Scheduled Tribes and Scheduled Castes of West Bengal,* Cultural Research Institute, Government of West Bengal, Calcutta.

Das, S. K., Majumder, P. P., and Basu, A., 1981, Demography and demographical genetics of two isolated mountain villages of Northern Sikkim, Eastern Himalayas, *J. Ind. Anthrop Soc.* **17:**155–162.

Donayre, J., 1966, Population growth and fertility at high altitude, in: *Life at High Altitude* (A. Hurtado, ed.), Sci. Publ. **140,** Pan American Health Organization, Washington D. C., pp. 74–79.

Donayre, J., Guerra-Garcia, R., Moncloa, F., and Sobrevilla, L. A., 1968, Endocrine studies at high altitude: IV. Changes in the semen of men, *J. Reprod. Fertil.* **16:**55–58.

Dutt, J. S., 1980, Altitude and fertility: The confounding effect of childhood mortality: A Bolivian example, *Soc. Biol.* **27:**101–113.

Encyclopaedia Britannica, *Macropaedia,* Volume 18, 1974, Encyclopaedia Britannica, Inc., Chicago.

Feigen, G. A., and Johnson, P. K., 1964, Blood volume and heart weights in two strains of rats during adaptation to a natural altitude of 12,470 feet, in: *The Physiological Effects of High Altitude* (W. H. Weihe, ed.), Pergamon Press, Oxford, pp. 45–58.

Frisancho, A. R., 1976, Growth and morphology at high altitude: I. Growth and functional development at high altitude, in: *Man in the Andes: A Multidisciplinary Study of High Altitude Quechua* (P. T. Baker and M. A. Little, eds.), Dowden, Hutchinson and Ross, Pennsylvania, pp. 180–200.

Frisancho, A. R., and Baker, P. T., 1970, Altitude and growth of a high altitude Peruvian Quechua population, *Am. J. Phys. Anthropol.* **32:**279–292.

Gazetteer of India, 1973, *Country and People,* Volume I, Publications Division, Government of India.

Goldstein, M. C., 1976, Fraternal polyandry and fertility in a high altitude Himalayan valley in northwestern Nepal, *Hum. Ecol.* **4:**223–235.

Goldstein, M. C., Tsarong, P., and Beall, C. M., 1983, High altitude hypoxia, culture and human fecundity/fertility: A comparative study, *Am. Anthrop.* **85:**28–49.

Gordon, A. S., Tornetta, F. J., D'Angelo, S. A., and Charipper, H. A., 1943, Effects of low atmospheric pressure on the activity of the thyroid, reproductive system and anterior lobe of the pituitary in the rat, *Endocrinology* **33:**366–383.

Gorer, G., 1967, *Himalayan Village: An Account of the Lepchas of Sikkim,* Joseph, London.

Government of India, 1960, *Climatological Tables of Observatories in India* (1931–1960), Meteorological Department, Government of India Press, Nasik.

Grahn, D., and Kratchman, J., 1963, Variation in neonatal death rate and birth weight in the United States and possible relations to environmental radiation, geology and altitude, *Am. J. Hum. Genet.* **15:**329–352.

Guerra-Garcia, R., Donayre, J., Sobrevilla, L. A., and Moncloa, F., 1965, Cambios en la testesterone urinaria en sujetos expuestos a la altura, in: *Proc. of the Sixth Pan American Congress of Endocrinology,* **130.**

Gupta, R., 1980, Altitude and demography among the Sherpas, *J. Biosoc. Sci.* **12:**103–114.

Haas, J. D., 1976, Prenatal and infant growth and development, in: *Man in the Andes: A Multidisciplinary Study of High Altitude Quechua* (P. T. Baker and M. A. Little, eds.) Dowden, Hutchinson and Ross, Pennsylvania, pp. 161–179.

Heath, D., and Williams, D. R., 1981, *Man at High Altitude,* Churchill Livingstone, Edinburgh.

His Majesty's Government of Nepal, 1975, *Climatological Records of Nepal,* Volume I, Department of Irrigation, Hydrology and Meteorology, Kathmandu.

Hock, R. J., 1970, The physiology of high altitude, *Sci. Am.* **222:**52–62.

Hoff, C., 1974, Altitudinal variations in the physical growth and development of Peruvian Quechuas, *Homo* 24:87–99.

Hu, S. T., 1981, Physiological comparison of the Tibetan (Tsan) highlanders and the Han lowlanders at moderate and great altitudes, in: *Environmental and Human Population Problems at High Altitude,* CNRS, Paris, pp. 47–48.

Lord, B. I., and Murphy, M. J., 1973, Haematopietic stem cell regulation, II. Chronic effects of hypoxia on C.F.U. kinetics, *Blood* **42:**89–98.

Lorimer, F., Fortes, M., Busia, K. A., Richards, A. I., Reining, P., and Mortara, G. (eds.), 1954, *Culture and Human Fertility,* UNESCO, Paris.

MacLennan, A. H., Sharp, F., and Shaw-Dunn, J., 1972, The ultrastructure of human trophoblast in spontaneous and induced hypoxia using a system of organ culture, *J. Obstet. Gynecol. Br. Common.* **72:**113–121.

Mamdani, M., 1972, *The Myth of Population Control: Family, Caste, and Class in an Indian Village,* Monthly Review Press, New York.

Mazess, R. B., 1965, Neonatal mortality and altitude in Peru, *Am. J. Phys. Antrhopol.* **23:**209–214.

Mirrakhimov, M. M., 1978, Biological and physiological characteristics of the high altitude natives of Tien Shan and the Pamirs, in: *The Biology of High Altitude Peoples* (P. T. Baker, ed.), Cambridge University Press, Cambridge, pp. 299–315.

Mueller, W. H., Schull, V. N., Schull, W. J., Soto, P., and Rothhammer, F., 1978, A multinational Andean genetic and health programme: Growth and development in an hypoxic environment, *Ann. Hum. Biol.* **5:**329–352.

Nag, M., 1962, *Factors Affecting Human Fertility in Nonindustrial Societies: A Cross-cultural Study,* Department of Anthropology, Yale University, New Haven.

Pawson, I. G., 1974, The Growth and Development in High Altitude Children with Special Emphasis on Populations of Tibetan Origin in Nepal, Ph.D. thesis, The Pennsylvania State University, University Park, Pennsylvania.

Pawson, I. G., and Jest, C., 1978, The high altitude areas of the world and their cultures, in: *The Biology of High Altitude Peoples* (P. T. Baker, ed.), Cambridge University Press, Cambridge, pp. 17–45.

Pugh, L. G. C. E., 1966, A programme for physiological studies of high altitude peoples, in: *The Biology of Human Adaptability* (P. T. Baker and J. S. Weiner, eds.), Clarendon Press, Oxford, pp. 521–532.

Rothhammer, F., and Spielman, R., 1972, Anthropometric variation in the Aymara: Genetic, geographic and topographic contributions, *Am. J. Hum. Genet.* **24:**371–380.

Schull, W. J., and Rothhammer, F., 1977, A multinational Andean genetic and health programme: Rationale and design for a study of adaptation to the hypoxia of altitude, in: *Physiological Variation and its Genetic Basis* (J. S. Weiner, ed.), Society for the Study of Human Biology, Symposia Volume 17, Taylor and Francis, London, pp. 139–169.

Stanhope, J. M., and Hornabrook, R. W., 1974, Fertility patterns of two. New Guinea populations: Karkar and Lufa, *J. Biosoc. Sci.* **6:**439–452.

Stycos, J. M., 1963, Culture and differential fertility in Peru, *Popul. Stud.* **16:**257–270.

Sundstroem, E. S., and Michaels, G. S., 1942, *The Adrenal Cortex in Adaptation to Altitude, Climate and Cancer,* University of California, Los Angeles, California.

Thakur, R., and Lepcha, S. W., 1981, Who are the Lepchas?, *East. Anthropol.* **34:**221–226.

Timiras, P. S., 1964, Comparison of growth and development of the rat at high altitude and at sea level, in: *The Physiological Effects of High Altitude* (W. H. Weihe, ed.), Pergamon Press, Oxford, pp. 21–44.

United Nations, 1980, *Population of Nepal,* ESCAP Country Monograph Series No. 6, ESCAP, Bangkok.

U. S. Bureau of Census, 1978, *World Populations: 1977, Recent Demographic Estimates for the Countries and Regions of the World,* Washington, D.C.

Ward, M., 1975, *Mountain Medicine,* Crosby, Lockwood and Staples, London.

Weihe, W. H. (ed.), 1964, *The Physiological Effects of High Altitude,* Pergamon Press, Oxford.

Weitz, C. A., 1973, The Effects of Aging and Habitual Activity Pattern on Exercise among a High Altitude Himalayan Population, Ph.D. thesis, The Pennsylvania State University, Pennsylvania.

Weitz, C. A., 1980, Biocultural Adaptations of the High Altitude Sherpas of Nepal, Paper presented at the 9th Wisconsin Conference on South Asia, November 1980.

Weitz, C. A., 1981, Letter to editor, *Ann. Hum. Biol.* **8**:383–385.

Weitz, C. A., Pawson, I. G., Weitz, M. V., Lang, S. D. R., and Lang, A., 1978, Cultural factors affecting the demographic structure of a high altitude Nepalese population, *Soc. Biol.* **25**:179–195.

Whelpton, P. K., and Kiser, C. V. (eds.), 1950, *Social and Psychological Factors Affecting Fertility,* Volume II, Milbank Memorial Fund, New York.

World Health Organization, 1971, Family planning in health services, *World Health Organization Technical Report Series* **476,** World Health Organization, Geneva.

Zodgekar, A. V., 1975, Maori fertility in transition, *J. Biosoc. Sci.* **7**:345–352.

CHAPTER 17

Aging and Growth at High Altitudes in the Himalayas

CYNTHIA M. BEALL

1. Introduction

The Himalayas and adjoining slopes and plateaus represent a unique setting for addressing a number of theoretical issues about the biological aging process. This chapter presents information on aspects of growth, development, and aging in a Himalayan population residing in a high altitude, rugged environment in Nepal and discusses this information in the context of several theories about factors influencing biological aging.

Biological aging is viewed as a progressive and irreversible morphological and functional change that gradually leads to a decline in adaptive and performance capacities (Bourliere, 1970; Shock, 1977; Comfort, 1979). Understanding the phenomenon of differential aging, the varying tempos at which individuals and populations show changes with age, is a challenging scientific problem. Two alternative time perspectives may be applied. One perspective limits the study of biological aging to changes occurring after the maturity of size or function has been attained. This may be difficult to apply to an entire organism because the various organ systems have different developmental timetables. Another perspective, the life span approach, has the premise that aging is a lifelong process beginning with conception and ending with death and it empha-

---

CYNTHIA M. BEALL • Department of Anthropology, Case Western Reserve University, Cleveland, Ohio 44106. The material from Upper Chumik is based upon work supported by the National Science Foundation under Grant No. BNS 80-14317. The material from Mugu, Helambu, and Pokhara, Nepal, is based upon work supported by grants from the Provost of Western Reserve College and the Office of Research Administration of Case Western Reserve University.

sizes the interrelatedness of the various stages of the life span. This may also be difficult to apply due to difficulties in assembling appropriate data relevant to several stages of the life cycle. Yet stages of the life cycle clearly are not isolated, self-contained events, and factors underlying differential aging theoretically may exert their influence at numerous times. Scientific interest in variation in the tempo of growth and development prior to attaining mature body size is longstanding (e.g., Sanders, 1934). For example, the accumulation of a large body of data on adolescent growth has permitted elaboration of hypotheses about its control (e.g., Frisch, 1978). Yet, despite documentation of variation in the patterns of change in morphology and function throughout adulthood (e.g., Bourlière, 1970), variation in the tempo of change after maturity has been subject to less scientific scrutiny, and systematic data collection in diverse populations and environments remains to be undertaken. There is no general agreement that certain populations, life-styles, cultural settings, or environments slow or accelerate the tempo of biological changes after maturity. There are, however, numerous hypotheses, and several especially pertinent ones for some Himalayan populations include those that focus on aspects of the physical environment and on certain biological characteristics of the populations. It is, however, possible to develop the competing theoretical arguments that high altitude Himalayan populations experience an accelerated tempo of biological changes before maturity and that they enjoy a slowed pace of biological change after maturity.

Some have reasoned that high altitude residents may lose function relatively rapidly after maturity is attained, that is, that the tempo is accelerated (McFarland, 1963, 1969, 1972; Frisancho, 1975). The environmental stress of high altitude hypoxia necessitates physiological adaptations to transport sufficient oxygen to the tissues. Throughout adulthood at sea level there is a progressively diminishing capacity to transport oxygen to the tissues (Davies, 1972). Noting the common physiological stress and a commonality between certain physiological aspects of old age and the response of young adults to acute high altitude hypoxia exposure led to an hypothesis implicating hypoxia as an etiologic agent of senescence (McFarland, 1963, 1969, 1972). Similar reasoning led to the hypothesis that the combined effects of high altitude hypoxia and an age-related diminished capacity to transport oxygen may accelerate the biological aging process (Frisancho, 1975).

On the other hand, several independent lines of reasoning argue that Himalayan populations may enjoy a slow pace of biological aging. One line emphasizes the rugged Himalayan physical environment. Leaf (1972) has hypothesized that life in rugged terrains where daily physical exertion is unavoidable leads to maintenance of a high level of physical fitness and functional capacity throughout the life span. Another line of reasoning focuses on slow growth in stature found among some Himalayan populations (Beall, 1981a, 1981b). Experimental work with laboratory animals finds that slower growth and a longer growing period prior to attaining maturity of body size is associated with later onset of some senescent changes and a longer life span (e.g., Goodrick, 1978). Furthermore, a purely theoretical line of reasoning argues that it is unusually disadvantageous from the standpoint of adaptive fitness for residents of an extreme environment to lose biological function and adaptive capacity. Thus, it might be hypothesized that biological aging is slowed in populations resident in rugged, high altitude environments.

The goal of this chapter is to explore the issue of the relative tempo of growth and development throughout the life cycle in Himalayan populations. The chapter adopts a life-span approach and features data from a single Himalayan population resident at high altitude in a rugged terrain in Nepal, comparing that population with other Himalayan populations and with sea-level Western populations. Four physiological systems easily and meaningfully measured over several stages of the life cycle are analyzed. Systems not involved in oxygen transport as well as those so involved are described because there is evidence from Andean high altitude populations that the growth of the two types is affected differently (Mueller *et al.*, 1978; Frisancho, 1981). Age differences in stature and in the development of the female reproductive system, neither of which is involved in oxygen transport, and age differences in pulmonary volumes and hemoglobin levels, both of which are involved in oxygen transport, are described and discussed first in a single Himalayan population and then in comparison with other Himalayan populations, an Andean high altitude population and Western sea-level populations (where data are available). The relative tempos of growth and development through several stages of the life cycle are evaluated. The question of whether the age differences truly represent aging phenomena or are instead artifacts of a secular trend is considered. This is a preliminary analysis and discussion of these data, one that illustrates utilities as well as difficulties of expanding the study of the varying tempos of growth and development to include processes occurring after mature size or function has been attained.

2. Description of Principal Population Samples and Comparative Samples

2.1. Principal Sample: Upper Chumik, Nepal

The principal sample for which data are presented is drawn from the population of Upper Chumik, Mustang District, Dhaulagiri Zone, Nepal—a small high altitude valley inhabited by native Tibetan-speaking Buddhists living in six villages ranging in altitude from 3250 to 3560 m. Agricultural fields and pastures range along steep slopes that are higher in altitude than the villages. Daily activity entails numerous climbs over uneven and steep trails between houses, fields, pastures, sources of water and fodder, other villages, and religious sites.

A 1977 census counted 1260 Tibetan residents, 8% of whom were over 60 years old. The present sample totaling 689 individuals is derived from all the villages and represents 56% of the 1977 census total, and 64% of those over 60. The sample consists of participants in a study of aging and high altitude adaptation conducted from June through September, 1981. At this time, the 1977 census was updated in four of the villages. The present sample represents 72% of the total population of these villages and 92% of those over 60. Essential to any study of biological age is accurate chronological age. The Tibetan system of assigning chronological age relies upon a 60-year cycle of named years. Individuals know the name of their birth year that is easily translated into the Western calendrical system to yield an accurate age in years.

A medical examination (collection of current medical complaints, a review of systems, and a physical exam) and anthropometric measurements were performed for each participant. A pulmonary function test was administered to those over 9 and a finger-stick blood sample obtained from those 14 and over. This chapter reports data on several subsamples isolated on the basis of age, sex and/or health status.

Means of stature are plotted for 1-year age intervals from 5 to 24, for 10-year intervals (25–34, etc.) through 64 and for one 15-year interval from age 65 to 79 (n = 600). The median age at menarche and menopause is estimated two ways, first by applying probit analysis to a status quo subsample of 80 females aged 12 to 25 and one of 49 females aged 39 to 53. Second, each woman who had attained menopause or menarche was asked to recall her age at the event. The mean and standard deviation of recalled age at menarche are presented for the sample of 207 women past menarche and the same for age at menopause for the sample of 61 women past menopause.

Pulmonary function data for a healthy subsample of people free of diseases, such as respiratory (e.g., chronic bronchitis, chronic obstructive pulmonary disease, tuberculosis) and cardiovascular diseases (e.g., congestive heart failure, valvular heart disease), known to affect pulmonary function adversely, is presented. Means of a volume, forced vital capacity (FVC) and a flow rate, forced expiratory volume at 1 second (FEV-1), are plotted for 503 people grouped into 5-year age intervals (10–14, etc., to 79). FVC is the largest volume of gas forcefully expired in one complete expiration following a full inspiration. FEV-1 is the volume expired during the first second of the FVC. The relation between FVC and FEV-1, age, and stature throughout adulthood is analyzed by multiple regression analysis performed on the samples of 142 males and 161 females aged 25 to 79.

Hemoglobin levels are reported for a subsample of 331 healthy individuals aged 14 to 79 years. Individuals in the sample were not pregnant and were free of respiratory and cardiovascular disease that might pathologically influence hematological parameters irrespective of the altitude of residence. Analysis of adolescent (n = 21, aged 14 to 19) and adult male (n = 126), adolescent (n = 30, aged 14 to 19), premenopausal (n = 100), and postmenopausal female (n = 44) samples is presented. Means and standard deviations are calculated for each subsample and the hypothesis of a relationship between hemoglobin and age, height, and weight is tested for each subsample using correlation regression analysis.

2.2. Comparative Samples

The Upper Chumik population is compared with three types of published samples. One type is published data on other Himalayan populations, principally Tibetans, Sherpas, and Bhutanese (who are of Tibetan origin), and Kirghiz living

Table I
Sources of Samples of Other Himalayan, Andean, and Western Populations Used to Compare Upper Chumik Statural Growth, Development, and Aging

Population	Altitude	Children	Adult	Source
Himalayan				
Tibetan				
Mugu, Nepal	3800 m	x	x	Beall, 1981a, Beall, unpublished ms.
Leh, India	3500 m	x	x	Malik and Singh, 1978; Bharadway *et al.*, 1973
Kulu Valley, India,	1500–2200 m	x		Malik and Singh, 1979
Jawalakhel, Nepal	1000 m	x	x	Frisancho, 1978; Weitz, 1973
Pokhara, Nepal	300 m	x	x	Beall, unpublished ms.
Sherpa				
Khumbu, Nepal	3475–4050 m	x	x	Frisancho, 1978; Weitz, 1973
Upper Khumbu, Nepal	3500–4500 m		x	Gupta, 1979
Kalimpong, India	1000–1500 m		x	Gupta, 1979
Phaplu, Nepal	2600		x	Sloan and Masali, 1978
Helambu, Nepal	2800 m		x	Beall, unpublished ms.
Kirghiz				
Kuzul Djar, U.S.S.R.	2300–2800 m	x		Miklashevskaia *et al.*, 1973
Kirov, U.S.S.R.	700 m	x		Miklashevskaia *et al.*, 1973
Andean				
Nuñoa, Peru	4000 m			Frisancho, 1978
U.S.				
Denver, Colorado	1500 m	x	x	Hansman, 1970
National Sample		x	x	Hammill *et al.*, 1977; Abraham *et al.*, 1979
Boston	sea level		x	Damon *et al.*, 1972
Michigan	sea level		x	Ohlson *et al.*, 1956

at a range of altitudes from 700 m to 4500 m. Table I summarizes the population samples used to compare stature—the measure for which the most comparative data exist. Using these comparisons, it is possible to assess the distinctiveness of the Upper Chumik population vis-à-vis other Himalayan populations. The second type of comparison is with a well-studied high altitude Andean population (Nuñoa, Peru). This comparison assesses the distinctiveness of two different high altitude populations. The third comparison is with Western industrial sea-level populations. These have been studied the most thoroughly and in the greatest detail, and many generalizations about "normal" processes are based on such populations. Thus, they provide a useful, reliable reference point against which the Upper Chumik population may be evaluated. The types of comparisons of necessity are very general due to lack of fully equivalent samples and data. For example, slightly different age ranges are often used, and this obviates precise statistical comparison. Authors may not indicate which age system is reported and this may reduce the accuracy of comparisons since use of the Tibetan system (also used by the Sherpas and Bhutanese) without transformation into the Western system overestimates age by an average of 18 months.

3. Growth, Development, and Aging from the Ages of 5 to 79 in Upper Chumik, Nepal, and Comparisons with Other Population Samples

First, the patterns of growth and development of two systems, stature, and the female reproductive system, not involved in oxygen transport are discussed and then the growth and development of the pulmonary and hematological systems, both involved in oxygen transport, are discussed.

3.1. Stature

Figure 1 depicts stature-for-age for Upper Chumik male and female children aged 5 to 24 and adults 25 to 79 years old. Upper Chumikbas are below the United States 10th percentile of stature-for-age throughout the entire age span (Hamill *et al.*, 1977; Abraham *et al.*, 1979). Sexual dimorphism in stature occurs after the age of 15. Regular increments in height continue through the late teens among males and early twenties among females, implying that growth continues at least this long. However, firm conclusions about the age at cessation of growth require longitudinal samples. A later age at cessation of growth reflects a longer growing period for achieving mature adult size and in this case is interpreted as reflecting slow growth, regardless of the absolute size of the growth increments. This interpretation permits comparison of populations of different body sizes and of different systems. Thus, in comparison, statural sexual dimorphism appears in

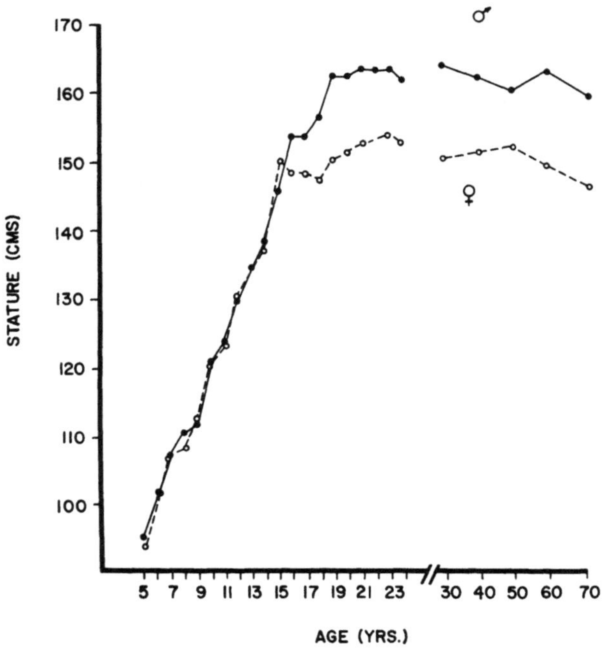

Figure 1. Mean stature-for-age for Upper Chumik male and female children aged 5–24 and adults 25–79.

the early teens, and statural growth ceases in North American and European sea-level populations at 17.5 years for males and 15.5 years for females (Tanner, 1978).

Statural growth of Upper Chumik children is graphically compared with that of other children at ages 5, 11, and 17 and of young adult individuals in Figure 2 (males) and Figure 3 (females). The average statures of published samples of several Himalayan, Andean (1), and American (1) low altitude populations are plotted. The Upper Chumik children are generally among the tallest Tibetans and Sherpas, but they are shorter than Kirghiz children. There is no apparent altitude-related pattern of growth and development among the Himalayan samples (Beall, 1981b). They are all short at early ages compared with the Andean reference sample, but this gradually shifts, and by young adulthood most are taller than the Andean reference. All the Himalayan samples of children are short at all ages compared with the U.S. reference.

To consider the relative tempos of growth, the percentage of expected young adult height at each age is graphed in Figure 4. At each age completion of a greater percentage of expected young adult stature is interpreted as indicative of faster growth tempo. Upper Chumik males and females are among the fastest

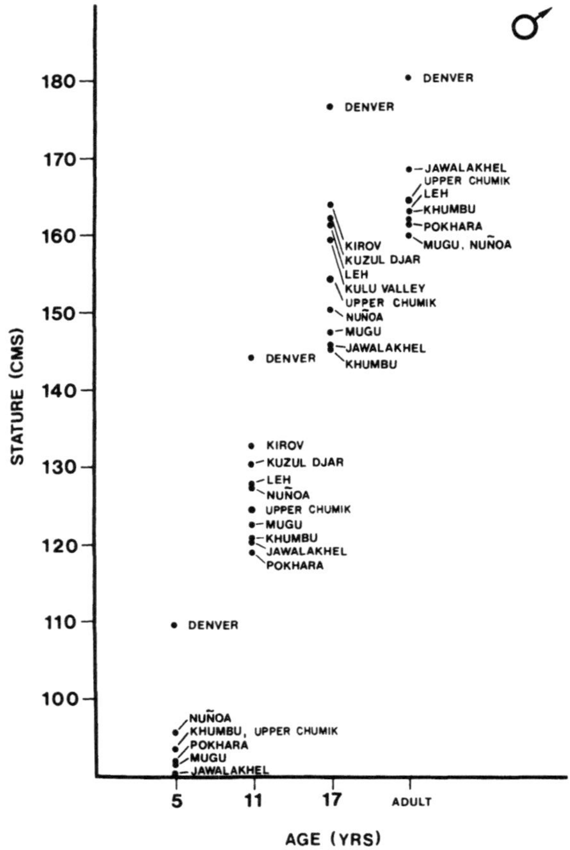

Figure 2. Mean stature at ages 5, 11, and 17 and young adulthood in Upper Chumik, several Himalayan, one Andean, and U.S. samples of males.

growing of Asian samples, nearly all of whom grow slowly compared with the Andean and the U.S. samples. The Upper Chumik sample of high altitude Tibetan children shares with other Himalayan samples the characteristics of small body size and delayed achievement of mature body size measured by young adult stature and a long growing period.

Old adults are shorter than young adults. There is a statistically significant inverse relationship between age (25–79) and stature ($r = -.21$ for both males and females, $p < .01$). Young adult male stature averages 164.2 ± 5.0 cm (n = 45) in the age range 25–34 compared with 159.9 ± 4.3 cm (n = 13) in the age range 65 to 79. Young adult female stature averages 150.7 ± 4.5 cm (n = 46) at the age range 25–34 compared with 146.7 ± 7.5 cm (n = 15) in the age range 65 to 79. This is an overall difference of 4.3 and 4.0 cm between young and old

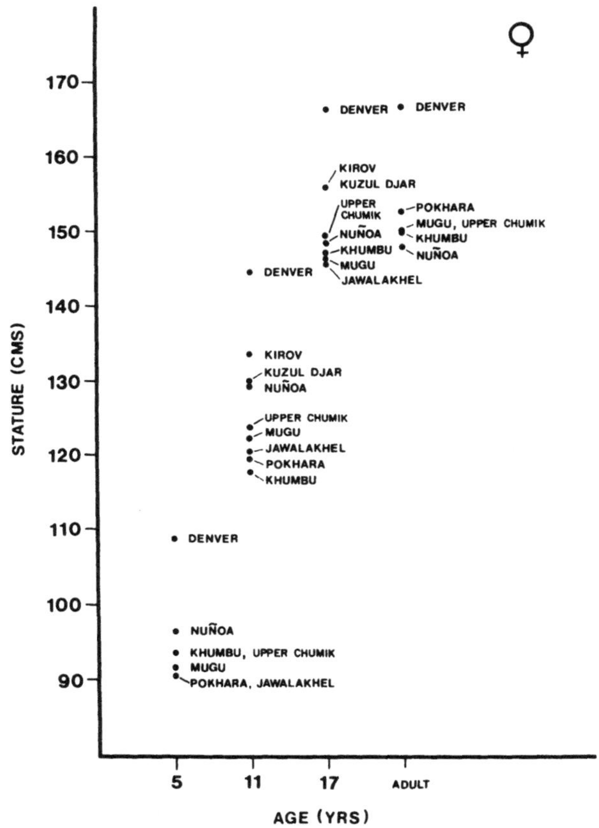

Figure 3. Mean stature at ages 5, 11, and 17 and young adulthood in Upper Chumik, several Himalayan, one Andean, and U.S. samples of females.

adult stature for males and females, respectively, or roughly 1 cm/decade, which is small in magnitude relative to the changes prior to young adulthood. In comparison, among U. S. sea-level populations, the height difference between young (aged 18–24) and elderly (65–74) adults is 6.4 cm for males and 5.1 cm for females, a difference of roughly 1.3 and 1.0 cm/decade (Abraham *et al.*, 1979). Thus, the stature difference/decade is roughly similar in the two populations.

Adult age differences in stature in Upper Chumik are compared with those for other Himalayan, Andean, and U.S. samples in Figure 5. Upper Chumik males and females conform to the general pattern of shorter stature in the older ages among both males and females, and neither they nor other Himalayan samples appear to depart from the general pattern of statural differences, nor do

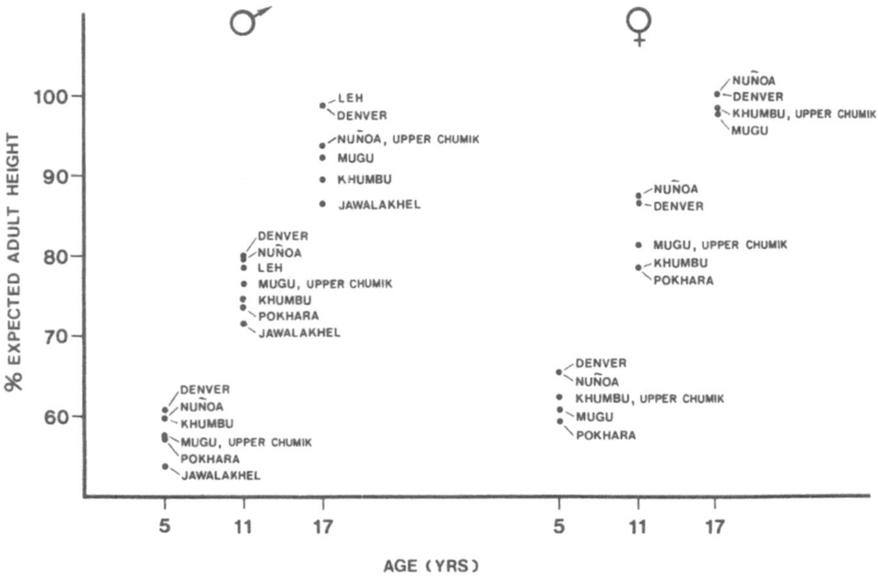

Figure 4. Percentage (%) of expected adult height at ages 5, 11, and 17 in Upper Chumik, several Himalayan, one Andean, and U.S. samples of males and females.

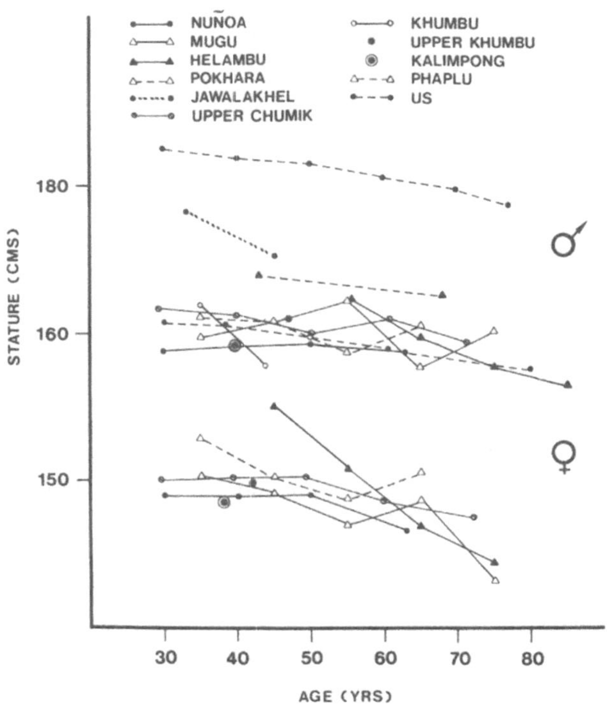

Figure 5. Adult age differences in stature in Upper Chumik, several Himalayan, one Andean, and U.S. samples of males and females.

they show unusually small or large age differences. Assuming that slow loss of stature with age would be reflected in relatively small age differences in a cross-sectional sample, it appears that the relatively slow tempo of statural change with age prior to young adulthood in Upper Chumik and other Himalayan populations does not persist during adulthood. Longitudinal samples are required to confirm or reject this observation.

3.2. Female Reproductive System

Menarche and menopause are single events, virtually universally experienced by females who survive long enough and thus are convenient markers of development of the female reproductive system marking the onset and end of the biological reproductive life span. The median age at menarche for Upper Chumik females is 16.2 years in the status quo subsample, and the mean recalled age at menarche is 17.2 ± 1.9 years. This is compared with a U.S. median of 12.8 (MacMahon, 1973) and a worldwide range from 12.3 to 18.4 (Eveleth and Tanner, 1978). Comparison with other Himalayan samples is problematic because authors do not indicate which age system was utilized and thus may be overstating ages. With this caveat in mind, medians of 14.4 and 15.2 for Kirghiz females at 700 and 2300 m, respectively, and mean recalled age at menarche of 16.2 for Tibetans at 1400 m, 18.2 for Sherpas at 3475–4050 m (Frisancho, 1978), 14.6 for Rajput females at 300 m, and 15.2 for Rajput females at 2300 m (Flint, 1974) have been reported.

The median age at menopause is 46.8 years, somewhat early compared with a U.S. median of 49.7 and with other Western industrial populations whose median age at menopause is around 50 (MacMahon and Worcester, 1966; Gray, 1976; Malina, 1979). It is also earlier than the medians of 48.9 and 47.3 reported for Indian Rajput women at 300 and 2300m (Flint, 1974). Since so few data are available it may be premature to conclude that late menarche and early menopause are general Himalayan caracteristics. In the Upper Chumik population relative to Western populations, age at menarche is delayed whereas age at menopause is accelerated. That is, delayed attainment of adult reproductive status is not followed by delayed attainment of postreproductive status, indicating that, on a population basis, slow development at an early life-cycle stage does not necessarily persist through later stages.

3.3. Pulmonary Function

FVC is a dimensional measure of the pulmonary portion of the oxygen transport system. Figure 6 presents average FVC and FEV-1 for 5-year age categories for male and female Upper Chumikbas aged 10 to 79. Both increase regularly through the 20s and then decline steadily with the exception of female FEV-1, which begins to decline slightly earlier, in the late 20s. In Andean high

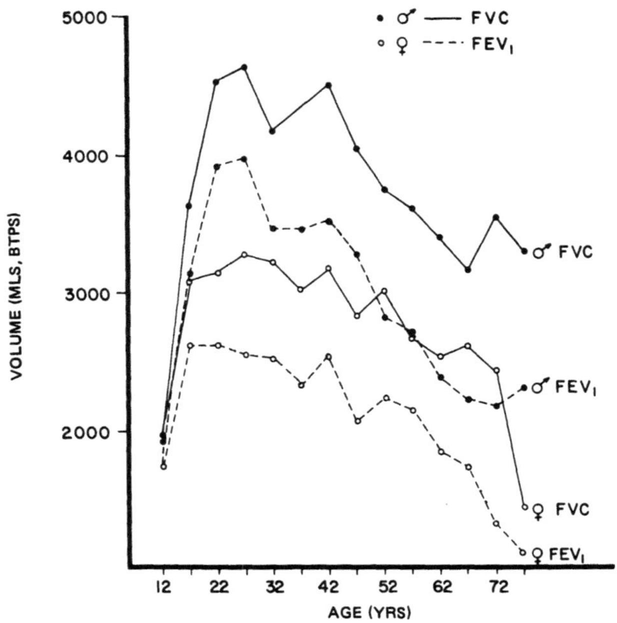

Figure 6. Mean FVC and FEV-1 among Chumik males and females aged 10–79.

altitude populations maximal FVC is attained during the 20s, whereas maximal FEV-1 is attained during the late teens (Mueller *et al.*, 1978). The general pattern of achievement and immediate commencement of loss of peak FVC in the Upper Chumik population parallels that found at sea level; however, the timing is slightly delayed. In Western populations, FVC increases into the early 20s (Hurwitz *et al.*, 1980), rather than the late 20s as in Upper Chumik. When the attainment of maximal mature function is delayed, its loss also begins later. However, the relative rate of loss compared with low altitude appears similar. This is demonstrated by regression equations predicting FVC and FEV-1 from stature and age, which were developed for adults aged 25–79 and summarized in Table II. This technique estimates that Upper Chumik male FVC declines 24.1 ml/year and female FVC declines 20.8 ml/year between the ages of 25 and 79. Male FEV-1 declines 33.2 ml/year and female 22.2 ml/year over the same time period. This conforms with some Himalayan samples. The decline in FVC with age among adult male Bhutanese residents at 3660 m is 22 ml/year (Cotes and Ward, 1966), although for a sample of adult Nepalese resident at 2000 m the decline is 57 ml/year among males and 22 ml/year among females (Bangham and Veale, 1977). The adult male Nepalese results appear anomalous. Otherwise, the Himalayan data compare with changes summarized for a large series of

Table II
Analysis of FVC and FEV-1 in Healthy Adult Male and Female Residents of Upper Chumik, Nepal, and Comparison with Other Himalayan Populations and a U.S. Sample

	Tibetan males	Tibetan females	Nepalese males	Nepalese fmeales	Bhutanese males	U.S. males	U.S. females
N	142	161	18	18	38	128	321
Age	25–79	25–79	25–55	25–68	20–69	25+	20+
Stature (cm)	162.8 ± 5.3	150.7 ± 5.1	161	152	168	—	—
FVC (ml, BTPS)	4123 ± 888	2941 ± 625	3860	2420	4920	4510 ± 1040	2960 ± 770
Regression for FVC							
Stature coefficient	60.8	52.5	45.7	44.4	58	65	37
Age coefficient	−24.1	−20.8	−57	−22	−20	−29	−22
Constant	−4724	−4048	−1590	−3410	−4050	−5459	−1774
FEV-1 (ml, BTPS)	3231 ± 931	2255 ± 664	3210	1850	3630	3680 ± 920	2460 ± 680
Regression for FEV-1							
Stature coefficient	48.7	29.3	29.7	34.6	37	52	27
Age coefficient	−33.3	−22.2	−44	−15	−22	−27	−21
Constant	−3254	−1196	−800	−2780	−1660	−4203	−794
Source	Present study		Bangham and Veale 1977[a]		Cotes and Ward, 1966 [a]	Knudson *et al.*, 1976[a]	

[a]Values multiplied to conform to units used in the analysis in the present study.

Western low altitude populations: A decrease in FVC of roughly 26 ml/year for males and roughly 22 ml/year for females and a decrease in FEV-1 of roughly 30 ml/years for males and roughly 26 ml/year for females between the ages of 20 and 60 (Muiesan *et al.*, 1971).

Another way of describing the loss of FVC with age is to ascertain how long it takes to lose a given proportion of FVC and to estimate FVC at various ages during adulthood. Using the prediction equations in Table II and the average stature of the 25–79-year age range to estimate a peak FVC at age 27 (the midpoint of the 5-year age category with the greatest average FVC), it is then possible to estimate the age at which 20% of this has been lost. By age 65, Upper Chumik males lose 20% of predicted FVC at age 27. By age 59, Upper Chumik females lose 20% of predicted FVC at age 27. Males lose 20% in 38 years and females in 32 years. The same procedure may be carried out for a low altitude Western population as well. Using prediction equations derived from a single U.S. population where males increase in FVC to age 27 and females to age 20, low altitude males have lost 20% of their peak FVC estimated at age 27 by age 57, whereas females have lost 20% of their peak FVC estimated at age 20 by age 51 (Knudson *et al.*, 1976). United States low altitude males lose 20% in 30 years and females in 31 years. It takes Upper Chumik males 8 years longer to lose the same proportion of estimated peak FVC. The estimated maximal mature function or peak FVC (at age 27) of Upper Chumik males is roughly 5% greater and of females is 2% less than that of their U.S. counterparts (controlling for stature and comparing males aged 27 in both populations, females age 20 at low altitude and 27 in Upper Chumik). This pattern of contrast changes so greatly, that by age 60 years FVC is 10% greater among males and 5% greater among females in Upper Chumik.

There are many uncertainties in estimating age at cessation of increase in FVC, (i.e., age at attaining peak or maximal mature function) and deriving the length of the growing period for measures such as FVC and FEV-1 that have large ranges of normal variation. Until recently, even in Western populations there was little information on the sequence of events of young adulthood (Hurwitz *et al.*, 1980), and there is conflicting information about the age at which FVC ceases to increase. Estimates range from 20 to 27 for males and 20 to 24 for females (e.g., Schmidt *et al.*, 1973; Knudson *et al.*, 1976; Schoenberg *et al.*, 1978). These uncertainties compound the difficulty of evaluating the tempo of Upper Chumik growth in FVC. Conservatively, males may experience a slight or no delay in age at achieving maximal mature function, whereas females appear to experience a delay of at least several years. Despite this delay in achieving peak or maximal mature function, the ensuing rate of loss is not atypical and results in a slightly higher average FVC at a given later age. The Upper Chumik population does not conform to expectations based on Andean high altitude populations—that functional measures of systems involved in oxygen transport will exhibit accelerated growth (Frisancho, 1981).

3.4. Hemoglobin Levels

The decline in the dimension and function of the pulmonary portion of the oxygen transport system suggests that additional strain may be placed on other portions, perhaps resulting in even greater hypoxic stress on the high altitude resident. Indeed, it has been argued that, among Andean high altitude populations, the age-related loss of pulmonary function results in a pathological hematological response in the form of regularly increasing high levels of hematological parameters (Whittembury and Monge, 1972; Sime *et al.*, 1975). This is not found in all Andean high altitude populations (Garruto, 1976). It does not occur in Upper Chumik where hemoglobin levels are maintained at a steady plateau throughout adulthood as in U.S. sea-level populations (Johnson and Abraham, 1979). At low altitudes an adult plateau of hemoglobin is attained earlier among females (aged 12–17) than among males (aged 18–19) (Advancedata, 1979). The truncated age span for which hemoglobin data are available for the Upper Chumik sample prevents thorough comparison. During the time span from 14 to 19 years, adolescent male hemoglobin averages 15.3 ± 1.4 gm/dl which is slightly less than that of adults, and females average 14.6 ± 0.7 gm/dl, which is similar to adults. The average hemoglobin for Upper Chumik males aged 20–79 is 16.1 ± 1.2 gm/dl. The average hemoglobin level for premenopausal females is 14.4 ± 1.4 and is 15.0 ± 1.1 gm/dl for postmenopausal females. There is no correlation between hemoglobin and age or height in any adult subsample. There is a slight but significant correlation between hemoglobin level and weight among adult males only (r .19, $p < .02$). A male whose weight is one standard deviation above the mean has a hemoglobin level 0.1 gm/dl above the estimate for a male of average weight. This suggests that the Upper Chumik females attain adult values earlier than males, just as they do at low altitudes and that adult values are attained by the early teens for females and the late teens among males as at sea level and do not increase throughout adulthood.

3.5. Aging versus Secular Trend

These are cross-sectional rather than longitudinal samples and therefore the differences between adults of different ages are not necessarily due to age changes. They may reflect true aging phenomena, that is, a consequence of the passage of time, or they may reflect a secular trend (cohort difference) or both. Secular trends occur if mature adults who grew up at different historical times, and therefore were potentially exposed to different congeries of factors influencing growth, have different biological characteristics. The possibility that a secular trend underlies these age differences cannot be absolutely discounted using cross-sectional samples; however, it is possible to evaluate that likelihood. One approach is to partition age differences into secular trend and aging phenomena by contrasting phenomena known to be influenced by a secular trend; but not by the passage of time (such as long-bone length), with those known to be influenced by the passage of time (such as height of the vertebral column) (Hertzog *et al.*, 1970; Rossman, 1977). Two parsimonious measures of long-bone length are tibial and forearm lengths. There are no age differences during adulthood (25–79) in these lengths, nor are there significant correlations with age for either in the Upper Chumik sample. In the present sample, stature declines significantly over the same age range ($r = -.21$, males and females, $p < .01$), as does trunk height (a measure of the vertebral column) ($r = -.33$, males, $r = -.35$, females, $p < .01$). At age 72 (midpoint of the oldest age category), elderly males' stature is 97.4% that of the young adult male (25–34), whereas trunk height is 94%. Elderly females' stature is 97.3% of the young adult, whereas trunk height is 94%. These data suggest that a secular trend toward increase in body size was not influencing child growth 30 to 79 years ago in Upper Chumik in such a way that longer long bones and taller young-adult stature resulted. Thus, the age differences in adult stature in the Upper Chumik population are probably due to degenerative changes of the vertebral colunn. Supporting evidence that the decline in stature is an aging phenomenon related to degenerative changes of the vertebral column derives from the observation that anteroposterior chest diameter (chest depth) increases significantly with age among both males and females ($r = .40$, males, $r = .23$, females, $p < .01$). This occurs in other populations as a result of progressive senile kyphosis of the spine due to collapse of vertebral bodies.

Further evidence that a secular trend has probably not been an important influence in the development of Upper Chumik females is provided by recalled ages at menarche and menopause. Recalled age at menarche for 201 women past that event averages 17.2 ± 1.9 years (the current median is 16.2), and there is no correlation between age and age at menarche. Recalled age at menopause for 58 postmenopausal women averages 46.2 ± 5.6 years (the current median is 48.6), and there is no correlation between age and age at menopause.

3.6. Tempo of Growth, Development, and Aging in Upper Chumik: Summary

Patterns of growth, development, and aging in the Upper Chumik samples described in this chapter have the following characteristics relative to the U.S. reference populations discussed.

1. Prior to achieving mature size as measured by young adult stature, there is a long growing period that is interpreted to indicate relatively slow statural growth. This pattern may be accentuated in females. After achieving mature size, the magnitude of statural change throughout adulthood is not unlike that reported for U.S. sea-level populations.

2. The development of the female reproductive system, as measured by age at menarche, is delayed. Its continued development as measured by age at menopause and the attainment of the postreproductive state is not delayed, but, instead, is accelerated relative to a U.S. reference.
3. There is a long growing period for FEV and FEV-1. Females have a relatively long growing period for FVC relative to United States reference populations and delayed attainment of maximal FVC that is interpreted to indicate relatively slow growth in FVC. Males may experience the same phenomenon, although this is less clear. The decline in FVC and FEV-1 throughout adulthood begins later and proceeds at a rate similar to that reported at low altitude.
4. The patterns of no age differences in hemoglobin levels during adulthood is similar in Upper Chumik and sea-level populations.

4. Conclusion

The data discussed in this chapter suggest many avenues of future research, although they do not lead to unequivocal conclusions about the tempos of growth and development from childhood through old age in Upper Chumik, Nepal. The age at attaining adult size or function is generally later than that in Western sea-level populations. The order of doing so appears the same: First menarche, then adult stature, then maximal FVC and FEV-1. It should be noted that a late age at menarche and a long period of slow statural growth are not limited to Himalayan or high altitude populations (e.g., Eveleth and Tanner, 1978; Frisancho *et al.*, 1970). It is unusual that the tempo of female growth and development in Upper Chumik may be more affected than that of males in Upper Chumik. Generally, among populations under environmental stress the opposite has been found (e.g., Stini, 1969). The relationship of growth prior to maturity and biological changes afterward appears to differ among physiological systems, and this confounds simple hypotheses such as those developed in the introduction. Whether the observed relationships are causal or are related to a third common factor is simply not known. Whether they are unique to this population is not known. The need for longitudinal and comparative studies is very evident. An anticipated contrast between systems involved and those not involved in oxygen transport did not appear in these data. Indeed, the prediction of accelerated growth and development of pulmonary and hematological systems was not confirmed.

The question of loss of size and function during adulthood requires further analysis and investigation. The late attainment of mature FVC and subsequently late commencement of FVC loss may place the elderly at a relative functional advantage in their later years. This question should be pursued using other physiological systems and relating physiological functional capacity to actual physical work capacity and to the social and economic function of adults in society.

Such issues and relationships are crucial ones in the biocultural study of aging. It is the remarkable capacity to continue to fill economic and social roles that has called attention to the Hunza of Pakistan, who are famous for being hale and hearty throughout adulthood (Leaf, 1972). Unfortunately, the Hunza data do not include chronological ages; they do not indicate what proportion of the elderly were sampled; and they do isolate the elderly analytically from the rest of the population. Yet the possibility of aging without debility and senility and the hypothesized reasons for such differential aging warrant serious investigation because these issues are important ones for the health and social welfare systems of developing countries also. In Nepal, India, and Pakistan, there were an estimated 12,286,000 people over 65 in 1950; this figure will increase to an estimated 43,388,400 by A.D. 2000 (United Nations, 1980). Life expectancy at birth in Nepal will have increased from 33.1 years in 1950 to 52.8 years in 2000, in India from 38.7 to 61.0, and in Pakistan from 39.1 to 61.3 (United Nations, 1980). There will be a slightly larger proportion of the elderly in these countries, and there will be vastly larger absolute numbers of elderly individuals as mortality and fertility control are successfully applied. The health and functional capacity of these individuals becomes increasingly critical social and biological/medical issue. Thus, the study of factors influencing the processes of biological aging among Himalayan populations has important social as well as scientific goals.

Acknowledgment

The author is grateful to S. Schuler who provided access to unpublished census materials from Upper Chumik.

References

Abraham, S., Johnson, C. L., and Najjar, M. F., 1979, Weight and Height of Adults 18–74 Years of Age: United States, 1971–1974. Data from the National Health Survey, Series 11, Number 211, DHEW Publication No. (PHS) 79-1659, USDHEW, Hyattsville, Maryland.

Bangham, C. R. M., and Veale, K. E. A., 1977, Ventilatory capacity in healthy Nepalese, *J. Physiol.* (London) **265**:31p–32p.

Beall, C. M., 1981a, Growth in a population of Tibetan origin at high altitude, *Ann. Hum. Biol.* **8**:31–38.

Beall, C. M., 1981b, Some aspects of the study of physical growth at high altitudes in Asia: in *Environmental and Human Population Problems at High Altitude*, Centre National de la Recerche Scientifique, Paris, pp. 49–54.

Beall, C. M., and Goldstein, M. C., 1982, Biological function, activity and dependency among elderly Sherpa in the Nepal Himalayas, *Soc. Sci. Med.* **16**:135–140.

Bharadway, H., Singh, A. P., and Malhotra, M. S., 1973, Body composition of the high latitude natives of Ladakh—A comparison with sea-level residents, *Hum. Biol.* **45**:423–434.

Bourliere, F., 1970, The Assessment of Biological Age in Man, Public Health Paper **37,** World Health Organization (WHO), Geneva.

Comfort, A., 1979, *The Biology of Senescence,* 3rd ed., Elsevier North Holland, Inc., New York.

Cotes, J. E., and Ward, M. P., 1966, Ventilatory capacity in normal Bhutanese, *J. Physiol.* (London) **186:**88P–89P.

Damon, A.; Seltzer, C. C., Stoudt, H. S. and Bell, B., 1972, Aging and physique in healthy white verterans at Boston, *Aging Hum. Dev.* **3:**202–208.

Davies, C. T. M., 1972, The oxygen transporting system in relation to age, *Clin. Sci.* **42:**1–13.

Eveleth, P. B., and Tanner, J. M., 1978, Worldwide Variation in Human Growth, International Biological Programme 8, Cambridge University Press, Cambridge.

Flint, M. P., 1974, Menarche and Menopause of Rajput Women., Ph.D. thesis, The City University of New York, New York.

Frisancho, A. R., 1975, Functional adaptation to high altitude hypoxia, *Science* **187:**313–320.

Frisancho, A. R., 1976, Growth and morphology at high altitude, in: *Man in the Andes: Multidisciplinary studies of High Altitude Quechua* (P. T. Baker and M. A. Little, eds.), Dowden, Hutchinson and Ross, Stroudsburg, Penn. pp. 279–292.

Frisancho, A. R., 1977, Developmental adaptation to high altitude hypoxia, *Int. J. Biometerol.* **21:**135–146.

Frisancho, A. R., 1978, Human growth and development among high altitude populations, in: *The Biology of High Altitude Peoples,* IBP Synthesis Volume 14 (P. T. Baker, ed.), Cambridge University Press, Cambridge, pp. 173–188.

Frisancho, A. R., 1981, Ecological interpretation of postnatal growth at high altitude, in: *Environmental and Human Population Problems at High Altitude,* Centre National de la Recherche Scientifique, Paris, pp. 87–96.

Frisancho, A. R., and Baker, P. T., 1970, Altitude and growth: A study of the patterns of physical growth of a high altitude population, *Am. J. Phys. Anthropol.* **32:**279–292.

Frisancho, A. R., Garn, S. M., Ascoli, W., 1970, Unequal influence of low dietary intakes on skeletal maturation during childhood and adolescence, *Amer. J. Clin. Nutr.* **23:** 1220–1227.

Frisch, R. E., 1978, Menarche and fatness: Reexamination of the critical body composition hypothesis, *Science* **200:**1509–1513.

Garruto, R. M., 1976, Hematology, in: *Man in the Andes. A Multidisciplinary Study of High-Altitude Quechua* (P. T. Baker and M. A. Little, eds.), Dowden, Hutchinson and Ross, Inc., Stroudsburg, Penn.

Gray, R. H., 1976, The Menopause—Epidemiological and demographic considerations, in: *The Menopause. A Guide to Current Research and Practice* (R. J. Beard, ed.), University Park Press, Baltimore, pp. 25–40.

Goodrick, C. L., 1978, Body weight increment and length of life: The effect of genetic constitution and dietary protein, *J. Gerontol.* **33:**184–190.

Gupta, R., 1979, *Altitude and Body Dimensions among the Sherpas,* Indian Statistical Institute, Calcutta.

Hamill, P. V. V., Johnson, C. L., Reed, R. B., and Roche, A. F., 1977, NCHS Growth Curves for Children Birth-18 Years. United States, Data from the National Health Survey, Series 11, Number 165, DHEW Publication No. (PHS) 78-1650, USDHEW, Hyattsville, Maryland.

Hansman, C., 1970, Section E., Anthropometry and related data, anthropometry, skinfold thickness measures, in: *Human Growth and Development* (R. W. McCammon, ed.), Chas. C. Thomas, Springfield, Ill., pp. 101–154.

Hertzog, K. P., Garn, S. M., Hempey, H. O. III, 1970, Partitioning the effects of secular trend and aging on adult stature, *Am. J. Phys. Anthropol.* **31:**11–17.

Hurwitz, S., Allen, J., Liben, A., and Becklake, M. R., 1980, Lung function in young adults: Evidence for differences in the chronological age at which various functions start to decline, *Thorax* **35:**615–619.

Johnson, C. L. and Abraham, S., 1979, Hemoglobin and Selected Iron-Related Findings of Persons 1–74 Years of Age: United States, 1971–1974. Advance data from Vital and Health Statistics, National Center for Health Statistics, Public Health Service Publication No. 46, January 26, 1979: 1–12, USDHEW, Hyattsville, Maryland.

Knudson, R. J., Slatin, R. C., Lebowitz, M. D., and Burrows, B., 1976, The maximal expiratory flor-volume curve. Normal standards, variability and effects of age, *Am. Rev. Respir. Dis.* **113**:587–600.

Korkushko, O. V., Ivanov, L. A., and Chebotarev, M. D., 1981, Changes in oxygen-binding properties of the blood in old age, *Hum. Physiol.* **7**:51–57.

Leaf, A., 1973, Unusual longevity: The common denominators, *Hosp. Pract.* **8**:75–86.

MacFarland, R. A., 1963, Experimental evidence of the relationship between ageing and oxygen want: In search of a theory of ageing, *Ergonomics* **6**:339–366.

McFarland, R. A., 1969, The problems of aging at altitude, *Yale Sci.* **43**:20–28.

McFarland, R. A., 1972, Psychophysiological implications of life at altitude and including the role of oxygen in the process of aging, in: *Physiological Adaptations* (M. Yousef, S. M. Horvath, and R. W. Bullard, eds.) Academic Press, New York, pp. 157–181.

MacMahon, B., 1973, Age at Menarche, United States, U.S. Vital and Health Statistics, Publication Number (HRA) 74-1615, Series 11, Number 133, USDHEW, U.S. National Center for Health Statistics, Rockville, Maryland.

MacMahon, B., and Worcester, J., 1966, Age at Menopause, United States—1960–1962, U.S. Vital and Health Statistics, Publication Number 1000, Series 11, Number 19, USDHEW, Washington, D.C.

Malik, S. I. and Singh, I. P., 1978, Growth trends among male Bods of Ladakh—A high altitude population, *Am. J. Phys. Anthropol.* **6**:471–476.

Malik, S. I. and Singh, I. P., 1979, Ventilatory capacity among highland Bods: A possible adaptive mechanism at high altitude, *Ann. Hum. Biol.* **6**: 471–476.

Miklashevskaia, M. M., Solovyeva, V. S., and Godina, E. Z., 1973, Growth and Development in High Altitude Regions of Southern Kirthizia, U.S.S.R., Field Research Projects, Miami, Fla.

Malina, R. M., 1979, Secular Changes in Maturity: Causes and Effects, in: *Secular Trends in Human Growth, Maturation and Development* (A. F. Roche, ed.), *Monog. Soc. Res. Child Dev.* **44**:59–91.

Mueller, W. H., Yen, R., Rothhammer, F., and Schull, W. J., 1978, A multinational Andean genetic and health program: VI. Physiological measurements of lung function in an hypoxic environment, *Hum. Biol.* **50**:489–514.

Muiesan, G., Sorbini, G. A., Grassi, V., 1971, Respiratory function in the Aged, *Bull. Europ. Physiopathol. Respir.* (*Nancy*) **7**:973–1009.

Ohlson, M. A., Biester, A., Brewer, W. D., Hawthorne, B. E., and Hutchinson, M. B., 1956, Anthropometry and nutritional status of adult women, *Hum. Biol.* **28**:189–202.

Palomino, H., Mueller, W. H., and Schull, W. J., 1979, Altitude, heredity, and body proportions in northern Chile, *Am. J. Phys. Anthropol.* **50**:39–50.

Pawson, I. G., 1976, Growth and development in high altitude populations: A review of Ethiopian, Peruvian and Nepalese studies, *Proc. R. Soc. London Ser. B* **194**:83–98.

Rossman, I., 1977, Anatomic and body composition changes with aging, in: *Handbook of the Biology of Aging* (C. E. Finch, and L. Hayflick, eds.), Van Nostrand Reinhold, New York, pp. 189–218.

Sanders, B., 1934, *Environment and Growth,* Warwick and York, Baltimore.

Schmidt, C. D., Dickman, M. L., Gardner, R. M., and Brough, F. K., 1973, Spirometric standards for healthy elderly men and women, 532 subjects, ages 55 through 94 years, *Am. Rev. Respir. Dis.* **108**:933–939.

Schoenberg, J. B., Beck, G. J., and Bouhuys, A., 1978, Growth and decay of pulmonary function in healthy blacks and whites, *Respir. Physiol.* **33**:367–393.

Shock, N. W., 1977, System Integration, in: *Handbook of the Biology of Aging* (C. E. Finch and L. Hayflick, eds.), Van Nostrand Reinhold, New York.

Sime, F., Monge, C., and Whittembury, J., 1975, Age as a cause of chronic mountain sickness (Monge's disease), *Int. J. Biometereol.* **19**:93–98.

Simmons, K., 1944, The Brush Foundation study of child growth and development, II. Physical growth and development, *Monogr. Soc. Res. Child Dev.* **9**(1):1–87.

Sloan, A. W., and Masali, M., 1978, Anthropometry of Sherpa men, *Ann. Hum. Biol.* **5**:453–458.

Stini, W. A., 1969, Nutritional stress and growth: Sex differences in adaptive response, *Am. J. Phys. Anthropol.* **31**:417–426.

Stoudt, H. W., Damon, A., and McFarland, R., 1965, Weight, height and selected body dimensions of adults, United States, 1960–1962, *Vital and Health Statistics* Series 11, Number 8, USDHEW, Washington, D.C.

Tanner J. M., 1978, *Fetus into Man. Physical Growth from Conception to Maturity*, Harvard University Press, Cambridge, Mass.

United Nations, 1980, Selected Demographic Indicators by Country, 1950–2000: Demographic Estimates and Projections as Assessed in 1978, ST/ESA/SER.R/38, New York, U. N.

Weitz, C. A., 1973, The effects of aging and habitual activity pattern on exercise performance among a high altitude Nepalese population, Ph.D. thesis, The Pennsylvania State University, University Park.

Whittembury, J., and Monge, C., 1972, High altitude, haematocrit and age, *Nature* (London) **238**:278–279.

Woodhull, M. C., 1977, An aging study of the Sherpas, M.A. thesis, Temple University, Philadelphia.

CHAPTER 18

Biocultural Adaptations of the High Altitude Sherpas of Nepal

CHARLES A. WEITZ

1. Introduction

There are a number of Tibetan-derived populations that inhabit the high altitude areas of the Nepal Himalayas. Collectively, they are referred to as *Bhotias,* which is from the Nepali word *Bhot,* meaning Tibet. Several of these groups are called *Sherpas,* a word derived from the Tibetan, *Sharp-pa,* meaning easterner. Perhaps the best-known group is the one living in the Khumbu region of eastern Nepal, which is adjacent to Mount Everest.

The Khumbu area consists of three narrow valleys that are created by the Dudh Kosi, Imja Kola, and Bhote Kosi rivers (see Figure 1). The Dudh Kosi originates in the Ngozumpa Glacier at an altitude of 4600 m and flows to the southeast for about 10 km. At that point, it meets the Imja Kola, a tributary that originates in the Khumbu, Lhotse, and Nuptse glaciers that are located about 12 km to the northeast of the confluence at an altitude of 5300 m. The combined waters of the two rivers flow in a southwesterly direction for 6 km until they meet the Bhote Kose River. This river originates in the Nangpa Glacier *ca.* 20 km to the northwest. The confluence of the Bhote Kosi and the Dudh Kosi rivers at 3000 m marks the southern limit of the Khumbu.

Environmentally, the Khumbu is a transitional zone between the moist, subtropical Dudh Kosi River valley to the south and the cold, dry Tibetan plateau to the north. The region's extreme altitude causes low air and ground temperatures and limits precipitation, despite its southerly location. The ground in most

CHARLES A. WEITZ • Department of Anthropology, Temple University, Philadelphia, Pennsylvania 19122

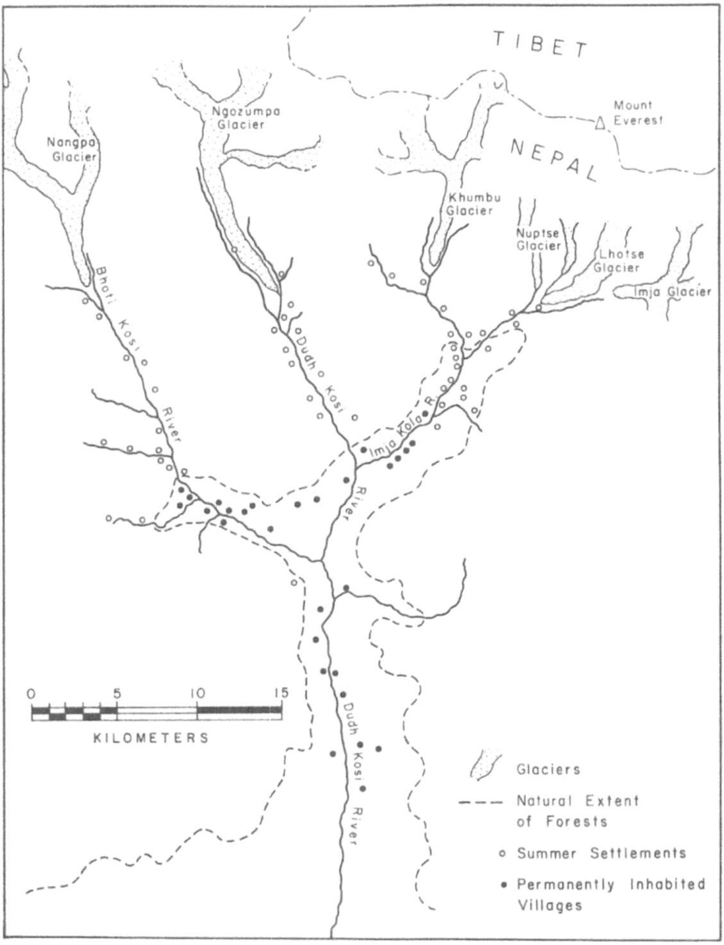

Figure 1. Map of the Khumbu region.

of the Khumbu region is frozen for 6 months out of the year, and air temperatures are at or below freezing for 4 to 6 months, depending upon the elevation. The amount of precipitation that falls in the Khumbu is inversely related to altitude. At Namche Bazar (3440 m), the lowest location in the Khumbu, the average annual precipitation (840 mm) is about twice that reported for the Khumbu Glacier at 5245 meters (Donner, 1972). On the other hand, just 12 km to the south of Namche Bazar in the Dudh Kosi River valley, Chaunrikarka (at 2700 m) receives almost 2300 mm annually.

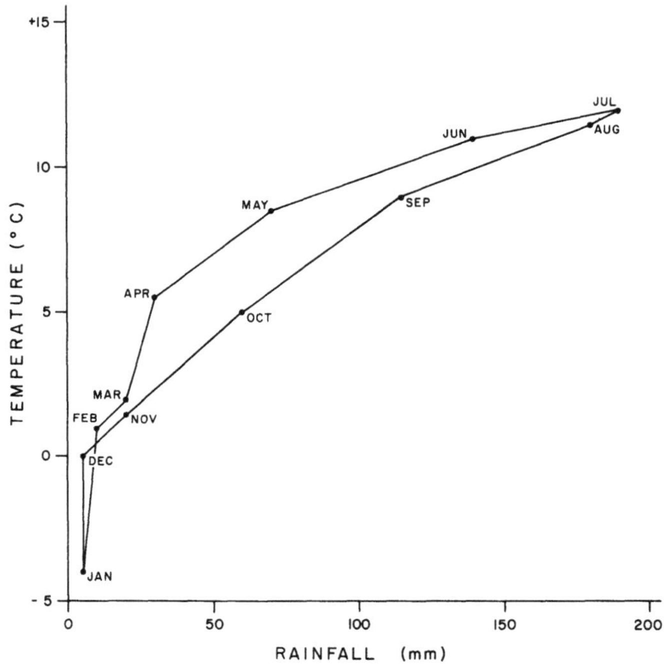

Figure 2. Climograph comparing monthly temperatures and precipitation.

There is considerable seasonal fluctuation in both temperature and precipitation. This is evident in Figure 2, a climograph based on data gathered over 25 years at Namche Bazar (Donner, 1972). From November through March, the temperatures are cold and precipitation is low. Between April and October, temperatures remain above freezing and the monsoon rains provide the bulk of the annual precipitation. Fogs and dews are also common at this time of the year and contribute to the very high humidity.

Only about 65 km^2 of the Khumbu region are covered by permanent vegetation, the distribution of which seems to be limited more by the availability of moisture than by the low temperatures. On the drier, sunny sides of the Khumbu's river valleys, the natural vegetation consists of juniper forests up to about 3800 m. The shaded sides of the river valleys where evaporation is lower support a more diverse birch forest fauna (*Betula utilis, Abies spectabilis, Rhododendron comparulatum,* and *Berberis angulosa*) up to between 4000 and 4200 m. Both types, but particularly the juniper forests, have been extensively denuded by human activity. During the summer monsoon season numerous wild flowers and wild grasses become abundant throughout the Khumbu, extending up to 5000 m.

2. History

The Khumbu Sherpa are derived from a population that originally emigrated from the eastern Tibetan province of Kham around A.D. 1400 (Oppitz, 1968). After settling for some years in the Tingri region of southern Tibet, the direct ancestors of the modern Sherpa emigrated to Nepal sometime after 1533 (Oppitz, 1968). These migrants were divided into four "protoclans" of a few families each. Two of these protoclans remained in the Khumbu temporarily, whereas the other two proceeded directly south to the Solu region. Solu was apparently uninhabited at the time (Oppitz, 1968), and it certainly possessed a milder climate and a greater potential for agriculture than the Khumbu region. After some indeterminate period, they were followed into the Solu by the majority of the two protoclans that had stayed in the Khumbu (Oppitz, 1968, 1974).

The size of the remaining settlements in the Khumbu must have been quite small, and it is possible that the region was used primarily during the summer time as high altitude pasturage for yaks owned by the larger population inhabiting the Pharak and Solu areas. In the years that followed, each of the Solu protoclans selected a clearly defined locality for settlement, originating the association between kinship and village membership. These small settlements gradually developed into the first identifiable clan villages (Oppitz, 1968). Then, as today, Solu villages were exogamous units composed primarily of nuclear families that were loosely organized into a patrilineal clan. When these villages grew beyond a few hundred inhabitants they split, and new settlements were then established in the clan's area. While new villages grew and became independent from the old villages, they began to develop their own clan identity and ultimately became independent social units.

Population size must have steadily increased during the 16th and 17th centuries because, by the early part of the 18th century, considerable emigration from the Solu and Pharak areas began to take place. Sherpa settlements are now found in the two river valleys immediately to the west of the Dudh Kosi River and along the upper reaches of the Sun Kosi River, north of Kathamndu. East of the Dudh Kosi, Sherpa settlements extend to the adjacent three river valleys and as far as Darjeeling where a particularly large number live. It is entirely possible that the first major occupation of the Khumbu also occured at this time. This might explain the contention of some Sherpas that their ancestors migrated from the Solu area (von Fürer-Haimendorf, 1964). It might also explain why Khumbu villages are not clan villages. Most include several Sherpa clans, and endogamy is more common than exogamy (Lang and Lang, 1971a).

The original Khumbu economy was probably based on yak herding and summer agriculture. Agriculture can only be practiced in the Khumbu during a single season—from April through September. Today, agriculture is practiced at all altitudes, but the earliest settlers probably grew crops like buckwheat and barley in forest clearings at the lower elevations (Hillary and Doig, 1962). Ownership of cattle was an integral part of the traditional Sherpa transhumanant pattern. The value of these animals, particularly purebred males (*yaks*) and purebred females (*naks*) lay not only in the supply of milk, meat, dairy products, fur, hides, and manure they provided for their owners but also in the prestige associated with ownership. However, maintenance of large herds required considerable attention. They were driven up to the summer villages during the warm weather to graze on the natural vegetation. During the winter, they were maintained in the areas adjacent to the permanent villages on fodder gathered during the summer, or they were driven to lower pasturages where they were able to eat the natural vegetation.

The limited Khumbu ecosystem may always have necessitated some participation in the extraregional economy. As early as 1828, the government in Kathamndu was interested sufficiently in the interregional trade centered at Namche Bazar to issue regulations controlling it (von Fürer-Haimendorf, 1975). Traditionally, the Khumbu Sherpa functioned as middlemen in the trade between Tibet and southern Nepal and India. While many Khumbu families made annual trips to the Tingri region to trade for salt and wool, the large-scale interregional trade in iron, butter, sugar, hides, paper, dyes, and cattle was carried out by the families of a single village—Namche Bazar (von Fürer-Haimendorf, 1964). Nevertheless, this system supported only a limited number of people in the harsh Khumbu environment. In 1836 the area was inhabited by about 750 people (Donner, 1972) living in 169 households (von Fürer-Haimendorf, 1964).

This early life-style was substantially altered during the middle of the 19th century when the potato was introduced into the Kumbu either from Kathmandu or Darjeeling (von Fürer-Haimendorf, 1964). This cultigen proved to be well adapted for growth in the poor Khumbu soil, and it produced a greatly superior per acre yield compared with buckwheat (von Fürer-Haimendorf, 1974). It became common to plant potatoes at the lower elevations near permanent villages, whereas buckwheat and barley were grown above 4000 m near summer settlements.

The increased productivity afforded by the potato undoubtedly contributed to population growth. First, it provided a caloric base for an increasing natural population. Second, it may have attracted settlers from southern Tibet (von Fürer-Haimendorf, 1964). Oppitz (1968) indicates that around this time small numbers of migrants from the Tingri region began arriving in the Khumbu. They were gradually absorbed into the Khumbu village structure, but they were normally organized into new clans rather than being integrated with those that already existed.

As the Khumbu population expanded, it too must have contributed to the continuing emigration to other areas. Basu *et al.* (1980) report that some of the Darjeeling Sherpas trace their ancestry to migrants from the Khumbu as well as from Solu and Pharak. By the end of the traditional period in Sherpa culture history, *ca.* 1957, the Khumbu contained a total of 2205 individuals (Donner, 1972) living in 596 households (von Fürer-Haimendorf, 1964).

The end of the traditional period was caused by the opening of Nepal to outsiders in the early 1950s and by the closing of the Tibetan border in the late 1950s. The former stimulated mountaineering and tourist interest in the Khumbu, whereas the latter effectively ended long-distance trading. Presently, almost all of the Khumbu's population participate to some extent in the cash economy created by the large number of mountain-climbing expeditions and tourists that pass through the Khumbu each year. The money that Sherpas earn as trekking guides, porters, and hotel keepers has been converted into luxuries unknown to most peasant populations.

The time spent in these pursuits has necessitated changes in the traditional agricultural/herding pattern. In the early 1970s, male absenteeism made the mobilization of females and children for many agricultural tasks necessary. By the late 1970s, the burgeoning service industry and the large cash flow made it both possible and necessary to recruit Sherpas from the Solu region and other workers from midaltitude zones to plant and harvest potatoes. Buckwheat and barley production have declined. Even the value of yaks seems to have been effected, and the size of yak herds is diminishing (Fisher, n.d.).

3. Population

3.1. Settlement

Most of the Khumbu population lives in villages located on the sunny flanks of the Bhoti Kosi and Dudh Kosi river valleys, within 6 to 8 km of the confluence of the two rivers. The altitude of these permanent habitation sites ranges between 3400 to 4000 m, but temporary settlements occupied during the warmer summer months exist up to 4800 m.

The settlement pattern of the Sherpa villages reflects the type of economy most prevalent in the area. In villages devoted primarily to agriculture, houses are arranged singly, with fields adjacent to, or surrounding the houses. In Namche Bazar, a village devoted primarily to trade, the houses are located in rows that are close together, often with adjoining walls. The fields are small and are not necessarily next to the houses. In monasteries or convents, the houses are situated close together, and arable land is practically nonexistant. Summer communities are characterized by a scatter of crude huts adjacent to large agricultural fields or near extensive grazing lands.

3.2. Demography

An extensive demographic study of the Khumbu population was carried out in 1970 and 1971. Two teams collected data independently, the second checking the accuracy of the first (see Weitz *et al.*, 1978). At the time, three identifiable groups resided in the Khumbu: Sherpas, recent Tibetan migrants, and mid-altitude Nepalis. The term *Sherpa* refers here to the descendants of the original 16th-century migrants as well as the descendants of the 19th- and 20th-century Tibetan migrants who have been integrated into Sherpa clan society. In 1970–1971, 2382 Sherpas were enumerated in the Khumbu. The most recent group of Tibetan migrants arrived *en masse* in 1959, when China formally annexed Tibet. At one time, more than 6000 Tibetan migrants were camped in the Khumbu (von Fürer-Haimendorf, 1964), but most moved on to Kathmandu or other midaltitude areas. In 1970–1971, only 287 remained in the Khumbu. Most of the 90 Nepalese listed in the Khumbu were involved in various governmental functions centered at Namche Bazar—a local subprovincial administrative center for the national government.

Figure 3 shows the 1970–1971 age and sex distribution of Sherpa and

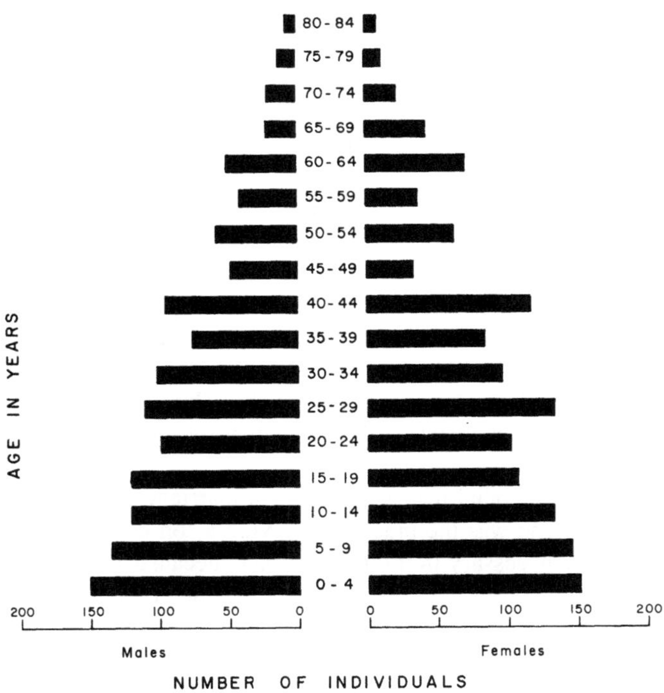

Figure 3. Age and sex distribution of the Khumbu's Sherpa and Tibetan inhabitants.

Tibetan residents in the Khumbu. Like most non-Western societies, the Khumbu population was fairly young: 32% were 14 years old and younger, 25% were 15 to 29 years old, 28% were 30 to 49 years old, and only 15% were 50 years old and older.

The sex ratio for the entire population was 89 (1259 males/1410 females), reflecting an excess of females at almost every age. It was very difficult to obtain any accurate idea of the primary and secondary sex ratios. However, the infant sex ratio was high (118), indicating a high secondary sex ratio as is reported among high altitude Andean populations (Baker and Dutt, 1972). The sex ratio of 15- through 49-year-old individuals, a group that includes reproductively active adults was considerably lower (638 males/682 females, or 94), and reflected early male mortality, male out-migration, and a high mortality among young adult males due to mountaineering accidents.

Despite the unequal sex ratio among reproductively aged Sherpas, marital arrangements like polyandry were rare, although this was clearly an option among other Tibetan-derived groups in Nepal (Goldstein, 1976). In 1957, 8% of the marriages in the three largest Khumbu villages were polyandrous (von Fürer-Haimendorf, 1964). By 1970–1971, only 4.9% of all Khumbu marriages were polyandrous. As might be expected from the low sex ratio, polygynous marriages were also uncommon (only 1.8% of the total). Apparently because of their greater number, many Sherpa women simply did not marry. Among 231 Sherpa women aged 30 and over who responded to a detailed fertility questionnaire, 12% reported never having been married. Some of these women were Buddhist nuns, but most of them were integrated into normal village life, frequently dwelling with their parents.

At the time of the survey, the Khumbu Sherpas were overwhelmingly endogamous. Over half of the Sherpa unions about which information was obtained in 1970–1971 ($n = 466$) occurred among individuals born in the same village, and nearly 90% occurred among individuals born in the Khumbu. Perhaps because of the uneven sex ratio, Sherpa women were more likely to marry outsiders than Sherpa men. About 10% of the ever-married Sherpa women were, or had been, married to men born outside the Khumbu—most frequently in Tibet. Only 6% of ever-married Sherpa men were, or had been, married to outsiders.

For a number of social reasons, the age at marriage among the Sherpa was traditionally late. One was the practice of giving a son his inheritance when he married. This was necessary in traditional times, because a son could not establish an independent household until his father provided him with land and cattle. However, these items were also the source of a man's wealth and prestige in the community. Therefore, relinquishing control to a son was resisted for as long as possible (Ortner, 1978).

Late marriage may have contributed to lowering Sherpa fertility. In

1970–1971, the crude birthrate was estimated to be between 30 and 35 per thousand, and completed fertility (number of live births to women aged 50 years and older) was 4.77 (Weitz *et al.*, 1978). The practice of prolonging premarital gift exchanges over many years, although not totally stopping sexual activity among the young, did seem to reduce early fertility. On the average, women aged 30 and over in 1970–1971 first became pregnant at age 24, about 1 year prior to their formal marriage. Indeed, pregnancy and childbirth seem to have been one factor accelerating the engagement process (von Fürer-Haimendorf, 1964). Women aged 29 years and younger in 1970–1971 tended to marry earlier, and those who were parous reported 22 as the age at which they first became pregnant. The younger age at marriage was probably related to changing economic conditions. Younger people could circumvent parental control by engaging in the cash economy and by using the money they earned to establish a neolocal life-style. In addition, young men and women would often work together, creating an opportunity for sexual access that would not have existed during traditional times.

The changing fertility pattern noted in 1970–1971 apparently has persisted. In those years, the highest age-specific fertility rates occurred among women aged 25 through 29, followed by women aged 30 through 34, and then by women aged 35 through 39. By 1976, peak fertility still occurred among women aged 25 through 29, but they were followed by nearly identical age-specific fertilities among women aged 20 through 24 and women aged 30 through 34 (Gupta, 1980). The 5½ years that lapsed between the two studies apparently witnessed an increase in live births among women in their early 20s and a general decline in live births among women in their 30s. A continuing trend toward greater sexual access prior to marriage and a younger age at marriage could account for the higher age-specific fertility among younger women, and an increasing acceptance of contraceptives (Fisher, n.d.) could account for the lower fertility among middle-aged women.

The low average fertility figures recorded in 1970–1971 masked considerable within-group variability. Tables I, II, and III show the average number of live births reported by women in different age, ethnicity, and marital categories. Sherpas in all age and most marital categories have more live births than Tibetans. Two circumstances may have contributed to this difference. First, women who migrated from Tibet apparently had smaller families than those who remained behind (Goldstein 1981a, 1981b), and second, Tibetan migrants living in the Khumbu had less access to health care and adequate nutrition than did the Sherpas (Weitz *et al.*, 1978). Women who were monogomously married tended to have the highest fertility, followed by widows and women engaged in serial monogamy. The fertility of women in polygamous marriages is difficult to interpret because of the small numbers—although the average number of live births reported by women in polyandrous unions seemed high. Never-married

Table I
Live Births Reported by Khumbu Women from Menarche to 29 years, Arranged by Ethnicity and Marital Type

Marital type	Sherpa women	Tibetan women	All women
Never married			
Total women in category	181	18	199
Number responding to fertility questionnaire	70	11	82
Total live births	16	2	18
Ave./respondent	0.23	0.17	0.22
Monogamous marriages			
Total women in category	64	6	70
Number responding to fertility questionnaire	38	3	41
Total live births	76	6	82
Ave./respondent	2.00	2.00	2.00
1 marriage, widowed			
Total women in category	4	1	5
Number responding to fertility questionnaire	2	—	2
Total live births	9	—	9
Ave./respondent	4.50	—	4.50
1 marriage, separated			
Total women in category	1	—	1
Number responding to fertility questionnaire	—	—	—
Total live births	—	—	—
Ave./respondent	—	—	—
Serial monogamy			
Total women in category	1	—	1
Number responding to fertility questionnaire	1	—	1
Total live births	2	—	2
Ave./respondent	2	—	2
Polyandrous marriages			
Total women in category	4	—	4
Number responding to fertility questionnaire	1	—	1
Total live births	2	—	2
Ave./respondent	2	—	2
Polygynous marriages			
Total women in category	—	1	1

Table I *Continued*

Marital type	Sherpa women	Tibetan women	All women
Number responding to fertility questionnaire	—	1	1
Total live births	—	3	3
Ave./respondent	—	3	3
All Women			
Total women in category	255	26	281
Number responding to fertility questionnaire	112	15	127
Total live births	105	11	116
Ave./respondent	1.07	0.73	0.91

women had very few children. Indeed, many were also nulliparous (Weitz, 1981).

Further subdivision based on residence and socioeconomic status indicate that some segments of Khumbu women have fertilities comparable to those reported among low altitude peasant populations (see Henry, 1961). For example, higher status, monogamously married Sherpa women aged 50 and over, who lived in villages that participated in the cash economy ($n = 12$) reported an average completed fertility of 7.17 live births (S.D. = 3.79)—indicating that the potential for high fertility existed in the Khumbu. Presumably, there is a casual relationship between the social characteristics that defined other groups of women in 1970–1971 and their lower fertility. Multiple regression analysis indicates that nearly half the individual variation in live births is statistically linked to differences in age, ethnicity, marital type, socioeconomic status, and residence ($R^2 = 0.47$). It is significant that a segregation of Sherpa women based on age and four rather crudely defined social characteristics can account for a large proportion of the total population variance in live births. This probably indicates that social differences within the Khumbu influence health, nutrition, and sexual access, thereby effecting fertility.

3.3. Nutrition

Traditionally, poor soil, low temperatures, and seasonal fluctuations in precipiation combined to limit the quantity and quality of food crops grown in the Khumbu, just as is the case with the natural vegetation. The effect of these environmental limitations on nutrition has been the subject of only one survey. In

Table II
Live Births Reported by Khumbu Women aged 30 to 49 Years, Arranged by Ethnicity and Marital Type

Marital type	Sherpa women	Tibetan women	All women
Never married			
Total women in category	66	16	82
Number responding to fertility questionnaire	19	9	28
Total live births	9	0	9
Ave./respondent	0.47	0.00	0.32
Monogamous marriages			
Total women in category	174	29	203
Number responding to fertility questionnaire	110	21	131
Total live births	490	81	571
Ave./respondent	4.45	3.86	4.36
1 marriage, widowed			
Total women in category	13	5	18
Number responding to fertility questionnaire	7	2	9
Total live births	16	6	22
Ave./respondent	2.29	3.00	2.44
1 marriage, separated			
Total women in category	11	—	11
Number responding to fertility questionnaire	4	—	4
Total live births	9	—	9
Ave./respondent	2.25	—	2.25
Serial monogamy			
Total women in category	4	—	4
Number responding to fertility questionnaire	3	—	3
Total live births	9	—	9
Ave./respondent	3	—	3
Polyandrous marriages			
Total women in category	8	2	10
Number responding to fertility questionnaire	3	2	5
Total live births	20	9	29
Ave./respondent	6.67	4.50	5.80
Polygynous marriages			
Total women in category	3	1	4

Table II *Continued*

Marital type	Sherpa women	Tibetan women	All women
Number responding to fertility questionnaire	2	1	3
Total live births	14	4	18
Ave./respondent	7.00	4.00	6.00
All women			
Total women in category	279	53	332
Number responding to fertility questionnaire	148	35	183
Total live births	567	100	667
Ave./respondent	3.83	2.86	3.65

the fall of 1974, a Japanese team studied the diets of 20 families (38 males and 56 females) in three large Khumbu villages (Hirai *et al.*, 1975). Food intake was measured for 1 or 2 days. Weights were then used to calculate protein, carbohydrate, fat, and calorie consumption.

Table IV shows average daily per capita food consumption in terms of weight. The average is considerably inflated by the inclusion of a fairly large consumption of rice beer (*chang*). There could be at least two reasons for this. First, this beverage is commonly served when guests (such as the Japanese survey team) are present; and second, this study was undertaken after the annual harvest when considerable celebration occurs anyway. Excluding beverages and liquors, 43.25% of the diet consisted of potatoes and another 34.1% was composed of cereals like millet, buckwheat, and rice (the latter is purchased at markets). Nearly 77% of the diet's total calories was derived from carbohydrates; 15% was derived from lipids and only 8% from protein.

Hirai *et al.* (1975) admit that a greater than normal consumption of special foods may have occurred during the survey and that the families who were examined had a high standard of living. Assuming this survey errs on the side of excess consumption, it is likely that any reported deficiencies indicate real nutritional problems for the population. For all age groups studied, the caloric consumption seemed adequate, although this assessment is biased by the large consumption of *chang* among adults and may therefore not be applicable to younger age groups. Protein consumption at or just above U.S. recommended dietary allowance levels (National Research Council, 1974) for most age and sex groups. However, it could have been marginal for adolescents and appeared to be slightly deficient for pregnant and lactating women. In other, less well-nourished

Table III
Live Births Reported by Khumbu Women aged 50 Years and Over, Arranged by Ethnicity and Marital Type

Marital type	Sherpa women	Tibetan women	All women
Never married			
Total women in category	37	8	45
Number responding to fertility questionnaire	9	4	13
Total live births	1	0	1
Ave./respondent	0.11	0.00	0.08
Monogamous marriages			
Total women in category	85	18	103
Number responding to fertility questionnaire	37	14	51
Total live births	239	58	297
Ave./respondent	6.46	4.14	5.82
1 marriage, widowed			
Total women in category	76	14	90
Number reponding to fertility questionnaire	25	6	31
Total live births	126	31	157
Ave./repondent	5.04	5.17	5.06
1 marriage, separated			
Total women in category	—	—	—
Number responding to fertility questionnaire	—	—	—
Total live births	—	—	—
Ave./respondent	—	—	—
Serial monogamy			
Total women in category	7	4	11
Number responding to fertility questionnaire	5	3	8
Total live births	19	16	35
Ave./respondent	3.80	5.33	4.38
Polyandrous marriages			
Total women in category	7	—	7
Number responding to fertility questionnaire	5	—	5
Total live births	28	—	28
Ave./respondent	5.60	—	5.60
Polygynous marriages			
Total women in category	4.00	—	4.00

Table III *Continued*

Marital type	Sherpa women	Tibetan women	All women
Number responding to fertility questionnaire	2	—	2
Total live births	7	—	7
Ave./respondent	3.50	—	3.50
All women			
Total women in category	216	44	260
Number responding to fertility questionnaire	83	27	110
Total live births	420	105	525
Ave./respondent	5.06	3.89	4.77

segments of the Khumbu population, protein intake was probably lower. In 1971, a survey of 137 schoolchildren indicated that 60% had never eaten eggs, 30% had never drunk milk, and 14% had never eaten meat (Lang and Lang, 1971a). Even in the well-nourished group studied by Hirai *et al.* (1975), most of the protein was from vegetables; only about 13% came from animal sources. Protein and chemical scores calculated by Hirai *et al.* (1975) indicate that the protein consumed was of low quality. They claim that methionine and cysteine

Table IV
Average Daily Per-Capita Food Consumption of 94 Sherpa Adults and Children[a]

Food group	Grams/day
Beverages and liquors	545.6
Starchy roots and tubers	494.8
Cereals	390.3
Milk and milk products	85.6
Leafy and yellow vegetables	59.3
Other vegetables	49.8
Sugar	19.7
Fats and oils	19.7
Fruits	5.5
Sweets	3.1
Pulses	0.6
Eggs	0.2

[a]From Hirai *et al.* (1975).

are the limiting amino acids (those available in the least amounts). Despite the apparently low protein intake, the incidence of clinical symptoms of protein-deficiency diseases, like kwashiorkor, is low (Lang and Lang, 1971a).

Hirai *et al.* (1975) found that intakes of vitamins B_1 and C were adequate, but that intakes of A and B_2 were low. Adams and Shresta (1974) inferred the presence of either folic acid or vitamin B_{12} deficiencies from blood studies carried out amont school-aged children in 1972. But clinical cases of vitamin deficiencies have rarely been diagnosed in the Khumbu (Lang and Lang, 1971b).

The diet seemed clearly deficient in at least two minerals. Hirai *et al.* (1975) noted extremely low levels of calcium consumption. This seems to correlate well with reports of extremely thin cortical bone among children (Pawson, 1977a, 1977b) and adults (Woodhull, 1977). Hirai *et al.* (1975) indicate that iron intakes were adequate, except for women aged 18 through 39. Lang and Lang (1971a, 1971b), however, felt that iron-deficiency anemias were common. They report that a fairly large proportion of 85 Khumbu schoolchildren had below normal hemoglobin concentrations and indicate that a few of the children had hypochromic films. One cause of iron-deficiency anemias in the face of apparently adequate iron intakes could have been diarrhea and other diseases that are known to reduce iron absorption. However, a systematic study of the extent to which iron deficiency might exist in the Khumbu has never been carried out.

Low iodine consumption was probably the most severe deficiency in the area. In 1969 a team of New Zealand physicians determined that 75.6% of a small Khumbu sample (n = 196) had protein-bound iodine levels below 4 mg/100 ml, and 43% had protein-bound iodine levels below 2 mg/100 ml. During a much larger study (n = 1,294), they determined that 92% had some form of goiter. In 63% of the cases, the goiter was clearly visible, and 30% were judged to be clinically hypothyroid (Ibbertson *et al.*, 1971). The high frequency of goiters may have been related to the presence of two potential goitregens: buckwheat and mustard greens (Ermans *et al.*, 1972). A fairly extensive depot iodine injection program was initiated in the late 1960s that by the mid-1970s had met with considerable success (Adams and Strang, 1975).

A weekly market has existed in the Khumbu since the late 1960s, but it has only recently begun to alter food paterns. Fisher (n.d.) believes that the consumption of market goods, particularly refined grains and sugar, has increased. He reports that traditional dietary items like Tibetan tea, buckwheat, and barley are being abandoned. Although it is difficult to assess these changes without further study, increased consumption of refined grains and sugar is not likely to improve apparent dietary efficiencies, and indeed, may even exaggerate them.

3.4. Disease and Mortality

Except for Ibbertson's survey of hypothyroidism, no systematic epidemiological studies have yet been carried out in the Khumbu. The records of a

Table V
Diagnoses Made at Kunde Dispensary from 1967 through 1971

Disease	Number of cases diagnosed	Percentage of total cases diagnosed
Dental disorders	310	19.1
Chronic respiratory disorders and pulmonary tuberculosis	181	11.1
Trauma	146	9.0
Eye disorders	139	8.5
Alimentary disorders	129	7.9
Chronic oititis media	125	7.7
Obstetrics	97	6.0
Genito–urinary and gynecology	76	4.7
Skin disorders	62	3.8
Nonpulmonary tuberculosis	60	3.7
Others[a]	301	18.5

[a]Includes, in descending order of frequency: contraception inquiries, viral illnesses, neurological disorders, tumors, cardiovascular diseases, musculo-skeletal disorders, psychiatric disorders, failure to thrive, leprosy, allergies, congenital disorders, and malaria.

dispensary established in 1967 (McKinnon, 1968; Lang and Lang, 1971a) provide the only information on the health of the Khumbu population. Table V shows the frequency with which certain categories of diseases were diagnosed during a 5-year period (1967 through 1971). During that time, 1125 Khumbu residents (about 40% of the total population) were examined (Lang and Lang, 1971b). About 40% of the diagnoses were made on young adults (aged 20 through 39), 24% of the diagnoses were made on middle-aged adults (aged 40 through 59), 23% were made on infants, children, and adolescents (aged 0 through 19), and 13% were made on the elderly (aged 60 years and over). The age distribution of diagnoses was not proportional to the age structure of the population as a whole, and the likelihood of visiting the dispensary varied greatly from village to village. Consequently, these data can only be used to provide a general understanding of the types of diseases that existed in the Khumbu.

Otitis media was the most commonly diagnosed disease among infants and children aged 1 through 4; it was followed closely by pulmonary diseases. The most commonly diagnosed pulmonary disorder was pneumonia; only about one quarter of the cases in this age group were diagnosed as pulmonary tuberculosis. Burns were also a common problem among infants and toddlers who frequently wandered too near to open fires. Viral diseases (mumps, measles, and chicken pox) and accidents were most commonly diagnosed among children and young adolescents (aged 5 through 14). Accidents commonly involved fractures, probably because of the thin cortical bone development among Khumbu children that, in turn, is probably a consequence of low calcium intake.

Among older adolescents (aged 15 through 19) and young adults (aged 20 through 39), tuberculosis, alimentary disorders, obstetrical consultations, and dental caries were the most frequent diagnoses. Only about half the tuberculosis cases were pulmonary in nature. Very frequently, bones and other organs were involved. Tapeworms seemed particularly common among Tibetans, perhaps because of the custom of eating uncooked dried meat. Otherwise, a fairly large number of young adults suffered from peptic ulcers that probably were caused by a fairly large intake of chiles.

About one third of the diagnoses made for middle-aged and elderly Sherpas concerned dental caries. The proportion of individuals diagnosed as having tuberculosis and alimentary disorders declined when compared with younger age groups. But other diseases, such as congestive heart failure and osteoarthritis, were more commonly diagnosed in these age groups than among younger people.

Among all age groups, mild chronic bronchitis and conjunctivitis were extremely common and were probably caused by the polluted microenvironment inside Sherpa houses (Lang and Lang, 1971b). Davidson *et al.* (1981) report high levels of lead and copper and excessive concentrations of aluminum, magnesium, and total suspended particulate matter. These levels are caused by the combustion of wood and dung for cooking and heating and are concentrated in the houses because chimneys and flues rarely exist.

Some diseases are significant by their apparent absence or their low frequency of diagnosis. No cases of thyphoid, cholera, smallpox, or rubella were diagnosed. Only 88 cases of pulmonary tuberculosis were diagnosed, a particularly low number out of over 1600 total diagnoses and one that may indicate a lower incidence of pulmonary disease in the Himalayas than in the Andes (Way, 1976). It is conceivable that some control of the disease resulted from B.C.D. vaccinations, which had been given to 60% of the total Khumbu population by 1971. Even so, the large number of new cases every year indicated a significant resevoir of the disease in the Khumbu and probably means that only a small number of the total cases of pulmonary tuberculosis were diagnosed. In many cases, the source of the infection was another family member (Lang and Lang, 1971a), but some tests on cattle yielded positive results, indicating that some infection may have been caused by bovines (Lang and Lang, 1971b).

Cardiovascular diseases were also rare. All of the 28 cases diagnosed between 1967 and 1971 were congestive heart failure due to valvar disease, and probably they were caused by rheumatic fever (Lang and Lang, 1971b). Atherosclerosis and strokes were rarely diagnosed. The generally nonpathological state of the vascular systems of Sherpa and Tibetan males is apparent in the absence of any significant increase in resting blood pressures with age (Weitz, 1982). Figure

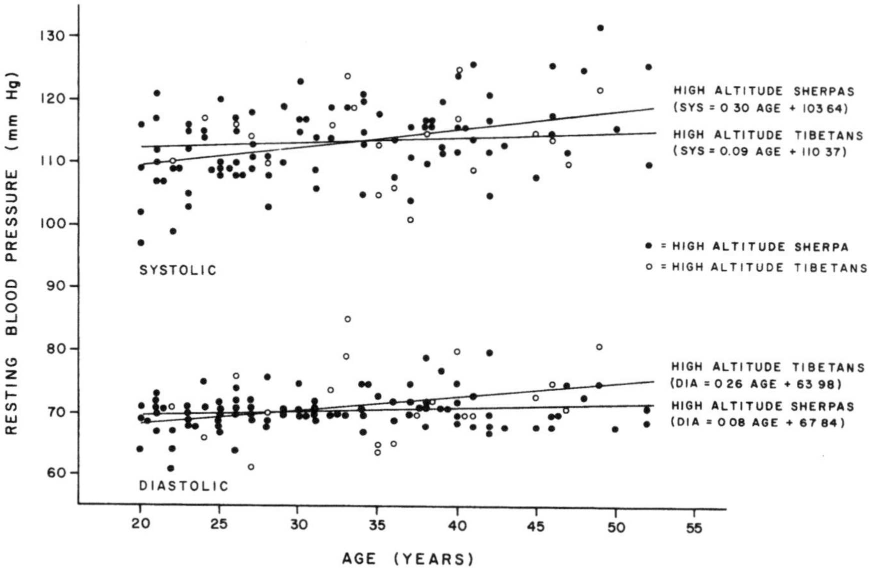

Figure 4. Age differences in resting blood pressure among Khumbu males.

4 shows the resting blood pressures of 110 Khumbu males aged 20 through 52. Mean systolic pressure, adjusted for age and weight, was 113.5 mm Hg for Sherpas and 113.0 mm Hg for Tibetans. Mean diastolic pressures adjusted by age and weight were 70.7 mm Hg for Sherpas and 71.5 mm Hg for Tibetans. Khumbu residents would consequently be classified as belonging to a low-blood-pressure population (Epstein and Eckoff, 1967).

Mortality during infancy and childhood is high in the Khumbu. Women in all age groups report, on the average, that 15.8% of their live births died during infancy. Unfortunately, it was extremely difficult to elicit the cause of infant deaths during reproductive history interviews. Data from the dispensary indicated that failure to thrive (commonly associated with low birth weight) may have been common. Occasionally, deaths due to pneumonia or severe burns were also noted. An analysis of maternal socioeconomic status and residence indicated that neither factor affected infant mortality. Consequently, altitude-related factors may have been involved (Weitz *et al.*, 1978).

Reports of childhood mortality varied, depending upon whether women resided in villages where Western contact was high or low. Women in traditional, isolated villages reported a frequency of child deaths nearly double that of women in more Westernized villages, where participation in the cash economy was high (Weitz *et al.*, 1978). Although the causes of death in this age group are no better known than are the causes of infant deaths, they are clearly influenced by social differences. This may suggest that access to medical attention or differences in nutrition played a role in childhood mortality.

Adolescent mortality seemed fairly low. Women aged 50 years and over reported that less than 4% of their live births died between 12 and 19 years of age. Males in this age group as well as those aged 20 through 39 were most likely to become involved in moutaineering accidents. From 1950 through mid-1974, 58 Sherpas had been killed while mountain climbing (Fisher, n.d.). For such a small population, two or three adult-male deaths per year contributes significantly to the total adult mortality. No other data are available on the causes of adult deaths.

The survivorship curve shown in Figure 5 is based on data from the 1970–1971 demographic survey. Figures for infant, child, and adolescent mortality are abstracted from the reproductive histories of individual women. Postadolescent mortality is crudely estimated from the age and sex structure of the population and assumed population stability. Survivorship through adolescence is very similar to that of the Nuñoa population living at high altitude in Peru (Baker and Dutt, 1972). Later survivorship appears lower in the Khumbu, but the method of calculation probably overestimates mortality by not considering factors like out-migration.

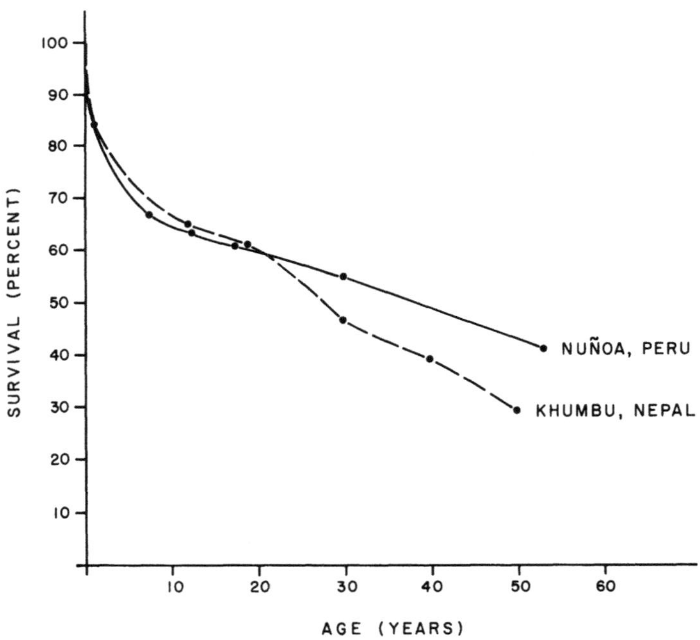

Figure 5. Survivorship estimates for two high altitude populations: Sherpas and Tibetans of the Khumbu (Nepal) and Quechua Indians of Nuñoa (Peru).

4. Sherpa Adaptations to Hypoxia

4.1. Oxygen Transport

Perhaps the most ubiquitous stress to which the Khumbu Sherpa must respond is the low partial pressure of oxygen. This condition results from low barometric pressure at altitude and causes a reduction in the amount of oxygen reaching the tissues, a condition referred to as *hypoxia*. To provide an adequate supply of oxygen to active tissues, a number of cardiovascular compensations may occur. Among these are large lung size, hyperventilation, an increased pulmonary-diffusing capacity, an increased number of red blood cells, an increased vascullarization of active tissues, and an increased utilization of oxygen by the tissues.

Not all human populations exposed to altitude rely on the same set of responses. Lowlanders tend to respond by increasing ventilation, red-blood-cell number, tissue vascularization, and compounds that facilitate the release of oxygen from hemoglobin in tissue capillaries. Unlike lowlanders, high altitude Andean natives possess large lung volumes relative to body size, a low hypoxic ventilatory response, and a greater pulmonary diffusion capacity. Like lowlanders, they also exhibit elevated red-blood-cell numbers, a high degree of tissue vascularization and increased concentrations of compounds that facilitate the release of oxygen from hemoglobin in tissue capillaries (Frisancho, 1975). Although there is still some debate, most of the differences between the responses of lowlanders and Andean highlanders seem to result from developmental, not genetic, adjustments to hypoxia (Frisancho *et al.*, 1973; Frisancho, 1975; Lahiri *et al.*, 1976a).

Much less research has been carried out among Himalyan highlanders. Of the studies that have been done, however, most have been focused on the Khumbu Sherpas. Taken together, this research seems to reveal a set of physical and physiological responses to hypoxia that are unlike those that exist among lowlanders or highland Andean natives. Although not all the literature on Sherpa adaptations is in agreement, the argument often seems to focus on how they differ from other highland groups—not *whether* they do.

Chest dimensions of the Khumbu Sherpas may not be as large as those of the Andean highlanders, although data on chest circumference do not always agree with those on width and depth. Children from both groups have similar chest circumferences to age 13. Between 14 and 20 years of age, Andean natives have larger chest circumferences, but they are also taller than Sherpas (Pawson, 1976). When chest circumference/stature ratios are compared, there are no differences to age 20. After 20, however, Sherpa males seem to have smaller chest circumferences, both absolutely (Gupta and Basu, 1981) (Table VI) and relative to stature (Pawson, 1976). Table VI shows that chest widths and depths of Sherpa and Quechua males aged 20 through 35 are not significantly different but

Table VI
Comparisons of Chest Measurements and Stature Between Khumbu Males and Males Tested at Nuñoa, Peru

	Khumbu, Nepal			Nuñoa, Peru[a]			
Age Group	*N*	$\bar{X}$	S.D.	*N*	$\bar{X}$	S.D.	*t* score
				Stature (cm)			
20–25	26	161.8	5.9	41	158.1	5.6	$2.51^{0.05}$
26–35	30	162.4	6.1	40	158.9	5.3	$2.47^{0.05}$
36–45	26	161.0	7.1	30	159.1	5.7	$1.07^{N.S.}$
46–55	8	156.6	5.5	14	159.3	5.6	$-1.04^{N.S.}$
				Chest width (cm)			
20–25	26	28.2	2.8	41	27.6	2.0	$0.93^{N.S.}$
26–35	30	28.0	1.4	40	27.6	1.8	$1.03^{N.S.}$
36–45	26	27.2	1.1	30	28.8	3.7	$-2.22^{0.05}$
46–55	8	27.5	2.0	14	28.2	0.9	$-0.88^{N.S.}$
				Chest depth (cm)			
20–25	26	20.0	1.3	41	20.5	2.0	$-0.73^{N.S.}$
26–35	30	20.6	1.0	40	20.6	1.7	0.00
36–45	26	21.0	1.0	30	21.4	2.2	$-0.88^{N.S.}$
46–55	8	20.7	1.2	14	21.5	1.2	$-1.42^{N.S.}$
				Chest circumference, maximum inspiration (cm)			
20–25	26	89.3	3.7	41	91.9	4.8	$-2.45^{0.05}$
26–35	30	89.1	4.6	40	93.9	3.7	$-4.62^{0.001}$
36–45	26	90.1	2.8	30	95.1	4.2	$-5.17^{0.001}$
46–55	8	89.8	4.4	14	94.8	4.1	$-2.48^{0.05}$

[a]Frisancho, 1976.

Sherpas are significantly taller. Among males aged 36 through 45, differences in stature are not significant, but Sherpas have significantly smaller chest widths. These data suggest that Sherpas have smaller chest dimensions relative to stature than do Andean males, but the difference between the two groups is much smaller than that indicated by a comparison of chest circumferences. The apparent contradiction could be attributable to differences in upper body muscle mass. Cross-sectional muscle areas determined from brachial radiographs are larger among the Quechua than among the Sherpa. A difference in muscle mass could effect the measurement of chest circumference but not the measurement of width and depth. It is also entirely possible that some Sherpa males did not inspire maximally during this measurement.

Table VII
Lung Volumes of Adult Male Highlanders

	Quechua Indians (Peru)[a]		Sherpas (Nepal)[b,c]	
	Vital capacity (BTPS)		Vital capacity (BTPS)	
Altitude	*n*	ml/M^2	*n*	ml/M^2
Sea Level	31	3070		
1377 m			25	2970
3400 m	40	3043		
3800 m			21	3021
3840 m	20	2916		
4000 m	12	3330		
4000 m	92	3210		
4243 m			10	3094
4540 m	185	3220		

[a]Modified from Velasquez, 1976.
[b]Hackett *et al.*, 1980.
[c]Lahiri, 1971.

Studies of lung function among the Sherpas support the impression obtained from chest width and depth measurements. Table VII shows that forced vital capacities, when corrected for body size (m/M^2) are not as large as those reported for most Quechua groups. Indeed, Hackett *et al.* (1980) report that the relationship between lung volume and body size is the same among Sherpas and lowland Europeans.

Compared with lowlanders, Andean highlanders ventilate less at high altitude (Lahiri *et al.*, 1969, 1970), but is not clear if the same reduced hypoxic ventilatory response occurs among Sherpas. Given the relatively small lung sizes of Sherpas compared with Andean natives, ventilatory differences between the two groups might be expected. Lahiri (1968) noted that resting alvoelar P_{CO_2} values among Khumbu Sherpas were slightly higher than those of high altitude Peruvians—a possible indication of different ventilatory responses to hypoxia. The differences were small, however, and it seemed clear to Lahiri that ventilation among both groups was reduced compared with lowlanders. Recently, Hackett *et al.* (1980) have criticized Lahiri's small samples (n = 4), and on a much larger group of subjects (n = 35) they indicate that Sherpas—unlike Andean natives—hyperventilate at rest compared with lowlanders. As in the Andes (Lahiri *et al.*, 1976a), Hackett *et al.* (1980) report that hypoxic ventilatory response was "blunted" among Sherpas who had spent most of their lives at high altitude. But, even when this "blunting" effect, age, and body size were considered, the hypoxic ventilatory response of the Sherpas was greater than among Andean natives or even among Americans raised above 3000 m in Colorado.

During exercise, the situation is reversed. On a fairly large sample tested at 3800 m, Lahiri *et al.* (1976b) report that Sherpas ventilate less relative to oxygen consumption than do lowlanders. At high levels of exercise, Sherpa ventilation was only 74% to 77% that of lowlanders at similar levels of oxygen consumption. In the Andes also, highland natives are known to ventilate less than newcomers during exercise (Buskirk, 1976), a condition that is usually interpreted as a consequence of a reduced hypoxic ventilatory drive (Lahiri *et al.*, 1970). Like Andean natives (Lenfant and Sullivan, 1971), Sherpa ventilation during exercise is positively correlated with altitude (Lahiri *et al.*, 1972; Weitz, 1973), indicating the existence of some hypoxic effect. But, at each altitude, the ventilation of Sherpas (Lahiri *et al.*, 1972) and their Andean counterparts is reduced compared with lowlanders.

Although the precise control of ventilation during exercise is not known, the ventilatory response to acute hypoxia seems to be mediated by peripheral chemoreceptors (Cunningham *et al.*, 1968). If exercise in hypoxic conditions merely enhances peripheral chemoreceptor control of ventilation (Cunningham *et al.*, 1968), then the ventilation of Sherpas relative to lowlanders ought to be the same during exercise as at rest. From this perspective, the results reported at rest by Hackett *et al.* (1980) and those reported during exercise by Lahiri *et al.* (1972, 1976b) and Weitz (1973) give contradictory indications of the Sherpa ventilatory response to hypoxia.

The hyperventilation among Sherpa subjects at rest reported by Hackett *et al.* (1980) could have been related to test anxiety. Personal experience on a fairly large sample of Sherpa/Tibetan subjects (n = 149) at both high and medium altitudes suggests that anxiety-related hyperventilation is common both with and without test apparatus in place. Anxiety-related hyperventilation could bias the calculation of hypoxic ventilatory response (HVR), because it was based on a regression equation in which ventilation was a major variable. Furthermore, the HVR of Sherpas was calculated on a sample (n = 23) that included 10 individuals born and raised at altitudes between 2200 and 2800m, where the nature of hypoxic stress is somewhat ambiguous. Finally, Hackett *et al.* (1980) indicate that their lowland subjects possessed relatively low HVR values, possibly due to high activity. No report of Sherpa activity patterns was given, although the very wide variation in Sherpa HVR values suggests that such differences could have existed. Indeed, differences in activity pattern are known to occur among high altitude Sherpas, and they do influence ventilation (Weitz, 1973). Until such problems can be properly addressed by more careful sampling and because Sherpa ventilation is lower than that of lowlanders during exercise, it is probably best to proceed on the notion that, like Andean natives, they possess a reduced ventilatory response to hypoxia.

Since hyperventilation increases alveolar PO_2, it is not unexpected that Hackett *et al.* (1980) also report high arterial-oxygen saturations among the Sherpas. In view of the sampling problems noted previously, however, this finding should be used cautiously. It is worth noting that Lahiri *et al.* (1967) report a value that is nearly identical to those found at high altitude in Peru (Velasquez, 1976).

Many researchers (Adams and Strang, 1975; Cerretelli, 1976; Morpurgo *et al.*, 1976; Samaja *et al.*, 1979), indicate that Sherpa hemoglobin concentrations (between 15 g/dl and 17 g/dl) are lower than those reported among high altitude Andean natives (Velasquez, 1976). The reason for this difference is not understood, but it is possible that anemias due to iron, folate, and/or vitamin B_{12} deficiencies may exist in the Khumbu and could be contributory factors (Lang and Lang, 1971a, 1971b; Adams and Strang, 1975).

The affinity between hemoglobin and oxygen also may be different among Sherpas. Samaja *et al.* (1979) report a P_{50} value (the oxygen pressure at which 50% of hemoglobin is saturated) for Sherpas that is similar to acclimatized lowlanders but lower than that of Andean natives. This condition is presumably not as advantageous as the higher Andean P_{50} values, which indicate a greater hemoglobin–oxygen dissociation at tissue-level PO_2. On the other hand, most studies of the oxygen dissociation curve have reported P_{50} values under a set of standardized, *in vitro* conditions (pH = 7.4, temperature = 37° C, P_{CO_2} = 40 torr). When a series of corrections are made for the effect of hematocrit on pH, the resulting *in vivo* P_{50} values of Andean highlanders are reduced and are also comparable to those of lowlanders (Winslow *et al.*, 1981). Winslow *et al.* (1981) suggest that there exists a trade-off between compensated respiratory alkalosis and increased 2,3 diphosphoglycerate concentrations. Increased 2,3 diphosphoglycerate concentrations are judged to be advantageous because they increase the Bohr effect and the slope of oxygen dissociation curve, both of which could augment oxygen delivery to the tissues.

The similarity in P_{50} values between Sherpas and lowlanders could indicate that the oxygen dissociation curves of highland populations in general are not different from lowlanders. While *in vivo* pH levels cannot be compared because the effect of hematocrit has not been assessed among Sherpas, 2,3 diphosphoglycerate concentrations are similar in both groups. This may suggest that the cause of similar P_{50} values between highlanders and lowlanders in the Himalayas is the same as in the Andes.

One way to determine how these characteristics effect the Sherpas' oxygen delivery capacity is to measure oxygen consumption during maximum exertion. Maximum oxygen consumption is an indication of the functional limits of the various systems involved in the exaction, transportation, and utilization of oxygen by the body. Studies of maximum oxygen consumption among the Sherpa have produced somewhat varied results. Samaja *et al.* (1979) and Cerritelli

(1976) report fairly low maximum oxygen consumption values at 3850 m (40.6 $ml \cdot kg^{-1} \cdot min^{-1}$), based on a fairly small sample ($n = 13$) of men aged 14 to 50 years. The only other published figure (Nag *et al.*, 1978) is based on an even smaller sample ($n = 7$) for which maximum oxygen consumption values are estimated rather than directly measured. The maximum of this group, tested at 3660 m, was projected to be 3.33 $l \cdot min^{-1}$ per 50 kg of body weight (66.6 $ml \cdot kg^{-1} \cdot min^{-1}$), a relatively high value.

A clearer indication of maximum oxygen consumption among Sherpa and Tibetans emerges from a much larger sample of males tested at altitudes above 3000 m in the Khumbu and adjacent Pharak regions of Nepal ($n = 122$). Analysis of these data indicate that the low average maximum oxygen consumption value reported by Samaja *et al.* (1979) and Cerritelli (1976) could have occurred by including a disproportionately high number of inactive and/or older subjects in the sample. Figure 6 shows that activity pattern effects maximum oxygen consumption at high altitudes in much the same way as it does at low altitudes. The maximum oxygen consumption of highly active Khambu and Pharak males in their 20s ($n = 32$) averaged 50.2 $ml \cdot kg^{-1} \cdot min^{-1}$, whereas the maximum oxygen consumption of relatively inactive males of the same age ($n = 13$) averaged 44.3 $ml \cdot kg^{-1} \cdot min^{-1}$. There also exists a decline in maximum oxygen consumption with age, comparable to that reported in cross-sectional studies at low altitudes (Dehn and Bruce, 1972). Among highly active Khumbu and Pharak males in their 40s and early 50s ($n = 24$), maximum oxygen consumption

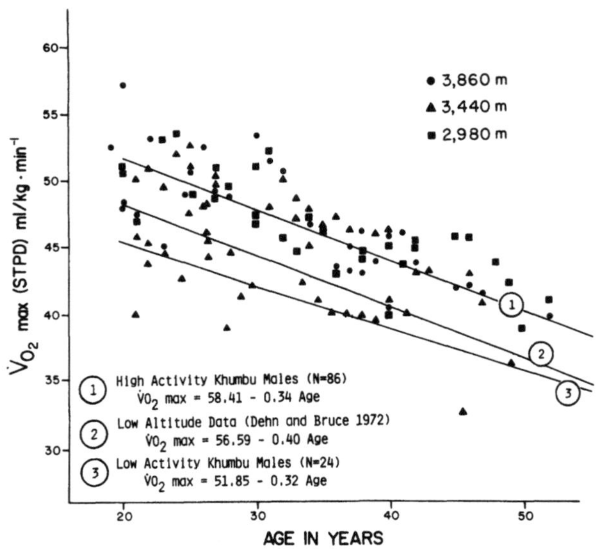

Figure 6. Age and activity differences in maximum oxygen consumption among high altitude Sherpas and Tibetans.

Table VIII
Pulmonary and Cardiovascular Responses of Young Males from High Altitude Regions of Nepal (Khumbu and Pharak) and Peru, Measured during Maximum Exertion

		Age (years)		Weight (kg)		$\dot{V}O_2$ (STPD) ($ml \cdot kg^{-1} \cdot min^{-1}$)		$\dot{V}_E$ (STPD) (liter/min)		$\dot{V}_E/\dot{V}O_2$		Heart rate (beats/min)		$\dot{V}O_2$/HR (ml/beat)	
Group	Number	$\bar{X}$	S.D.	$\bar{X}$	S.D.	$\bar{X}$	S.D.	$\bar{X}$	S.D.	$\bar{X}$	S.D.	$\bar{X}$	S.D.	$\bar{X}$	S.D.
Active Nepalese males	32	24.2	3.0	53.5	5.6	50.2	2.4	70.8	5.1	26.4	1.2	183.6	6.3	14.6	1.1
Inactive Nepalese males	13	24.6	2.9	59.2	4.6	44.3	1.4	74.8	6.7	28.5	0.8	180.0	6.2	14.6	1.0
Quechua males[a]	25	25.0	—	57.0	—	49.1	—	75.0	—	27.3	—	171.0	—	16.0	—
Quechua males[b]	10	23.8	—	59.8	—	46.8	—	72.0	—	25.8	—	188.0	—	14.8	—
Quechua males[c]	8	25.0	—	57.3	—	51.8	3.4	75.3	13.4	26.5	3.4	176.0	9.0	16.8	2.3
Quechua males[d]	20	23.4	1.7	58.6	4.6	46.3	5.0	—	—	—	—	196.1	6.6	13.9	1.8

[a]Baker, 1969.
[b]Mazess, 1969.
[c]Kollias *et al.*, 1968.
[d]Frisancho *et al.*, 1973.

averaged 43.5 $ml \cdot kg^{-1} \cdot min^{-1}$, whereas for similarly aged inactive males, the average was only 36 $ml \cdot kg^{-1} \cdot min^{-1}$.

Table VIII shows the average maximum oxygen consumption, ventilation, ventilation/oxygen consumption ratios, heart rate, and oxygen consumption/heart rate ratios of young males tested at altitudes above 3000 m in Nepal and Peru. The small variation that exists among different groups is more likely associated with differences in habitual activity patterns than with any fundamental differences in functional capacities. The oxygen consumption of the Peruvian groups falls within the range of active and inactive Sherpa/Tibetan males. This is also the case for ventilation and for the ventilation/oxygen consumption ratio, a measure of oxygen-extraction efficiency. Variable activity patterns produce similar differences in oxygen extraction efficiency at low altitudes (Astrand and Rodahl, 1970) and probably contribute to the differences that exist in Table VIII. Maximum heart rate values are similar, except for the high value reported by Frisancho *et al.* (1973) and the low value reported by Baker (1969). Variations in body weight effect the oxygen consumption/heart rate ratio because weight is correlated with oxygen consumption. In Nepal, highly active males weigh about 6 kg less than inactive males. Consequently, they have a significantly higher average weight-controlled oxygen consumption/heart rate ratio than inactive males (0.274 ± 0.015 $ml \cdot kg^{-1} \cdot beat^{-1}$ versus 0.244 ± 0.013 $ml \cdot kg^{-1} \cdot beat^{-1}$), probably indicating differences in caridac output caused by variations in habitual activity patterns. It is likely, then, that the group differences in oxygen consumption/heart rate ratios are due to variations in body weight and activity patterns.

Because the Sherpa and Quechua seem to have similar functional potentials although apparently possessing different lung volumes, hemoglobin concentrations, and oxy-hemoglobin affinity, explaining the similar oxygen consumption values becomes rather problematic. Presuming the existing data to be accurate, one or two factors may be involved: (1) an increase in pulmonary diffusion due to a unique oxygen transport factor or to a more favorable ventilation/perfusion ratio; and/or (2) differences in the utilization of available oxygen at the tissue level.

4.2. Effect of Hypoxia on Fertility and Postnatal Growth

Integrated into the research on the hypoxic responses of high altitude populations are studies of fertility and growth. Although obviously not concerned with the transport of oxygen to the tissues, questions of fertility and growth have been linked with hypoxia because pre- and postnatal growth and development are thought to be retarded by limited oxygen availability.

To date it has not been possible to demonstrate clearly any hypoxic effect on the fertility of indigenous high altitude populations, either in the Andes or in the Himalayas. In the Andes, reports of a negative association between altitude and the number of live births are common (Baker and Dutt, 1972; Abelson *et al.*, 1974; Hoff and Abelson, 1976). However, Dutt (1980) indicates that socioeconomic status is a major confounding variable. He concludes that much of the altitude variation in live births is due to altitude-related scioeconomic differences.

In the Khumbu, the low completed fertility reported by Weitz *et al.* (1978) has been interpreted as a consequence of hypoxia (Bangham and Sacherer, 1980). However, as noted previously, nearly 50% of the individual variation in live births reported by Khumbu women is related to differences in marital type, residence pattern, socioeconomic status, and ethnicity. This is not to say that hypoxia has no effect on fertility. However, it may not be easily detectable if only live-birth data are analyzed.

Studies of newborns may help to determine if any antenatal hypoxic stress exists, and, if it does, whether it is severe enough to effect fertility. A small sample of Sherpa newborns were weighed at delivery by physicians at the Kunde dispensary between 1967 and 1971. Table IX shows that the birth weights of this group are fairly low. Haas *et al.* (1980) report similarly low birth weights at high altitude among the children of non-Indian women, but much higher birth weights among the children of native Andean women. Haas (1980) and Haas *et al.* (1980) interpret this difference to be a consequence of a superior adaptation to hypoxia among high altitude Andean women. The low male birth weights noted among the Sherpa may occur because male fetuses have a reduced buffering capacity for environmental insults, like hypoxia (Stini, 1969; Haas *et al.*, 1977). If true, this would also indicate that the oxygen transport systems of Sherpa women do not completely compensate for environmental hypoxia. Depending upon the ubiquity of less-than-adequate compensations for hypoxia as well as on how severe an

Table IX
Birth Weights of Children Born of Indian and Non-Indian Mothers in the Andes and of Sherpa Mothers in Nepal

	Offspring of Indian women (La Paz, Bolivia[a])			Offspring of non-Indian women (La Paz, Bolivia[a])			Offspring of Sherpa women (Khumbu, Nepal)		
	n	$\bar{X}$	S.D.	*n*	$\bar{X}$	S.D.	*n*	$\bar{X}$	S.D.
Males	20	3251 g	417 g	25	3030 g	407 g	11	2903 g	441 g
Females	31	3149 g	438 g	29	3083 g	377 g	10	3087 g	366 g

[a]From Haas *et al.* (1980).

hypoxic stress this produces *in utero,* a negative effect on Sherpa fertility is conceivable.

A more definitive statement must await more controlled sampling, however. The small sample reported here is not accompanied by data on gestational length, parity, or maternal size. Small birth weight might also be related to the low protein intake reported for Sherpa women (Hirai *et al.*, 1975) as well as to the development problems associated with hypothyroidism, because these data were gathered prior to, or in the first stages of, the depot iodine injection program.

As among the high altitude Quechua of Peru (Frisancho, 1976), growth following birth among the Sherpa is reported to be retarded relative to low altitude standards (Pawson, 1976, 1977a, 1977b). But, growth in stature and weight is even slower among the Sherpa than among high altitude Andeans. This is also true for skeletal development and for growth in cortical bone thickness. Pawson posits a genetic hypothesis for this because a similar growth pattern occurs among Tibetans at midaltitude (1440 m) in Nepal. But other Khumbu environmental elements may be equally important. Hypothroidism might have been involved, because many of the children measured by Pawson were born prior to the beginning of the depot iodine injection program. Low calcium intake as well as low levels of protein in the diet may also be implicated (Hirai *et al.*, 1975). Ongoing research among the Khumbu Sherpas should help to resolve many of these problems (Pawson, personal communication).

5. Conclusion

Much of the present research among Himalayan populations seems to challenge the understanding of high altitude adaptations that has been developed in the Andes. Some important physical/physiological characteristics of the oxygen transport system (such as lung volume, red-blood-cell number and oxygen–hemoglobin affinity) appear to be different. Antenatal development among the Serpas may be more effected by hypoxia than among Andean natives. The rate of growth and development appears to be even more retarded among the Sherpas than it is among Andean groups, and adult body proportions (e.g., chest dimensions) also seem to vary. Yet the documentation of these differences as well as unambiguous tests of hypotheses concerning their cause is often made difficult by poor sampling, poor control of contributing variables, or poor techniques. For the most part, present research knowledge of Himalayan populations is similar to what existed for Andean populations prior to the 1960s. It is carried out among groups in widely different circumstances and is often difficult to compare. Even in the Khumbu, most of the research consists of uncoordinated, one-time-only studies. It is possible that a long-term, multidisciplinary study of a single group would be as beneficial to understanding life in the Himalayas now as the study of the Nuñoa (Peru) Quechua was in the mid-1960s (Baker, 1976). At the very least, more studies of the oxygen transport system, of growth *in utero*, of growth and development after birth, of fertility, and of the influences exerted by social factors, diet, disease, and hypoxia are needed.

References

Abelson, A. E., Baker, T. S., and Baker, P. T., 1974, Altitude, migration and fertility, *Soc. Biol.* **21**:12–27.

Adams, W. H., and Shresta, S. M., 1974, Hemoglobin levels, vitamin B_{12}, and folate status in a Himalayan village, *Am. J. Clin. Nutr.* **27**:217–219.

Adams, W. H., and Strang, L. J., 1975, Hemoglobin levels in persons of Tibetan ancestry living at high altitude, *Proc. Soc. Exp. Biol. Med.* **149**:1036–1039.

Astrand, P. O., and Rodahl, K., 1970, *Textbook of Work Physiology,* McGraw-Hill Book Company, New York.

Baker, P. T., 1969, Human Adaptation to high altitude, *Science* **163**:1149–1156.

Baker, P. T., 1976, Evolution of a project: Theory, method, and sampling, in: *Man in the Andes* (P. T. Baker and M. A. Little, eds.), Dowden, Hutchinson and Ross, Inc., Stroudsburg, Penn., pp. 1–20.

Baker, P. T., and Dutt, J. S., 1972, Demographic variables as measures of biological adaptation: A case study of high altitude human populations, in: *The Structure of Human Populations* (G. A. Harrison and A. J. Boyce, eds.), Clarendon Press, Oxford, pp. 352–378.

Bangham, C. R. M., and Sacherer, J. M., 1980, Fertility of Nepalese Sherpas at moderate altitudes: Comparison with high altitude data. *Ann. Hum. Biol.* **7**:323–330.

Basu, A., Bharati, P., Mukhopadhyay, B., and Gupta, R., 1980, A Microlevel Study of Fertility Differences and Decline in Relation to Physical and Cultural Environmental Factors in Some Communities of West Bengal, India and Upper Khumbu, Nepal, Indian Statistical Institute Technical Report Number Anthrop/8/80 (November, 1980), p. 24.

Buskirk, E. R., 1976, Work performance of newcomers to the Peruvian highlands, in: *Man in the Andes* (P. T. Baker and M. A. Little, eds.), Dowden, Hutchinson and Ross, Inc., Stroudsburg, Penn., pp. 283–299.

Ceretelli, P., 1976, Metabolismo ossidativo ed anaerobico nel soggetto acclimatato all'altitudine, *Suppl. Minerva Med.* **67**:1–26.

Cunningham, D. J. C., Spurr, D., and Lloyd, B. B., 1968, The drive to ventilation from arterial chemoreceptors in hypoxic exercise, in: *Arterial Chemoreceptors* (R. W. Torrance, ed.), Blackwell Scientific Publishers, Oxford, pp. 301–321.

Davidson, C. I., Grimm, T. C., and Nasta, C., 1981, Airborne lead and other elements derived from local fires in the Himalayas, *Science* **214**:1344–1346.

Dehn, M. M., and Bruce, R. A., 1972, Longitudinal variation in maximal oxygen uptake with age and activity, *J. Appl. Physiol.* **33**:805–807.

Donner, W., 1972, *Nepal: Raum, Mensch und Wirtschaft,* Otto Harassowitz, Wiesbden.

Dutt, J. S., 1980, Altitude and fertility: The confounding effect of childhood mortality—A Bolivian example, *Soc. Biol.* **27**:101–113.

Epstein, F. H., and Eckoff, R. D., 1967, The epidemiology of high blood pressure—Geographic distributions and etiologic factors, in: *Epidemiology of Hypertension* (J. Stamler, R. Stamler, and T. M. Pullman, eds.), Grune & Stratton, New York, pp. 155–166.
Ermans, A. M., Delange, F., Van Der Velden, M., and Kinthart, J., 1972, Possible role of cyanine and thiocyanate in the etiology of endemic cretinism, in: *Human Development and the Thyroid Gland: Relation to Endemic Cretinism* (J. B. Stanbury and R. L. Kroc, eds.), Plenum Press, New York, pp. 455–486.
Fisher, J., n.d., Tourists and Sherpas, unpublished ms.
Frisancho, A. R., 1975, Functional adaptation to high altitude hypoxia, *Science* **187**:313–319.
Frisancho, A. R., 1976, Growth and morphology at high altitude, in: *Man in the Andes* (P. T. Baker and M. A. Little, eds.), Dowden, Hutchinson and Ross, Inc., Stroudsburg, Penn., pp. 180–207.
Frisancho, A. R., and Baker, P. T., 1970, Altitude and growth: A study of the pattern of physical growth of a high altitude Peruvian Quechua population, *Am. J. Phys. Anthropol.* **32**:279–292.
Frisancho, A. R., Martinez, C., Velasquez, T., Sanchez, J., and Montoye, H., 1973, Influence of developmental adaptation on aerobic capacity at high altitude, *J. Appl. Physiol.* **34**:176–180.
Goldstein, M. C., 1976, Fraternal polyandry and fertility in a high Himalayan valley in northwest Nepal, *Hum. Ecol.* **4**:223–233.
Goldstein, M., 1981a, High-altitude Tibetan populations in the remote Himalaya: Social transformation and its demographic, economic and ecological consequences, *Mountain Res. Dev.* **1**:5–18.
Goldstein, M. C., 1981b, New perspectives on Tibetan fertility and population decline, *Am. Ethnol.* **8**:721–739.
Gupta, R., 1980, Altitude and demography among the Sherpas, *J. Biosoc. Sci.* **12**:103–114.
Gupta, R., and Basu, A., 1981, Variation in body dimensions in relation to altitude among the Sherpas, *Ann. Hum. Biol.* **8**:145–151.
Haas, J. D., 1980, Maternal adaptation and fetal growth at high altitude in Bolivia, in: *Social and Biological Predictors of Nutritional Status* (L. S. Greene and F. E. Johnston, eds.), Academic Press, New York, pp. 255–288.
Haas, J. D., Baker, P. T., and Hunt, E. E., 1977, The effects of high altitude on body size and composition of the newborn infant in southern Peru, *Hum. Biol.* **49**:611–628.
Haas, J. D., Frongello, E. A., Stepick, C. D., Beard, J. L., and Hurtado, L., 1980, Altitude, ethnic and sex differences in birth weight and length in Bolivia, *Hum. Biol.* **52**:459–477.
Hackett, P. H., Reeves, J. T., Reeves, C. D., Grover, R. F., and Rennie, D., 1980, Control of breathing in Sherpas at low and high altitude, *J. Appl. Physiol.* **49**:374–379.
Henry, L., 1961, Some data on natural fertility, *Eug. Q.* **8**:81–91.
Hillary, E., and Doig, D., 1962, *High in the Thin, Cold Air,* Doubleday and Company, Inc., Garden City, New York.
Hirai, K., Okuda, T., and Fukuwatari, M., 1975, Observations of living of the Sherpa tribe in Nepal and their dietary survey, *Rep. Sci. Liv.* **23**: 27–34.
Hoff, C. J., and Abelson, A. E., 1976, Fertility, in: *Man in the Andes* (P. T. Baker and M. A. Little, eds), Dowden, Hutchinson and Ross, Stroudsburg, Penn., pp. 128–146.
Ibbertson, H. K., Perl, M., McKinnon, J., Tait, J., Lim, T., and Gill, M. B., 1971, Endemic cretinism in Nepal, in: *Endemic Cretinism* (B. S. Hetzel and P. O. Pharoah, eds.), Institute of Human Biology, Papua New Guinea, pp. 71–88.
Kollias, J., Buskirk, E. R., Akers, R. F., Prokop, E. K., Baker, P. T., and Picon-Reategui, E., 1968, Work capacity of long-time residents and newcomers to altitude, *J. Appl. Physiol.* **24**:792–799.
Lahiri, S., 1968, Alveolar gas pressures in men with life-time hypoxia, *Resp. Physiol.* **4**:373–386.
Lahiri, S., 1971, Cardio-Respiratory Function and Physical Performance Capacity of Native Resi-

dents of Nepal at Various Altitudes: A Study of the Effect of High Altitude, Research Report to the World Health Organization.
Lahiri, S., Milledge, J. S., Chattophdhyay, H. P., Bhattacharyya, A. K., and Sinha, A. K., 1967, Respiration and heart rate of Sherpa highlanders during exercise. *J. Appl. Physiol.* **23**:545–554.
Lahiri, S., Kao, F. F., Velasquez, T., Martinez, C., and Pezzia, W., 1969, Irreversible blunted respiratory sensitivity to hypoxia in high altitude natives, *Resp. Physiol.* **6**:360–374.
Lahiri, S., Kao, F. F., Velasquez, T., Martinez, C., and Pezzia, W., 1970, Respiration of man during exercise at high altitude: Highlander vs. lowlander, *Resp. Physiol.* **8**:361–375.
Lahiri, S., Milledge, J. S., and Sorenson, S. C., 1972, Ventilation in man during exercise at high altitude, *J. Appl. Physiol.* **32**: 766–769.
Lahiri, S., Delaney, R. G., Brody, J. S., Simpser, M., Velasquez, T., Motoyama, E. K., and Polgar, C., 1976a, Relative role of environmental and genetic factors in respiratory adaptation to high altitude, *Nature* **261**:133–135.
Lahiri, S., Weitz, C. A., Milledge, J. S., and Fishman, M. C., 1976b, Effects of hypoxia, heat and humidity on physical performance, *J. Appl. Physiol.* **40**:206–210.
Lang, S. D. R., and Lang, A., 1971a, The Kunde Hospital and a demographic survey of the Upper Khumbu, Nepal, *N. Z. Med. J.* **74**:1–8.
Lang, S. D. R., and Lang, A., 1971b, Kunde hospital Annual Report for the Year Ending 31st October 1971—Including an analysis of cases for the first five years (1967–1971), p. 21.
Lenfant, C., and Sullivan, K., 1971, Adaptation to high altitude, *N. Engl. J. Med.* **284**:1298–1309.
Mazess, R. B., 1969, Exercise performance at high altitude in Peru, *Fed. Proc.* **28**:1301–1306.
McKinnon, J. R., 1968, Health problems of Khumbu in Nepal: The work at the Kunde hospital, *N. Z. Med. J.* **67**:140–143.
Morpurgo, G., Arese, P., Bosia, A., Pescarmona, G. P., Luzzana, M., Modiano, G., and Ranjit, S. K., 1976, Sherpas living permanently at high altitude: A new pattern of adaptation, *Proc. Natl. Acad. Sci. (U.S.A.)* **73**:747–751.
Nag, P. K., Sen, R. N., and Ray, U. S., 1978, Optimal rate of work for mountaineers, *J. Appl. Physiol.* **44**:952–955.
National Research Council, 1974, *Recommended Dietary Allowances*, 8th ed., National Academy of Sciences, Washington, D.C.
Oppitz, M., 1968, *Geschichte und Sozialordnung der Sherpa*, Universitäts verlag Wagner, Innsbruck and Munich.
Oppitz, M., 1974, Myth and facts: Reconsidering some data concerning the clan history of the Sherpa, *Kailash* **2**:121–131.
Ortner, S. B., 1978, *Sherpas through Their Rituals*, Cambridge University Press, New York.
Pawson, I. G., 1976, Growth and development in high altitude populations: A review of Ethiopian, Peruvian and Nepalese studies, *Proc. R. Soc., Lond.* [Biol.] **194**:83–98.
Pawson, I. G., 1977a, The effects of high altitudes on child growth and development, *Int. J. Biometerol.* **21**:171–178.
Pawson, I. G., 1977b, Growth characteristics of populations of Tibetan origin in Nepal, *Am. J. Phys. Anthropol.* **47**:473–482.
Samaja, M., Veicsteinas, A., and Cerretelli, P., 1979, Oxygen affinity of blood in altitude Sherpas, *J. Appl. Physiol.* **47**:337–341.
Stini, W. A., 1969, Nutritional stress and growth: Sex differences in adaptive response, *Am. J. Phys. Anthropol.* **31**:417–426.
Velasquez, T., 1976, Pulmonary function and oxygen transport, in: *Man in the Andes* (P. T. Baker and M. A. Little, eds.), Dowden, Hutchinson and Ross, Stroudsburg, Penn., pp. 237–260.
von Fürer-Haimendorf, C., 1964, *The Sherpas of Nepal*, University of California Press, Berkeley, California.

von Fürer-Haimendorf, C., 1975, *Himalyan Traders,* St. Martin's Press, New York.

Way, A., 1976, Morbidity and postneonatal mortality, in: *Man in the Andes* (P. T. Baker and M. A. Little, eds.), Dowden, Hutchinson and Ross, Stroudsburg, Penn., pp. 147–160.

Weitz, C. A., 1973, The effects of aging and habitual activity pattern on exercise performance among a high altitude Nepalese population, Ph.D. thesis, The Pennsylvania State University, University Park, Penn., p. 175.

Weitz, C. A., 1981, Response to Bangham and Sacherer, *Ann. Hum. Biol.* **8:**383–385.

Weitz, C. A., 1982, Blood pressure at rest and during exercise among Sherpas and Tibetan migrants in Nepal, *Soc. Sci. Med.* **16:**223–231.

Weitz, C. A., Pawson, I. G., Weitz, M. V., Lang, S. D. R., and Lang, A., 1978, Cultural factors affecting the demographic structure of a high altitude Nepalese population, *Soc. Biol.* **25:**179–195.

Winslow, R. M., Monge, C. C., Statham, N. J., Gibson, C. G., Charache, S., Whittembury, J., Moran, O., and Berger, R. L., 1981, Variability of oxygen affinity of blood: Human subjects native to high altitude, *J. Appl. Physiol.* **51:**1411–1416.

Woodhull, M. E., 1977, An aging study of the Sherpas, M.A. thesis, Temple University, Philadelphia, Penn.

CHAPTER 19

Ecology and Human Physiology in Ladak

S. L. MALIK AND INDERA P. SINGH

1. Ecological Considerations

Situated at lat. 34°09′ and long. 77°34′, the Ladak Plateau is the most westwardly region of the Indian subcontinent occupied by the Tibetan people. It is surrounded by China in the northeast and southeast, by Lahaul and Spiti in the south, and by Kashmir in the west. It consists of several snow-covered parallel mountain ranges running southeast to northwest. These ranges and the plateau support very scanty vegetation that is concentrated along the Indus River. This sacred river originates between the ranges of Kabas and Tibet and flows about 370 km before it reaches Leh, the capital of Ladak.

Ladak is situated in one of the most elevated reaches of the earth with permanent human habitation, and it is fairly isolated from the rest of the subcontinent. Its elevation, isolation, and heavy snowfall make it one of the most unusual climatic zones. The climate of Ladak is characterized by a marked difference in diurnal temperature, mainly because the dry and highly evaporative breezes exhaust the little moisture present in the atmosphere and dry air becomes intensively cold because of great terrestrial radiation under a cloudless sky. Cunningham (1970), while discussing the climate of Ladak, said that "the rarefied atmosphere offers but little impediment to the sun's rays, which during short summers are sufficiently powerful to ripen barley at an elevation of 15,000 ft. although temperature falls below freezing point every night." Apart from the

S. L. MALIK AND INDERA P. SINGH • Department of Anthropology, University of Delhi, Delhi 110 007.

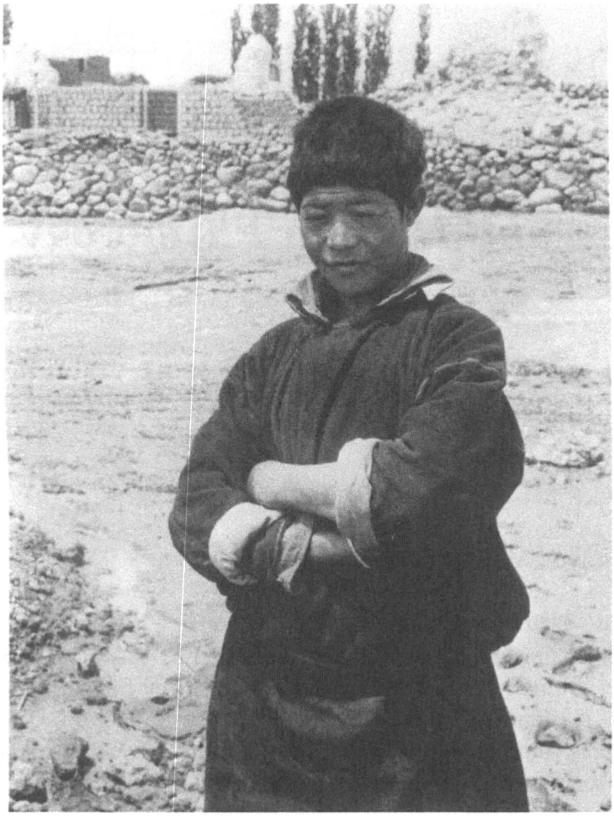

Figure 1. Adolescent Ladaki boy wearing traditional dress.

wide variation in diurnal temperature, there is also a large variation in temperature between shaded areas and those with direct sunlight.

The climate of Ladak thus presents a number of complex and interlinked environmental stresses that include reduced atmospheric pressure, cold, aridity, and local environmental conditions that directly or indirectly effect the human body. Some of the key factors associated with a high altitude environment are summarized as follows.

1. Increase in altitude reduces the atmospheric pressure and oxygen pressure, although the fall in atmospheric pressure is not uniform with increase of altitude.
2. Reduced atmospheric pressure results in high transparency of air favoring atmospheric cold.
3. Reduced atmospheric pressure also leads to reduced water vapor tension, and this directly favors atmospheric aridity.

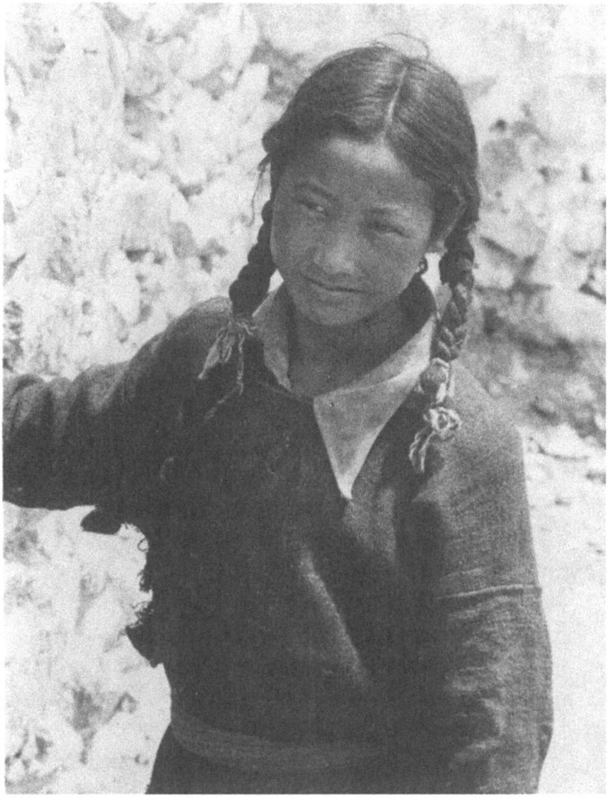

Figure 2. Young Ladaki girl in traditional dress.

4. High transparency of air and low water vapor tension result in greatly increased intensity of ultraviolet solar radiation.
5. The rarefied and arid atmosphere increases the rate of insulation and radiation that produces wide differences in diurnal temperature.

The present study was conducted in Leh and its surrounding villages. At an average altitude of 3514 m above the mean sea level, the mean barometric pressure at Leh is of 480 mm of mercury. The average annual rainfall is as low as 9.6 mm with a low relative humidity of 50%. The temperature varies from a minimum of −28.3°C to a maximum of 33.9°C with a mean temperature of 3.1°C.

The Chinese pilgrim Fa Hian recorded in A.D. 400 that "Ladak is inhabited by a peculiar race of people, who call themselves 'Bot-pa' who speak a peculiar language called Tibetan and who profess the religion of Budha, under the peculiar Hierachy of monks called Lamas" (Cunningham, 1970). Bods or Bodhs

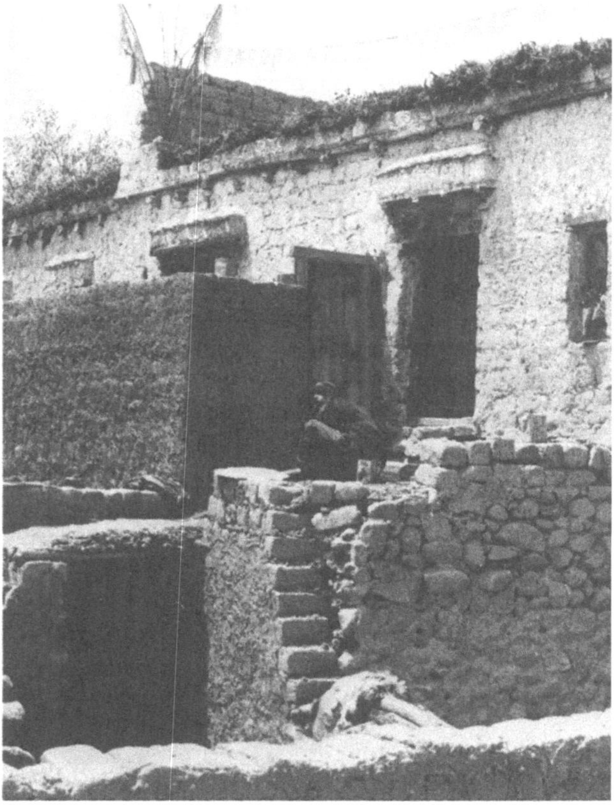

Figure 3. Typical Ladaki house showing characteristic flatness of the roof and entrance to the animals' quarters in the basement (dark entrance, lower left).

(pronounced *Bots*) are sometimes also known by the name of *Botis* (Cunningham, 1970). *Bods* is a term that seems to have originated from the Tibetan and means *strong* (Herra and Vergara, 1899).

The Bod community has lived in isolation in Ladak for a long time but the exact date of their settlement is unknown. The only evidence of contact is recorded by Sherring, (1906), who described a trade route connecting Tibet via Ladak and western Nari to Lahaul. The principal trade goods are wool and pasham (a superior quality of wool). Bods are basically agriculturists, although pastoralism is not uncommon. The common crops grown in the area are wheat, barley, millet, oilseeds, and some fruit and vegetables. Some of the common animals of the region are goats, sheep, horses, ponies, yaks, and donkeys. Few persons are engaged in business; they run tea shops, stationary businesses or places that sell other items of daily use. Only a few individuals are employed in the state services, but this is a recent phenomenon. Though agriculture is their major occupation, they have to import essential commodities often—wheat, flour, sugar, salt, and kerosene oil.

A quantitative nutritional study of the Bods unfortunately has not been conducted. A generalized inquiry into the dietary habits revealed that the average food of the common Bod consists of a preparation of wheat or barley cake or barley moistened in water to which turnips and few peas may be added. They relish *Thupa,* a particular type of chopped meat preparation to which spaghetti is sometimes added. Butter tea is the traditional hot drink; the quantity of butter and frequency of intake generally varies with the economic status of the individual.

Bods are very sociable and cheerful people and at the slightest pretext make an occasion for feasting. *Chhang* (undistilled wine) drinking, singing, and occasionally dancing by females are the characteristic features of any feast. Almost all families celebrate several feasts, according to their means: birth feasts (*tsas-ton*), naming feasts (*ming-ton*), marriage feasts (*bag-ton*), and funeral feasts (*shid-ton*). These are important occasions that are observed by all the Bods. The system of polyandry that was prevalent in Ladak in the past is now dying out. If such a system is prevalent anywhere at all, the wife is shared only by brothers in a family.

The finest buildings of Ladak are the monasteries that are invariably built on mountaintops. The monastery or *Gompa* is a sacred place and commands supernatural powers. The lamas (or priests) have high prestige in the society and have a number of traditional sanctions. The most common *mantra* in the Buddhist religion in Ladak is *Om mani Padme hum* (Oh Jewel in the lotus)—a representation for the Lord Buddha. Bods of Ladak frequently live in two-or three-story houses; the lower portion of their buildings is made up of stones whereas the walls of the upper story are made of large sun-dried bricks. The doors are nothing more than rough planks of wood; some of the houses have balconies also.

The traditional dress of men in Ladak is a woolen cloak (*La-pa-sha*) with woolen leggings of felt (*r-kang-phying*). Quilted skullcaps or caps of sheepskin with the wool inside serve as their headgear. The traditional women of Ladak wear woolen jackets that are studded with many colored pieces of torquois that hang to the waist. Recently Bods, specially youngsters, wear dresses that are common in other parts of India.

Ladak is divided into three *tehsils,* namely Leh, Kargil, and Zanskar. The Leh tehsil consists of 107 villages and the town of Leh. The town of Leh is the most thickly populated area in Ladak and had a total estimated population of 5466 in 1971, according to the district census report. Cunningham (1970) reported that in Ladak the population remains nearly stable, not because of an unhealthy climate but because the system of polyandry most effectively checks any population increase. According to the district census report published from the office of the deputy commissioner in Leh, the population in Ladak in

1970–1971 was 105,291, whereas it was 88,651 in 1960–1961. This indicates that the population of Ladak is not stabilized but is increasing. A spurt in the population growth was expected with the disintegration of the system of polyandry, coupled with minimization of the number of individuals becoming lamas. However, no such increase was observed, and the average number of children per family is still as low as two. Cunningham (1970) reported that Bods of Ladak have a low longevity, and persons reaching over 70 years of age are less than 1.3%. These factors should be examined in detail for determing the effect of hypoxia on reproductive performance, infant mortality, and longevity at high altitude. A detailed study of demographic variables reveals patterns that are caused by the multiple environmental stresses of living at high altitude.

2. Cultural Adaptation

All living organisms have the ability to modify themselves in response to changes in the environment. Most of the animals rely exclusively on their biological makeup and basic instincts to make such adjustments. Short-term physiological changes may allow relaxation, but modifications in the biological makeup occur slowly through processes such as natural selection.

Unlike other animals, human beings do not rely solely on their ability to adapt biologically. Human beings make ample use of extrasomatic characteristics, that is, culture, in meeting the demands of environmental stress. In many situations, it is much easier and more economical to use technology to avert stress. This need not imply that people meet all their ecological stresses through culture and that genetics has no role to play. An example from the Ladak amply illustrates this point. To meet the stress of cold, Bods wear woolens, but simultaneously morphological and functional alterations have occurred in their biological makeup. In contrast, the stress of reduced oxygen/atmospheric pressure is difficult to overcome through cultural factors and in most of the natives of the area several biological modifications have developed in response to this stress. Adaptation in humans is neither solely because of their genetical makeup nor is it entirely dependent on cultural factors. Adaptation in human populations is a matter of constant interaction between biology and culture.

The Bods of Ladak also adapt to environmental stresses through culture, and many cultural practises may be deciphered as buffers of environmental stress. Houses are constructed in such a manner that they preserve maximum heat. Built along the sloping terrain of mountain cliffs, they also register a minimum impact to high winds. The chimney is set in the center of the sitting room thus keeping the room amply warm in the chilling cold. Cattle are kept on the ground floor and their body heat keeps the floor of the first story—where Bods live—warm. Usually at the back portion of the first floor is the laterine, which is a small room with a hole so that waste is collected on the ground floor.

The cold climate of Ladak is such that the waste does not produce a foul odor. Each year soil is put on this waste and kept for few months, producing good manure. The housetops are neither gabled, nor are they made of tin; rather, they are flat and are prepared from a mixture of thatch and soil. In the first instance, one wonders why they have not wanted to alter this, and therefore have a heavy work load of removing ice in the winter. But the reasons are many, according to the Bods. First, tin must be imported, which is an extremely difficult process because transport facilities are either absent or prohibitively costly. Second, tin roofs become cold because they are good conductors of heat. Finally, the top of the house provides space for carrying out most of the activities in the summer months and the costly fuel is saved.

Flower gardens are rarely found around the houses and the casual onlooker may think that Bods have no asthetic sense. However, many colorful flowers hang from the balconies or are kept on the roof to save agricultural space that cannot be spared for flower gardens. In the space available around their houses, they grow vegetables. Many initially incomprehensible practices can later be interpreted as economically efficient adaptations to the harsh environment of Ladak. For example, Bods prefer to wear their new dresses underneath and old ones outside, and they reverse the order on special occasions thereby saving the new one from dust, yet using their warmth.

Their diet is also well suited to their environment. A detailed nutritional survey in the area has not been conducted, but their dietary patterns indicate that they have sufficient quantities of proteins and fat. Butter tea and *Thupa* are good examples of such a diet. They try to consume as much meat as possible, particularly in winter. The snow acts as a refrigerator where they store their meat for nearly a month by digging up ice, keeping the meat by covering it with ice and placing a heavy stone on it so that the animals may not dig it up. Other than this, Bods are known to consume certain local medicinal herbs and roots that yield energy as well as heat.

There are many other examples that could be cited from their day-to-day life indicating the cultural adaptation of Bods to the environment. Cultural adaptations serve to buffer environmental stress, but they do not eliminate them; therefore unbuffered stresses have a definite effect on the biological makeup of the Bods. Stresses such as low oxygen/atmospheric pressure cannot be met by cultural factors, and they depend upon alteration in the biological/physiological functions of human organisms.

3. Ecology and Growth

Adaptation to the ecological component of exogenous factors is an important and vital characteristic of all living beings, especially mammals including human beings. Beginning with the physiological respones to acclimation, acclimatization, and genetic adaptation, numerous and varied changes are brought about in the functions and structures of the human body. Initially, in the process of adaptation, functional alterations occur to encounter the external stress and then, according to these altered functions, related structures are modified or moulded over time.

The development of individuals of a population reflects to quite an extent the degree to which a population is adapted. As a case study, we investigated the impact of ecological factors on growth patterns among Bods with a view to understanding adaptation among them.

Results of previous studies indicate a poorly defined adolescent spurt in stature among male native highlanders from the Himalayas (Malik, 1976; Malik and Singh, 1978; Malik, 1979) and the Andes (Baker *et al.*, 1966; Frisancho, 1966, 1968, 1969; Baker, 1969; Frisancho and Baker, 1970, Baker, 1971). Similarly, Rothammer and Spielmann (1972) concluded that the Peruvian Aymara anthropometric variability is due to high altitude environmental factors. This finding, however, is equivocal, and Hoff (1972) suggested that the distinctive Quechua growth patterns are not strongly influenced by the environmental factors but by some undetermined metabolic forces that are operating in both the high and low altitude Quechua populations.

The study by Clegg *et al.* (1970) on Ethiopian highlanders indicated that they grow faster and are taller and heavier than the lowlanders in all age groups. A year later, Pawson (1971) observed that the highlanders from Debarek are taller and heavier than the genetically similar populations living in the low altitude area of Adi Arkai. Their differences were shown to be caused by the unfavorable conditions of living at low altitude (Clegg *et al.*, 1970; Pawson, 1976). On the other hand, in the eastern Himalayas, Pawson (1974) revealed that the Tibetans (1125 m) are larger, especially males above the age of 12 years, than the highland Sherpas living at altitudes between 3475 m and 4050 m. He (Pawson, 1976) accords this difference to the unfavorable conditions of high altitude.

This section describes the effect of altitude on human physical development and in particular on the adolescent spurt on a high altitude population of Ladak. For this purpose, a cross-sectional sample of 457 apparently healthy male Bods was collected, out of which 257 were from the high altitude ranges (3354 m) of Ladak, and the rest (n = 183) were from Kulu Valley.

In brief, the origin of the Bods can be traced back to the strains that reflect their links with Tibetans. Historical records say that the Tibetans had a trade route from Tibet via western Nari and Ladak to Lahaul—which in present times is well connected with the Kulu Valley. Though observations on the genetic material of the two groups were not available, their morphological features suggests their ethnic similarity. Moreover, the oral traditions of the Bods of Kulu document their ancestoral links with those of Ladak.

Table I
Age Changes in Stature (cm) among Male Bods of Ladak (Highland Population) and Male Bods of Kulu (Lowland Population)[a]

	Bods of Ladak, highland population				Bods of Kulu, lowland population			
Age group (midvalue)	Number of individuals	Mean	Standard deviation	Annual increment	Number of individuals	Mean	Standard deviation	Annual increment
11	21	128.0	7.4		14	131.5	6.4	
12	24	133.7	3.5	5.7	16	135.9	5.0	[illegible] 4
13	24	135.9	5.7	2.2	20	137.0	7.0	1.1
14	33	143.4	5.3	7.5	19	140.4	8.0	3.4
15	41	150.3	7.7	6.9	18	147.6	8.2	7.2
16	59	157.9	5.9	7.6	27	155.7	7.9	8.1
17	31	161.1	5.9	3.2	24	158.3	9.7	2.6
18	21	163.7	3.9	2.6	25	163.5	5.7	5.2
19	20	167.8	2.8	4.1	20	164.6	5.4	0.9

[a]Bods of Ladak and Bods of Kulu are significantly different only in 19-year-old age group (analysis of variance).

The mean values, standard deviations, and annual increments in stature for Bods of Ladak and Bods of Kulu are shown in Table I. Stature in both the groups increases with advancement in age. Analysis of variance shows that the two groups do not differ significantly (at a 5% probability level) in stature in any of the age groups except at 19 years when highlanders tend to be taller than the lowlanders. This difference may be attributed largely to the still-increasing growth at 19 years among the highland population (Figure 4; Table I).

In stature, the highest peak velocity (Figure 4) or maximum annual increment (Table I) occurs between 15 and 16 years among the Bods of Kulu, whereas, there are two peak velocities, that is, between 13 and 14 and 15 and 16 years of age, indicating a biadolescent spurt among the Bods of Ladak. The absence of a clear adolescent spurt may be largely due to hypoxia and malnutrition because these two factors may restrict the required energy output needed at this stage of ontogenic development. In view of the similar food habits of both groups studied, low oxygen pressure seems to play a vital role in this situation. However, this is not to dismiss the contributing effects of genetic factors, general living conditions, disease patterns, and the differential responses to the exogenous factors. The role of hypoxia has been emphasized, keeping in mind that in the oxygen-deficient environment, the physiological changes that occur as a result of acclimatization may not be sufficient to meet the increased demand of oxygen for growth at puberty, thereby resulting in an unclear adolescent spurt at high altitude.

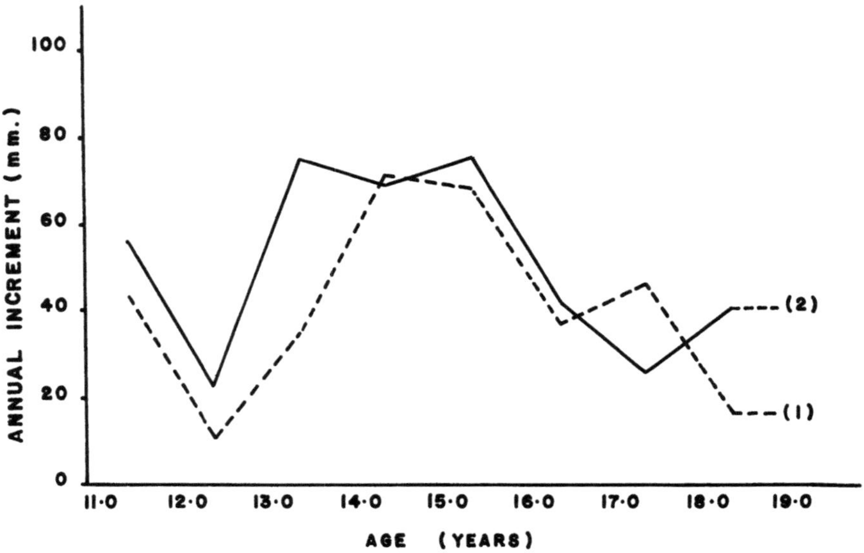

Figure 4. Growth in stature among Male Bods of Ladak (1) and Bods of Kulu (2).

In Table II, mean values, standard deviations, and annual increments of body weight are shown with respect to age for both Bods of Ladak and Bods of Kulu. The analysis of variance suggests that the two groups do not differ in body weight with respect to age *per se* except at 19 years when the Bods of Ladak are heavier than the Bods of Kulu. The increasing trend in both stature (Figure 4) and body weight (Figure 5) in the highland group forces one to hypothesize that the development in the high altitude group is not completed, even at the age of 19 years. This is specially interesting in view of the earlier reports that growth in highland groups is not completed even at 22 years of age (Frisancho, 1966; Malcolm, 1970). Because the data for adults (older than 19 years) is not available yet, the authors cannot comment on this issue. Though the differences are not significant statistically (except at 19 years) before 13 years of age, Bods of Kulu are taller and heavier than Bods of Ladak, but thereafter the trend is reversed. This demonstrates that highlander Bods have a tendency to have greater body sizes than the lowlanders, but only after 13 years of age.

It has been established previously that high altitude populations have greater chest dimensions than lowlanders (Hurtado, 1932; Monge, 1948; Frisancho, 1969; Frisancho and Baker, 1970; Baker, 1969, 1971; Pawson, 1971; Hoff, 1972; Frisancho *et al.*, 1973a; Pawson, 1976). Hurtado (1932) suggested that larger chest size and lowered diaphragm allowed larger space for lungs and heart and that that facilitated acclimatization to high altitude. Bods of Ladak have

Table II
Age Changes in Body Weight (kg) among Male Bods of Ladak (Highland Population) and Male Bods of Kulu (Lowland Population)[a]

	Bods of Ladak, highland population				Bods of Kulu, lowland population			
Age group (midvalue)	Number of individuals	Mean	Standard deviation	Annual increment	Number of individuals	Mean	Standard deviation	Annual increment
11	21	24.5	1.6		14	25.9	1.9	
12	24	26.9	1.9	2.4	16	28.1	2.5	2.2
13	24	27.8	3.0	0.9	20	28.3	3.6	0.2
14	33	32.2	4.0	4.4	19	30.3	3.4	2.0
15	41	37.7	6.9	5.5	18	37.0	6.9	6.7
16	59	43.9	5.8	6.2	27	43.0	7.1	6.0
17	31	46.8	6.0	2.8	24	45.2	8.9	2.2
18	21	51.6	4.6	4.8	25	49.8	5.5	4.6
19	20	57.5	2.5	5.9	20	51.4	4.9	1.6

[a]Bods of Ladak and Bods of Kulu are significant only in 19-year-old age group (analysis of variance).

significantly greater chest circumferences at all ages than do the Indians. This seems to be a morphological adaptation to the thin atmosphere of high altitude as has been suggested previously (Frisancho, 1969; Frisancho and Baker, 1970; Frisancho *et al.*, 1975). Pawson (1974) stated that the high chest circumference may be a result of higher body mass and suggested the use of chest circum-

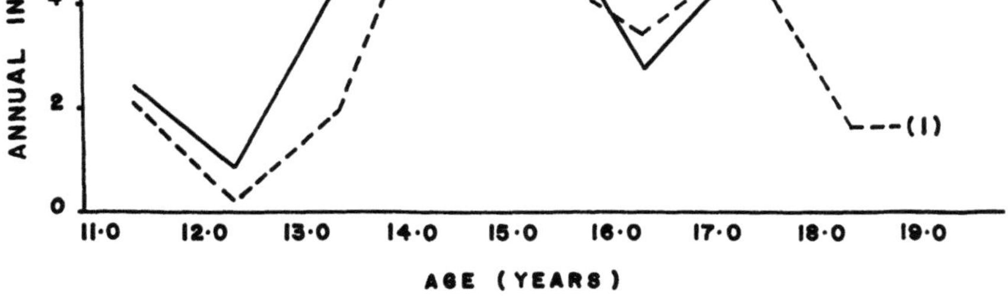

Figure 5. Growth in weight among Male Bods of Ladak (1) and Bods of Kulu (2).

Table III
Age Change in Stature (cm) and Body Weight (kg) among Female Bods of Ladak

Age group (midvalue)	Number of individuals	Stature			Weight		
		Mean	S.D.	Annual increment	Mean	S.D.	Annual increment
10	13	127.6	4.1		23.7	6.3	
11	10	134.3	5.7	6.7	27.2	5.3	3.5
12	11	140.8	7.2	6.5	30.0	11.3	2.8
13	16	148.7	6.2	7.9	36.7	13.3	6.7
14	23	148.9	5.7	0.2	38.1	13.3	1.4
15	23	150.0	4.7	1.1	40.7	13.0	2.6
16	27	150.3	4.8	0.3	43.6	12.0	2.9
17	15	153.8	5.5	3.5	44.6	9.6	1.0
18	10	156.5	3.7	2.7	46.2	8.7	1.6

ference/stature ratio. When the ratio of chest circumference/stature was compared between Bods of Ladak and Indians, the former showed higher values in all the age groups, thereby establishing that the greater chest dimension is one of the natural acclimatization factors among Bods.

Singh and Malik (1977) showed that female Bods exhibit a clear adolescent spurt in stature and weight (Table III). Previously, Baker (1969) reported the absence of a well-defined growth spurt for males, but not in the case of females. This may be partially because females are more resistant to the environmental stress than are males (Wolanski and Malik, 1979).

These investigations on the Bods of Ladak when compared with All India pooled data (ICMR, 1972) show that the former have greater body weight/body-surface-area ratio than the later (Singh and Malik, 1977; Malik and Singh, 1978). It is widely held that the production of heat is directly proportional to its mass, and loss of heat through radiation, to surface area; therefore individuals with higher body weight/surface-area ratio can produce more heat as well as conserve more heat, which facilitates adaptation to cold climates (Schreider, 1951; Newman, 1953, 1955; Scholander, 1955; Garn, 1961; Walter, 1971). The higher body weight/body-surface-area ratio among Bods may be interpreted as adaptation to the cold climate of Ladak.

4. Respiratory Adaptation

To release energy, people require continuous delivery of oxygen to the tissues. How this process occurs in the thin atmosphere of the high altitude has attracted the attention of numerous biologists. Among the highlanders, high vital capacity has been observed frequently from the Andes (Hurtado, 1932; Choidi, 1963; Frisancho, 1969; Baker, 1971; Boyce *et al.*, 1974), Nepal (Bangham and Veale, 1976), Bhutan (Cotes and Ward, 1966), Poland (Pyzuk and Wolanski, 1972), and the U.S.S.R. (Mikleschewskaya *et al.*, 1976).

We reported previously (Malik and Singh, 1979a) that male Bods of Ladak have higher forced vital capacity (FVC), forced expiratory volume 1st second (FEV_1) and maximal voluntary ventilation (MVV) than do the Indians. Subsequently, we (Malik and Singh, 1979b) compared the Bods of Ladak with the Bods of Kulu after developing regression equations between respiratory functions and age. The results indicated that FVC and FEV_1 have faster rates of development among highland Bods than among the lowland Bods. It was also clear that greater differences between the two groups began only after 12 years of

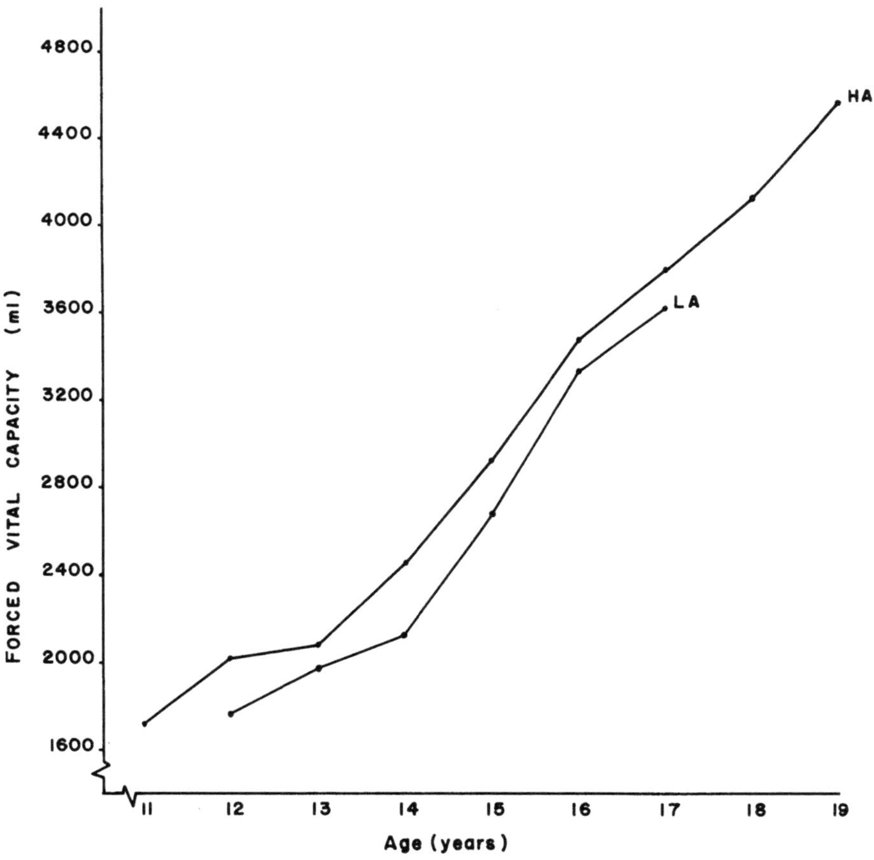

Figure 6. Comparison of forced vital capacity between highland (HA) and lowland (LA) Bods (after adjusting height and weight).

age as was suggested earlier by Boyce and associates (Boyce *et al.*, 1974). If an outsider settles at high altitude before he or she reaches puberty—a period associated with both greater activity and development—he or she may acclimatize much faster than the individual who is exposed to a high altitude environment after reaching adulthood. This has been explained as a developmental response by Frisancho and his co-workers (Frisancho *et al.* 1973a). By comparing the regression lines for maximal voluntary ventilation it was observed that the highland Bods have significantly higher MVV than do the lowland Bods.

In Figures 6, 7, and 8 the FVC, FEV_1, and MVV have been presented for the Bods of Ladak and the Bods of Kulu after making adjustment for stature and body weight by linear interpolation. These figures show that the Bods of Ladak have higher respiratory functions in all age groups than do the Bods of Kulu. The higher ventilatory capacity of highland Bods in comparison to the ethnically

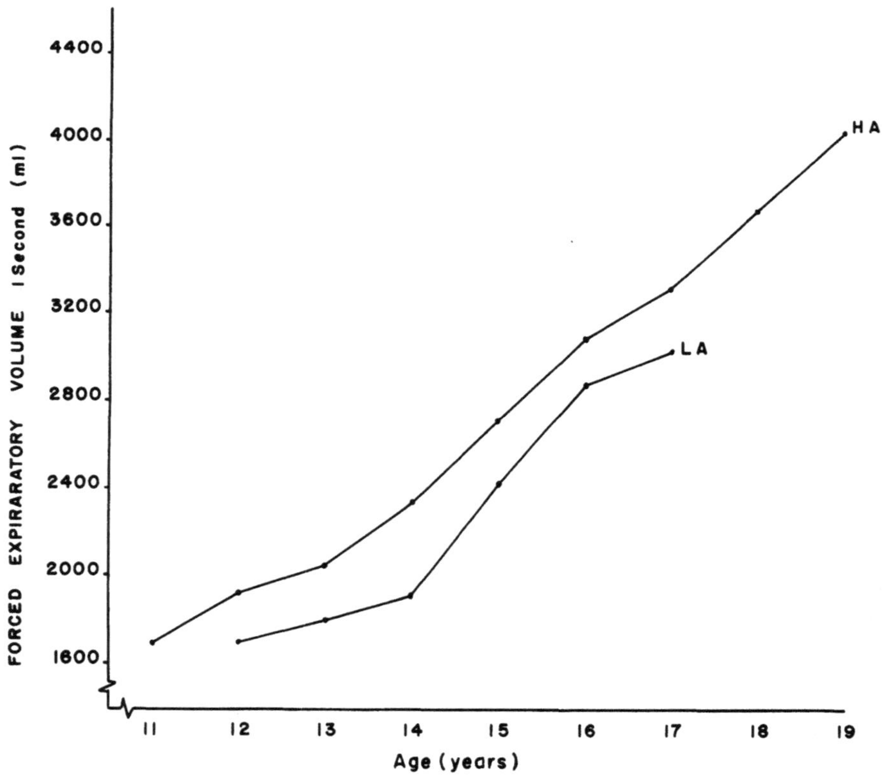

Figure 7. Comparison of forced expiratory volume 1 second between highland (HA) and lowland (LA) Bods (after adjusting for height and weight).

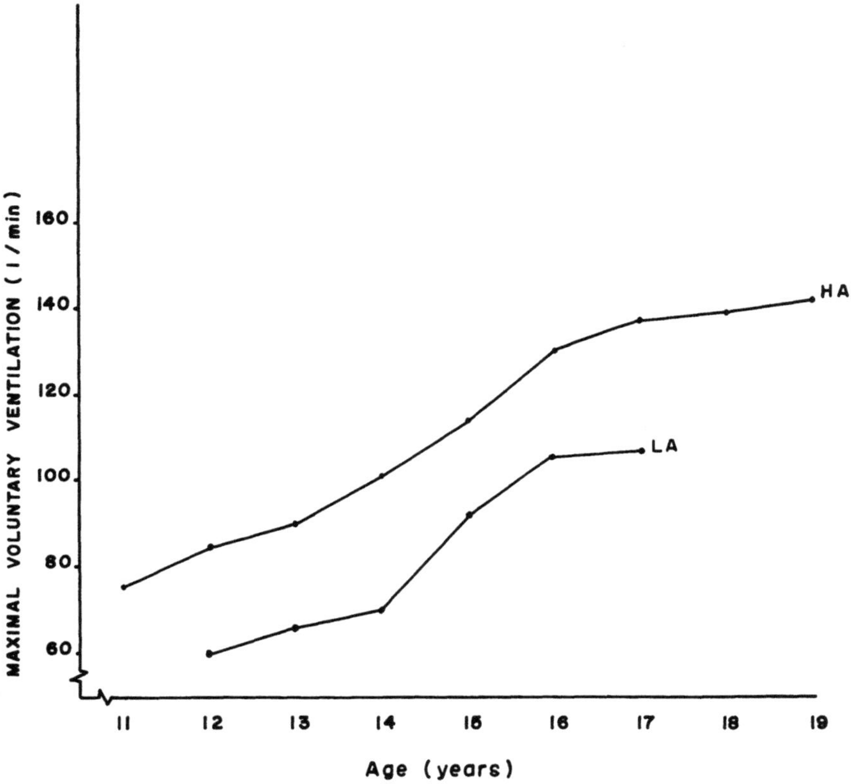

Figure 8. Comparison of maximal voluntary ventilation between highland (HA) and lowland (LA) Bods (after adjusting for height and weight).

similar population of lower altitudes may be attributed to low oxygen pressure, increased work load, or minimal air pollution of the high altitude environment.

The values of coefficient of correlation (r), presented in Table IV, show that the lung volumes (FVC, FEV_1, MVV) are significantly associated with all the body measurements considered in this study. In populations from the plains, lung volumes are significantly correlated with stature, weight, body surface area, and age (Ferris and Smith, 1953; Rao *et al.*, 1961; Ferris *et al.*, 1962; Lyons and Tanner, 1962; Bhattacharya, 1963; Jain and Gupta, 1967; Jain and Ramiah, 1968, 1969; Huizinga and Glanville, 1968; Boyce *et al.*, 1974). The relationship between the chest dimensions and respiratory functions, if any, is generally low. In highlander Bods, all the chest measurements are significantly associated with the three respiratory functions (Table IV). Frisancho (1969) reported previously that among Peruvian highlanders FVC has the highest association with chest

Table IV
Values of Coefficient of Correlation (*r*) and Coefficient of Partial Correlation (*pr*) between Respiratory Functions and Body Measurements[a]

Body measurements	Respiratory functions					
	FVC		FEV_1		MVV	
	r	*pr*	*r*	*pr*	*r*	*pr*
Body weight	0.885	0.654	0.850	0.605	0.721	0.439
Stature	0.886	0.589	0.831	0.546	0.726	0.450
Sitting height	0.869	0.613	0.844	0.593	0.734	0.473
Trunk height	0.840	0.529	0.820	0.529	0.649	0.273
Total upper extremity length	0.712	0.441	0.683	0.402	0.591	0.312
Total lower extremity length	0.794	0.472	0.759	0.383	0.663	0.320
Biacromial breadth	0.838	0.572	0.795	0.503	0.705	0.428
Anteroposterior depth of chest	0.786	0.534	0.757	0.471	0.617	0.290
Transverse diameter of chest	0.799	0.539	0.758	0.474	0.650	0.357
Biiliocristal breadth	0.777	0.480	0.755	0.461	0.661	0.375
Chest circumference (I)	0.865	0.636	0.828	0.577	0.724	0.574
Chest circumference (N)	0.859	0.617	0.823	0.562	0.708	0.429
Chest circumference (E)	0.847	0.599	0.808	0.537	0.693	0.405
Abdominal circumference	0.715	0.447	0.694	0.424	0.559	0.257
Head length	0.516	0.224	0.482	0.184	0.362	0.163
Head breadth	0.276	0.153	0.248	0.112	0.249	0.133
Nasal height	0.621	0.271	0.584	0.288	0.481	0.141
Nasal breadth	0.576	0.328	0.559	0.310	0.477	0.229

[a]Partial coefficient of correlation is between respiratory functions and body measurements, keeping age as intermediate variable.

circumference of maximal inspiration. The stress of low oxygen pressure added to a greater work load seems to be the vital reason for the larger lung volumes (Malik and Singh, 1979a). Probably as a consequence, larger chests were developed among natives of Ladak (Malik and Singh, 1978) and the Andes (Frisancho, 1969; Baker, 1969, 1971). The increased association between respiratory functions and chest measurements further strengthens the view that chest development at high altitude is a by-product of increased respiratory volumes.

As lung volumes and body measurements are both age dependent in our sample, it was thought desirable to eliminate the effect of age and then examine the association between the respiratory volumes and anthropometric measurements. The values of the partial correlation (age as an intermediate variable) between lung functions and body measurements, though reduced from the values of coefficient of product moment correlations, were significant at a 5% probability level except between FEV_1 and head breadth (Table IV). Henceforth, it may be inferred that the relationship between the respiratory volumes and body measurements is not merely due to the effect of age.

5. Concluding Remarks

Ladak is the largest district of India with the least population density. In spite of the harshness of the climate, the Bods of Ladak are extremely sociable and cheerful people and the slightest pretext is an occasion for feasting. The environment of Ladak presents a number of complex and interlinked environmental factors, such as low oxygen/atmospheric pressure and cold atmospheric aridity that directly or indirectly affects the human body.

The Bods of Ladak have higher respiratory functions, greater chest dimensions, and a greater correlation between respiratory functions and chest measurements, which may be adaptive in nature in the low atmospheric pressure of the area. They have a higher ratio of body mass/body surface area, which has practical adaptiveness in the cold climate. The male Bods do not have a clear adolescent spurt in stature, indicating that the growth at high altitude may be curbed under unfavorable conditions. The clear adolescent spurt in stature among females, however, indicates the stronger resistance of females to environmental stress.

ACKNOWLEDGMENT

The photographs accompanying this article were taken by Dr. John R. Lukacs during a visit to Ladak in August 1982. The authors express their thanks for his cooperation in providing these photos.

References

Baker, P. T., 1969, Human adaptation to high altitude, *Science* **163:**1149–1156.

Baker, P. T., 1971, Adaptation problems in Andean human population, in: *Ongoing Evolution of Latin American Populations* (F. M. Salzano, ed.), Charles C. Thomas, Springfield, Ill.

Baker, P. T., Frisancho, A. R., and Thomas, R. B., 1966, A priliminary analysis of human growth in the Peruvian Andes, in: *Human Adaptability to Environment and Physical Fitness* (M. S. Malhotra, ed.), DIPAS, Madras.

Bangham, C. R. M., and Veale, K. E. A., 1976, Ventilatory capacity in Napalese health, *J. Physiol.* **265;**31–32.

Bhattacharya, D. K., 1963, Vital capacity of Jat males of Punjab: A modification of the formula existing for its computation, *Ind. J. Med. Res.* **51:**361–365.

Boyce, A. J., Haight, J. S. J., Rimmer, D. B., and Harrison, G. A., 1974, Respiratory function in Peruvian Quechua Indians, *Ann. Hum. Biol.* **1:**137–148.

Choidi, H., 1963, Respiratory adaptation to high altitude, in: *The Regulation of Human Respiration* (D. J. C. Cunningham and B. B. Lloyd, eds.), Blackwell, Oxford.

Clegg, E. J., Harrison, G. A., and Baker, P. T., 1970, The impact of high altitude on human populations, *Hum. Biol.* **42:**486–518.

Cotes, J. E., and Ward, M. P., 1966, Ventilatory capacity in normal Bhutanese, *J. Physiol.* **186:**88–89.

Cunningham, A., 1970, *Ladak: Physical, Statistical and Historical with Notes on the Surrounding Countries,* Sagar Publications, New Delhi.

Ferris, B. F., Jr., and Smith, C. W., 1953, Maximum breathing capacity and vital capacity in female children and adolescents, *Pediatrics* **12:**341–352.

Ferris, B. F., Jr., Whittenberger, J. L., and Gallagher, J. R., 1962, Maximum breathing capacity and vital capacity of male children and adolescents, *Pediatrics* **9:**659–670.

Frisancho, A. R., 1966, Human Growth in High Altitude Peruvian Population. M. S. thesis, Pennsylvania State University (unpublished).

Frisancho, A. R., 1968, *Growth, Physique and Pulmonary Functions of a High Altitude Peruvian Quechua Population,* Ph.D. thesis, Pennsylvania State University.

Frisancho, A. R., 1969, Human growth and pulmonary function of a high altitude Peruvian Quechua population, *Hum. Biol.* **41:**365–379.

Frisancho, A. R., and Baker, P. T., 1970, Altitude and growth: A study of patterns of physical growth of a high altitude Peruvian Quechua Population, *Am. J. Phys. Anthropol.* **32:**279–292.

Frisancho, A. R., Velasquez, T., and Sanchez, J., 1973a, Influence of developmental adaptation on lung function at high altitude, *Hum. Biol.* **45:**583–594.

Frisancho, A. R., Martinez, C., Velasquez, T., Sanchez, J., and Monotype, H., 1973b, Influence of developmental adaptation of aerobic capacity at high altitude, *J. Appl. Physiol.* **34:**176–180.

Frisancho, A. R., Borkan, G. A., and Klayman, J., 1975, Pattern of growth of lowland and highland Peruvian Quechua of similar genetic composition, *Hum. Biol.* **47:**233–244.

Garn, S. M., 1961, *Human Races,* Charles C Thomas, Springfield, Ill.

Herra, A. L., and Vergara, D., 1899, *La Vie Sur hauts Plateaux,* Smithsonian Institute, Washington, D.C.

Hoff, C. J., 1972, Preliminary Observation on Altitudinal Variations in the Physical Growth and Development of Peruvian Quechua, Ph.D. thesis, Pennsylvania State University (unpublished).

Huizinga, J., and Glanville, E. V., 1968, Vital capacity and timed vital capacity in the Kurumba from Upper Volta, *S. Afr. J. Sci.* **64:**125–133.

Hurtado, A., 1932, Respiratory adaptation in the Indian natives of the Peruvian Andes, Studies at high altitude, *Am. J. Phys. Anthropol.* **17:**137–323.

ICMR, 1972, Growth and Physical Development of Indian Infants and Children ICMR Technical Report No. 18, ICMR, New Delhi.

Jain, S. K., and Gupta, G. K., 1967, Age height and body weight as determinants of ventilatory "norms" in health: Men above fifty years of age, *Ind. J. Med. Res.* **55:**599–619.

Jain, S. K., and Ramiah, T. J., 1968, Lung volumes and mechanisms of breathing in healthy boys 7–14 years old, *Ind. J. Chest Dis.* **10:**63–68.

Jain, S. K., and Ramiah, T. J., 1969, Normal standards of pulmonary function tests for healthy Indian men, 15–40 year old: Comparison of different regression equation, *Ind. J. Med.* Res. **57:**1453–1466.

Lyons, H. A., and Tanner, R. W., 1962, Total lung volume and its subdivisions in children: Normal standards, *J. Appl. Physiol.* **17:**601–604.

Malcolm, L. A., 1970, Growth and development of Bundi children of New Guinea highlands, *Hum. Biol.* **42:** 293–328.

Malik, S. L., 1976, Age Changes and Few Biological Responses at High Altitude: A Study among Male Bods of Ladak, Ph.D. thesis, Delhi University (unpublished).

Malik, S. L., 1979, Effect of altitude on physical development: Comparison of highland and lowland Bods, *Spectra of Anthropolog. Prog.* **2**:45–50.
Malik, S. L., and Singh, I. P., 1978, Growth trends among male Bods of Ladak—A high altitude population, *Am. J. Phys. Anthropol.* **48**:171–176.
Malik, S. L., and Singh, I. P., 1979a, Lung function in highlander Bods of Ladak, *Am. J. Phys. Anthropol.* **51**:383–388.
Malik, S. L., and Singh, I. P., 1979b, Ventilatory capacity among highland Bods: A possible adaptive mechanism at high altitude, *Ann. Hum. Biol.* **6**;471–476.
Miklaschewskaya, N. N., Solovyeva, V. S., and Godina, E. J., 1976, The effect of climatic factors on growth processes in man, in: GROWTH AND DEVELOPMENT: *Physique* (O. G. Eiben, ed.), Akademiai Kiado, Hungary.
Monge, C., 1948, *Acclimatization in the Andes: Historical Confirmation of Climatic Aggression in the Development of Andean Man,* John Hopkins Press, Baltimore.
Newman, M. T., 1953, The application of ecological rules applied to the racial anthropology of the aborginals of the New World, *Am. Anthropolog.* **55**:311–327.
Newman, M. T., 1955, Application of man to cold climates, *Evolution* **9**:101–105.
Pawson, I. G., 1971, The Effects of Altitudinal Variation on Growth in Ethiopian Populations, M.A. thesis, Pennsylvania State University (unpublished).
Pawson, I. G., 1974, The Growth and Development of High Altitude Children with Special Emphasis on Populations of Tibetan Origin, Ph.D. thesis, Pennsylvania State University (unpublished).
Pawson, I. G., 1976, Growth and development in high altitude populations: A review of Ethiopian, Peruvian and Nepalese studies, *Proc. R. Soc. Lond.* [Biol.], **194**:83–98.
Pyzuk, M., and Wolanski, N., 1972, *Uklad oddychanla i. kranzenia ulzeici u Roznorodnych Uarunkachi Sorodowiskowych,* Panstwowe Wydawnictwo Naukowe, Warsaw.
Rao, M. N., Sengupta, A., Saha, P. N., and Devi, S., 1961, Physiological Norms in Indians: Pulmonary Capacity in Health, pecial Report Series No. 38, ICMR, New Delhi.
Rothammer, F., and Spielmann, R. S., 1972, Anthropometric variation in the Aymara: Genetic, geographic and topographic contributions, *Am. J. Hum. Genet.* **24**:371–380.
Scholander, P. F., 1955, Evolution of climatic adaptation in homeotherm, *Evolution* **9**:15–26.
Schreider, E., 1951, Anatomical factors of body heat regulation, *Nature* **167**:823–824.
Sherring, C. A., 1906, *Western Tibet and the British Borderlands,* Edward Arnold, London.
Singh, I. P., and Malik, S. L., 1977, A study of human growth among high altitude female Bods of Ladak with remarks on morphological adaptation, *Anthropol. Kozl.* **21**:63–70.
Walter, H., 1971, Remarks on the environmental adaptation of man, *Humangenetik* **13**:85–97.
Wolanski, N., and Malik, S. L., 1979, Modern environment and future of man, *Acta Anthropogenet.* **3**:157–162.

CHAPTER 20

Subsistence Strategies among the Pastoralists of Maharashtra, India

KAILASH C. MALHOTRA AND *MADHAV GADGIL*

1. Introduction

Indian society consists of more than 4000 endogamous castes, tribes, and religious communities (Malhotra, 1979a). Of these, some 500 groups, constituting about 7% of India's population are nomads (Malhotra, 1983). These nomads are in various stages of nomadism; some are completely sedentary; others are seminomads, and still others are true nomads. True nomads are the ones who move during the year in a cyclical rhythmic manner in a more or less fixed territory and who have no permanent dwellings and practice no agriculture (Bacon, 1954). The seminomads have permanent dwellings and may engage in agriculture or other persuits, but they migrate only during part of the year.

1.1. Pastoral Nomads

Structurally and functionally, the Indian nomads are of two very different types—pastoral and nonpastoral. The pastoral nomads are animal herders and breeders. Pastoral nomadism is perhaps 10,000 years old, and it has been practiced in India since at least 4000 B.C. (Allchin, 1963). Pastoral nomadism continues to be practiced in almost all parts of India, the notable exception being the

KAILASH C. MALHOTRA • Indian Statistical Institute, Calcutta 700 035, India and ***MADHAV GADGIL*** • Indian Institute of Science, Center for Theoretical Studies, Bangalore 560 012, India.
The work was supported by the University Grants Commission, New Delhi, the Indian Statistical Institute, Calcutta, the Indian Institute of Science, Bangalore, the Karnataka State Council for Science and Technology, Bangalore, and the Maharashtra Association for the Cultivation of Science, Pune.

northeastern hill states. India is unique in the world in terms of the diversity of animals that are associated with pastoral nomadism: There are examples of herders of camels in Rajasthan, Gujarat, of donkeys in Maharashtra, yaks in Ladakh and Sikkim, pigs in Andhra Pradesh, sheep, goats, cattle, and buffaloes in most parts of the country, especially in the semiarid and arid regions and in the western Himalayas. Ducks are found in Tamilnadu, Kerala, Andhra Pradesh, Karnataka, and Goa, and guinea fowl in Uttar Pradesh and so forth (Malhotra, 1983).

Traditionally each group maintained a herd of a single animal; for example, the Gujjars of Kashmir were buffalo keepers and the Kurubras of Karnataka were sheep keepers. A few groups—especially shepherds and goatherds—also practice weaving (for example, the Khutekar Dhangars of Maharashtra). In contrast to the settled pastoralists who depend heavily on the husbanded fodder base, the nomads depend almost entirely on the natural-growing vegetation. Due to the nonavailability of a sustained supply of fodder and water at a given place, or due to the rigors of the environment (heavy rainfall, snow), nomads move continually in search of viable pastures. The pastoral nomads are primarily food producers, and they provide the sedentary society with a number of products—milk, butter, ghee, eggs, meat, hides, wool, and manure. These people thus directly add to the food inventory.

It is estimated that some 200 endogamous population groups in India are associated with pastoral nomadism; this would constitute nearly 5 to 6 % of India's population (Malhotra, 1983).

1.2. Nonpastoral Nomads

The nonpastoral nomads comprise of more than 300 endogamous groups (in Maharashtra and Karnataka they number about 105 and 90, respectively) and they constitute about 1 to 2% of India's population. They embrace a great variety of specialized occupations, namely, they are hunters, trappers, fishermen, artisans, entertainers, dancers, singers, fortune-tellers, folktale narraters, genealogists, palmists and medicinemen (Misra, 1967, 1969; Misra *et al.*, 1971; Malhotra, 1974). Each of these nomad groups has a characteristic traditional mode of subsistence, and they have at least some distinguishing features—the manner in which they dress, the portable dwellings they raise, and the shape and beat of their drums. Another characteristic feature these nomads display is multiplicity of occupation. Nearly all of these groups engage in subsidiary activities in addition to their main occupation (Misra *et al.*, 1971; Malhotra *et al.*, 1982). In contrast to the pastoral nomads, the nonpastoral nomads thus depend heavily on settled peasants and other sedentary groups. Several of these groups also depend substantially on wild animal and plant resources (Malhotra *et al.*, 1982). It is quite surprising that until recently no serious attempts were made to study the subsistence pattens of the pastoral nomads in particular and the pastoralists in general (Sopher, 1975). Even now, given the extent and variety of pastoral nomadism that is being particed in India, our understanding of pastoral peoples is far from adequate. Since Misra's classic work among the nonpastoral Gaudulia Lohars of Rajasthan (Misra, 1966), several other nonpastoral nomadic groups have been studied (Malhotra, 1974; Kolte *et al.*, 1982; Khomne *et al.*, 1982; Mohanty, 1982; Morab, 1982).

Since 1969 we have been studying several pastoral and nonpastoral population groups in western India. As part of these multidisciplinary projects, data on subsistence strategies were also generated. In this chapter we shall describe and interpret the subsistence strategies adopted by two pastoral groups—the Gavli Dhangars, a buffalo-keeping group, and the Hatkar Dhangars, a sheep-keeping group.

2. Methods and Materials

The materials reported in this chapter have been generated over a 13-year period from 1969 through 1982 as part of an ongoing project on pastoral nomads in the state of Maharashtra. The Gavli and the Hatkar Dhangars were studied as part of a major biosocial investigation of the entire Dhangar pastoral caste-cluster of Maharashtra led by the senior author from 1969 until the present. This involved visits to selected *tehsils* (administrative geographical units) of every district in Maharashtra, which was followed by extensive interviews of over 4000 households (for more details on sampling techniques, etc., see Malhotra, 1979b and Malhotra *et al.*, 1977). The Gavli Dhangars of the state of Karnataka were investigated independently by the junior author in 1972–1973. Additional ecological investigations of 10 Gavli settlements were jointly carried out by us in 1979 (for details, see Gadgil and Malhotra, 1982).

3. Subsistence Strategies: Case Study I

3.1. The Gavli Dhangars

The Gavlis, with an estimated population of 85,000 (1977, personal estimate), are one of the 23 endogamous castes belonging to the Dhangar (pastoral) caste-cluster of Maharashtra in western India. Presently they are distributed over the forested hill tracts of the western Ghats from 19°N to 13° 30′N latitudes covering 11 districts and 47 *tahsils* of the three states of Maharashtra, Goa, and Karnataka (Figure 1). Today this entire tract is free of malaria. The northern limit of the distribution of the Gavli Dhangars near Panvel coincides with the begin-

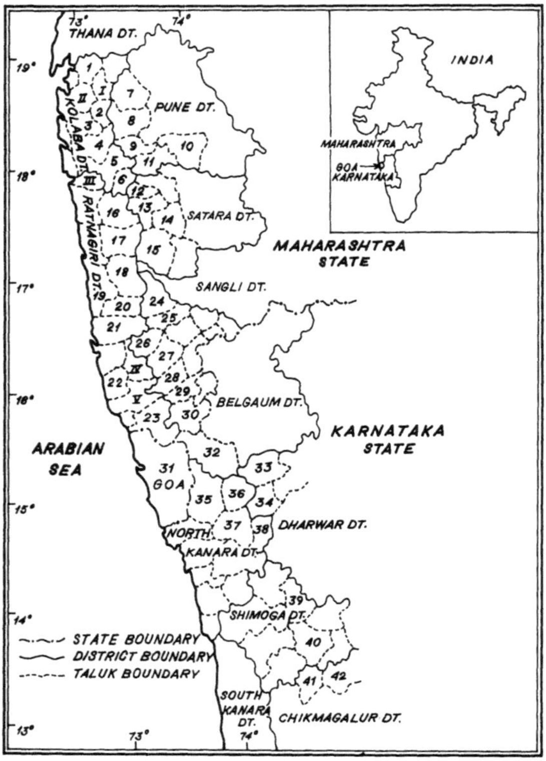

Figure 1. Geographical distribution of the Gavli populations.

ning of the currently somewhat malarial forest of Thana district that harbors a large tribal population. Until recent times, the southern limit of the Gavli distribution was at 16°N near Sawantwadi. This was the northern limit of the forested tracts of the western Ghats of Karnataka that were highly malarial until 1949. Interestingly enough, the Gavlis migrated into this tract in large numbers soon after the control of malaria in 1949. The Gavlis themselves lack any known genetic defense against malaria (Undevia *et al.*, 1973), and their distribution seems to have been regulated by the incidence of malaria (Vishwanathan, 1950; Gadgil and Malhotra, 1982).

In Maharashtra, the Gavlis are restricted to the rainfall zone of 2000 to 6000 mm, whereas in Karnataka they live in the rainfall zone of 800–2500 mm. The dry deciduous forest in the rainfall limit of 800–1500 mm offers the best habitat for buffalo and cattle under climax conditions. The moist deciduous forest in the rainfall zone of 1500–2500 mm with an open canopy has excellent grass and bamboo growth. The tree growth on the Karnataka western Ghats has been largely preserved, except for extraction of larger trees and the slight opening of the canopy that has created ideal conditions for the Gavli animals in the deciduous forest zone of 800–2500 mm rainfall. The Karnataka Gavli populations are largely restricted to this zone.

3.1.1. Traditional subsistence patterns. The Gavlis traditionally have been primarily buffalo-keeping pastorals. They live in small settlements away from the peasant villages and have very little social interaction, apart from economic exchanges, with the rest of the rural population. Traditionally, they exchanged the butter derived from their animals in exchange for cereal, oil and clothing.

It is possible to reconstruct the distribution and subsistence pattern of the Gavlis before the modern era of population growth and deforestation beginning in the 1860s. The Gavli population was then distributed on the upper plateaus of the western Ghats between Panvel and Sawantwadi. Duff (1826) mentions that all the valleys were under paddy cultivation by the Kunbis—a cultivator caste of western Maharashtra—whereas the entire upper reaches of the hills were under a thick forest cover. Duff also records that the means of communication were practically nonexistent and that these higher reaches of hills were very difficult to reach.

The Gavlis then inhabited the thickly forested upper hill plateaus. They shared this habitat with a variety of wild animals, including a substantial population of panthers and tigers. With the highly seasonal rainfall of the region, good grass growth is confined to about 6 months of the year, from May to October. The forest, however, harbors a number of tree species with highly palatable browse, for example, *Grewia tilifolia, Dalbergia latifolia, D. Sympathetica, Ochlandra scriptoria, Eriolaena Quinquelocularis, Ficus hispida, Albizzia procera, Trema orientalis,* and *Ehretia laevis*. The Gavli animals could browse on these during the dry months. The forest also had a number of perennial springs.

3.1.2. Herd size. The Gavlis report that traditionally the ideal herd of a household included 60 buffaloes and 20 head of cattle. In none of the regions visited by us did they report the absence of buffaloes in their traditional husbandry practices, whereas absence of cattle in earlier times was reported from nearly all the localities.

The Gavlis report that buffaloes were the animals most ideally adapted to their traditional habitat because of their abilities to defend themselves against panthers and tigers. The buffalo is more heavily built than the Gavli cattle and has the natural behavior of communal defense against predators. When threatened, the adults form a circle facing outward keeping the calves in the center, thus effectively protecting themselves. In contrast, the Gavli cattle are much smaller, and their natural response to predation is to scatter and run, thereby falling easy prey to the predators. The buffaloes, of course, require plentiful water, shade, and much more browse than the cattle do. These provisions were readily available in the forested habitat. The buffalo was, therefore, the mainstay of the traditional subsistence pattern of Gavlis.

3.1.3. Household requirements. Traditionally and until 1960–1970 for most localities, the Gavlis used to curdle all their milk, churn it, and convert it into buttermilk for domestic consumption and butter or clarified butter (especially during rainy months) for marketing. This butter was accummulated for a week or so and then was sold at a weekly market in a nearby village (*Bombay Gazetteer Kanara* 1883). As mentioned previously, the Gavli settlements are located away from peasant villages, high up in the hills. There was no ready market for the fresh milk, and butter was the only marketable commodity. Gavli subsistence then depended on the exchange of butter for cereal, basically *ragi* (*Elusine coracana*) or *jowar* (*Sorghum vulgare*). The per capita daily requirement for cereal by the rural population in India is *ca.* 0.5 kg per adult (Indian Council of Medical Research ([ICMR] 1951), and this was also the reported requirement of over 50 Gavli households from 10 widely scattered settlements that were interviewed by us. Apart from their cereal requirements, the Gavlis need edible oil, lentils, jaggery, oil for lighting (now kerosene), clothes, condiments, salt, tobacco, dried fish, and so forth. The given estimates for all these items based on interviews of 37 households for a household of six adult equivalents are in Table I. The total annual requirement of a household equals 2263 kg of cereal equivalents.

3.1.4. Butter production. The butter production from Gavli milk ranges from 50 to 80 g/liter, which agrees with the known high fat contents of 6–9% in buffalo milk. The exchange rate of butter to cereal ranges from 12 to 20 kg of

Table I
Annual Consumption of Basic Requirements by 37 Gavli Households Normalized for a Household Size of 6 Adults[a]

Item	Annual consumption: Mean	Annual consumption: S.D.	Equivalent in kg of cereals for the mean
Cereals kg	1100.00	—	1100.00
Oil kg	13.85	6.96	103.87
Lentils kg	40.92	27.84	136.40
Jaggery kg	48.96	35.40	122.40
Kerosene liter	39.00	17.52	65.00
Clothes Rs.	521.90	335.15	434.92
Miscellaneous Rs.	360.00	—	300.00
Total	—	—	2262.59

[a]The expenditure on clothing and miscellaneous items at 1979 price levels.

Table II
Mean Per Capita Daily Consumption of Major Items in the Diet of Gavlis and Their Protein and Calorific Value

Item	Daily consumption in g	Protein content in g	Calorific value (kcal)
Ragi	500.00	35	1700
Vegetable oil	6.67	0	58
Lentils	18.33	4	58
Jaggery	21.67	0	84
Total	—	39	1900
Buttermilk	1000	35	350
Total	—	74	2250

cereal for 1 kg of butter and has remained largely stable, although the absolute prices have increased greatly. This implies that 1 liter of milk could produce enough butter for the purchase of 1 kg of cereal; in addition, buttermilk will be available for household consumption. In a buffalo herd, about one half the buffaloes will be adults, and, with an intercalving interval of 2 years, half of these will yield milk in any given year. Thus, one buffalo (or cow) out of four will be yielding milk in a given year. The annual milk yield per buffalo in optimal conditions will be 200 liters, and some 70 liters per cow. Thus, a herd of 11 buffaloes or 32 cows would be required just to meet the subsistence requirements of a Gavli household.

A herd of 11 buffaloes or 32 cows required for the subsistence of a Gavli household would provide 1 litre of buttermilk per day per head along with the other food items mentioned in Table II. This gives an estimate of the basic nutritional intake of a Gavli at this subsistence level. Such a diet implies a daily protein intake of 74 g and caloric intake of 2250 kcal (Ranganathan, *et al.*, 1937).

Because this represents the average consumption of a household including adult males, females, and children, the nutrition is evidently adequate. This diet would be further supplmented by eggs from domestic poultry, honey, and wild edible plants resulting in a fairly adequate diet. In a good habitat, a herd of 11 buffaloes or 32 cows would then provide a Gavli family with very adequate nutrition and other basic necessities. As noted previosuly, the Gavlis report a herd of 60 buffaloes and 20 cows per household as the traditional norm; such herds are even today maintained by some households of Haliyal *tehsil*.

3.1.5. Lack of hunting tradition. It may be noted that the Gavlis completely lack any tradition of hunting. They have lived in a habitat rich in wild animals, including mouse deer, barking deer, sambar, wild pig, porcupine, blacknapped hare, junglefowl, and peafowl—all animals that are regularly hunted by the Kunbi peasants who share these hill tracts with the Gavlis. The Kunbis cultivate only cereal crops in addition to some lentils. They traditionally kept very few milk animals. The peasants depended heavily on wild animals for their protein requirements. Because Gavlis' protein requirements were met by their buttermilk consumption, they did not have to depend on wild animals for protein and therefore did not develop a tradition of hunting.

3.1.6. Carrying capacity. We shall now consider the amount of grazing land required for a Gavli herd of 60 buffaloes and 20 cattle per household. The weight of a Gavli buffalo is about 150 kg and of a Gavli cow 100 kg. The herd of a single household would then represent a biomass of 11,000 kg. Eisenberg and Seidensticker (1976) have reviewed the known biomasses of large grazing herbivores in Asian tropical and subtropical forests. The estimates per km^2 for a moist deciduous forest, the optimal habitat for such animals, are about 1500 kg of wild and 4500 kg of domestic livestock. The levels of domestic stock show considerable overgrazing and a level of perhaps half this total biomass, namely, 3000 kg/km^2, reflects sustainable levels in a very good habitat. Consequently, the traditional herd of a single Gavli household would need 3.66 km^2 of grazing land. Gavli animals utilize an area of up to 3 km around their settlement for grazing. Thus, if the terrain was flat and all the land in a circle of a 3-km radius was available for grazing, about 8 Gavli households could keep their livestock together on a sustainable basis. However, the terrain is typically in the form of narrow valleys with steep hills forming stepped terraces leading to the flat hilltops. The Gavlis can utilize the upper slopes and the hilltops. In this terrain, the available grazing land tends to be in strips of ½ to 1 km width. Thus, the average area available for grazing around a settlement would be 3–6 km^2, which is sufficient for utilization on a sustained basis by 1 or 2 households maintaining herds of traditional size. However, the distribution of the number of households/settlement at the present time is between 5 to 10. This implies livestock densities of 2 to 10 times what can be sustained on a long-term basis. The traditional pattern in the past was to shift camp to a new locality every 3 to 4 years.

4. Pattern of Change

The nonsustainable commercial exploitation of forests, submersion of river valleys, and growth of the population through eradication of epidemics has drastically reduced, over much of the Gavli range, the carrying capacity of the habitat for Gavli animals. Our investigation of 433 households, spread over eight *tehsils,* representing nearly the entire range of the Gavli habitat, shows that the

Table III
Average Strength of Livestock Per Household in Different Parts of the Gavli Range

Tahsils Districts	Haliyal North Kanara	Jaoli, Patan, Satara Satara	Poladpur Kolaba	Mulshi Pune	Mahad Kolaba	Mahabaleshwar Satara	Shahuwadi Kolhapur	Ratnagiri Ratnagiri
Buffaloes	15.01	7.61	3.29	3.26	3.10	2.06	1.7	1.17
Cattle	8.42	5.39	4.29	9.32	4.57	2.53	2.81	4.50
Goats	0.30	0.39	1.14	2.94	1.33	0.00	3.56	6.40
Number of households sampled	188	18	7	34	42	24	87	33

present-day herd sizes and composition fall drastically short of the traditional ideal (Table III). The Gavli herds show two kinds of changes; the biomass of the herd declines with degradation of habitat, and the composition of the herd shifts from buffalo to cattle and then to goat. The Gavlis relate these changes to two major factors, namely, deterioration of tree growth and substantial decline in predation pressure. In comparison with cattle, buffalo require better grazing, more water and shade, and can defend themselves better against predators. Today, in many degraded habitats the browse is not readily accessible to animals themselves, and in the dry season the Gavlis have to search out palatable browse, lop off the trees, and bring the foliage to their animals. With the lack of shade, the buffaloes are now kept indoors and are stall-fed throughout summer in many localities. Cattle and especially goats are hardier and can better tolerate scarcity of fodder and water, particularly in the dryer season.

Earlier we demonstrated that in a good habitat, a herd of 11 buffaloes or 32 cows is adequate to meet the subsistence requirements of a Gavli household. This requirement may be reduced further if we allow for the income generated by selling the male buffaloes and/or bullocks and marketing the milk (in recent times many Gavlis supply milk to the dairies) instead of butter. Selling the male animals would reduce the minimal herd by about 20%. Marketing of milk enables the Gavli to exchange 1 liter of milk for 1.5 kg of cereal instead of 1 kg exchanged for the butter produced from 1 liter of milk. Thus, completely forgoing the protein provided by buttermilk, the milk-selling Gavlis can meet their basic needs with 66% of the herd necessary for the butter sellers.

The minimal required herd will then be 5 to 6 buffaloes or 12 to 18 cows, or a mixture thereof. Table III reveals that only in Haliyal *tahsil* the buffalo and cattle holdings are comfortably above the minimum levels. They are close to this minimal level in Satara district and are considerably below this in the other six localities from Maharashtra.

In the absence of adequate subsistence from the animals, the Gavlis have turned to two other major activities: keeping goats and shifting cultivation for millet. The goats breed twice a year, and a herd of four goats allows the mar keting of one goat a year, which can generate an income of Rs. 100–150 at 1979 prices or the equivalent of marketing almost 14 kg of butter, which would require the maintenance of one buffalo.

The overall picture that emerges is one in which buffalo and cattle keeping, even when supplemented by goats, is very inadequate to sustain the Gavlis over much of their ancestral habitat in Maharashtra. In response, the Gavlis have adopted shifting cultivation. Shifting cultivation is a highly intensive labor operation with animal power playing almost no role. Only about 2 to 3 hectares can be cultivated in the hill slopes by a household producing some 600–800 kg of cereals, which is enough to meet one half to two thirds of the household's requirement for cereal. A large number of Gavli households (57.6%) do practice such shifting cultivation. With the supplement from shifting cultivation, the animal requirements of the Gavlis would be further reduced, perhaps to 2 to 3 buffaloes and 7 to 10 cows or 2 buffaloes, 6 cows and 8 to 10 goats. The herds of the Gavlis in most of the areas of their distribution are inadequate to meet the basic subsistence requirements in spite of shifting cultivation.

This of course is the reason that a number of Gavlis are engaged in various and sundry jobs, including the one Gavli household in our survey that has reported begging as a means of livelihood.

In conclusion, if the present trend of depletion of tree cover, increasing encroachment on the forestland for cultivation, overgrazing by domestic livestock, a shift to the maintenance of goats, and no efforts whatsoever to increase the fodder base continue, the Gavlis will progressively pass through the stages of buffalo keeping to cow keeping to goatherding to being cultivators of marginal land to landless laborers, thus inflating the already staggering number of rural unemployed. In fact, in absence of alternative viable means of subsistence in their own traditional but now degraded habitat, over 10,000 Gavlis have migrated to Bombay and are working as unskilled workers. Also, some 8000 have moved to cities like Kolhapur, Satara, and Pune, where they are working as laborers and are living in slums.

5. Subsistence Strategies: Case Study II

5.1. The Hatkar Dhangars

The Hatkar Dhangars, with an estimated 573,000 persons (personal estimate, 1971), are found distributed in 19 districts of Maharashtra: Ahmednagar, Akola, Amraoti, Aurangabad, Bhir, Buldhana, Dhulia, Jalgaon, Kolhapur,

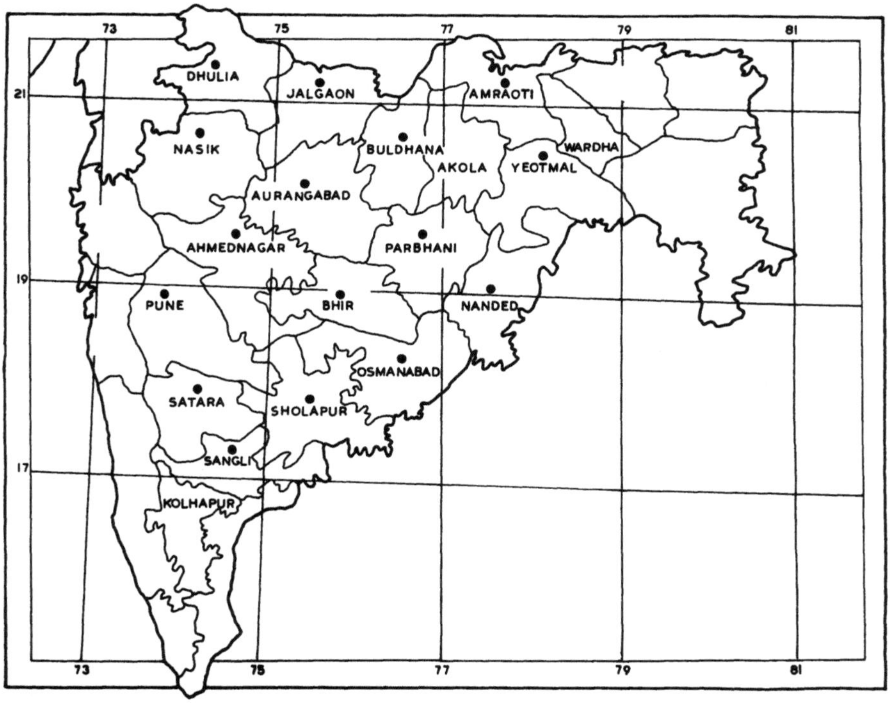

Figure 2. Geographical distribution of the Hatkar Dhangars in 19 districts of Maharashtra. The 16 sampled districts are shown with a black dot.

Nanded, Nasik, Osmanabad, Parbhani, Pune, Sangli, Satara, Sholapur, Wardha, and Yeotmal (Figure 2). Their main concentration, however, is in the semiarid tract of central Maharashtra which has rainfall of 800 mm or less per year. Only the river valleys of this region can sustain agriculture on a long-term basis. There are vast tracts of uncultivated land available for grazing sheep in this geographical region.

The Hatkars traditionally maintained sheep and were true nomads. During the dry period they grazed their animals in a mutually agreed-upon territory, and in the rainy season (about 3 to 4 months, from July to October) they returned to their rainy season campsites.

The entire Dhangar household, including old women and children, moved. In some areas where they lived, they used horses as pack animals and maintained some dogs to protect the sheep against predators. The usual spatial strategies adopted were to stay at a given place until the fodder and water were available for the animals and then move to another site.

At each camp site, which was generally far away from the peasant villages, the adult males would set out for grazing in the morning and return to camp by sunset. The young lambs would be left behind.

The median size of a band Hatkar Dhangar is about 20 households, composed mostly of a single clan. During the dry period the herd starts moving toward the band's traditionally owned grazing territories. Initially the movement of the band would be quite rapid, covering some 10 km/day. After reaching the destination, various families, mostly nuclear ones who owned the herd, would then move away and reassemble at a fixed place just before the onset of monsoon weather and return quickly to their base camps.

Quite often, at the base camp as well as during movement, the herd of different families would get mixed up. In order to identify one's own herd (or a single animal) each family in the band used an exclusive symbol, which usually consisted of cutting the ear in a particular fashion.

In the territory of their operation, the herds during the night are usually made to stay in the farmers' fields within an enclosure which was usually a net. At times they did not use a net. The adult males and the dog(s) stay with the herd. The night droppings and the urine of the animals provide excellent organic manure. Like other pastoral nomads, the Hatkars depend entirely on natural vegetation, and because they do not stay at a place long enough (the maximum length is 3 to 4 months at rainy-season camps), they did not develop any tradition of husbanding fodder for their animals. While migrating the shepherds usually avoided grazing their animals in the farmers' grazing fields; the peasants usually maintained a few animals for draft purposes, and each village had some grazing area of its own.

The Hatkars lack a tradition of drinking sheep milk, and they do not engage in hunting wild animals. For all their needs, they exchanged sheep and products derived from the herd. Tbe shepherds report that traditionally a herd of 100 sheep was necessary to meet the bare minimum need of a household of six persons.

The products they exchanged were wool, sheep manure, and hides of dead animals. For a herd of 100 sheep, some four rams would be kept for breeding purposes, and the remaining males and barren females would be marketed every year.

These pastoralists are now at a cultural crossroad and are undergoing a traumatic experience. Our extensive investigations have established beyond doubt that the developmental strategies persued so far—in particular, the expansion of agriculture to marginal lands (earlier grazing fields), urbanization, industrial projects, and the destruction of the traditional land-tenure systems—have drastically reduced pasture areas and rendered spatial strategies of livestock production totally maladaptive.

The results of our investigations summarized as follows would amply support our conclusions.

A total of 536 Hatkar households were interviewed for the assessment of their mode of subsistence, livestock and land holdings, pattern of migration and level of sedentary life. The sampled households were in 16 of the 19 districts in which the Hatkars live (see Figure 2). The data were generated using a multistage stratified random sampling design.

5.1.1. Main occupation. The responses with respect to main occupations were grouped into five categories: sheep-keeping, agriculture, labor, service (professional), and trade. It is noteworthy that 74.7% of the Hatkars reported agriculture as their main occupation; only 7% maintained sheep, 7.64% were in service, 2% were petty traders, and 9.5% were working as landless laborers.

5.1.2. Subsidiary occupation. Nearly one third of the Hatkars (61.89%)

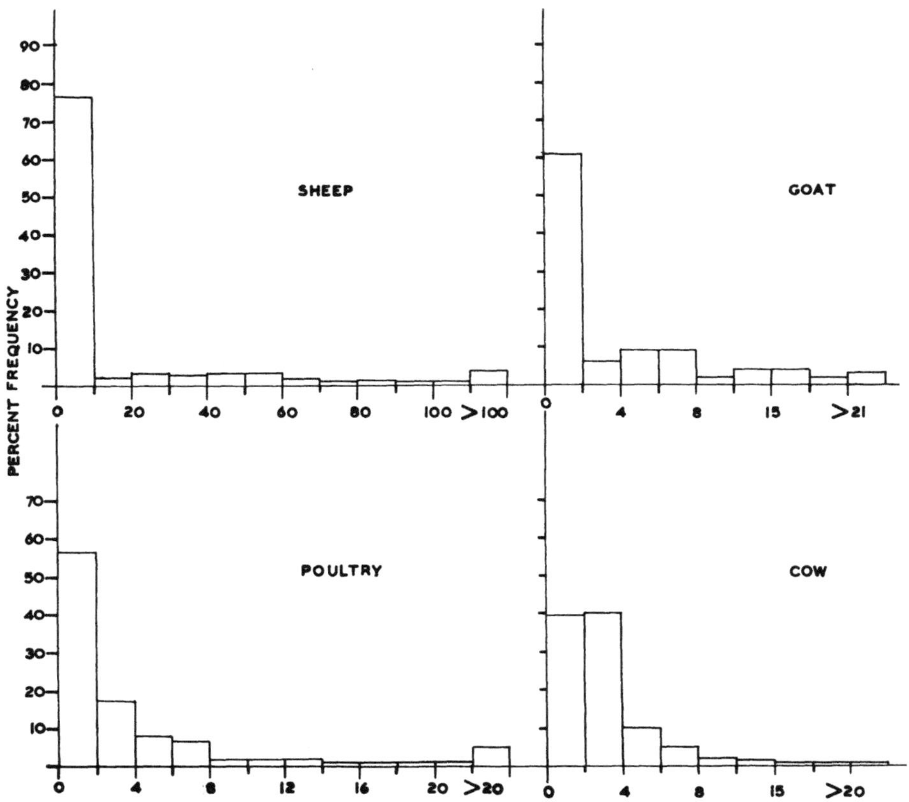

Figure 3. Distribution of sheep, goats, cows, and poultry among the Hatkar Dhangars. The distributions in all cases, as expected, are leptokurtic and highly positively skewed.

had no subsidiary occupation. Of the remaining ones, 11.7% reported sheep keeping as a subsidiary occupation, 8.36% labor, 10.03% agriculture, 4.08% service, and 4% trade.

It is thus quite obvious that only about 19% of the Hatkars at the time of investigation (1971–1973) were engaged in their traditional occupation of sheep keeping.

5.1.3. Livestock holdings. An inventory of the various animals possessed by the Hatkars revealed that they now maintain sheep, goats, buffaloes, poultry, horses, and dogs. The mean number of animals per household (of 6.7 persons) are sheep (11.9), goats (2.74), cattle (4.11), buffaloes (0.91), horses (0.16), and dogs (0.54). The distribution of various animals among the Hatkar households is shown in Figure 3. Of those who possessed sheep, 47.06% had up to 40, 29.31% between 41 and 80, 8.4% between 81 and 100, and 15.13% in excess of 100.

About 61% of the Hatkar households did not maintain any goats. Of those who did, 38.6% had up to 4, 28.4% between 5 and 8, 5.1% between 9 and 20, and 7.11%, over 21 goats.

Nearly 40% of Hatker households did not possess a cow. Of the households that did, 82.1% had up to 4, 11% between 5 and 8, 3.6% between 9 and 15, 2% between 16 and 20, and 1.3%, over 20 cows. The bulk of the Hatkar households (40.9%) did not possess any bullocks; 69.1% of the households possessed up to 2, 21.26% between 3 and 4, 5.98% between 5 and 6, and 3.65% above 6 bullocks. Approximately half of the Hatkar households did not possess poultry (56.2%). Among those who did a majority (72.2%) had up to 6 fowls and the remaining 27.8% had more than 6 fowls. The average dog, horse, and buffalo holdings per household are rather small and therefore no further analysis was attempted.

5.1.4. Land holdings. About 60% of the Hatkar households did not own any irrigated land. Of thoose that did, 37.7% had up to 2 acres, 38.4% had 3–6 acres, and the remaining 24% had 7 or more acres (Figure 4).

On the other hand, about 80% of the households owned some nonirrigated land (entirely dependent on rain); 34.5% of these had up to 6 acres, 36% had 7 to 15 acres, and the remaining 29.5% owned 16 or more acres (Figure 4).

5.1.5. Levels of sedentary life. About 80% of the surveyed households reported a complete sedentary mode of existence. A majority of these households depended for their sustenance on agriculture and a few on petty trade. A negligible proportion of these households that are located near the irrigated tracts of the region also maintain sheep. Of the 20% who lead a nomadic way of life, about 3% even now do not have permanent dwellings, practice no agriculture or any other occupation, and are thus true nomads. The remaining 17% are seminomads; during dry months they migrate in search of pasture and water for their animals and in rainy months they stay in their base villages.

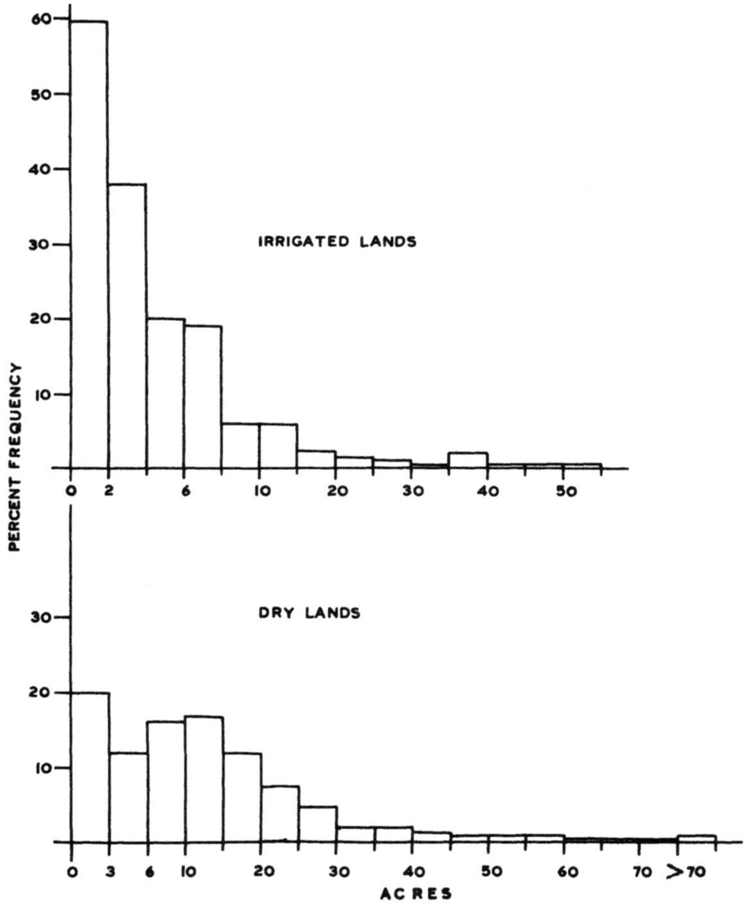

Figure 4. Distribution of land holdings among the Hatkar Dhangars; the distribution for irrigated land holdings is leptokurtic and positively skewed, whereas it is platykurtic and positively skewed for dry land holdings.

5.1.6. Migration pattern. The present-day pattern of migration of the true nomads and seminomads, generally speaking, is the same as that described previously. A few major departures from the traditional pattern that have taken place are as follows.

1. The rules of rigid territoriality within the group, which were followed meticulously earlier, have largely eroded leading to an increased number of between-band conflicts.
2. The duration of stay-at-base villages has reduced from 4 to 5 months a year to 2 to 3 months a year.

3. The distances traveled during the annual migration cycle have increased by 50%.
4. Due to the reduced pasture lands and an increased need for farmers to maintain more animals, the conflicts between the Hatkars and the peasants have assumed alarming proportions.
5. In the case of seminomads, usually only adult males migrate with the herd.

6. Pattern of Change

From the results presented in the previous section the following main points emerge as important changes in subsistence strategies of the Hatkars:

1. Due to the depletion of a natural fodder base, an increasing number of Hatkars are unable to retain their traditional occupation of sheep keeping.
2. There is an increasing tendency to replace sheep by goats.
3. The earlier pattern of a single occupation has drastically changed, and nearly 40% of the Hatkars have more than one occupation.
4. A large number of Hatkars have begun to cultivate degraded marginal lands; 74.1% of the sampled households reported agriculture as the main occupation and another 10% as a subsidiary occupation.
5. Although we have as yet not worked out detailed conversion of land holdings and livestock holdings to caloric equivalents, preliminary assessment shows that a majority of the Hatkar households are unable to meet their basic minimum requirements.
6. Cultivation of marginal lands and the introduction of goats and overgrazing have accelerated the process of the deterioration of the semiarid ecosystem.
7. If the present-day development policies are continued, this mode of production—the most adaptive and potentially viable economic system in semiarid land ecosystems—will not only disappear but will result in the destruction of pastoral societies.

7. Conclusions

In the preceding pages we have described the traditional subsistence strategies followed by two pastoral groups, the Gavlis and the Hatkars of Maharashtra. We have shown the extent and nature of changes that have occurred in their subsistence patterns since modern developmental policies were introduced.

Our investigations have clearly demonstrated that the developmental policies being persued by the government have totally neglected the various aspects associated with fodder base, the single most vital component of pastoralism.

Because it is well established that this mode of production is the most adaptive and potentially viable in environmentally marginal areas, immediate efforts should be taken to develop long-term approaches to rational land use and livestock management with an emphasis on genetic improvement of livestock, grass, and fodder tree species. All the marginal lands in the semiarid and arid regions should, with immediate effects, be brought under pasture development. The pastoralists must be fully involved in the design and implementation of programs. The introduction and development of community pastures and rotational grazing holds the best hope for the future of pastoralist people.

References

Allchin, F. R., 1963, Cattle and economy in neolithic South India, in: *Man and Cattle* (A. E. Mourant and F. E. Zeuner, eds.), University Press, Glasgow, pp. 149–155.

Bacon, E. E., 1954, Types of nomadism in central and south-west Asia, *S. W. J. Anthropol.* **10**:44–68.

Bombay Gazetteer Kanara, 1883, Volume XXV, Part I, Government Central Press, Bombay.

Duff, J. G., 1826, *A History of Maharattas,* Volume I., Longman, Rees, Orme, Brown and Green, London.

Eisenberg, J. F., and Sedensticker, J., 1976, Ungulates in southern Asia: A consideration of biomass estimates for selected habitats, *Biol. Conser.* **10**:293–308.

Gadgil, M., and Malhotra, K. C., 1982, Ecology of a pastoral caste: Gavli Dhangars of Peninsular India, *Hum. Ecol.* **10**:107–143.

Indian Council of Medical Research, 1951, Results of Diet Survey in India 1935–48, Special Report, New Delhi.

Khomne, S. B., Hulbe, S. K., and Vetschera, T., 1982, An ethnographic account and economic activities of the Kevats—A semi-nomadic group of weavers in Maharashtra, in: *Nomads in India* (P. K. Misra and K. C. Malhotra, eds.).

Kolte, S. B., Khomne, S. B., Hulbe, S. K., and Vetschera, T, 1982, A brief note on the Vaidus of Maharashtra, in: *Nomads in India* (P. K. Misra and K. C. Malhotra, eds.), Anthropological Survey of India, Calcutta.

Malhotra, K. C., 1974, Socio-biological investigations among the Nandiwallas—a nomadic caste-cluster in Maharashtra, *Bull. Urgt. Anthrop. Ethnol. Res.* (Austria) **16**:63–102.

Malhotra, K. C., 1979a, Excommunication as a process leading to the formation of new groups, *The Eastern Anthropol.* **32**:49–53.

Malhotra, K. C., 1979b, Inbreeding Among Dhangar castes of Maharashtra, India., *J. Biosoc. Sci.* (U.K) **11**:397–410.

Malhotra, K. C., 1983, Future of pastoral peoples in India, in: *State of Environment in India,* Centre for Science and Environment, New Delhi.

Malhotra, K. C., Chakraborty, R., and Chakravartti, A., 1977, Gene differentiation among the Dhangar caste-cluster of Maharashtra, India, *Heredity* **28**:26–36.

Malhotra, K. C., Hulbe, S. K., Khomne, S. B., and Kolte, S. B., 1982, Economic organization of the Nandiwallas and Deowallas of Maharashtra, in: *Nomads in India* (P. K. Misra and K. C. Malhotra, eds.), Anthropological Survey of India, Calcutta.

Misra, P. K., 1966, *The Economy of a Nomadic Artisan Community; A Study of the Economy and Society among the Nomadic Gadulia Lohars of Eastern Rajasthan*, Ph.D. thesis, Lucknow University.

Misra, P. K., 1967, Study of nomads, in: *Proc. Seminar on Research Programmes in Cultural Anthropology and Related Disciplines*, (S. C. Sinha, ed.), Anthropological Survey of India, Calcutta.

Misra, P. K., 1969, Nomadism in India, *J. Ind. Anthropol. Soc.* **4**:79–87.

Misra, P. K., Rajalakshmi, C. R., and Verghese, I, 1971, *Nomads in Mysore City*, Anthropological Survey of India, Calcutta.

Mohanty, U. C., 1982, The social organization of the semi-nomadic snake charmers of Orissa, in: *Nomads in India* (P. K. Misra and K. C. Malhotra, eds.), Anthropological Survey of India, Calcutta.

Morab, S. G., 1982, Values and world view of the nomadic Killekyatha, in: *Nomads in India* (P. K. Misra and K. C. Malhotra, eds.), Anthropological Survey of India, Calcutta.

Ranganathan, S., Sundarajan, A. R., and Swaminathan, M., 1937, Survey of the nutritive value of Indian foodstuffs. Part I. The chemical composition of 200 common foods, *Ind. J. Med. Res.* **24**:689–706.

Sopher, D. E., 1975, Indian pastoral castes and livestock ecologies: A geographic analysis, in: *Pastoralists and Nomads in South Asia* (L. S. Leshnik and G. Sontheimer, eds.), Otto Harrassowitz, Weisbaden, Heidelberg.

Undevia, J. V., Malhotra, K. C., and Dundhwalla, F., 1973, G-6-PD deficiency and abnormal hemoglobin among the Dhangars of Maharashtra, in: *Proc. Conf. of the Indian Physicians*, Udaipur. Abstract No. 41, Udaipur.

Vishwanathan, D. K., 1950, *Malaria and its Control in Bombay State*, Chitrasala Press, Pune.

Index

MIX
Papier aus verantwortungsvollen Quellen
Paper from responsible sources
FSC® C105338

If you have any concerns about our products,
you can contact us on
ProductSafety@springernature.com

In case Publisher is established outside the EU,
the EU authorized representative is:
Springer Nature Customer Service Center GmbH
Europaplatz 3, 69115 Heidelberg, Germany

Printed by Libri Plureos GmbH
in Hamburg, Germany